Crystal-Induced Arthropathies

Crystal-Induced Arthropathies

Gout, Pseudogout and Apatite-Associated Syndromes

edited by

Robert L. Wortmann
University of Oklahoma College of Medicine
Tulsa, Oklahoma, U.S.A.

H. Ralph Schumacher, Jr.
University of Pennsylvania and VA Medical Center
Philadelphia, Pennsylvania, U.S.A.

Michael A. Becker
University of Chicago School of Medicine
Chicago, Illinois, U.S.A.

Lawrence M. Ryan
Medical College of Wisconsin
Milwaukee, Wisconsin, U.S.A.

Taylor & Francis
Taylor & Francis Group
New York London

Taylor & Francis is an imprint of the
Taylor & Francis Group, an informa business

Published in 2006 by
Taylor & Francis Group
270 Madison Avenue
New York, NY 10016

Printed in the United States of America on acid-free paper
10 9 8 7 6 5 4 3 2 1

International Standard Book Number-10: 0-8493-9382-5 (Hardcover)
International Standard Book Number-13: 978-0-8493-9382-2 (Hardcover)
Library of Congress Card Number 2006040382

Library of Congress Cataloging-in-Publication Data

Crystal-induced arthropathies : gout, pseudogout and apatite-associated syndromes / edited by Robert L. Wortmann ... [et al.]
p. cm.
ISBN-13: 978-0-8493-9382-2 (alk. paper)
ISBN-10: 0-8493-9382-5 (alk. paper)
1. Gout--Etiology. 2.Hyperuricemia. I. Wortmann, Robert.

RC629.3.C795 2006
616.3'999--dc22 2006040382

informa
Taylor & Francis Group
is the Academic Division of Informa plc.

Visit the Taylor & Francis Web site at
http://www.taylorandfrancis.com

Preface

When most people hear the term "crystal-induced arthropathy," they think of gout, the disease that results from the body's response to monosodium urate crystals. Furthermore, they usually envision a patient with acute, intensely inflammatory monoarthritis, the cardinal feature of gout. However, gout is not the most common crystal-induced arthropathy. The arthropathies that result from the body's response to calcium-containing crystals, those of calcium pyrophosphate dihydrate or basic calcium phosphates, occur more frequently. In fact, it is likely that everyone will develop some sort of calcium-containing arthropathy if they live long enough. Furthermore, although each crystal type can induce an acute monoarticular disease, each can also be associated with a variety of other clinical presentations. Thus, the crystal-induced arthropathies are common and complex diseases.

Whereas gout has been recognized for centuries, not until 1960 was it appreciated that monosodium urate crystals were present in the synovial fluid in patients with attacks of gout. It was at that same time that calcium pyrophosphate dihydrate crystals were identified in joint fluids from patients who were previously believed to suffer from gout and the term "pseudogout" was coined. Our present understanding of basic calcium phosphate arthropathies began to unfold in the early 1980s with the description of Milwaukee shoulder syndrome.

Motivation for this work stemmed from the editors' long-standing interest in the crystal-induced arthropathies, each of us having been actively investigating various elements of these diseases for the last 30 to 40 years. It was our desire to produce a concise but comprehensive review of this large field, recognizing that much of the present understanding of these diseases is the result of observations that have occurred during the span of our careers. In addition to reviewing the present state of understanding regarding the clinical presentations of the various diseases, their respective underlying pathogeneses, and current approaches to management, our goals included providing a sound basis for understanding the discoveries that will be made in the future, both in etiology and in therapy. If we have accomplished our goals, this book will be helpful to clinicians, teachers, and scientists.

The authors who have contributed to this text share the editors' interest and enthusiasm for the field. We were particularly pleased that Dan McCarty was willing to share his perspective on the history of the crystal-induced arthropathies. As one of the individuals who identified monosodium urate crystals in gouty synovial fluids, recognized pseudogout, and described Milwaukee shoulder syndrome, he has contributed greatly to our knowledge of the field. In addition, he has provided training and influenced a large number of investigators, many of whom authored chapters for this edition. Although most authors of this text can not match Dr. McCarty's breadth of observations, each of the senior authors has been involved in original research in the area about which they wrote and is widely recognized for their individual expertise. We are also pleased to have involved younger individuals who will become future leaders in this field.

Robert L. Wortmann
H. Ralph Schumacher, Jr.
Michael A. Becker
Lawrence M. Ryan

Contents

Contributors

Joel Abbott Division of Clinical Immunology and Rheumatology, University of Alabama at Birmingham, Birmingham, Alabama, U.S.A.

Michael A. Becker Rheumatology Section, Department of Medicine, University of Chicago School of Medicine, Chicago, Illinois, U.S.A.

Guillermo F. Carrera Department of Radiology, Medical College of Wisconsin, Milwaukee, Wisconsin, U.S.A.

Lan X. Chen Division of Rheumatology, Department of Medicine, University of Pennsylvania, Philadelphia, Pennsylvania, U.S.A.

Herman S. Cheung Department of Biomedical Engineering, University of Miami and Miami VA Medical Center, Miami, Florida, U.S.A.

Jill C. Costello Division of Rheumatology, Department of Medicine, Medical College of Wisconsin, Milwaukee, Wisconsin, U.S.A.

Bruce N. Cronstein Divisions of Clinical Pharmacology and Rheumatology, Department of Medicine, NYU School of Medicine, New York, New York, U.S.A.

Nicola Dalbeth Faculty of Medicine, Eric Bywaters Centre, Imperial College London, London, U.K.

Kevin D. Deane Division of Rheumatology, University of Colorado Health Sciences Center, Denver, Colorado, U.S.A.

N. Lawrence Edwards Section of Rheumatology, Department of Medicine, University of Florida and VA Medical Center, Gainesville, Florida, U.S.A.

Adel G. Fam Sunnybrook and Women's College Health Sciences Centre, University of Toronto, Toronto, Ontario, Canada

Daniel I. Feig Renal Section, Department of Pediatrics, Baylor College of Medicine, Houston, Texas, U.S.A.

Paul B. Halverson Division of Rheumatology, Department of Medicine, Medical College of Wisconsin, Milwaukee, Wisconsin, U.S.A.

Dorian O. Haskard Faculty of Medicine, Eric Bywaters Centre, Imperial College London, London, U.K.

Iñaki Hernando Rheumatology Section, Hospital de Cruces, Baracaldo, Vizcaya, Spain

Ana M. Herrero-Beites Rehabilitation Division, Hospital de Gorliz, Vizcaya, Spain

Michael S. Hershfield Division of Rheumatology and Immunology, Departments of Medicine and Biochemistry, Duke University School of Medicine, Durham, North Carolina, U.S.A.

Kanyakorn Jaovisidha Division of Rheumatology, Department of Medicine, Bangkok Hospital, Bangkok, Thailand

Richard J. Johnson Section of Nephrology, Hypertension, and Transplantation, University of Florida, Gainesville, Florida, U.S.A.

John Kanellis Department of Nephrology, Monash Medical Centre, Clayton, Melbourne, Victoria, Australia

Duk-Hee Kang Division of Nephrology, College of Medicine, Ewha Women's University and Ewha Research Center, Seoul, Korea

Brian F. Mandell Department of Medicine and Rheumatic and Immunologic Diseases, Cleveland Clinic Lerner College of Medicine of Case Western Reserve University, Cleveland, Ohio, U.S.A.

Geraldine M. McCarthy Department of Molecular and Cellular Therapeutics, Royal College of Surgeons of Ireland and Mater Misericordiae University Hospital, Dublin, Ireland

Daniel J. McCarty Department of Medicine, Medical College of Wisconsin, Milwaukee, Wisconsin, U.S.A.

Ted R. Mikuls Section of Rheumatology and Immunology, University of Nebraska and Omaha VA Medical Center, Omaha, Nebraska, U.S.A.

Eamonn S. Molloy Department of Molecular and Cellular Therapeutics, Royal College of Surgeons of Ireland, Dublin, Ireland

Fernando Perez-Ruiz Rheumatology Section, Hospital de Cruces, Baracaldo, Vizcaya, Spain

Ann K. Rosenthal Division of Rheumatology, Department of Medicine, Medical College of Wisconsin, Milwaukee, Wisconsin, U.S.A.

Lawrence M. Ryan Division of Rheumatology, Department of Medicine, Medical College of Wisconsin, Milwaukee, Wisconsin, U.S.A.

Kenneth G. Saag Division of Clinical Immunology and Rheumatology, University of Alabama at Birmingham and Center for Education and Research on Therapeutics (CERTs) of Musculoskeletal Disorders, Birmingham, Alabama, U.S.A.

H. Ralph Schumacher, Jr. Division of Rheumatology, Department of Medicine, University of Pennsylvania and VA Medical Center, Philadelphia, Pennsylvania, U.S.A.

Peter A. Simkin Division of Rheumatology, Department of Medicine, University of Washington School of Medicine, Seattle, Washington, U.S.A.

John S. Sundy Division of Rheumatology and Immunology, Department of Medicine, Duke University School of Medicine, Durham, North Carolina, U.S.A.

R. Swamy Venuturupalli Division of Rheumatology, Department of Medicine, Cedars Sinai Medical Center and David Geffen School of Medicine at UCLA, Los Angeles, California, U.S.A.

Michael H. Weisman Division of Rheumatology, Department of Medicine, Cedars Sinai Medical Center and David Geffen School of Medicine at UCLA, Los Angeles, California, U.S.A.

Sterling G. West Division of Rheumatology, University of Colorado Health Sciences Center, Denver, Colorado, U.S.A.

Charlene J. Williams Division of Rheumatology, Department of Medicine, Thomas Jefferson University, Philadelphia, Pennsylvania, U.S.A.

Robert L. Wortmann Division of Rheumatology, Department of Medicine, University of Oklahoma College of Medicine, Tulsa, Oklahoma, U.S.A.

Raihana Zaka Division of Rheumatology, Department of Medicine, Thomas Jefferson University, Philadelphia, Pennsylvania, U.S.A.

1

Crystal-Induced Arthropathies—Historical Aspects

Daniel J. McCarty
Department of Medicine, Medical College of Wisconsin, Milwaukee, Wisconsin, U.S.A.

INTRODUCTION

It is now widely accepted that microcrystals are associated with both joint inflammation and degeneration. This volume deals with the three most common types of crystal-induced arthropathy, monosodium urate (MSU) monohydrate (MSU), calcium pyrophosphate dihydrate (CPPD), and basic calcium phosphate (BCP), associated with gout, pseudogout, and calcific periarthritis/osteoarthritis, respectively. Selected historical contributions to the development of this field are reviewed here.

MONOSODIUM URATE CRYSTAL DEPOSITION

Antoni Van Leeuwenhoek described the morphologic characteristics of MSU crystals obtained from a draining tophus of one of his relatives (1) about a century before uric acid was identified by Scheele (as urolithic acid) in 1776 (2). A. B. Garrod wrote that MSU crystals were a constant feature of gout in 1867 (3) and attributed this deposition to over-saturation of body fluid uric acid as demonstrated by his famous "thread" test. But as late as 1960 it was widely believed that urate crystals were *not* causally related to acute gouty inflammation, although crystal aggregates were held responsible for the destruction of chronic tophaceous gouty arthritis.

In 1961 McCarty and Hollander described MSU crystals in gouty synovial fluid using compensated polarized light microscopy (4) followed by digestion with the specific enzyme, uricase. Crystals were found in polymorphonuclear leukocytes in fluids from acutely inflamed joints (5), raising the question of causality. Working independently, Faires and McCarty in Philadelphia (6) and Seegmiller, Howell, and Malawista in Bethesda (7) synthesized MSU crystals and injected suspensions of them into normal human knee joints, canine stifle joints, and joints of gouty patients (6,7). An acute self-limited, dose-related, inflammatory response followed every injection. Aspirated synovial fluid showed phagocytosis of crystals by neutrophilic and mononuclear phagocytes. The experiments using normal joints fulfilled Koch's postulates for proof of etiology.

A literature review at that juncture revealed that a Viennese dermatologist, Gustave Riehl, had described MSU crystals in phagocytic cells in two fresh skin tophi in 1897 (8). He speculated that the crystals might be the cause of the inflammation, but stated that further work would be left to the internists. In 1899, Max Freudweiler, a young internist and native of Zurich, working in the laboratory of a fellow Swiss internist (famous for his description of the conducting "bundles" in heart muscle), Wilhelm His, Jr., at the University of Leipzig, synthesized MSU crystals and injected them under the skin of rabbits (about 200 times) and into his own skin on two occasions (9). The resulting inflammatory response was followed histologically by serial biopsy, including polarized light examination of frozen sections. The deposits eventually became the nidus of tophi identical to those found in gouty patients. Professor His reported in 1900 that MSU and control crystals injected into rabbit joints or peritoneal cavities also produced inflammation (10). He expressed reluctance to inject crystals in human subjects, stating that the most appropriate subject, "a gouty physician possessing moderate heroism had not yet been placed at his disposal." Subsequently Freudweiler established his own laboratory in the basement of the medical school of the University of Zurich and performed further work in rabbits and chickens with ligated ureters (11). He refuted the work of VonNoorden, Klemperer, and Ebstein (referred to in Refs. 9 and 11), whose data suggested that necrosis preceded MSU crystal deposition and whose histological examination of gouty tissues often failed to show crystals. Freudweiler found that MSU crystals did not deposit in tissue made necrotic by heat, but that crystals caused both inflammation and necrosis. His, Freudweiler, and Riehl disputed the thought that necrosis preceded crystal deposition, claiming that the watery tissue fixatives used by VonNoorden, Klemperer, and Epstein had dissolved the MSU crystals from gouty lesions. Simkin et al. have shown that formalin is an excellent solubilizer of MSU crystals (12).

Why these data were lost to medical science remains unclear. Professor His became a German national to qualify for the top university chair in internal medicine in that country (Berlin) and subsequently became Colonel His when

World War I broke out. He wrote the classic history of German military medicine in that war and died in 1936. His only other contribution to gout was a postwar description of the increased uricosuria invariably preceding spontaneous acute attacks in gouty subjects hospitalized in the clinical research center at Berlin for up to a year! Freudweiler died, virtually unknown, in September 1901 at the age of 30 years. In summary, conclusive proof linking MSU crystals to both acute inflammation and tophus formation was published but apparently forgotten as most investigators interested in gout focused their attention on the metabolic mechanisms leading to hyperuricemia.

CALCIUM PYROPHOSPHATE DIHYDRATE (CPPD) CRYSTAL DEPOSITION

CPPD crystals are of the same size range as MSU crystals (1–20 microns) but are parallelpiped or rod-like rather than needle-shaped (13). They have completely different characteristics by compensated polarized light microscopy and, as they contain calcium, are radiopaque. They are seen as linear deposits in fibrocartilagenous structures such as the menisci of the knee, glenoid and acetabular labra, symphysis pubis, anulus fibrosus of the intervertebral discs, the articular disc of the distal radioulnar joint, and to a lesser extent in the hyaline articular cartilage, especially of the larger joints. This distinctive appearance led to many case reports [summarized in Ref. (13)] including Zitnan and Sitaj's classic paper describing hereditary disease in five Hungarian families living in Slovakia (14). Their serial radiographic studies showed calcific deposits in normal appearing joints that invariably underwent progressive degeneration (15). The optical characteristics of the crystals were described by McCarty and collaborators (13), and the nature of the deposits was established crystallographically in 1962 (16).

Hyaline cartilage from the distal humerus of William Hunter's original case of osteitis fibrosa cystica was found to have a fine line of calcification paralleling the radiodensity of the underlying bone (17). This radiographic appearance is very suggestive of CPPD crystal deposits, and hyperparathyroidism is one of the associated metabolic diseases. A mummy from the Field Museum in Chicago with ochronosis was shown to have homogentisic acid deposits and had cartilaginous calcification compatible with CPPD crystal deposits (18). Bennett of Dublin's Sir Patrick Dun's Hospital described calcific deposits in cartilage in 1903 (19), but he provided no microscopic description. He found that the deposits released bubbles when he added acid, suggesting that they were calcium carbonate. Unfortunately, definitive crystal identification was not done in any of these reports.

In summary, CPPD crystals, like MSU, can be associated with acute inflammatory attacks of arthritis, with chronic devolutionary joint change, and in some cases, with antecedent metabolic diseases. These similarities prompted the neologism "pseudogout" (13).

BASIC CALCIUM PHOSPHATE CRYSTAL DEPOSITION

"Apatite" derives from a Greek word meaning "deceiver." In mineral form it has a calcium to phosphorus molar ratio of 1.67. Biological apatite, however, has a lower molar ratio. Apatite crystals are ultramicroscopic in size. Synovial fluid specimens were first shown to contain "apatite" crystals by Schumacher et al. using transmission electron microscopy (20) and, independently, by Dieppe et al. (21) using scanning electron microscopy. Because apatite can form from amorphous calcium phosphate precipitated when biological fluids lose CO_2 to the atmosphere, a process augmented by cooling (refrigeration or freezing will always cause this to happen), Halverson and McCarty attempted to reproduce their findings in synovial fluid specimens handled anaerobically (under oil), using (^{14}C) bisphosphonate binding, followed by scanning electron microscopy of the centrifuged pellet with X-ray energy dispersive analysis to determine the calcium/phosphorus molar ratio (22). Bisphosphonate does not bind to other particulates or crystals found in joint fluid. The binding of unknown compared to that of synthetic apatite standards was used to quantify the amount of mineral per unit volume of synovial fluid. Virtually all specimens from joints with radiographically narrowed joint spaces contained detectable mineral with calcium to phosphorous (Ca/P) ranging from 1.4 to 1.6. The most extensive binding occurred in fluid from the shoulder joints of elderly women with complete loss of the rotator cuff and extensive glenohumeral joint degeneration, a condition later designated as the "Milwaukee Shoulder Syndrome" (MSS) (23).

Fourier transform infrared spectophotometric analysis (FTIR) of washed synovial fluid pellets containing (^{14}C) bisphosphonate binding mineral showed mixtures of octacalcium phosphate (OCP) and heavily carbonate-substituted apatite (for both hydroxyl and phosphate groups), accounting for the "calcium deficient" Ca/P molar ratios (24). A biopsy specimen of calcific periarthritis from Israel contained only OCP (25). Another specimen from a calcinosis lesion accompanying scleroderma showed pure carbonate apatite. The vast majority of pathologic calcifications contain mixtures of OCP and carbonate-substituted hydroxy apatite. The use of the generic term "BCP" crystal deposition was proposed because all crystals identified were basic (as opposed to acidic) calcium phosphates (24). An acidic calcium phosphate and (a dimorph of brushite), dicalcium phosphate dehydrate, was described in specimens of anatomical cadaver fibrocartilaginous menisci as multiple punctate deposits, but has never been identified definitively in synovial fluid (26). Such deposits may be postmortem artifacts, possibly due to local tissue alkalinity accompanying loss of CO_2 as already described for synovial fluid.

In summary, BCP crystals are always found in synovial fluid when radiographic evidence of cartilage degeneration is present (narrowed joint spaces and subchondral bony changes). Like MSU and CPPD, they are biologically active and could accelerate devolutionary joint changes as described elsewhere in this volume. As the mechanism of such activity of calcium-containing crystals becomes clear, prevention of the associated degenerative joint changes might become a reality.

REFERENCES

1. McCarty DJ. A historical note: Van Leuwenhoek's description of crystals from a gouty tophus. Arthritis Rheum 1970; 3:414–418.
2. Scheele CW, Analysis of the calculus vesicae 1776. The chemical essays of Charles William Sheele. Translated from the Transactions of the Academy of Sciences at Stockholm. London: J Murray, 1787: p199.
3. Garrod AB. A Treatise on Gout and Rheumatic Gout (Rheumatoid Arthritis). 3rd ed. London: Longmans, Green & Co., 1867.
4. McCarty DJ, Hollander JL. Identification of urate crystals in gouty synovial fluid. Ann Intern Med 1961; 54:452–460.
5. McCarty DJ. Phagocytosis of urate crystals in gouty synovial fluid. Am J Med Sci 1963; 243:288–295.
6. Faires JS, McCarty DJ. Acute arthritis in man and dog after intrasynovial injection of sodium urate crystals. Lancet 1962; 2:682–685.
7. Seegmiller JE, Howell RR, Malawista S. The inflammatory reaction to sodium urate. JAMA 1962; 180:469–473.
8. Riehl G. Zur Anatomie der Gicht. Wiener Klin Wochenschr 1897; 10:761–774
9. Brill JM, McCarty DJ. Studies on the nature of gouty tophi, an abridged translation with comments, Freudweiler M. Dtsch Arch Klin Med 1899; 63:266–272. Ann Intern Med 1964; 60:485–505.
10. His W, Jr. Schicksal und Wirkungen des Sauren Harnsauren Natrons in Bauch und Gelenkhöhale des kanimchens. Dtsch Arch Klin Med 1900; 67:82.
11. Brill JM, McCarty DJ. An abridged translation of "Experimental investigations into the origin of gouty tophi" by Max Freudweiler. Dtsch Arch für Klin Med 1901; 69:155. Arthritis Rheum 1965; 8:167–188.
12. Simkin PA, Bassett JE, Lee QP. Not water, but formalin, dissolves urate crystals in tophaceous tissue samples. J Rheumatol 1994; 21:2320–2321.
13. McCarty DJ, Kohn NN, Faires JS. The significance of calcium phosphate crystals in the synovial fluid of arthritis patients: the "pseudogout syndrome," I. Clinical aspects. Ann Intern Med 1962; 56:711–737.
14. Zitnan D, Sitaj S. Chondrocalcinosis polyarticularis (familiaris) rentgenologicky a klinicky rozelor. Cesk Rentgenol 1960; 14:27.
15. Zitnan D, Sitaj S. Chondrocalcinosis articularis, Section I. Clinical and radiologic study. Ann Rheum Dis 1963; 22:142–152.
16. Kohn NN, Hughes RE, McCarty DJ, Faires JS. The significance of calcium phosphate crystals in the synovial fluid of arthritis patients: The "psuedogout syndrome," II Identification of crystals. Ann Intern Med 1962; 56:738–745.
17. Buchanan WW, Kraag GR, Palmer DG, Cockshott WP. The first recorded case of osteitis fibrosa cystica. Can Med Assoc J 1981; 124:812–815.
18. Lee SL, Stenn FC. Characterization of mummy bone ochronotic pigment. JAMA 1978; 240:136–138.
19. Bennett EH. Abnormal deposits in joints. Dublin J Med Sci 1903; 65:161–163.

20. Schumacher HR, Smolyo AP, Tse RL, Maurer K. Arthritis associated with apatite crystals. Ann Intern Med 1977; 87:411–416.
21. Dieppe PA, Huskisson EC, Crocker P, Willoughby DA. Apatite deposition disease. Lancet 1976; 1:266–269.
22. Halverson PB, McCarty DJ. Identification of hydroxyapatite crystals in synovial fluid. Arthritis Rheum 1979; 22:389–395.
23. McCarty DJ, Halverson PB, Carrera GF, Brewer BJ, Kozin F. "Milwaukee Shoulder": association of microspheroids containing hydroxyapatite crystals, active collagenase and neutral protease with rotator cuff defects. I Clinical aspects. Arthritis Rheum 1981; 24:464–473.
24. McCarty DJ, Lehr JR, Halverson PB. Crystal populations in human synovial fluid. Identification of apatite, octacalcium phosphate and beta tricalcium phosphate. Arthritis Rheum 1983; 26:1220–1224.
25. Caspi D, Rosenbach TO, Yaron M, McCarty DJ, Graff E. Periarthritis associated with basic calcium phosphate crystal deposition and low levels of serum alkaline phosphatase—Repeat of three cases from one family. J Rheumatol 1988; 15:823–827.
26. McCarty DJ, Gatter RA. Identification of calcium hydrogen phosphate dihydrate crystals in human fibrocartilage. Nature 1963; 201:391–392.

2

The Epidemiology of Gout and Calcium Pyrophosphate Dihydrate Deposition Disease

Kenneth G. Saag

Division of Clinical Immunology and Rheumatology, University of Alabama at Birmingham and Center for Education and Research on Therapeutics (CERTs) of Musculoskeletal Disorders, Birmingham, Alabama, U.S.A.

Ted R. Mikuls

Section of Rheumatology and Immunology, University of Nebraska and Omaha VA Medical Center, Omaha, Nebraska, U.S.A.

Joel Abbott

Division of Clinical Immunology and Rheumatology, University of Alabama at Birmingham, Birmingham, Alabama, U.S.A.

INTRODUCTION—GOUT

The study of gout epidemiology dates to antiquity, to Hippocrates' first descriptions of disease risk factors including advancing age, female menopause, and male sex. Thomas Sydenham, a 17th century English physician and infamous gout sufferer, made seminal contributions to our understanding of gout as an entity distinct from other forms of "rheumatism." In the latter half of the 18th century, uric acid was isolated from select bladder stones and found to be the primary constituent of gouty tophi. In the middle part of the 19th century, Sir Alfred Barring Garrod devised the first qualitative test for serum urate (the so-called "string test") and, in the process, defined the association of hyperuricemia with gout. Perhaps in response to the work of his contemporary (Robert Koch, who published his postulates in 1884), Freudweiler reproduced acute gout attacks by injecting monosodium urate crystals into the knee joints of otherwise healthy "volunteers."

Despite these early advances, a precise and reproducible method of gout diagnosis remained elusive until the 1960s, with McCarty and Hollander's initial description of crystal analysis using polarized microscopy (1). Although crystal diagnosis remains the "gold standard" for diagnosis, progress in gout epidemiology has been hampered by the lack of a standardized approach in defining case status. Findings of one recent study showed that the practice of performing needle aspiration and microscopic crystal analysis is done infrequently in the general practice setting (2), indicating that the sole reliance on microscopic crystal diagnosis leads to inappropriately low estimates of gout burden. Other groups of investigators have relied on patient self-report (3–5), periodic physical examination (6,7), physician diagnostic codes, and analyses of administrative claims database (8) to define gout status, each method with its own inherent limitations.

As with other rheumatic conditions, classification criteria have been developed to define gout status, including the American College of Rheumatology (ACR; formerly American Rheumatism Association) (9), Rome (10) and New York (11) criteria (Table 1). As with other means of defining case status, there are advantages and disadvantages to the application of such criteria. Applied in retrospective fashion, the use of such criteria often mandates the availability of

Table 1 American College of Rheumatology[a] Preliminary Classification Criteria for the Acute Arthritis of Primary Gout

Clinical setting[b]	Survey setting[c]
More than 1 attack of acute arthritis	More than 1 attack of acute arthritis
Maximum inflammation developed within 1 day	Maximum inflammation developed within 1 day
Monoarticular attack	Oligoarthritis attack
Redness observed over joint(s)	Redness observed over joint(s)
First MTP joint painful or swollen	First MTP joint painful or swollen
Unilateral first MTP joint attack	Unilateral first MTP joint attack
Unilateral tarsal joint attack	Unilateral tarsal joint attack
Tophus (suspected)	Tophus (proven or suspected)
Hyperuricemia	Hyperuricemia
Asymmetric swelling within a joint on X-ray	Asymmetric swelling within a joint on X-ray
Subcortical cysts without erosion on X-ray	Complete termination of an attack
Joint fluid culture negative for organisms during an attack	

[a]Formerly the American Rheumatism Association.
[b]Gout diagnoses in a clinical setting require (1) the presence of urate crystals in joint fluid, (2) the presence of a proven tophus, or (3) the presence of at least 6 of the 12 criteria.
[c]Gout diagnoses in the survey setting require the presence of 6 of the 11 criteria.
Abbreviation: MTP joint, metatarsophalangeal joint.

well-documented medical records for case validation, a process that can be both labor- and time-intensive. However, the ACR criteria have been reported to have a favorable sensitivity (85%) and specificity (93%, vs. patients with pseudogout) for gout diagnosis in the context of a population-based survey (9).

Despite persistent problems with defining gout status, it is important to recognize that substantial progress has been made in furthering our understanding of gout over the last four decades. Taken together, epidemiologic investigations suggest that gout frequency is on the rise worldwide. Moreover, recent investigations have shed important insight on the complex relationships of hyperuricemia, gout, and comorbid conditions, including hypertension, atherosclerosis, and the metabolic syndrome. In this chapter, we review our current knowledge of gout epidemiology with an emphasis on recent trends in disease frequency and an evolving understanding of factors associated to disease onset and resultant comorbidity.

ESTIMATES OF FREQUENCY OF GOUT

Prevalence

Results of several population-based investigations of gout prevalence are summarized in Table 2. Recognizing the substantial limitations in comparing results across different studies (based on differences in case definition, the use of point prevalence vs. period prevalence, different populations studied, etc.), results of these investigations suggest that gout prevalence has increased over the last 3 decades. Using a large U.K. practice registry in the mid-1970s, Currie observed an overall gout prevalence of 2.6 cases per 1000 (13) among the adult population. Employing a similar study methodology in 1993, Harris and

Table 2 Gout Prevalence (per 1000 Persons) and Incidence Rates (per 1000 Patient-Years) from Select Population-Based Investigations

Author(s) (Ref.)	Year(s)	Country	Population	Prevalence	Incidence
O'Sullivan (12)	1972	U.S.	Adults, >15 yr	3.0	–
Currie (13)	1975	U.K.	Adults, >15 yr	2.6	0.30
Aromdee, et al. (2)	1977–78	U.S.	All ages	–	0.45
Stewart, Silman (14)	1981–82	U.K.	Adults, >25 yr	–	1.40
Abbott, et al. (6)	1988	U.S.	Adults, >30 yr	–	0.84
Lawrence, et al. (15)	1992	U.S.	Adults, >18 yr	8.6	–
Harris, et al. (16)	1993	U.K.	All ages	9.5	–
Aromdee, et al. (2)	1995–96	U.S.	All ages	–	0.62
Klemp, et al. (17)	1997	New Zealand	Adults, >15 yr	47.2	–
Mikuls, et al. (18)	1999	U.K.	All ages	13.9	1.31

colleagues found that overall gout prevalence had increased by approximately three-fold (9.5 cases per 1000) from the time of Currie's prior report (16). In a more recent study examining enrollees of the U.K. General Practice Research Database (GPRD), investigators observed the overall gout prevalence to be even higher at 13.9 cases per 1000 (18).

Similar trends in disease prevalence have been reported in other geographic regions. In a population-based survey from New Zealand, investigators observed the overall gout prevalence (in patients over 15 years of age) to be 4.7% (17), an estimate that had nearly doubled over the previous thirty years (19).

U.S. data on gout prevalence comes from the National Health Interview Survey (NHIS; from 1969 to 1992) (3,15,20) and the Framingham study (6,7). In the late 1960s, investigators from the Framingham study reported a gout prevalence for adults over the age of 32 years of 28.5 and 3.9 cases per 1000 among adult men and women, respectively (7). The NHIS, based on patient self-report, showed that the overall gout prevalence doubled during the interval from 1969 to the mid-1980s before reaching a nadir of 8.6 cases per 1000 in 1992 (15,20). Relying on gout self-report to establish prevalence is problematic, with 44% of cases from the Sudbury study of 1972 failing to be confirmed using the Rome and New York criteria (12). A descriptive analysis utilizing an administrative claims database for a managed care population throughout the United States demonstrated that the prevalence of gout and/or hyperuricemia increased in the overall study population during the 10-year period between 1990 and 1999 (8). The increase was greatest in those over 65 years of age. In those under 65, men had four times higher prevalence than women (4:1). This gender gap narrowed for those over 65 (3:1).

Incidence

Available data examining disease incidence support the concept that gout frequency has risen over recent times (Table 2). Using the Rochester Epidemiology Project database and ACR Classification Criteria for gout diagnosis, investigators compared the age-adjusted gout incidence in 1995–1996 with that of 1977–1978 (2). Over this twenty-year interval, gout incidence increased 1.5 fold from a baseline of 45.0 per 100,000 person-years (95% CI: 31.7–59.3) to 62.3 per 100,000 (95% CI: 48.4–76.2). Notably, investigators observed a two-fold increase in the incidence of primary gout (i.e., no history of diuretic exposure) ($p=0.002$ for difference) over the same time period. A similar temporal trend has been noted by investigators from the U.K. Using data from the Second (1971–1972) and Third (1981–1982) National Morbidity Survey, Stewart and Silman noted an approximate 30% increase in gout incidence over one decade (14). Gout incidence in men increased from 1.6 cases per 1000 to 2.1 per 1000. Similarly, gout incidence increased among women from a baseline of 0.4 cases per 1000 in the early 1970s to 0.7 per 1000 over the next ten years.

As with disease prevalence, incidence rates vary based on the case definitions used and the populations examined. Investigators from the Framingham Study, using biennial physical examination, observed an annualized incidence rate (based on the number of new cases per person-bienniums at risk) of 0.84 per 1000 person-years (6). In a study of the U.K. GPRD using physician diagnostic codes, the overall 1999 gout incidence was found to be 1.31 cases per 1000 patient-years of follow-up (95% CI: 1.26–1.37) (18). Among men in the Framingham Study (6), the overall gout incidence rate was 1.6 cases per 1000. Roubenoff and colleagues (5), using patient self-report, observed a similar incidence rate (1.7 cases per 1000 patient-years) among male participants in the Johns Hopkins Precursors Study, a prospective cohort study involving medical students. In comparison, gout incidence among otherwise healthy male veterans over a 15-year follow-up period was found to be 2.8 cases per 1000 patient-years (21). The higher disease incidence noted in the latter study may relate to the relatively older population that was studied or differences in the frequency of select comorbidity or medication use that may have predisposed this population to gout. The role of emerging and changing risk factors in the incidence of gout is discussed below.

Factors Potentially Associated with an Increased Gout Risk

In 1726, Richard Blackmore, in his Discourse on the Gout, a Rheumatism, and the King's Evil, defined gout risk in stating, "The disease (gout)…owes its production to the tables of epicure and the abuse of delicious wine. It is the dissolute and voluptuous indulgence of sensual appetites that administer to the blood the seeds of gout by oppressing nature with too great plenty of rich supplies, and not those methods of life that enfeeble her faculties." Today, we know that gout is not just a disease of royalty or the over-indulgent but that a number of diverse factors lead to a higher risk and may partially explain the apparent increased prevalence of gout observed in the past two decades (Table 3). Evidence associating these risk factors with an increased prevalence of gout is summarized below. It is important to note that the direction of causality for certain associations, such as between gout and hypertension, is often controversial and difficult to accurately determine, due to the cross-sectional nature of many of the studies.

Hyperuricemia

A sustained elevation in serum urate represents the primary risk factor for the development of gout. In men, serum urate levels begin to increase during adolescence and, for most men, remain stable throughout adulthood. For men with gout and persistent, untreated hyperuricemia tophi develop on average 11 years later. In contrast, serum urate levels remain relatively low in women until menopause when levels increase before reaching a plateau during the postmenopausal years (23). The association of hyperuricemia with gout risk was confirmed in both the Framingham Study (7) and Normative Aging Study (21). In

Table 3 Proposed Principal Contributory Factors to the Increased Prevalence of Gout and Subsets of Refractory Disease Over the Last Two Decades in the United States

Increased longevity
Increased prevalence of hypertension
Dietary trends
Increased prevalence of obesity and metabolic syndrome
Changing demographic trends and high prevalence of hypertension or metabolic syndrome in specific racial and ethnic population subgroups
Increased prevalence of end-stage renal disease
Improved survival from congestive heart failure and coronary artery disease
Increased prevalence of diuretic and low-dose acetylsalicylic acid therapy
Limitations in the current armamentarium of antihyperuricemic agents, particularly in the allopurinol-hypersensitive patient with renal insufficiency
Increases in major organ transplantation linked with cyclosporine-induced gout

Source: From Ref. 22.

both investigations, there was a dramatic dose-response relationship of baseline serum urate levels with subsequent gout risk. In the Normative Aging Study, for instance, gout incidence was >40 cases per 1000 patient-years among men with baseline serum urate levels above 9.0 mg/dL. In contrast, incidence rates were <1 case per 1000 in men with baseline serum urate values less than 7.0 mg/dL (21).

Sociodemographic Factors

Sociodemographic factors, including male sex and older age, serve as important determinants of gout risk. As noted above, gout frequency increases in linear fashion with advancing age (2,3,14,18) and is relatively rare in younger age groups, particularly among younger women (Fig. 1). Of nearly 10,000 women under the age of 50 enrolled in the Framingham Study, only 2 developed incident gout (6). Likewise, in the recently published GPRD study (18) only 42 (<0.01%) of more than 500,000 at-risk women under the age of 45 years developed gout during the 1999 calendar year. This compares to 305 (0.06%) of over 500,000 at-risk men who developed incident gout during the same follow-up period.

Epidemiologic studies have consistently shown that men are three to six times more likely than women to develop gout (2,3,13,14,16,18). However, male-to-female prevalence ratios decrease appreciably with advancing age, possibly reflecting the loss of the uricosuric effect of estrogen in postmenopausal women (24). Of gout patients older than 60, one-third to one-half are women (18). With dramatic declines in the use of estrogen replacement therapy, it has been predicted that gout incidence will continue to rise in older women (22), resulting in an even lower male-to-female sex ratio among older gout patients.

As with age and sex, geographic residence and race/ethnicity may also serve as important correlates of gout risk. For instance, as opposed to urban residence,

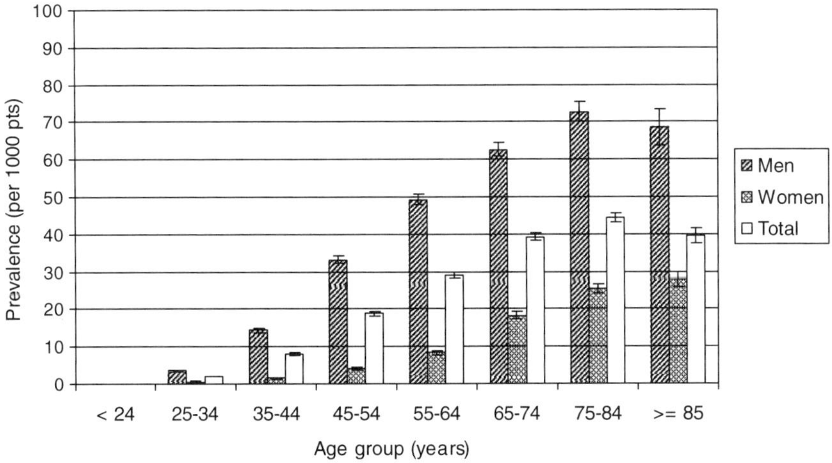

Figure 1 Gout prevalence (1999) among enrollees in the U.K. General Practice Research Database (GPRD). Ninety-five percent CIs (*shown with bars*) were calculated using normal approximation. *Source*: From Ref. 18.

several early European studies suggested a "protective effect" associated with rural residence (25–27). In a national U.K. study, Currie found important regional variations in gout prevalence, with higher gout rates found in England compared to the rest of Great Britain and higher rates in Wales compared to Scotland (13).

In a population-based New Zealand study (using ACR Classification Criteria), gout was found to be far more prevalent among patients of Maori descent than those of European descent (6.4% vs. 2.9%) (17). Among Maori men the cumulative incidence was noted to be as high as 13.9%, compared to a rate of 5.8% among European men. These very high rates of gout are greatest in those Polynesians who migrate to more urban centers where exposure to western diet and alcohol may contribute to an already enhanced genetic predisposition. Rates of hyperuricemia over 25% have been noted in men living in Kin-Hu, Kinmen, islands very close to southern mainland China (28). In contrast to the high gout frequency in many Asian and Polynesian cultures, Native American populations (including the Blackfeet and Pima) appear to have a lower gout burden than Caucasians (29). Of note, there is an almost a complete absence of gout in certain African populations (30–33).

A survey of gout in 36 Korean women revealed the onset after menopause (mean age 54.3 years) for the majority (34). Earlier onset was associated with the use of cyclosporin or renal insufficiency. Risk factors included hypertension (61%), renal insufficiency (47%), and diuretic use (28%). Compared to a cohort of Korean men with gout, hypertension and renal insufficiency were more common in women.

To date, there has been only one reported case of crystal-proven gout in an Australian Aborigine, despite a high rate of hyperuricemia in that population (35).

That individual was found to have "excessive alcohol consumption" and was taking furosemide. The prevalence of gout in a rural community in Western Maharashtra, India, is 0.12% (36). Finally, a review of Saudi Arabian individuals, a population with rare alcohol consumption, revealed a prevalence of hyperuricemia of 8.42% and no cases of gout (37).

Hyperuricemia is significantly increased in African Americans compared to Caucasians (38). One study found that African Americans were substantially more likely than Caucasians to develop incident gout (RR = 1.7; 95% CI 1.0–2.8) (4). The excess number of gout cases observed among African Americans was attributed to a higher prevalence of hypertension in this group compared to Caucasians. This is important because hypertension is strongly associated with gout (see below). This racial/ethnic disparity in disease burden may also relate to an increased prevalence of obesity (39) and renal disease (40) among African Americans compared to Caucasians, both factors also closely associated with gout.

Diet and Alcohol Consumption

Based on the results of numerous metabolic studies (41–44), a purine-rich diet has long been implicated as a potential risk factor for gout onset. This was recently corroborated by investigators from the Health Professionals Follow-up Study (45). In this study, gout incidence was significantly associated with the daily intake of meats and seafood, foods with relatively high purine contents (Fig. 2). During a twelve-year follow-up period, investigators identified 730 confirmed new cases of gout using self-reported satisfaction of the ACR Classification Criteria. After adjusting for potentially confounding factors including age, alcohol intake, body mass index, diuretic use, and comorbidity (including hypertension and renal insufficiency), men in the highest quintile of meat intake (>1.92 daily servings) were more likely than those in the lowest quintile to develop gout (RR=1.41; 95% CI 1.07–1.86). Compared to those in

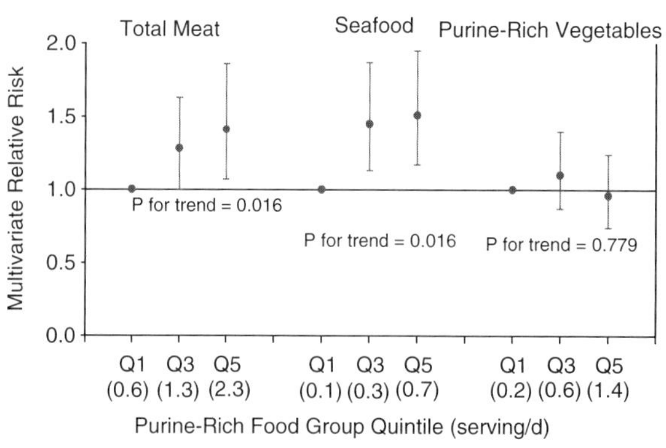

Figure 2 Associations of purine-rich food groups with gout. *Source*: Data from the Health Professionals Follow-up Study in Ref. 45.

the lowest quintile, men in the highest quintile of seafood intake (>0.56 servings) were also at increased risk of gout (RR=1.51; 95% CI 1.17–1.95). The reported association of seafood intake with gout was more pronounced among men who were not overweight, suggesting that there may be important subgroup differences to consider in dietary risk factor assessment. Notably, there was no increased risk of gout with greater consumption of purine-rich vegetables or total protein intake.

In the same study, gout incidence was found to be lower among men with the highest levels of dairy product consumption. Compared to those in the lowest quintile, men in the highest quintile of dairy product intake (>2.88 daily servings) were only half as likely to develop gout (RR=0.56; 95% CI 0.42–0.74). The perceived protective effect of these foods appeared to be most pronounced for low-fat dairy products, as opposed to those with high-fat content. Although its biologic plausibility remains to be defined, the association of lower gout incidence with a high intake of dairy foods may relate to the uricosuric effect of milk proteins including casein and lactalbumin (46). It is important to recognize, however, that an increased intake of milk proteins failed to show a significant urate-lowering effect in a controlled trial involving postmenopausal women (47). Other foods have also been reported to have a potent uricosuric effect and, as such, have been hypothesized to have a beneficial effect on gout (48). In a metabolic study of young women (age 22–40 years), the daily consumption of 280 grams of cherries (2 servings) was associated with significant declines in plasma urate levels with concomitant increases in urinary urate excretion (49).

As has been long suspected (50), alcohol consumption is a major determinant of gout risk. Recent data also from the Health Professionals Follow-up Study has provided important insight into alcohol related risk in gout (51). Compared to prior cohort studies examining the association of alcohol use with gout (4–6,21,52), this investigation was relatively large in size (n=730 incident gout cases) and had ample data available to allow investigators to adjust for multiple potential confounders of gout risk. Referent to men who did not drink alcohol, investigators observed a significant association of gout risk with total daily alcohol intake, and there was a marked dose-response across categories of consumption ($p < 0.0001$ for trend) (51). The relative risk for every 10 g increase in daily alcohol intake (approximately one drink/day) was 1.17 (95% CI 1.11–1.22). Investigators found differences in gout risk based on the type of alcohol consumed (Fig. 3). Gout risk appeared to be most strongly associated with beer intake, perhaps related to its greater purine content (guanosine) relative to other alcoholic beverages (53). The relative risk for each daily 12 oz. beer serving was 1.49 (95% CI 1.32–1.70) while the relative risk for a single daily serving of liquor (one shot) was 1.15 (95% CI 1.04–1.28). In contrast, there was no association of daily wine consumption with gout risk (RR per 4 oz. serving per day 1.04; 95% CI 0.88–1.22).

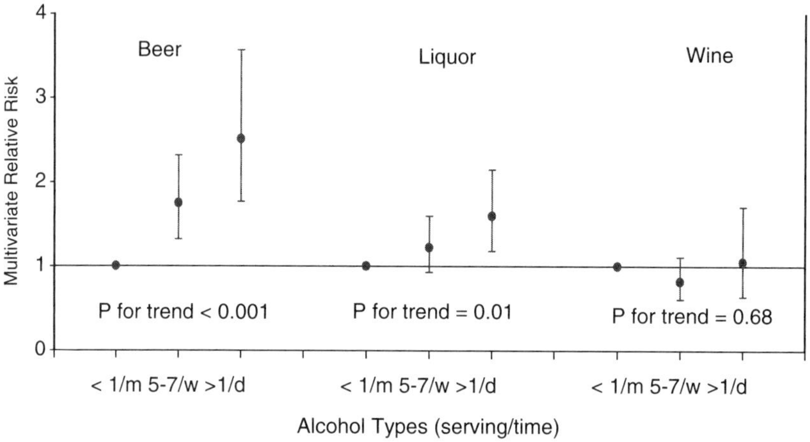

Figure 3 Gout risk based on the type of alcoholic beverage consumed. *Source*: Data from the Health Professionals Follow-up Study in Ref. 51.

Lead Exposure

Lead intoxication has long been recognized as a cause of secondary gout, commonly referred to as saturnine gout. Indeed, overt lead intoxication (predominantly via the consumption of tainted food and wines) has been intimately linked to two historical epidemics of gout, the first involving ancient Roman aristocrats and the second occurring during the European Renaissance (54). There have been two recent investigations examining the influence of chronic low-level environmental lead exposure on urate excretion and gout risk. Taken together, these studies suggest that subclinical exposures to lead enhance the risk of hyperuricemia and gout. In a cross-sectional study involving 111 otherwise healthy Taiwanese (27 with a history of gout), gouty subjects had a significantly higher total body lead burdens and lower measures of urate clearance (55). Additionally, increased blood lead levels were significantly related to higher serum urate values. In a large retrospective cohort study, high bone lead levels were significantly correlated with elevations in serum urate (52). However, perhaps related to the relatively low blood lead levels encountered in this latter study, investigators found no association of either bone or blood lead levels with the development of gout.

Genetics

The incidence of gout and hyperuricemia appear to have a substantial genetic component (see also Chapter 3). It is estimated that the heritability of gout ranges from between 60% and 90% (56). Gout heritability is predominantly polygenic with multiple genes conferring risk. Monogenic disorders account for only rare gout cases and include both X-linked (i.e., complete or partial hypoxanthine-guanine phosphoribosyltransferase deficiency causing Lesch-Nyhan Syndrome and increased phosphoribosyl pyrophosphate synthetase activity) and autosomal dominant (i.e., Familial Juvenile Hyperuricemic Nephropathy) forms (57). With data emerging from the Human Genome Project (58), it is likely that our understanding of genetic influences in gout will expand substantially in the near future.

Post-Surgery

Acute gout, often in atypical joints, commonly presents in patients who have recently undergone surgical procedures. This affects both those with a known history of gout as well as persons who post-operatively develop their initial attack (59). Differentiating post-surgical gout attacks, which are often accompanied by fever, from infectious sequelae can present a diagnostic challenge. Dehydration, catabolism, changes in medications, general anesthesia, and starvation are postulated as mechanisms responsible for a urate flux and precipitation of acute post-operative gout attacks.

Medication Use

Certain drugs are associated with secondary gout due to their effects on renal reabsorption, secretion, and excretion of uric acid. Although hypertension is associated with gout (see below), thiazide diuretics increase uric acid reabsorption leading to hyperuricemia and ultimately gout for many individuals (60). Despite a rising incidence of gout over the past two decades, there was not an increase in gout associated with thiazide diuretic use in the Rochester Epidemiology Project (6), perhaps corresponding to a declining use in diuretics in the 1990s. Of note, this trend could change based partially on the results of a large randomized controlled trial showing that hydrochlorothiazide is a low cost hypertension therapy that significantly lowers the risk of stroke (61).

Hyperuricemia occurs in the vast majority of post-transplant patients and gout is thus very common (62). Among renal transplant patients the prevalence of gout is estimated at 2% to 13% (63,64). In post-transplant patients gout may present with an accelerated clinical course. Manifestations more typically seen in the advanced stages of gout, such as tophi and polyarticular involvement, can develop within 6 months to 4 years (62). Cyclosporine, typically prescribed for transplant patients, inhibits uric acid excretion (65). Cyclosporin can predispose to gout via a number of mechanisms that include: (1) hypertension, (2) decreased renal clearance of urate, (3) decreased glomerular filtration, and (4) interstitial nephropathy (64–66).

High doses of aspirin (>3 g/day) are uricosuric. Low doses, however, cause uric acid retention. Aspirin doses as low as 75 mg/day caused a 15% decrease in the rate of uric acid excretion and a corresponding increase in serum urate (67).

Pyrazinamide, ethambutol, and niacin are associated with gout due to their suppressive effects on uric acid secretion.

GOUT COMORBIDITIES, OTHER ASSOCIATIONS, AND PROGNOSIS

Metabolic Syndrome

The metabolic syndrome (previously referred to as syndrome X) is a highly prevalent condition defined by high fasting glucose, abdominal obesity, hypertriglyceridemia, low HDL-C, hypertension, and increased risk for atherosclerotic events (68). The metabolic syndrome, as well as its components, is independently associated with hyperuricemia, and evidence supporting these associations are reviewed individually below.

Obesity

Gout is more common in those with obesity, particularly among men with an endomorphic body habitus (69). Excessive weight gain in young adulthood is also a risk factor independent of obesity (5). Similarly, a reduction in weight may also lower gout risk (70). As body mass index has risen in the U.S. and certain other nations, so has the prevalence of gout (71). High body mass index is directly associated with hyperuricemia and an increased risk of gout, even in adolescents, and this risk decreases with weight loss (72–74). Many obese persons meet the definition for metabolic syndrome summarized above. It has recently been suggested that leptin may be a link between obesity and hyperuricemia (72).

Hypertension

The association of hypertension and hyperuricemia has been well described for many decades (75). Half of untreated hypertensive patients have hyperuricemia (76). Elevated serum urate (concentration >5.5 mg/dL) may precede hypertension and correlates with blood pressure in children with primary hypertension (77) and in adults (78). In the Normative Aging Study, gout was 3-fold more common in hypertensives compared with normotensive adults, although a large proportion of this increased risk was suspected to be due to thiazide diuretic use (21). Hypertension has increased in the US, particular among African Americans, and along with other risk factors may contribute to a higher frequency of gout, observed among African Americans in comparison to Caucasians (4,34).

Hyperlipidemia

Hyperuricemia is strongly correlated with serum triglycerides, with a weaker correlation with serum cholesterol (74).

Diabetes Mellitus

An increased incidence of impaired glucose tolerance and diabetes in normal glucose tolerant patients was associated with hyperuricemia (79). Insulin resistance may lead to overactivity of Na+/H+exchange in the kidney resulting in more urate reabsorption (80). Alternative mechanisms include increased intracellular availability of esters of long chain fatty acids, which may promote renal vasoconstriction, renal uric acid retention, and up-regulated uric acid (81).

Hypothyroidism

A higher prevalence of hypothyroidism has been observed among men and women with gout (82,83). Thyroid replacement therapy is associated with a decrease in serum urate perhaps mediated by uric acid diuresis. It has been speculated that urate homeostasis is partially controlled by thyroid-stimulating hormone receptors in extrathyroidal tissues including the kidney.

Renal Insufficiency

Although renal insufficiency clearly leads to hyperuricemia, the converse, whether gout results in chronic renal disease, has been debated for many years (84). Interpretations are confounded by a more robust relationship between gout and hypertension, a clear confounder for a gout renal disease association. As summarized above, elevated urate can reduce renal blood flow (85). Thus, hyperuricemia, found in up to a third of patients with hypertension, could lead to early renal vascular involvement, specifically nephrosclerosis.

Examination of a large group-practice cohort found that azotemia attributable to hyperuricemia is generally mild and not problematic until serum urate levels reach 13 mg/dL in men (86). The Normative Study of Aging found no deleterious effects of gout on renal function (21). It is likely that hypertension, chronic lead exposure, ischemic heart disease, and preexistent renal insufficiency play important roles in the pathogenesis of "urate" nephropathy.

Nephrolithiasis

Cross sectional studies have suggested a 15% to 22% prevalence of nephrolithiasis among individuals with gout (87) and a nearly 50% higher risk of stones in the National Health and Nutrition Examination Survey (NHANES), an association that persisted even after accounting for race, hypertension, body mass index, sex, and age (88). In the Health Professionals Follow-up Study, there was a 15% prevalence of kidney stones among men with a history of gout compared to an 8% prevalence in those with no gout history. This nearly two fold increased risk was maintained after adjustment for age and body mass index

(OR = 1.9, 95% CI 1.7 to 2.1). Gout also increased the risk of incident kidney stone disease (OR = 2.1 95% CI 1.2 to 3.7) in that study (89).

Cardiovascular Disease

Past U.S. and multinational epidemiologic studies have both supported (6,34,90–93) and refuted (94–96) an association of elevated serum urate with cardiovascular disease (reviewed in Alderman, 2004). Furthermore, associations may be seen in only particular patient subgroups, such as for women (91,97) and those with particular body physiques (69). Contrasting results from longitudinal analyses of two large and well-designed U.S. studies, the NHANES and the Framingham study, have fueled controversy about whether serum urate is a causal factor in cardiovascular disease. For example, in NHANES I, a 60 micromol/L increase in serum urate level was associated with a 48% increase in the risk of ischemic heart disease among women (34). There was higher all-cause mortality and greater ethnic diversity in NHANES compared to Framingham, suggesting possible greater external validity (generalizability) of NHANES. On the other hand, critics contend that serum urate may simply be a confounder for hypertension, diuretic use, dyslipidemia, disordered glucose metabolism and/or renal insufficiency (95,98).

Evidence supporting an association of serum urate with cardiovascular disease can be drawn from randomized clinical trials. The Losartan Intervention For Endpoint Reduction in Hypertension (LIFE) study compared the effects of losartan and atenolol for reduction in cardiovascular morbidity and mortality among over 9000 subjects with confirmed hypertension and left ventricular hypertrophy. Losartan, an angiotensin II receptor antagonist, interferes with urate reabsorption in the proximal tubule, thereby lowering serum urate. Atenolol, a beta-blocker, has no known effect on serum urate concentration. Although patients were not hyperuricemic upon entry into the study, the baseline serum urate was significantly associated with an increase in future cardiovascular events (hazard ratio 1.02, 95% CI 1.02 to 1.03). The estimated contribution of serum urate to the treatment effect of losartan on the composite endpoint (i.e., cardiovascular death, nonfatal and fatal MI, nonfatal and fatal stroke) was 29%, suggesting that attenuating serum urate could reduce cardiovascular events in a high-risk population (99). Stroke may also occur more frequently among diabetics who have higher serum urate levels, even after other cardiovascular risk factors were considered (100). Despite an absent association with cardiovascular outcomes, in one Scandinavian study serum urate level was positively correlated with 12-year overall mortality (90).

Beyond coronary artery disease, hyperuricemia was a strong, independent marker of impaired prognosis in heart failure (101). After analytically accounting for renal disease, heart failure patients with a serum urate level > 800 micromol/L had a relative risk of mortality that was 18-times higher than in patients with urate < 400 micromol/L.

Table 4 Diagnostic Criteria and Categories for Calcium Pyrophosphate Dihydrate Crystal Deposition Disease (Pseudogout)

Criteria	
I	Demonstration of CPPD crystals obtained by biopsy, necropsy, or aspirated synovial fluid, by definitive means, e.g., characteristic "fingerprint" by X-ray diffraction powder pattern or by chemical analysis
II	A. Identification of monoclinic or triclinic crystals showing a weakly positive, or a lack of, birefringence by compensated polarized light microscopy B. Presence of typical calcifications on radiographs[a]
III	A. Acute arthritis, especially of knees or other large joints, with or without concomitant hyperuricemia B. Chronic arthritis, especially of knee, hip, wrist, carpus, elbow, shoulder, and metacarpophalangeal joints, particularly if accompanied by acute exacerbations; the chronic arthritis shows the following features to be helpful in differentiating it from osteoarthritis: 1. Uncommon site for primary osteoarthritis, e.g., wrist, metacarpophalangeal joints, elbow, or shoulder 2. Radiographic appearance, e.g., radiocarpal or patellofemoral joint space narrowing, especially if isolated (patella "wrapped around" the femur)[b], femoral cortical erosion superior to the patella on the lateral view of the knee 3. Subchondral cyst formation 4. Severe progressive degeneration with subchondral bony collapse (microfractures), and fragmentation with formation of intra-articular radiodense bodies 5. Variable and inconstant osteophyte formation 6. Tendon calcifications, especially of Achilles, triceps, and obturator tendons 7. Involvement of the axial skeleton and subchondral cysts of apophyseal and sacroiliac joints, multiple levels of disc calcification and vacuum phenomenon, and sacroiliac vacuum phenomenon
Categories	
A	Definite—criteria I or II(A) or II(B) must be fulfilled
B	Probable—criteria II(A) or II(B) must be fulfilled
C	Possible—criteria III(A) or III(B) should alert the clinician to the possibility of underlying CPPD deposition

[a]Heavy punctuate and linear calcifications in fibrocartilages, articular (hyaline) cartilages, and joint capsules, especially if bilaterally symmetric; faint or atypical calcifications may be due to dicalcium phosphate dehydrate (CDPD) ($CaHPO_4 \cdot 2H_2O$) deposits or to vascular calcifications; both are also often bilaterally symmetric.

[b]Also described as a feature of the arthritis of hyperparathyroidism.

Abbreviation: CPPD, calcium pyrophosphate dehydrate.

Source: From Ref. 103.

CALCIUM PYROPHOSPHATE DIHYDRATE DEPOSITION DISEASE

Diagnostic criteria for CPPD diseases have been proposed and generally include demonstration of CPPD crystals by synovial biopsy or synovial fluid analysis (102) and the presence of calcifications on radiographs (Table 4) (104). Given the heterogeneity of the clinical presentations of CPPD diseases and the nomenclature used to characterize them, defining their epidemiology is difficult. For example, there is minimal data available to define the incidence of the syndrome of pseudogout. Most of the epidemiologic characterization of CPPD diseases is therefore derived from prevalence studies utilizing post-mortem and radiographic surveys of chondrocalcinosis (105). The prevalence of chondrocalcinosis found in these surveys is quite variable, ranging from 2% to 35%.

ESTIMATES OF FREQUENCY OF CPPD DISEASES

Prevalence

Post-Mortem Analyses

In post-mortem analyses, prevalence data may be influenced by the methods used to identify articular calcifications (105). Menisci from 215 cadavera of all ages were analyzed radiographically for calcifications between 1963 and 1964 (106). CPPD deposits were found in at least one meniscus in 35% of cadavers studied. Similarly, a more recent study identified calcifications radiographically in menisci and knee articular cartilage in 20.7% of 130 consecutive autopsies (107). In contrast, at least two post-mortem analyses employing histological means of identifying CPPD crystals have yielded prevalence rates of less than 10% (106,108). This suggests that the sensitivity of histologic identification of CPPD crystals versus radiographic identification of calcifications differs in post-mortem analyses. To what extent the presence of calcifications in these series correlated with clinical CPPD disease is also unclear.

There are numerous studies investigating the radiographic prevalence of chondrocalcinosis with variable results (Table 5). Direct comparisons are hindered by differences in sample sizes, radiographic techniques, choice of joints examined, patient age, and populations surveyed. Some of these studies, for example, are taken from geriatric patient populations that may not be representative of the general aging population. Still, it is reasonable to conclude that the prevalence of chondrocalcinosis increases with age. Prevalence is quite high among subjects 80 years of age or older in some series. In the Framingham Osteoarthritis Study, chondrocalcinosis of the knee was found in 27.1% of subjects greater than 85 years of age compared to 3.2% of those 65 to 69 years of age (109). Among a cohort of 261 subjects in north east Spain, articular chondrocalcinosis was noted in 43% of patients greater than 80 years of age compared to 7% of those between the ages of 60 and 69 (110).

Table 5 Prevalence of Radiographic Chondrocalcinosis Based on Population Surveys

Authors (Ref.)	Year	Country	Number	Age	Joints	Articular chondrocalcinosis (%)		Overall (%)
						Women	Men	
Bocher, et al. (113)	1965	U.S.	455	>59	Knee	8	6	7
Cabanel, et al. (114)	1970	France	360	>60	Knee	6	6	6
Trentham, et al. (115)	1975	U.S.	100 men	>50	Wrist	–	–	2
Ellman, Levin (116)	1975	U.S.	58	>70	Knee/wrist/pelvis	32	–	28
Leonard, et al. (117)	1977	France	272	>50	Knee, wrist	19	7	16
Delauche, et al. (118)	1977	France	62	>80	Knee/wrist/pelvis	28	41	32
Memin, et al. (119)	1978	France	108	>80	Knee	23	–	23
Ellman, et al. (120)	1981	U.S.	574	>50	Knee	8	12	10
Mégard, et al. (121)	1983	France	120	>68	Knee	–	–	13
Wilkins, et al. (122)	1983	U.K.	100	>65	Knee/wrist/pelvis	39	23	34
Gordon, et al. (123)	1984	Australia	127	>55	Knee/wrist/pelvis	24	4	16
Bergstrom, et al. (111)	1986	Sweden	81	All 79	Knee/wrist	23	6	16
Felson, et al. (109)	1989	U.S.	1402	>63	Knee	9	7	8
Sanmarti, et al. (110)	1993	Spain	261	>60	Knee, wrist	14	6	10

Source: From Ref. 110.

Factors Potentially Associated with an Increased CPPD Risk

As chondrocalcinosis and CPPD deposition occur in a significant proportion of the adult population (Table 5), associations should be interpreted with caution. However, it appears that gender, genetic factors, and certain metabolic diseases influence CPPD risk.

Gender and Ethnic Influences

In many of the prevalence surveys listed in Table 5, chondrocalcinosis was found more commonly in women than in men, an observation that may be reflective of the increasing ratio of women to men in an aging population. In one series, the female to male prevalence ratio increased almost four-fold from ages 70 to 79 (111). Though methods of data collection differ between ethnic populations, making comparisons difficult, there does not appear to be an obvious ethnic influence on the development of chondrocalcinosis as prevalence is similar among a number of North American and European populations (Table 5).

Genetic Factors

The prevalence of familial CPPD not associated with metabolic or endocrine diseases is uncertain (112). Familial aggregation has been described in certain populations such as in southern Chile, where a high incidence of articular chondrocalcinosis has been reported among the Chiloe Islanders (124). There are numerous reports of familial aggregation among Spanish families (125–127). In one study, 44 Spanish kindreds with CPPD were compared to 16 kindreds with other inflammatory or noninflammatory arthritides (126). Familial aggregation of two or more members was found among 21 of the CPPD kindreds with a further 10 kindreds having relatives without definite CPPD but a history of "pseudogout-like attacks" or radiographic evidence of MCP arthropathy. Two additional Spanish surveys noted a similar familial prevalence of articular chondrocalcinosis (26% and 28%) among family members of CPPD disease patients (125,127). Kindreds have also been described in other European countries (128–130), Argentina (131), and the United States (132). These CPPD kindreds differ with respect to age of onset, severity of clinical or radiographic manifestations, and frequency of endogamous marriages (112,133). For further information, see Chapter 3.

Hypomagnesemia

Magnesium is an important cofactor for pyrophosphatase activity rendering the association between hypomagnesemia and CPPD deposition theoretically plausible (134,135). There are numerous case reports of this association in the literature (136–139). Patients are typically young with polyarticular chondrocalcinosis and disease characterized by recurrent episodes of pseudogout rather than chronic pyrophosphate arthropathy (136). Renal magnesium wasting appears to be the mechanism in most cases, and association of chondrocalcinosis with genetic abnormalities of magnesium conservation including Bartter's syndrome

(137,140) and Gitelman syndrome (141) have been reported. In a controlled trial, chronic pyrophosphate arthropathy patients given oral magnesium demonstrated significant improvement in articular signs and symptoms at six months without radiographic improvement in chondrocalcinosis (142).

Hypothyroidism

The association of CPPD arthropathy and hypothyroidism is controversial. In a study of 105 patients with pyrophosphate arthropathy, 11% were found to be hypothyroid compared to 3% of a matched group of acute medical admissions (143). In a cohort of 100 hypothyroid patients, 17% were found to have chondrocalcinosis compared to 10% of age and gender-matched controls (144). Another study did not support a relationship between hypothyroidism and chondrocalcinosis. In a cohort of 49 hypothyroid patients, only two patients were found to have chondrocalcinosis of the knee compared to one euthyroid patient (145). Data collected from 1375 members of the Framingham Osteoarthritis Cohort demonstrated no evidence of an association between high levels of thyroid stimulating hormone (TSH) and knee chondrocalcinosis (146).

Hyperparathyroidism

The relationship between CPPD deposition diseases and hyperparathyroidism was initially described in case reports in the late 1950s and early 1960s (147–150). There are few comparator studies evaluating the relationship between hyperparathyroidism and CPPD deposition. A small study comparing the frequency of hyperparathyroidism and other metabolic parameters in 28 subjects with pseudogout and 22 controls with osteoarthritis failed to demonstrate statistical intergroup differences (151). In another study, eight of 26 patients (31%) with documented hyperparathyroidism were found to have chondrocalcinosis compared to four of 104 controls (4%) ($p<0.01$) (152). Similar findings of increased chondrocalcinosis were observed among 41 hyperparathyroid patients compared to 100 geriatric controls (153). The proposed mechanism for the development of chondrocalcinosis in hyperparathyroidism is the increased ionic product of calcium pyrophosphate owing to increased extracellular calcium concentrations. Interestingly, there are numerous case reports of pseudogout attacks after parathyroidectomy (154–156). Postoperative hypocalcemia is felt to promote the solubility of CPPD crystals and their subsequent shedding into the synovial space (136).

Hemochromatosis

The original report of arthritis occurring in hemochromatosis was published in 1964 and included an example of chondrocalcinosis (157). An association between hemochromatosis and articular chondrocalcinosis has since been well-described.

In one series of 63 patients with iron overload, an arthropathy was present in 55%, and of these, chondrocalcinosis was present in approximately half (158). Compared to patients with idiopathic chondrocalcinosis, a male predominance and younger age has been described among patients with hemochromatosis and chondrocalcinosis (159). Distinct radiographic features in hemochromatosis compared to idiopathic pyrophosphate arthropathy include metacarpophalangeal joint involvement, hook-like osteophytes on the radial aspect of the metacarpal heads, and maintenance of the scapholunate space (160). Treatment of iron overload in patients with established chondrocalcinosis does not appear to prevent progression of the arthropathy (161).

EPIDEMIOLOGY OF BASIC CALCIUM PHOSPHATE ARTHROPATHIES

Basic calcium phosphate (BCP) crystals are the crystals associated with the most common forms of crystal associated arthropathies. The term BCP includes crystals of partially carbonated substituted hydroxyapatite, octacalcium phosphate, and tricalcium phosphate. Clinically these crystals can occur in a wide variety of clinical presentations ranging from calcific periarthritis to intra-articular deposition with osteoarthritis (see Chapter 3 for more information).

Few systematic studies of the incidence of prevalence of juxta-articular deposits of BCP crystals have been performed. Because the deposits are often asymptomatic, they may be discovered as an incidental finding on shoulder radiographs. One large study of predominantly white North Americans found a prevalence of calcific periarthritis in the shoulders of 2.7%, only 34% to 45% of which were symptomatic (162). Calcific periarthritis occurred more commonly in females, with the highest prevalence found between ages 31 and 40 years (19.5%). Others report periarticular calcifications to occur most commonly between ages 40 and 70 years, with prevalence to be as high as 7.5%, and to affect each sex equally. The joints most commonly involved are the shoulder (60%), followed by the hip, knee, elbow, wrist, and ankle (163,164). This complication has been reported in a 3-year-old and appears to be less common in the elderly (165).

The prevalence of intra-articular BCP crystal deposition is not established. Apatite crystals were present in 50% of osteoarthritic knees evaluated prior to surgery and, and in other studies, were found in 26% to 60% of synovial fluid samples for osteoarthritic knees (166–168). The most severe form of BCP crystal-associated arthropathy is Milwaukee shoulder syndrome (although this arthropathy affects other joints as well) in a condition found in the elderly (169). Although its true prevalence is unknown, it is likely that prevalence of intra-articular BCP crystal deposition correlates with the severity of osteoarthritis.

BCP crystals can also be found in the tumorous deposits seen in chronic renal failure, especially in patients on chronic dialysis as well as in scleroderma, systemic lupus erythematosus, dermatomyositis, and hyperparathyroidism. The true prevalence of BCP crystals in these conditions is not certain.

REFERENCES

1. McCarty D, Hollander J. Identification of urate crystals in gout synovial fluid. Ann Intern Med 1961; 54:452–460.
2. Aromdee E, Michet C, Crowson C, O'Fallon M, Gabriel S. Epidemiology of gout: is the incidence rising? J Rheumatol 2002; 29:2403–2406.
3. Benson V, Marano M. Current estimates from the National Health Interview Survey. Vital Health Stat 1992; 189:1–269.
4. Hochberg M, Thomas J, Thomas D, Mead L, Levine D, Klag M. Racial differences in the incidence of gout: the role of hypertension. Arthritis Rheum 1995; 38:628–632.
5. Roubenoff R, Klag M, Mead L, Liang K, Seidler A, Hochberg M. Incidence and risk factors for gout in white men. JAMA 1991; 266:3004–3007.
6. Abbott RD, Brand FN, Kannel WB, Castelli WP. Gout and coronary heart disease: the Framingham Study. J Clin Epidemiol 1988; 41:237–242.
7. Hall A, Barry P, Dawber T, McNamara P. Epidemiology of gout and hyperuricemia: a long-term population study. Am J Med 1967; 42:27–37.
8. Wallace KL, Riedel AA, Joseph-Ridge N, Wortmann R. Increasing prevalence of gout and hyperuricemia over 10 years among older adults in a managed care population. J Rheumatol 2004; 31:1582–1587.
9. Wallace S, Robinson H, Masi A, Decker J, McCarty D, Yu T-F. Preliminary criteria for the classification of the acute arthritis of primary gout. Arthritis Rheum 1977; 20:895–900.
10. Kellgren JH. In: Jeffrey MR, Ball J, eds. The Epidemiology of Chronic Rheumatism. In: A symposium organized by the Council for International Organizations of Medical Sciences (1961: Rome), Vol. 1. Oxford: Blackwell, 1963.
11. Bennett PH, Wood PHN. In: Population Studies of the Rheumatic Diseases: Proceedings of the Third International Symposium, New York, June 5th–10th, 1966. Amsterdam: Excerpta Medica Foundation, 1968:457–458.
12. O'Sullivan J. Gout in a New England town: a prevalence study in Sudbury, Massachusetts. Ann Rheum Dis 1972; 31:166–169.
13. Currie W. Prevalence and incidence of the diagnosis of gout in Great Britain. Ann Rheum Dis 1979; 38:101–106.
14. Stewart O, Silman A. Review of UK data on the rheumatic diseases-4 Gout. Br J Rheumatol 1990; 29:485–488.
15. Lawrence R, Helmick C, Arnett F, et al. Estimates of the prevalence of arthritis and selected musculoskeletal disorders in the United States. Arthritis Rheum 1998; 41:778–799.
16. Harris C, Lloyd C, Lewis J. The prevalence and prophylaxis of gout in England. J Clin Epidemiol 1995; 48:1153–1158.
17. Klemp P, Stansfield S, Castle B, Robertson M. Gout is on the increase in New Zealand. Ann Rheum Dis 1997; 56:22–26.
18. Mikuls T, Farrar J, Bilker W, Fernandes S, Schumacher H, Saag K. Gout epidemiology: results from the U.K. General Practice Research Database, 1990–1999. Ann Rheum Dis 2005; 64:267–272.
19. Prior I, Rose B. Uric acid, gout and public health in the South Pacific. NZ Med J 1966; 65:295–300.

20. Lawrence R, Hochberg M, Kelsey J, et al. Estimates of the prevalence of selected arthritic and musculoskeletal diseases in the United States. J Rheumatol 1989; 16:427–441.
21. Campion E, Glynn R, DeLabry L. Asymptomatic hyperuricemia. Risks and consequences in the Normative Aging Study. Am J Med 1987; 82:421–426.
22. Bieber J, Terkeltaub R. On the brink of novel therapeutic options for an ancient disease. Arthritis Rheum 2004; 50:2400–2414.
23. Mikkelsen W, Dodge H, Valkenburg H. The distribution of serum uric acid values in a population unselected as to gout or hyperuricemia, Tecumseh, Michigan 1959–1960. Am J Med 1965; 39:242–251.
24. Fam A. Gout in the elderly: clinical presentation and treatment. Drugs Aging 1998; 13:229–243.
25. De Blecourt J. Screening the population for rheumatic diseases. Ann Rheum Dis 1954; 13:338–340.
26. Isomaki H, Takkunen H. Gout and hyperuricemia in a Finnish rural population. Acta Rheumatol Scand 1969; 15:112–120.
27. Popert A, Hewitt J. Gout and hyperuricemia in rural and urban populations. Ann Rheum Dis 1962; 21:154–163.
28. Lin KC, Lin HY, Chou P. Community based epidemiological study on hyperuricemia and gout in Kin-Hu, Kinmen. J Rheumatol 2000; 27:1045–1050.
29. Bennett P, Burch T. Serum Uric Acid and Gout in Blackfeet and Pima Indians. In: Bennett P, Wood P, eds. Population studies of the rheumatic diseases: proceedings of the third international symposium, New York, June 5th–10th, 1966. Amsterdam: Excerpta Medica Foundation, 1968:358–364.
30. Beighton P, Daynes G, Soskolne CL. Serum uric acid concentrations in a Xhosa community in the Transkei of Southern Africa. Ann Rheum Dis 1976; 35:77–80.
31. Beighton P, Soskolne CL, Solomon L, Sweet B. Serum uric acid levels in a Nama (Hottentot) community in South West Africa. S Afr J Sci 1974; 70:281–283.
32. Beighton P, Soskolne L, Soskolne CL, Sweet B. Serum uric acid concentrations in a rural Tswana community in Southern Africa. Ann Rheum Dis 1973; 32:346–350.
33. Muller AS. Population Studies on the Prevalence of Rheumatic Disease in Liberia and Nigeria. University of Leiden, 1970.
34. Park YB, Park YS, Lee WK, Suh CH, Lee SK. Clinical manifestations of Korean female gouty patients. Clin Rheumatol 2000; 19:142–146.
35. Chin G, Segasothy M. Gouty arthritis in Australian Aborigines. Aust NZ J Med 2000; 30:639–640.
36. Chopra A, Patil J, Billempelly V, Relwani J, Tandle HS. Prevalence of rheumatic diseases in a rural population in western India: a WHO-ILAR COPCORD study. JAPI 2001; 49:240–246.
37. Al-Arfaj AS. Hyperuricemia in Saudi Arabia. Rheumatol Int 2001; 20:61–64.
38. Fang J, Alderman M. Serum uric acid and cardiovascular mortality: NHANES I epidemiologic follow-up study, 1971–1992. JAMA 2000; 283:2404–2410.
39. Burke G, Jacobs D, Sprafka J, Savage P, Sidney S, Wagenknecht L. Obesity and overweight in young adults: the CARDIA study. Prev Med 1990; 19:476–488.
40. US Renal Data System. USRDS 1999 annual data report. National Institutes of Health, National Institute of Diabetes and Digestive and Kidney Diseases; 1999.

41. Clifford A, Story D. Effect of oral purines on serum and urinary uric acid of normal, hyperuricemic and gouty humans. J Nutr 1976; 106:428–434.
42. Clifford A, Story D. Levels of purines in foods and their metabolic effects in rats. J Nutr 1976; 106:435–442.
43. Zollner N. Influence of various purines on uric acid metabolism. Bibl Nutr Dieta 1973; 19:34–43.
44. Zollner N, Griebsch A. Diet and gout. Adv Exp Med Biol 1974; 41:435–442.
45. Choi H, Atkinson K, Karlson E, Willett W, Curhan G. Purine-rich foods, dairy and protein intake, and the risk of gout in men. N Engl J Med 2004; 350:1093–1103.
46. Garrel D, Verdy M, PetitClerc C, Martin C, Brule D, Hamet P. Milk- and soy protein ingestion: acute effect on serum uric acid concentration. Am J Clin Nutr 1991; 53:665–669.
47. Ghadirian P, Shatenstein B, Verdy M, Hamet P. The influence of dairy products on plasma uric acid in women. Eur J Epidemiol 1995; 11:275–281.
48. Blau L. Cherry diet control for gout and arthritis. Tex Rep Biol Med 1950; 8:309–311.
49. Jacob R, Spinozzi G, Simon V, et al. Consumption of cherries lowers plasma urate in healthy women. J Nutr 2003; 133:1826–1829.
50. Gordon T, Kannel WB. Drinking and its relation to smoking, BP, blood lipids, and uric acid: the Framingham study. Arch Intern Med 1983; 143:1366–1374.
51. Choi H, Atkinson K, Karlson E, Willett W, Curhan G. Alcohol intake and risk of incident gout in men: a prospective study. Lancet 2004; 363:1277–1281.
52. Shadick N, Kim R, Weiss S, Liang M, Sparrow D, Hu H. Effect of low level lead exposure on hyperuricemia and gout among middle aged and elderly men: the normative aging study. J Rheumatol 2000; 27:1708–1712.
53. Gibson T, Rodgers A, Simmonds H, Toseland P. Beer drinking and its effect on uric acid. Br J Rheumatol 1984; 23:203–209.
54. Ball G. Two epidemics of gout. Bull Hist Med 1971; 45:401–408.
55. Lin J-L, Tan D-T, Ho H-H, Yu C-C. Environmental lead exposure and urate excretion in the general population. Am J Med 2002; 113:563–568.
56. Brown M, Newton J, Wordsworth B. In: Hatchwell E, ed. Genetics for Rheumatologists: The Molecular Genetic Basis of Rheumatic Disorders. London: Remedica, 2002.
57. Davidson B, Tarle S, Van Antwerp M, et al. Identification of 17 independent mutations responsible for humanb hypoxanthine-guanine phosphoribosyltransferase (HPRT) deficiency. Am J Hum Genet 1991; 48:951–958.
58. Austin C. The impact of the completed human genome sequence on the development of novel therapeutics for human disease. Annu Rev Med 2004; 55:1–13.
59. Craig MH, Poole GV, Hauser CJ. Postsurgical gout. Am Surg 1995; 61:56–59.
60. Langford HG, Blaufox MD, Borhani NO, et al. Is thiazide-produced uric acid elevation harmful: analysis of data from the hypertension detection and follow-up program. Arch Intern Med 1987; 147:645–649.
61. The ALLHAT Officers and Coordinators for the ALLHAT Collaborative Research Group. Major outcomes in high-risk hypertensive patients randomized to angiotensin-converting enzyme inhibitor or calcium channel blocker vs diuretic: the anti-hypertensive and lipid-lowering treatment to prevent heart attack trial (ALLHAT). JAMA 2002; 288:2981–2987.

62. Burack DA, Griffith BP, Thompson ME, Kahl LE. Hyperuricemia and gout among heart transplant recipients receiving cyclosporine. Am J Med 1992; 92:141–146.
63. Chapman JR, Harding NGL, Griffiths D, Morris PJ. Reversibility of cyclosporin nephrotoxicity after three months' treatment. Lancet 1985; 325:128–130.
64. Clive DM. Renal transplant-associated hyperurecemia and gout. J Am Soc Nephrol 2000; 11:974–979.
65. Lin HY, Rocher LL, McQuillan MA, Schmaltz S, Palella TD, Fox IH. Cyclosporine-induced hyperuricemia and gout. N Engl J Med 1989; 321:287–292.
66. Ahn KJ, Kim YS, Lee HC, Park K, Huh KB. Cyclosporine-induced hyperuricemia after renal transplant: clinical characteristics and mechanisms. Transplant Proc 1992; 24:1391–1392.
67. Caspi D, Lubart E, Graff E, Habot B, Yaron M, Segal R. The effect of mini-dose aspirin on renal function and uric acid handling in elderly patients. Arthritis Rheum 2000; 43:103–108.
68. Ford ES, Giles WH, Dietz WH. Prevalence of the metabolic syndrome among U.S. adults. Findings from the Third National Health and Nutrition Examination Survey. JAMA 2002; 287:356–359.
69. Gertler MM, Gam SM, Levine SA. Serum uric acid in relation to age and physique in health and coronary heart disease. Ann Intern Med 1951; 34:1421–1431.
70. Scott JT, Sturge RA. The effect of weight loss on plasma and urinary uric acid and lipid levels. J Clin Chem Clin Biochem 1976; 14:319.
71. St-Onge MP, Keller KL, Heymsfield SB. Changes in childhood food consumption patterns: a cause for concern in light of increasing body weights. Am J Clin Nutr 2003; 78:1068–1073.
72. Bedir A, Topbas M, Tanyeri F, Alvur M, Arik N. Leptin might be a regulator of serum uric acid concentrations in humans. Jpn Heart J 2003; 44:527–536.
73. Denzer C, Muche R, Mayer H, Heinz E, Debatin KM, Wabitsch M. Serum uric acid levels in obese children and adolescents: linkage to testosterone levels and pre-metabolic syndrome. J Pediatr Endocrinol Metab 2003; 16:1225–1232.
74. Nakanishi N, Tatara K, Nakamura K, Suzuki K. Risk factors for the incidence of hyperuricaemia: a 6-year longitudinal study of middle-aged Japanese men. Int J Epidemiol 1988; 28:888–893.
75. Breckenridge A. Hypertension and hyperuricaemia. Lancet 1966; 1:15–18.
76. Gavin AR, Struthers AD. Hyperuricemia and adverse outcomes in cardiovascular disease: potential for therapeutic intervention. Am J Cardiovasc Drugs 2003; 3:309–314.
77. Feig DI, Johnson RJ. Hyperuricemia in childhood primary hypertension. Hypertension 2003; 42:247–252.
78. Tykarski A. Evaluation of renal handling of uric acid in essential hypertension: hyperuricemia related to decreased urate secretion. Nephron 1991; 59:364–368.
79. Boyko EJ, de Courten M, Zimmet PZ, Chitson P, Tuomilehto J, Alberti KG. Features of the metabolic syndrome predict higher risk of diabetes and impaired glucose tolerance: a prospective study in Mauritius. Diabetes Care 2000; 23:1242–1248.
80. Ruiz-Palomo F, Toledo T. Primary Na+/H+exchanger dysfunction: a possible explanation for insulin resistance syndrome. Med Hypotheses 1993; 41:186–189.

81. Bakker SJ, Gans RO, ter Maaten JC, Teerlink T, Westerhoff HV, Heine RJ. The potential role of adenosine in the pathophysiology of the insulin resistance syndrome. Atherosclerosis 2001; 155:283–290.
82. Erickson AR, Enzenauer RJ, Nordstrom DM, Merenich JA. The prevalence of hypothyroidism in gout. Am J Med 1994; 97:231–234.
83. Giordano N, Santacroce C, Mattii G, Geraci S, Amendola A, Gennari C. Hyperuricemia and gout in thyroid endocrine disorders. Clin Exp Rheumatol 2001; 19:661–665.
84. Johnson RJ, Kivlighn SD, Kim YG, Suga S, Fogo AB. Reappraisal of the pathogenesis and consequences of hyperuricemia in hypertension, cardiovascular disease, and renal disease. Am J Kidney Dis 1999; 33:225–234.
85. Messeril FH, Frohlich ED, Dreslinski GR, Suarez DH, Aristimuno GG. Serum uric acid in essential hypertension: an indicator of renal vascular involvement. Ann Intern Med 1980; 93:817–821.
86. Fessel WJ. Renal outcomes of gout and hyperuricemia. Am J Med 1979; 67:74–82.
87. Yu T, Gutman AB. Uric acid nephrolithiasis in gout: predisposing factors. Ann Intern Med 1967; 67:1133–1148.
88. Mattix HJ, Curhan GC. The association between gout and nephrolithiasis: The National Health and Nutrition Examination Survey III. Am J Kidney Dis 2002; 40:37–42.
89. Kramer HJ, Choi HK, Atkinson K, Stampfer M, Curhan GC. The association between gout and nephrolithiasis in men: The Health Professionals' Follow-Up Study. Kidney Int 2003; 64:1022–1026.
90. Bengtsson C, Lapidus L, Stendahl C, Waldenstrom J. Hyperuricaemia and risk of cardiovascular disease and overall death. A 12-year follow-up of participants in the population study of women in Gothenburg, Sweden. Acta Med Scand 1988; 224:549–555.
91. Freedman DS, Williamson DF, Gunter EW, Byers T. Relation of serum uric acid to mortality and ischemic heart disease. The NHANES I Epidemiologic Follow-up Study. Am J Epidemiol 1995; 141:637–644.
92. Levine W, Dyer AR, Shekelle RB, Schoenberger JA, Stamler J. Serum uric acid and 11.5-year mortality of middle-aged women: findings of the Chicago Heart Association Detection Project in Industry. J Clin Epidemiol 1989; 42:257–267.
93. Woo J, Swaminathan R, Cockram C, Lau E, Chan A. Association between serum uric acid and some cardiovascular risk factors in a Chinese population. Postgrad Med J 1994; 70:486–491.
94. Brand FN, McGee DL, Kannel WB, Stokes J, III, Castelli WP. Hyperuricemia as a risk factor of coronary heart disease: the Framingham study. Am J Epidemiol 1985; 121:11–18.
95. Culleton BF, Larson MG, Kannel WB, Levy D. Serum uric acid and risk for cardiovascular disease and death: the Framingham Heart Study. Ann Intern Med 1999; 131:7–13.
96. Gelber AC, Klag MJ, Mead LA, et al. Gout and risk for subsequent coronary heart disease. The Meharry-Hopkins Study. Arch Intern Med 1997; 157:1436–1440.
97. Persky VW, Dyer AR, Idris-Soven E, et al. Uric acid: a risk factor for coronary heart disease? Circulation 1979; 59:969–977.

98. Rathmann W, Funkhouser E, Dyer AR, Roseman JM. Relations of hyperuricemia with the various components of the insulin resistance syndrome in young black and white adults: the CARDIA study. Ann Epidemiol 1998; 8:250–261.
99. Høieggen A, Alderman MH, Kjeldsen SE, et al. The impact of serum uric acid on cardiovascular outcomes in the LIFE study. Kidney Int 2004; 65:1041–1049.
100. Lehto S, Niskanen L, Ronnemaa T, Laakso M. Serum uric acid is a strong predictor of stroke in patients with non-insulin-dependent diabetes mellitus. Stroke 1998; 29:635–639.
101. Anker SD, Doehner W, Rauchhaus M, et al. Uric acid and survival in chronic heart failure: validation and application in metabolic, functional, and hemodynamic staging. Circulation 2003; 107:1991–1997.
102. McCarty DJ, Jr. Crystal-induced inflammation; syndromes of gout and pseudogout. Geriatrics 1963; 18:467–478.
103. Rosenthal AK, Ryan L. Calcium pyrophosphate crystal deposition disease, pseduogout, and articular chondrocalcinosis. In: Koopman, Moreland, eds. Arthritis and Allied Conditions. 15th ed. Lippincott Williams and Wilkins, 2005:2373–2396.
104. Resnick D, Niwayama G, Goergen TG, et al. Clinical, radiographic and pathologic abnormalities in calcium pyrophosphate dihydrate deposition disease (CPPD): pseudogout. Radiology 1977; 122:1–15.
105. Silman AJ. Calcium pyrophosphate dihydrate (CPPD) deposition disease. In: Silman AJ, Hochberg MC, eds. Epidemiology of the Rheumatic Diseases. New York: Oxford University Press, 2001:247–258.
106. Carty DJ, Jr., Hogan JM, Gatter RA, Grossman M. Studies on pathological calcifications in human cartilage. I. Prevalence and types of crystal deposits in the menisci of two hundred fifteen cadavera. J Bone Joint Surg Am 1966; 48:309–325.
107. Mitrovic DR, Stankovic A, Iriarte-Borda O, et al. The prevalence of chondrocalcinosis in the human knee joint. An autopsy survey. J Rheumatol 1988; 15:633–641.
108. Lagier R, Baud CA. Pathological calcifications of the locomotor system. Status of articular chondrocalcinosis. In: Milhaud GOM, Blackwood H, eds. Reports and communications of the IV European symposis of calcified tissues. Bordeaux 1967. Paris: Sedes, 1968.
109. Felson DT, Anderson JJ, Naimark A, Kannel W, Meenan RF. The prevalence of chondrocalcinosis in the elderly and its association with knee osteoarthritis: the Framingham Study. J Rheumatol 1989; 16:1241–1245.
110. Sanmarti R, Panella D, Brancos MA, Canela J, Collado A, Brugues J. Prevalence of articular chondrocalcinosis in elderly subjects in a rural area of Catalonia. Ann Rheum Dis 1993; 52:418–422.
111. Bergstrom G, Bjelle A, Sorensen LB, Sundh V, Svanborg A. Prevalence of rheumatoid arthritis, osteoarthritis, chondrocalcinosis and gouty arthritis at age 79. J Rheumatol 1986; 13:527–534.
112. Reginato AJ, Tamesis E, Netter P. Familial and clinical aspects of calcium pyrophosphate deposition disease. Curr Rheumatol Rep 1999; 1:112–120.
113. Bocher J, Mankin HJ, Berk RN, Rodnan GP. Prevalence of calcified meniscal cartilage in elderly persons. N Engl J Med 1965; 272:1093–1097.

114. Cabanel G, Phelip X, Verdier JM, Gras JP. [Frequency of meniscal calcifications and their pathological signification]. Rhumatologie 1970; 22:255–262.
115. Trentham DE, Masi AT, Hamm RL. Letter. Roentgenographic prevalence of chondrocalcinosis. Arthritis Rheum 1975; 18:627–628.
116. Ellman MH, Levin B. Chondrocalcinosis in elderly persons. Arthritis Rheum 1975; 18:43–47.
117. Leonard A, Solnica J, Cauvin M, Houdent G, Mallet E, Brunelle P, Deshayes P. [Chondrocalcinosis: study of its radiologic frequency and its relation to arthrosis. Study of the level of parathyroid homone]. Rev Rhum Mal Osteoartic 1977; 44:559–564.
118. Delauche MC, Stehle B, Cassou B, Verret JM, Kahn MF. [Frequency of radiologic chondrocalcinosis in patients over 80 years of age. A prospective study] . Rev Rhum Mal Osteoartic 1977; 44:555–557.
119. Memin Y, Monville C, Ryckewaert A. [Articular chondrocalcinosis after 80 years of age]. Rev Rhum Mal Osteoartic 1978; 45:77–82.
120. Ellman MH, Brown NL, Levin B. Prevalence of knee chondrocalcinosis in hospital and clinic patients aged 50 or older. J Am Geriatr Soc 1981; 29:189–192.
121. Mégard M, André Fouet E. La chondrocalcinose chez les personnes agées. Rhumatologie 1983; 35:249–252.
122. Wilkins E, Dieppe P, Maddison P, Evison G. Osteoarthritis and articular chondrocalcinosis in the elderly. Ann Rheum Dis 1983; 42:280–284.
123. Gordon TP, Smith M, Ebert B, McCredie M, Brooks PM. Articular chondrocalcinosis in a hospital population: an Australian experience. Aust N Z J Med 1984; 14:655–669.
124. Reginato AJ, Hollander JL, Martinez V, et al. Familial chondrocalcinosis in the Chiloe Islands, Chile. Ann Rheum Dis 1975; 34:260–268.
125. Balsa A, Martin-Mola E, Gonzalez T, Cruz A, Ojeda S, Gijon-Banos J. Familial articular chondrocalcinosis in Spain. Ann Rheum Dis 1990; 49:531–535.
126. Fernandez Dapica MP, Reginato AJ. Familial and sporadic calcium pyrophosphate deposition disease (CPPDD) in Spain: a unified hypothesis about an Iberian mutation. Arthritis Rheum 1992; 35:S119.
127. Fernandez Dapica MP, Gomez-Reino JJ. Familial chondrocalcinosis in the Spanish population. J Rheumatol 1986; 13:631–633.
128. Andrew LJ, Brancolini V, de la Pena LS, et al. Refinement of the chromosome 5p locus for familial calcium pyrophosphate dihydrate deposition disease. Am J Hum Genet 1999; 64:136–145.
129. Doherty M, Hamilton E, Henderson J, Misra H, Dixey J. Familial chondrocalcinosis due to calcium pyrophosphate dihydrate crystal deposition in English families. Br J Rheumatol 1991; 30:10–15.
130. Gaucher A, Faure G, Netter P, et al. Hereditary diffuse articular chondrocalcinosis. Dominant manifestation without close linkage with the HLA system in a large pedigree. Scand J Rheumatol 1977; 6:217–221.
131. Caeiro F, Babini A, Marchegiani A, et al. Familial calcium pyrophosphate deposition disease and marfanoid features in a kindred of northern Italian-Argentinean ancestry. Arthritis Rheum 1994; 37:S413.
132. Richardson BC, Chafetz NI, Ferrell LD, Zulman JI, Genant HK. Hereditary chondrocalcinosis in a Mexican-American family. Arthritis Rheum 1983; 26:1387–1396.

133. Reginato AJ, Reginato AM, Fernandez-Dapica MP, Ramachandrula A. Familial calcium pyrophosphate crystal deposition disease or calcium pyrophosphate gout. Rev Rheum Engl Ed 1995; 62:376–391.
134. McCarty DJ, Pepe PF. Erythrocyte neutral inorganic pyrophosphatase in pseudogout. J Lab Clin Med 1972; 79:277–284.
135. McCarty DJ, Solomon SD, Warnock ML, Paloyan E. Inorganic pyrophosphate concentrations in the synovial fluid of arthritic patients. J Lab Clin Med 1971; 78:216–229.
136. Jones AC, Chuck AJ, Arie EA, Green DJ, Doherty M. Diseases associated with calcium pyrophosphate deposition disease. Semin Arthritis Rheum 1992; 22:188–202.
137. Milazzo SC, Ahern MJ, Cleland LG, Henderson DR. Calcium pyrophosphate dihydrate deposition disease and familial hypomagnesemia. J Rheumatol 1981; 8:767–771.
138. Runeberg L, Collan Y, Jokinen EJ, Lahdevirta J, Aro A. Hypomagnesemia due to renal disease of unknown etiology. Am J Med 1975; 59:873–881.
139. Smilde TJ, Haverman JF, Schipper P, et al. Familial hypokalemia/hypomagnesemia and chondrocalcinosis. J Rheumatol 1994; 21:1515–1519.
140. Salvarani C, Rossi F, Macchioni PL, et al. Bartter's syndrome and chondrocalcinosis: a possible role for hypomagnesemia in the deposition of calcium pyrophosphate dihydrate (CPPD) crystals. Clin Exp Rheumatol 1989; 7:415–420.
141. Cobeta-Garcia JC, Gascon A, Iglesias E, Estopinan V. Chondrocalcinosis and Gitelman's syndrome. A new association? Ann Rheum Dis 1998; 57:748–749.
142. Doherty M, Dieppe PA. Double blind, placebo controlled trial of magnesium carbonate in chronic pyrophosphate arthropathy [abstract]. Ann of Rheum Dis 1983; 42s:106–107.
143. Alexander GM, Dieppe PA, Doherty M, Scott DG. Pyrophosphate arthropathy: a study of metabolic associations and laboratory data. Ann Rheum Dis 1982; 41:377–381.
144. Job-Deslandre C, Menkes CJ, Guinot M, Luton JP. Does hypothyroidism increase the prevalence of chondrocalcinosis? Br J Rheumatol 1993; 32:197–198.
145. Komatireddy GR, Ellman MH, Brown NL. Lack of association between hypothyroidism and chondrocalcinosis. J Rheumatol 1989; 16:807–808.
146. Chaisson CE, McAlindon TE, Felson DT, Naimark A, Wilson PW, Sawin CT. Lack of association between thyroid status and chondrocalcinosis or osteoarthritis: the Framingham Osteoarthritis Study. J Rheumatol 1996; 23:711–715.
147. Aitken RE, Kerr JL, Lloyd HM. Primary hyperparathyroidism with osteosclerosis and calcification in articular cartilage. Am J Med 1964; 37:813–820.
148. Bywaters EG, Dixon AS, Scott JT. Joint lesions of hyperparathyroidism. Ann Rheum Dis 1963; 22:171–187.
149. Bywaters EGL. Discussion of simulation of rheumatic disorders by metabolic bone diseases. Ann Rheum Dis 1959; 18:64.
150. Zvaifler NJ, Reefe WE, Black RL. Articular manifestations in primary hyperparathyroidism. Arthritis Rheum 1962; 5:237–249.
151. McCarty DJ, Silcox DC, Coe F, et al. Diseases associated with calcium pyrophosphate dihydrate crystal deposition. Am J Med 1974; 56:704–714.
152. Rynes RI, Merzig EG. Calcium pyrophosphate crystal deposition disease and hyperparathyroidism: a controlled, prospective study. J Rheumatol 1978; 5:460–468.

153. Pritchard MH, Jessop JD. Chondrocalcinosis in primary hyperparathyroidism. Influence of age, metabolic bone disease, and parathyroidectomy. Ann Rheum Dis 1977; 36:146–151.
154. Bilezikian JP, Connor TB, Aptekar R, et al. Pseudogout after parathyroidectomy. Lancet 1973; 1:445–446.
155. Glass JS, Grahame R. Chondrocalcinosis after parathyroidectomy. Ann Rheum Dis 1976; 35:521–525.
156. O'Duffy JD. Clinical studies of acute pseudogout attacks: comments on prevalence, predispositions, and treatment. Arthritis Rheum 1976; 19:349–352.
157. Schumacher HR, Jr. Hemochromatosis and Arthritis. Arthritis Rheum 1964; 26:41–50.
158. Dymock IW, Hamilton EB, Laws JW, Williams R. Arthropathy of haemochromatosis. Clinical and radiological analysis of 63 patients with iron overload. Ann Rheum Dis 1970; 29:469–476.
159. Atkins CJ, McIvor J, Smith PM, Hamilton E, Williams R. Chondrocalcinosis and arthropathy: studies in haemochromatosis and in idiopathic chondrocalcinosis. Q J Med 1970; 39:71–82.
160. Adamson TC, 3rd, Resnik CS, Guerra J, Jr., Vint VC, Weisman MH, Resnick D. Hand and wrist arthropathies of hemochromatosis and calcium pyrophosphate deposition disease: distinct radiographic features. Radiology 1983; 147:377–381.
161. Hamilton EB, Bomford AB, Laws JW, Williams R. The natural history of arthritis in idiopathic haemochromatosis: progression of the clinical and radiological features over ten years. Q J Med 1981; 50:321–329.
162. Bosworth BM. Calcium deposits in shoulder and subacromial bursitis. A survey of 12,222 shoulders. JAMA 1941; 116:2477–2482.
163. Resnick D. Calcium hydroxyapatite crystal deposition disease. In: Resnick D, ed. Diagnosis of Bone and Joint Disorders. 3rd ed. Philadelphia: W.B. Saunders, 1955:1615–1648.
164. Chow HY, Recht MP, Schils J, et al. Acute calcific tendinitis of the hip: case report with magnetic resonance imaging findings. Arthritis Rheum 1997; 40:974–977.
165. McCarthy G. Basic calcium phosphate crystal deposition desease. In: Hochberg MC, Silman AJ, Smolen JS, Weinblatt ME, Weisman H, eds. Rheumatology. 3rd ed. Edinburgh: Mosby, 2003:1952.
166. Kerian J, Daft L, Carerra GF, Derfus B. The high prevalence of calcium crystals in pre-operative knees. Arthritis Rheum 1999; 42:S145.
167. Dieppe PA, Crocker PR, Corke CF, et al. Synovial fluid crystals. Q J Med 1979; 192:533–553.
168. Gibilisco PA, Schumacher HR, Hollander JL, Soper KA. Synovial fluid crystals in osteoarthritis. Arthritis Rheum 1985; 28:511–515.
169. McCarty DJ, Halverson PB, Carerra GF, et al. "Milwaukee shoulder"—association of microspheroids containing hydroxyapatite crystals, active collagenase, and neutral protease with rotator cuff defects. I. Clinical aspects. Arthritis Rheum 1981; 24:464–473.

3

Genetics of the Crystal-Induced Arthropathies

Raihana Zaka and Charlene J. Williams

Division of Rheumatology, Department of Medicine, Thomas Jefferson University, Philadelphia, Pennsylvania, U.S.A.

INTRODUCTION

Familial forms of the crystal-induced arthropathies occur in almost all ethnic groups and are frequently characterized by early onset and severe clinical manifestations. Despite their relative rarity, inherited forms of these arthropathies often provide insights into critical mechanisms important in the development of idiopathic as well as familial varieties of these diseases. The purpose of this chapter is to review the current status of gene discovery in the crystal-induced arthropathies and to describe the putative role of these genes in the pathogenesis of the corresponding diseases.

FAMILIAL GOUT SYNDROMES

Gout, or monosodium urate crystal deposition disease, has long been recognized as resulting from a variety of environmental and genetic abnormalities favoring hyperuricemia. Earlier reviews of studies of inherited gout concluded that the disorder was likely due to polygenic rather than monogenic influences (1–5). In recent years, understanding of the role of inheritance in gout has rapidly accelerated due, in part, to the identification of hyperuricemic disorders that exhibit Mendelian patterns of inheritance. Since uric acid is the end-product of purine metabolism, most of the early reports of families with inherited hyperuricemia and gout concentrated on identifying and characterizing defects in purine metabolic pathways. These reports documented familial defects in the regulation of purine nucleotide synthesis transmitted as autosomal as well as sex-linked traits (6–15). Of particular interest were the X-linked disorders hypoxanthine phosphoribosyltransferase (HPRT) deficiency and phosphoribosylpyrophosphate (PRPP) synthetase overactivity, each of which is characterized by purine nucleotide and uric acid overproduction and distinct infantile and later-onset phenotypes.

By the late 1970s, however, it was clear that inherited abnormalities in the regulation of uric acid production accounted for only a small proportion of individuals with familial gout. Moreover, a number of reports appeared in which hyperuricemia preceded the development of renal failure in affected members of families in which purine nucleotide and uric acid production were normal. For example, in 1978, a multi-generation kindred in which hyperuricemia, acute gouty arthritis, and renal medullary cystic disease were co-morbid as an autosomal dominant trait was reported. In this family, hyperuricemia was attributable to impaired renal excretion of uric acid (16). Other reports described the concurrence of precocious gout and renal failure in teenage children in some families and even in a young girl of nine years of age in one family (17,18). By 1983, the concordance of dominantly inherited interstitial nephropathy and hyperuricemia and gout with impaired renal uric acid excretion was recognized as a distinct clinical entity (19), and the term familial hyperuricemic nephropathy was coined (20). Patients with familial hyperuricemic nephropathy showed diminished renal tubular net excretion of uric acid unaccompanied by evidence for accelerated purine synthesis de novo, and these findings were confirmed in a large Japanese family with autosomal dominant gouty arthritis and renal disease (20,21).

Thus, pathogenetic mechanisms underlying familial gout are heterogeneous and now include disorders characterized by primary increases in purine nucleotide and uric acid production and those characterized by altered renal uric acid handling. Much of the recent literature devoted to the genetics of familial gout has concentrated on the latter disorders that are transmitted as autosomal dominant traits, usually presenting with interstitial nephropathy and progressing to end-stage renal failure. The major disorders of this type include familial juvenile hyperuricemic nephropathy (FJHN) and medullary cystic kidney disease. A summary of the genetics of gout and gout-related familial disorders is presented in Table 1.

FAMILIAL JUVENILE HYPERURICEMIC NEPHROPATHY

FJHN, sometimes termed familial juvenile gouty nephropathy, was described in 1960 (22). This disorder is inherited as an autosomal dominant trait with a high degree of penetrance and is usually, although not always, associated with gout. Renal disease usually develops in the second decade of life and progresses to

Table 1 Summary of the Genetics of Gout and Gout-Related Disorders

Locus (MIM #)	Chromosomal location	Inheritance	Gene (symbol)
Xanthinuria, type I (278300)	2p23–p22	AR	Xanthine dehydrogenase (XDH)
Gout, HPRT-related (300323)	Xq26–q27.2	XD	Hypoxanthine guanine phosphoribosyl transferase 1 (HPRT1)
Gout, PRPS-related (311850)	Xq22 q24	XD	Phosphoribosyl pyrophosphate synthetase 1 (PRSP1)
Hyperuricemic nephropathy, familial juvenile (FJHN; 162000)	16p12.3 17cen–q21.3	AD AD	Uromodulin (UMOD) Hepatocyte nuclear factor 1β (HNF-1β; also TCF2)
Medullary cystic kidney disease, type 1 (MCKD1; %174000)	1q21	AD	?
Medullary cystic kidney disease, type 2 (MCKD2; 603860)	16p12.3	AD and AR	Uromodulin (UMOD)
Gout susceptibility 1 (GOUT1; %138900)	4q25	Complex	?

Abbreviations: MIM, Mendelian Inheritance in Man; AR, autosomal recessive; AD, autosomal dominant; XD, X-linked dominant; Complex, polygenic (assigned locus probably is one of several susceptibility loci).

end-stage renal failure by mid-life. Histological examination of renal biopsies shows tubulointerstitial inflammation and splitting of thickened tubular basement membranes. The primary diagnostic criterion is a reduced fractional excretion of urate (FEur), regardless of the gender or age of the patient. FEur, defined as uric acid clearance factored by creatinine clearance X 100, ranges from about 8% to 18% in normal subjects of all ages and both genders, with FJHN patients usually having values of 5% or less (23). The dramatically low FEur and the early onset of the disease are conspicuous characteristics of FJHN and distinguish it from other autosomal dominant hyperuricemic disorders that usually appear later in life (see below). Following the initial report of FJHN, additional families with this disease were described (17,19,21,24–30). The availability of large families and the obvious Mendelian pattern of transmission of the disorder in these families made it possible to utilize the tools of parametric linkage analysis in the search for the FJHN gene.

In 2000 the results of a genome wide screen for linkage performed on affected and unaffected members of a Japanese family were described (21,31).

Affected family members developed gout and hyperuricemia after adolescence, although uric acid excretion abnormalities were apparent before puberty. The investigators genotyped 343 markers covering all autosomes at approximately 10 cm intervals and obtained linkage between the disease trait and a marker on the short arm of chromosome 16. By performing refined linkage mapping within 30 cm of the linked marker, a candidate interval for the FJHN gene was localized to a region of approximately 9 cm at 16p12. Confirmation of this observation was reported in 2003 when five additional European families with FJHN were linked to chromosome 16p12-p11 (32). One FJHN family, however, was not linked to the 16p locus, thus suggesting genetic heterogeneity for this disorder.

AUTOSOMAL DOMINANT MEDULLARY CYSTIC KIDNEY DISEASE

Autosomal Dominant Medullary Cystic Kidney Disease (ADMCKD) is another hereditary nephropathy that usually, although not always, includes gout among its constellation of symptoms. Five generations in a family suffering from this disorder were described in 1966 (33). Affected members showed numerous corticomedullary and intramedullary cysts in the kidneys and an increase in medullary connective tissue and an onset of disease later than for FJHN. In two unrelated families, the average ages at onset were 23 years and 35 years (34). Subsequently symptoms manifesting after age 50 years have been observed (35). Owing to the availability of large families and the advantages of a defined mode of inheritance, genetic linkage analysis was utilized to identify a chromosomal locus for this disorder. A genome wide screen identified a locus on the long arm of chromosome 1 that was linked to the disorders in two Cypriot families (35). Refined linkage mapping and haplotype analyses suggested a founder effect for the disorder in the two Cypriot families and placed the locus within an 8 cm interval on chromosome 1q21. Successive refinements of the interval were performed using recombination mapping in a Belgian kindred to refine the interval for ADMCKD1 to a 2.1 Mbp interval on chromosome 1q21 (36,37).

Analysis of an Italian family with ADMCKD, however, excluded linkage between the disease phenotype and the 1q21 locus (38). A genome-wide genetic linkage analyses was performed on the four generation kindred, and linkage to the short arm of chromosome 16 was established—the same region which had previously been linked to FJHN. These studies imply at least two loci for ADMCKD: a chromosome 1 locus for what is now termed ADMCKD1, and a 16p locus for ADMCKD2. Since ADMCKD2 and FJHN loci mapped to approximately the same region of chromosome 16p, the possibility was raised that these two syndromes might be allelic variants (39,40). A more recent study has further refined the FJHN/ADMCKD2 locus to a region of approximately 1.7 Mbp (41).

CANDIDATE GENES FOR FJHN AND ADMCKD1 AND 2

Refinement of loci for the hyperuricemic nephropathies permitted examination of positional candidate genes for these disorders. The chromosome 16p12 locus that harbored the candidate interval for FJHN and ADMCKD2 contained six candidate genes, including the uromodulin gene (UMOD), which was of particular interest because of the abundance of its gene product in normal urine (42). UMOD encodes the Tamm-Horsfall protein, a glycosylphosphatidylinositol anchored glycoprotein with expression localized to the thick ascending limb of the loop of Henle (43). Amorphus deposits of uromodulin were present in the renal interstitium of patients with medullary cystic kidney disease (44,45). Sequencing of this gene from affected members of three families with FJHN and one family with ADMCKD2 led to the identification of four different mutations in exon 4 of the gene (41). The finding that mutations in the same gene were responsible for both FJHN and ADMCKD2 confirmed allelism between these disorders and reinforced the hypothesis that mutation in UMOD result in decreased urinary concentrations of Tamm-Horsfall protein with resulting hyperuricemia and progressive renal failure.

The initial report of mutations in UMOD was rapidly followed by a series of studies in which additional mutations in UMOD were observed in other families with either FJHN or ADMCKD2 (46–49). In a recent study of a large consanguineous Spanish kindred with ADMCKD2, three affected family members were homozygous for a UMOD mutation at Cys255 (C255Y), thus permitting a comparison of phenotypes associated with homozygosity and heterozygosity. Patients with homozygous UMOD mutations had more severe disease, earlier onsets of hyperuricemia and gout and more rapid progression to end-stage renal failure than those heterozygous for the UMOD mutation (50).

The function of the Tamm-Horsfall protein remains unknown. It may be important for the integrity of the loop of Henle, forming a gel-like structure that blocks urinary tract infections by preventing the binding of Escherischia coli to kidney cells (51). Uromodulin is also reported to have an anti-oxidant effect and to inhibit calcium oxalate crystallization (52,53). The majority of mutations in UMOD in FJHN and ADMCKD2 patients are missense mutations that substitute a Cys for another amino acid (Fig. 1). UMOD contains 48 cysteine residues which can potentially form 24 intramolecular disulfide bonds. It has been suggested that mutations in UMOD may disrupt the tertiary structure of the gene product, permitting accumulation of the Tamm-Horsfall protein in tubular cells. Mutations in UMOD result in profound reduction of Tamm-Horsfall protein excretion (55). Several studies have shown that aggregated Tamm-Horsfall protein has a proinflammatory potential, including activation of neutrophils, stimulation of monocytes, and release of cytokines and proteinases. A pro-inflammatory effect of Tamm-Horsfall protein aggregation may be responsible for the tubulointerstitial nephritis seen in FJHN and ADMCKD2 patients (56–60). Furthermore, it has been suggested that the hyperuricemic manifestations of these disorders, characterized by reduced urate fractional excretion

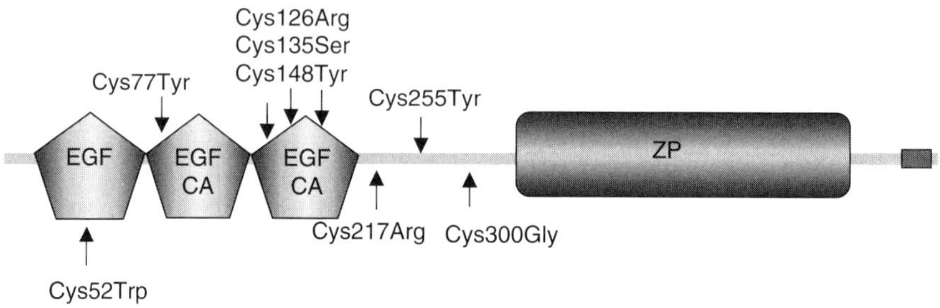

Figure 1 Domain structure of the Tamm-Horsfall protein (THP), the product of the UMOD gene. Depiction is reproduced from SMART (Simple Modular Architecture Research Tool). Some reported mutations involving cysteine substitutions in families with FJHN are depicted (41,46,49); many of the mutations in the UMOD gene fall within the EGF and EGF_CA domains of THP. *Abbreviations*: EGF, epidermal growth factor-like domain; EGF_CA, calcium-binding EGF-like domain; ZP, zona pellucida domain. *Source*: Adapted from Ref. 54.

may result from a contraction of extracellular volume as a result of the loss of Tamm-Horsfall protein function in renal salt and water transport (61).

Unlike the rapid success encountered in identifying mutations in patients with FJHN and ADMCKD2, progress in the search for the gene responsible for ADMCKD1 has been hampered by the lack of viable candidate genes in the 2.1 Mbp region that has been genetically refined by linkage analysis to chromosome 1q21. The current positional genes in this region include a variety of interesting candidates that may be relevant to the pathophysiological mechanisms underlying this and other hyperuricemic disorders. One candidate gene, mucin 1 (MUC1), encodes a cell surface glycoprotein that is expressed by a variety of epithelial cells including those of the urinary tract. The MUC1 gene product interacts with several cell adhesion proteins that also interact with polycystin-1 and inversin, two proteins in which mutations can give rise to polycystic kidney disease 1 and nephronophthisis type 2, respectively (62,63). Another candidate gene, thrombospondin 3 (THBS3), is also important in cell adhesion and is expressed in mouse kidney (64). THBS3 is known to interact with TGF-β, a cytokine involved in renal fibrosis (65). Other potential candidates exist in this region, but no single positional candidate gene is as established as UMOD at chromosome 16p12 in ADMCKD2 and FJHN (see Ref. 37 for discussion). Systematic sequencing of several of the candidates in the 1q21 will be required in order to identify the gene altered in ADMCKD1.

GENETIC HETEROGENEITY IN FJHN

Not all families with FJHN and ADMCKD2 are linked to the chromosome 16p12 locus of the UMOD gene. For example, the 16p12 locus has been excluded as pertinent in a family with FJHN presenting with underexcretion-type hyperuricemia, gouty arthritis, and precocious and progressive renal disease (66). In a follow-up study, the possibility that mutations in the organic anion transporter 1 gene (hOAT1), whose gene product transports urate, might be responsible for the phenotype of this atypical family was examined and no mutations were found in the hOAT1 gene in affected members of this family (67). This report highlighted the potential for genetic heterogeneity in the hyperuricemic nephropathy syndromes and suggested that aberrant function of organic anion transporters such as hOAT1, solute carrier family 22, member 12 (SLC22A12), human urate/anion transporter 2 (hUAT2), and human urate/anion transporter (hUAT) might also be responsible in some families with these disorders. Homozygous mutations in SLC22A12, the gene encoding the urate transporter URAT1, are responsible for renal hypouricemia in some patients (68,69). hUAT is the gene encoding galectin 9, which can function as a selective urate channel when inserted into lipid bilayers (70); hUAT and hUAT2 are 96% homologous (71).

Finally, a mutation in the hepatocyte nuclear factor 1β gene (HNF-1β) has been identified in a family with FJHN (72). Mutations in this gene had previously been associated with several disorders of renal development and with renal cystic disease and precocious diabetes, and in some families, with hyperuricemia. The mutation is a base substitution that produces a splice site mutation, presumably resulting in premature termination of translation (72). Most affected members of this family exhibited hyperuricemia and three members had early onset gout, suggesting that gout and hyperuricemia are general features of HNF-1β mutations. However, the mechanism by which HNF-1β mutations results in hyperuricemia is still unknown. HNF-1β is homologous to HNF-1α, a transcription factor that is expressed in the renal proximal tubule (73). Both HNF-1α and -1β are expressed during tubular differentiation (74). It has been speculated that reduced activity of HNF-1β might reduce the transcription of the urate transporters URAT1 and hUAT.

TREATMENT OF THE HYPERURICEMIC NEPHROPATHIES

The effectiveness of allopurinol in the treatment of the hyperuricemic nephropathies has been disputed. Most studies of allopurinol therapy have focused on single families, and it has been suggested that disparities among studies might result from patient heterogeneity and differences in the course of treatment utilized in each study. Studies of eight separate FJHN families with a strong history of renal disease and early mortality due to end-stage renal failure were undertaken. In these families long-term follow-up of progression of renal disease indicated that allopurinol reduced the morbidity and mortality from renal failure in treated family members compared to untreated members and previous generations of untreated individuals (75). This effect, however, was most evident when treatment was begun before compromise of renal function. These studies suggest that early diagnosis and treatment, as well as conscientious patient compliance, can result in long-term prevention of renal damage in at least some FJHN patients.

OTHER GENETIC STUDIES OF GOUT

Although gout affects about 1% of the United States population, its prevalence can be significantly higher in certain ethnic and racial groups. Among these groups are Pacific Islanders. It has been suggested that the genetic relationship among Pacific Islanders and the high morbidity of gout in these populations may be due to a founder effect, perhaps compounded by environmental influences. A genome-wide linkage study of an isolated population of Taiwanese aborigines presenting with primary gout has been conducted (76). This population was selected because, as an isolated group, the Taiwanese aborigines might be more homogeneous than other populations and thus might provide better statistical power for a non-parametric analysis of linkage. Analyses detected significant linkage on the long arm of chromosome 4. When corrected for certain co-variates, the statistical significance for linkage at chromosome 4q25 increased (76).

A subset of this same population was used to evaluate possible linkage of the hyperuricemia/gout phenotype to the ADMCKD1 locus on chromosome 1q21 (77). Marginally significant linkage was detected, suggesting that an additional susceptibility locus for this population may be located on chromosome 1q21. These studies are a reminder of the complex genetic nature of primary gout and that several susceptibility loci may define the genetic landscape of the idiopathic disorder.

With regard to potential positional candidates at chromosome 4q25, it has been noted that the region of strongest linkage is a relatively short distance from a previously identified longevity locus (78). This led to speculation that a common gene in this region might be responsible for both gout and longevity traits, in light of the positive correlation between the concentration of urate in serum, where it presumably acts as an antioxidant, and lifespan among mammalian species (79).

FAMILIAL CALCIUM PYROPHOSPHATE DIHYDRATE (CPPD) DEPOSITION DISEASE

The history of the non-urate, calcium crystal arthropathies dates to 1958 when Zitnan and Sitaj presented case studies of 27 patients, most of whom were members of five families, with what was referred to as articular chondrocalcinosis (80,81). The nature of the crystal deposition in affected patients was clarified by McCarty and Hollander, who studied two cases of non-urate associated crystal deposition in the joints of patients thought to have gout (82). Radiographic examination of the joints in these and other patients revealed distinctive and abnormal calcifications in and around articular hyaline cartilage and fibrocartilage. Following the initial description of chondrocalcinosis in

Czech families, multiple series of affected families from around the world were reported (83–99). Most familial cases appeared to be inherited in an autosomal dominant manner with precocious onset, variable clinical expression, and deposition of calcium-containing crystals occurring before the development of frank degenerative joint disease (Fig. 2). The most common radiographic features included crystal deposition in the knee, symphysis pubis, and triangular fibrocartilage of the wrist (85,102,103). Atypical osteoarthritis with involvement of metacarpophalangeal and wrist joints and with numerous and large subchondral cysts and beak-like osteophytes was also observed.

The primary crystals that are observed in chondrocalcinosis are CPPD. With few exceptions family studies of chondrocalcinosis demonstrate the presence of CPPD crystals in synovial aspirates. The mechanisms responsible for the deposition of these crystals are not known. Some studies have reported that structural changes in articular cartilage extracellular matrix might promote

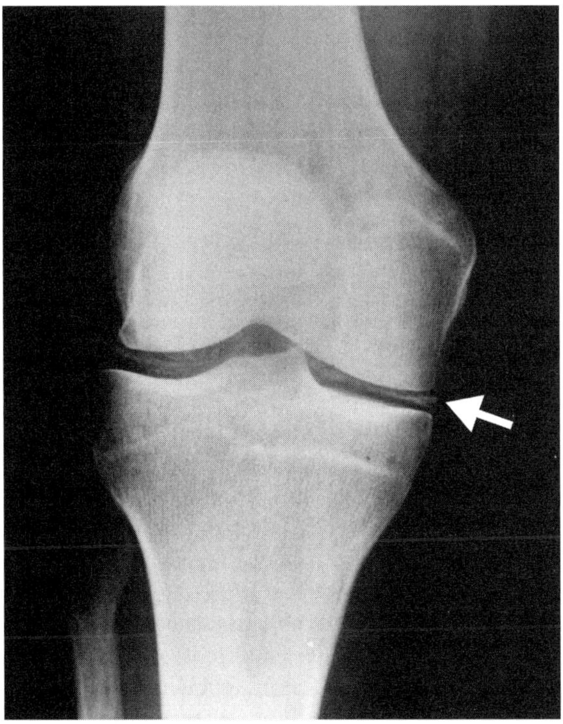

Figure 2 Radiograph of patient with familial calcium pyrophosphate dihydrate (CPPD) disease. The knee of a 42-year-old patient, a member of an Argentine CPPD disease kindred (100,101), is shown. Note that there is minimal compromise of joint space and structure of the tibial plateau and femoral condyle at the early stage of disease in this individual; however, chondrocalcinosis is clearly visible in the joint (*indicated by arrow*).

crystal formation (104,105), thus prompting an exploration of genes encoding cartilage extracellular matrix proteins as candidate genes for chondrocalcinosis. In a large family from the Chiloe Islands with a clinical phenotype of severe, precocious osteoarthritis with ankylosis, late-onset spondyloepiphyseal dysplasia, and chondrocalcinosis in multiple joints and fibrocartilages, a heterozygous mutation in the COL2A1 gene that resulted in an Arg to Cys substitution at amino acid 75 in the gene product was identified (106,107). It is likely, however, that the chondrocalcinosis phenotype in this kindred is a secondary consequence of advanced and severe osteoarthritis.

Numerous studies of a chondrocyte nucleoside triphosphate pyrophosphohydrolase (NTPPPH) suggested that the biochemical pathway responsible for the generation of inorganic pyrophosphate (PPi) may play a role in the crystal deposition (108–110). Altered levels of intracellular inorganic pyrophosphate have been observed in cultured fibroblasts and lymphoblasts of patients affected with familial CPPD disease (111,112), and in synovial fluids from a British family (98), thus strengthening the suspicion that abnormalities in pyrophosphate metabolism may underlie crystal deposition in these families.

GENETIC LINKAGE ANALYSES IN FAMILIAL CPPD DISEASE

The availability of numerous families presenting with CPPD disease as a Mendelian trait has permitted the use of parametric methods of linkage analysis to define potential disease loci. A study of a large family from Maine, in which the CPPD disease phenotype was associated with severe, non-dysplastic osteoarthritis, excluded linkage to the COL2A1 locus (113). In this family, genetic linkage was demonstrated between the disease phenotype and a locus on the long arm of chromosome 8, now referred to as the CCAL1 locus. The locus on chromosome 8q, although statistically significant, was broad and spanned a genetic interval of approximately 30 cm, or a physical distance of over 25 Mbp.

Linkage analysis on a British CPPD disease family subsequently identified a second chondrocalcinosis locus on the short arm of chromosome 5 (114) that was confirmed in genetic studies of two other families from France and Argentina (100). All of the families presented with typical symptoms of CPPD disease. In addition, the large kindred from the Alsace region of France, like the British family, had also been extensively characterized with respect to abnormalities in PPi metabolism (100,111,112). The chromosome 5p15 locus, referred to as CCAL2, has now been shown to be linked to the CPPD disease phenotype in five apparently unrelated families, confirming the fact that CCAL2 is an important locus for familial chondrocalcinosis.

CANDIDATE GENES FOR FAMILIAL CPPD DISEASES

The chromosome 5p15 locus contained a number of positional genes that could serve as candidates for familial CPPD disease. However, in a timely stroke of intersecting research efforts, a gene for an animal model of aberrant calcification was identified on mouse chromosome 15 in a region of the chromosome that was syntenic to human chromosome 5p (115). The animal model was the *progressive ankylosis* (*ank*) mouse, a naturally occurring autosomal recessive mutant whose phenotype included the deposition of hydroxyapatite in articular spaces and synovial fluid. In affected animals, disease progression includes joint space narrowing, cartilage erosion and formation of osteophytes that cause joint immobility and eventual fusion. Complete rigidity and death occurs at around 6 months of age (116–120). Although the phenotype of the mouse model was considerably different from that seen in human chondrocalcinosis, the abnormal articular calcification and the fact that the human homologue of the gene, referred to as ANKH, was located at the CCAL2 locus made it a viable positional candidate gene. Furthermore, the gene product of *ank* functioned to regulate PPi levels in cells (115).

Mutational analyses of ANKH detected four mutations in the five families in which linkage to the CCAL2 locus had been confirmed. A heterozygous base substitution at position -11 of the 5′ untranslated region (UTR) that introduced a new methionine (ATG) codon was identified in one family (121). In vitro translation studies and mass determination of the resultant protein by electrospray ionization mass spectrometry demonstrated that the upstream ATG sequence was recognized as a new translational start site. In the Argentine and French families, heterozygous missense mutations were observed in highly conserved amino acids in the first and second exons, respectively (101,121). Two families with CPPD disease in the United States have mutations at the same amino acid position as that observed in the Argentine kindred (122). However, the sequence variants in the two United States families are transversion mutations, while that in the Argentine family is a transition mutation. Haplotype analyses of microsatellite and single nucleotide polymorphic markers in all three families demonstrate that they are not related, suggesting that the mutations at the same amino acid arose independently of each other, and that this site may represent a hot spot for mutations in CPPD disease families (see Table 2 for compilation of ANKH mutations).

Table 2 ANKH Gene Mutations in Families with Calcium Pyrophosphate Dihydrate Deposition Disease

Family	Amino acid position	Type of mutation
British	NA	INS+4[a]
French	48	Met↔Thr
Argentinean	5	Pro↔Leu
U.S.	5	Pro↔Thr
U.S.	5	Pro↔Thr

[a]INS+4: insertion of 4 amino acids at the N-terminus of ANK.

Ninety-five patients from the United Kingdom with CPPD disease were studied to evaluate the relevance of mutations in ANKH to idiopathic CPPD disease (121). One patient, who presented with late-onset CPPD deposition in several joints, displayed a 3 bp in-frame deletion in exon 12 that eliminated a glutamic acid at amino acid position 490. This change, like those observed in the familial mutations, was not observed in any controls. The same change was observed in the sister and nephew of the patient, although CPPD disease could not be confirmed in these individuals.

GENETIC HETEROGENEITY IN FAMILIAL CPPD DISEASE

Not all families with CPPD disease are linked to the CCAL1 or CCAL2 loci that have been identified by linkage analyses. For example, the multi-generation family previously described (97) failed to exhibit linkage to either locus when genotyped with markers selected from the two candidate regions, CCAL1 and CCAL2 (Baldwin C and Williams CJ, unpublished data). These findings suggest that another uncharacterized locus may be responsible for the familial CPPD disease phenotype.

ANK AND CPPD DEPOSITION DISEASE

Studies of *ank* function in cells from the *progressive ankylosis* mouse and in COS cells transfected with normal and mutant Ank suggest that the protein may regulate transport of PPi. Intracellular PPi levels in fibroblasts from mutant mice were increased about two-fold over that of wild-type controls, and extracellular levels of PPi were dramatically reduced in fibroblast cultures mice compared to wild-type controls (115). This observation was consistent with the postulated role of PPi as a potent inhibitor of hydroxyapatite deposition in cartilage and bone. An abnormally functioning Ank would fail to inhibit hydroxyapatite deposition and could conceivably account for the excessive calcification phenotype seen in *ank/ank* mice.

Further experiments showed that fibroblasts from mutant mice could be restored to normal levels of intracellular and extracellular PPi when transfected with wild-type (115) and overexpression of wild-type Ank in COS cells resulted in a dramatic decrease in intracellular PPi levels and a concomitant increase in extracellular PPi levels. Finally, the decreased levels of intracellular PPi resulting from over-expression of Ank in COS cells could be restored by the addition of probenecid, a nonspecific anion transport inhibitor, suggesting that Ank functioned via an ion channel transport mechanism (see Fig. 3 for proposed structure and function for Ank/ANK).

In order to evaluate the impact of mutations in ANKH observed in two families on the function of the gene product, COS cells were transfected with constructs containing the INS+4 and M48T mutants (121). Interestingly, the familial mutations did not appreciably change intracellular PPi levels. To explain

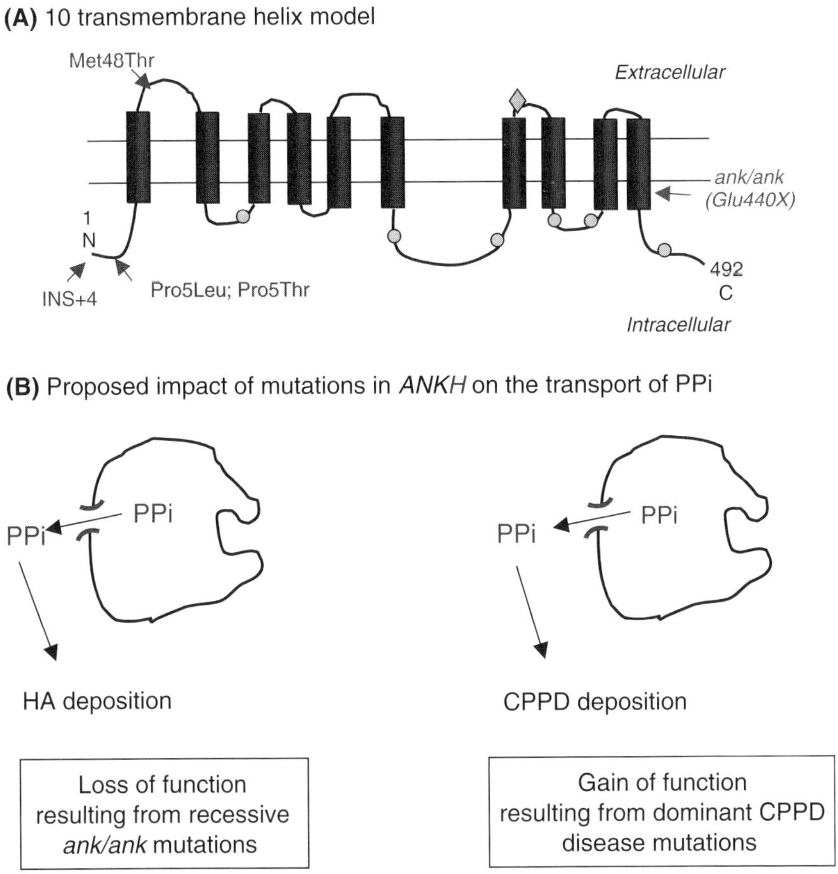

Figure 3 Putative structure and function of ANK. (**A**) The transmembrane prediction algorithm, TMpred1 (123), suggests that ANK, the 492 amino acid gene product of ANKH, is a multipass transmembrane protein with 10 transmembrane helices. The positions of mutations in familial calcium pyrophosphate dihydrate deposition (CPPD) disease, relative to the position of the naturally occurring recessive mutation in the *ank/ank* mouse (which occurs at amino acid 440, changing a glutamic acid residue to a stop codon), are shown. *Symbols*: ◈, potential N-glycosylation site; ◉, potential phosphorylation sites by protein kinase C or cAMP/cGMP-dependent protein kinase. (**B**) Proposed impact of mutations on PPi generation. ANK appears to act as a channel or transporter for the inorganic anion, PPi. Recessive mutations in the *ank/ank* mouse produces decrease in extracellular PPi (115), permitting deposition of hydroxyapatite. It has been postulated that dominant mutations in humans may lead to excess efflux of PPi, resulting in the deposition of CPPD crystals. *Source*: From Refs. 101, 115, 121.

this result, it was hypothesized that, in contrast to the *ank* mouse mutant, human CPPD disease mutations might act as gain-of-function alleles which would moderately increase extracellular PPi levels over time, leading to subtle abnormalities that have cumulative impact on articular cartilage homeostasis.

FAMILIAL CONDITIONS INVOLVING BASIC CALCIUM PHOSPHATE (APATITE) CRYSTALS

There are few reports of the deposition of hydroxyapatite and other basic calcium phosphate crystals as a heritable disorder in the medical literature, and the earliest descriptions were of calcific periarthritis in multiple joints of identical twins and in relatives of a proband presenting with intervertebral disc calcification (124,125). In a case where the primary crystal type was determined to be basic calcium phosphate, the phenotype mainly involved the dorsolumbar spine, with intervertebral disc calcification primarily in the nucleus polpulsus, as well as the peripheral joints with periarticular calcific deposits in the hand joints. This phenotype was displayed by a family in which no affected members showed calcific deposits in the knees, pubic symphysis, or triangular ligament of the carpus, thus distinguishing the hydroxyapatite arthropathy in this family from the condition seen in patients with familial CPPD disease (126). In three members of another family in which periarthritis of multiple joints was observed, the exclusive crystal type was octacalcium phosphate, an observation confirmed by Fourier transform infrared spectrophotometry of an open biopsy of a calcification of a proximal interphalangeal joint (127). This crystal type often accompanies deposits of carbonate substituted hydroxyapatite, but the finding of octacalcium phosphate alone in a biopsy specimen is unique to this family. Another unusual observation in this kindred was the fact that affected individuals displayed low serum alkaline phosphatase activity, a finding not seen in other families with basic calcium phosphate arthropathies.

Milwaukee shoulder syndrome is an erosive arthritis of the shoulder associated with apatite crystal deposition (128). Manifestations of this syndrome begin with limited shoulder joint mobility and stability accompanied by joint effusion, and progresses to degenerative changes in the scapula humeral head, and acromioclavicular joint, and calcification of the rotator cuff. Rotator cuff tear is common. A family of four members with calcific periarthritis of the shoulder was described (129).

A more detailed description of a large Italo-Argentine kindred with Milwaukee shoulder syndrome was recently reported (130). This family displayed an unusual type of osteoarthritis with secondary intraarticular and periarticular calcification in numerous joints, including the shoulder in the most severely affected elderly members and evidence of superior shoulder subluxation in younger members. Examination of synovial fluid from the shoulders of two affected family members showed the presence of both hydroxyapatite and calcium pyrophosphate dihydrate crystals.

ANALYSES OF GENETIC LINKAGE AND CANDIDATE GENES IN FAMILIAL BASIC CALCIUM PHOSPHATE ARTHROPATHIES

Studies of the Italo-Argentine kindred described above indicated that the disorder was inherited in an autosomal dominant manner in this family. While the phenotype in the family was not consistent enough to warrant a genome-wide search for linkage to a putative disease-causing locus, it was sufficient for analysis of potential candidate loci. The loci that were targeted included the chondrocalcinosis loci on chromosomes 8q and 5p15, and the COL2A1 locus on chromosome 12q. These loci were definitively excluded in the family. Several other loci that have been implicated in normal skeletal patterning and cartilage differentiation, the HOX A,B,C, and D gene cluster and the PAX 1 and 9 genes, were also analyzed. These loci were either excluded or were uninformative in terms of their linkage to the disease phenotype of Milwaukee shoulder/subluxation in the affected kindred (130).

Finally, observations of mineralization defects in the *ank* mutant mouse indicated that hydroxyapatite deposition was the crystal type deposited in articular spaces. Therefore, two other families displaying autosomal dominant hydroxyapatite deposition disease that have not been reported in the literature but have been studied by us were screened for mutations in ANKH. No sequence variants in the coding regions of the ANKH gene were observed in these families (Kingsley D and Williams CJ, unpublished observations).

CONCLUSIONS

This review has attempted to recapitulate the development of the genetic studies of the inherited crystal arthropathies. As the above discussion indicates, this is a very active area of study in which considerable progress has been made, especially in the last decade. The progress in our understanding of these disorders is in large part due to the identification of families in which the crystal-associated arthropathies are inherited in a Mendelian manner, thus permitting the use of traditional methods of parametric linkage analysis to establish loci that are linked to the phenotype in these families. Also, the availability of high-throughput techniques for genotype analyses and candidate gene analysis has significantly increased the speed with which suitable kindreds can be analyzed. Furthermore, intriguing animal models presenting with skeletal abnormalities associated with pathological mineralization have also proved to be an outstanding resource for providing suggestions of potential candidate genes that may warrant analysis in families suffering from crystal arthropathies. At this time, there is every reason to believe that population-based studies of susceptibility genes for the crystal arthropathies will, likewise, contribute to our understanding of the complexity of inheritance of these disorders.

REFERENCES

1. Hauge M, Harvald B. Heredity in gout and hyperuricemia. Acta Med Scand 1955; 152:247–257.
2. Emmerson B. Heredity in primary gout. Aust Ann Med 1960; 9:168–175.
3. Neel J, Rakic M, Davidson R, Valkenburg H, Mikkelson W. Studies on hyperuricemia. II. A reconsideration of the distribution of serum uric acid values in the families of Smyth, Cotterman, and Freyburg. Am J Hum Genet 1965; 17:14–22.
4. Healey L, Skeith M, Decker J, Bayani-Sioson P. Hyperuricemia in Filipinos: interaction of heredity and environment. Am J Hum Genet 1967; 19:81–85.
5. Morton N. Genetics of hyperuricemia in families with gout. Am J Med Genet 1979; 4:103–106.
6. Auscher C, Pasquier C, deGery A, Weissenbach R, Delbarrer F. Xanthinuria: study of a large kindred with familiar urolithiasis and gout. Biomedicine 1977; 27:57–59.
7. Kelley W, Rosenbloom F, Henderson F, Seegmiller E. A specific enzyme defect in gout associated with overproduction of uric acid. PNAS (USA) 1967; 57:1735–1739.
8. Sperling O, Boer P, Persky-Brosh S, Kanarek E, deVries A. Altered kinetic property of erythrocyte phosphoribosylpyrophosphate synthetase in excessive purine production. Eur J Clin Biol Res 1972; 17:703–706.
9. Becker M, Kostel P, Meyer L, Seegmiller E. Human phosphoribosylpyrophosphatase synthetase:Increased enzyme specific activity in a family with gout and excessive purine synthesis. Proc Natl Acad Sci USA 1973; 70:2749–2752.
10. Becker MA, Meyer LJ, Wood AW, Seegmiller JE. Purine overproduction in man associated with increased phosphoribosylpyrophosphate synthetase activity. Science 1973; 179:1123–1126.
11. Akaoka I, Fujimori S, Kamatani N, et al. A gouty family with increased phosphoribosylpyrophosphate synthetase activity: case reports, familial studies, and kinetic studies of the abnormal enzyme. J Rheumatol 1981; 8:563–574.
12. Roessler BJ, Nosal JM, Smith PR, et al. X-linked phosphoribosylpyrophosphate synthetase superactivity is associated with distinct point mutations in the PRPS1 gene. J Biol Chem 1993; 268:26476–26481.
13. Christen H-J, Hanefeld F, Duley JA, Simmonds HA. Distinct neurological syndrome in two brothers with hyperuricemia. Lancet 1992; 340:1167–1168.
14. Becker M, Taylor W, Smith P, Ahmed M. Overexpression of the normal phosphoribosylpyrophosphate synthetase 1 isoform underlies catalytic superactivity of human phosphoribosylpyrophosphate synthetase. J Biol Chem 1996; 271:19894–19899.
15. Becker M, Smith P, Taylor W, Mustafi R, Switzer R. The genetic and functional basis of purine nucleotide feedback-resistant phosphoribosylpyrophosphate synthetase superactivity. J Clin Invest 1995; 96:2133–2141.
16. Thompson G, Weiss J, Goldman R, Rigg G. Familial occurrence of hyperuricemia, gout, and medullary cystic disease. 1978; 138:1614–1617.
17. Simmonds HA, Warren DJ, Cameron JS, Potter CF, Farebrother DA. Familial gout and renal failure in young women. Clin Nephrol 1980; 14:176–182.
18. Warren D, Simmonds H, Gibson T, Naik R. Familial gout and renal failure. Arch Dis Child 1981; 56:699–704.

19. Leumann EP, Wegmann W. Familial nephropathy with hyperuricemia and gout. Nephron 1983; 34:51–57.
20. MacDermot K, Allsop J, Watts R. The rate of purine synthesis de novo in blood mononuclear cells in vitro from patients with familial hyperuricaemic nephropathy. Clin Sci (Lond) 1984; 67:249–258.
21. Yokota N, Yamanaka H, Yamamoto Y, Fujimoto S, Eto T, Tanaka K. Autosomal dominant transmission of gouty arthritis with renal disease in a large Japanese family. Ann Rheum Dis 1991; 50:108–111.
22. Duncan H, Dixon ACJ. Gout, familial hyperuricemia and renal disease. Q J Med 1960; 29:127–136.
23. McBride MB, Simmonds HA, Moro F. Genetic gout in childhood:familial juvenile hyperuricemic nephropathy or "familial renal disease". J Inher Metab Dis 1997; 20:351–353.
24. Rosenbloom FM, Kelley WN, Carr AA, Seegmiller JE. Familial nephropathy and gout in a kindred. Clin Res 1967; 15:270.
25. Van Goor W, Kooiker CJ, Mees FJD. An unusual form of renal disease associated with gout and hypertension. J Clin Path 1971; 24:354–359.
26. Massari PU, Hsu CH, Barnes RV, Fox IH, Gikas PW, Weller JM. Familial hyperuricemia and renal disease. Arch Intern Med 1980; 140:680–684.
27. Calabrese G, Simmonds HA, Cameron JS, Davies PM. Precocious familial gout with reduced fractional urate clearance and normal purine enzymes. Quart J Med 1990; 277:441–450.
28. Cameron JS, Ogg CS, Moro F, Chantler C, Simmonds HA. Precocious familial gout. Lancet 1990; 336:745.
29. Moro F, Ogg CS, Simmonds HA, et al. Familial juvenile gouty nephropathy with renal urate hypoecretion preceeding renal disease. Clin Nephrol 1991; 35:263–269.
30. Saeki A, Hosoya T, Okabe H, et al. Newly discovered familial juvenile gouty nephropathy in a Japanese family. Nephron 1995; 70:359–366.
31. Kamatani N, Mortiani M, Yamanaka H, Takeucji F, Hosoya T, Itakura M. Localization of a gene for familial juvenile hyperuricemic nephropathy causing under-excretion type gout to 16p12 by genome-wide linkage analysis of a large family. Arthritis Rheum 2000; 43:925–929.
32. Stacey JM, Turner JJO, Harding B, et al. Genetic mapping studies of familial juvenile hyperuricemic nephropathy on chromosome 16p13-p11. J Clin Endocr Metab 2003; 88:464–470.
33. Goldman SH, Walker SR, Merigan TC, Jr., Gerdner KD, Bull JMC. Hereditary occurrence of cystic disease of the renal medulla. New Engl J Med 1966; 274:984–992.
34. Gardner KD, Jr. Evolution of clinical signs in adult-onset cystic disease of the renal medulla. Ann Intern Med 1971; 74:47–54.
35. Christodoulou K, Tsingis M, Stavrou C, et al. Chromosome 1 localization of a gene for autosomal dominant medullary cystic kidney disease (ADMCKD). Hum Mol Genet 1998; 7:905–911.
36. Fuchshuber A, Kroiss S, Karle S, et al. Refinement of the gene locus for autosomal dominant medullary cystic kidney disease type 1 (MCKD1) and construction of a physical and partial transcriptional map of the region. Genomics 2001; 72:278–284.

37. Wolf MTF, Van Vlem B, Hennies HC, et al. Telomeric refinement of the MCKD1 locus on chromosome 1q21. Kidney Int 2004; 66:580–585.
38. Scolari F, Puzzer D, Amoroso A, et al. Identification of a new locus for medullary cystic disease on chromosome 16p12. Am J Hum Genet 1999; 64:1655–1660.
39. Dahan K, Fuchshuber A, Adamis S, et al. Familial juvenile hyperuricemic nephropathy and autosomal dominant medullary cystic kidney disease type 2. Two facets of the same disease? J Am Soc Nephrol 2001; 12:2348–2357.
40. Scolari F, Viola BF, Ghiggeri GM, et al. Towards the identification of (a) gene(s) for autosomal dominant medullary cystic kidney disease. J Nephrol 2003; 16:321–328.
41. Hart TC, Gorry MC, Hart PS, et al. Mutations of the UMOD gene are responsible for medullary cystic kidney disease 2 and familial juvenile hyperuricemic nephropathy. J Med Genet 2002; 39:882–892.
42. Malagolini N, Cavallone D, Serafini-Cessi F. Intracellular transport, cell-surface exposure and release of recombinant Tamm-Horsfall glycoprotein. Kidney Int 1997; 52:1340–1350.
43. Hoyer JR, Sisson SP, Vernier RL. Tamm-Horsfall glycoprotein: ultrastructural immunoperoxidase localization in rat kidney. Lab Invest 1979; 41:168–173.
44. Zager RA, Coltran RS, Hoyer JR. Pathologic localization of Tamm-Horsfall protein in interstitial deposits in renal disease. Lab Invest 1978; 38:52–57.
45. Resnick JS, Sisson S, Vernier RL. Tamm-Horsfall protein: abnormal localization in renal disease. Lab Invest 1978; 38:550–555.
46. Turner JJ, Stacey JM, Harding B, et al. Uromodulin mutations cause familial juvenile hyperuricemiz nephropathy. J Clin Endocrinol Metab 2003; 88:1398–1401.
47. Wolf MTF, Mucha BE, Attanasio M, et al. Mutations in the uromodulin gene in MCKD type 2 patients cluster in exon 4 which codes three EGF-like domains. Kidney Int 2003; 64:1580–1587.
48. Bleyer AJ, Trachtman H, Sandhu J, Gorry MC, Hart TC. Renal manifestations of a mutation in the uromodulin (Tamm Horsfall protein) gene. Am J Kidney Dis 2003; 42:20–26.
49. Kudo E, Kamatani N, Tezuka O, et al. Familial juvenile hyperuricemic nephropathy: detection of mutations in the uromodulin gene in five Japanese families. Kidney Int 2004; 65:1589–1597.
50. Rezende-Lima W, Parreira KS, Garcia-Gonzalez M, Riveira E, Banet JF, Lens XM. Homozygosity for uromodulin disorders: FJHN and MCKD-type 2. Kidney Int 2004; 66:558–563.
51. Dulawa J, Rambausek M, Jann K, Ritz E. Tamm-Horsfall glycoprotein interferes with bacterial adherence to human kidney cells. Eur J Clin Invest 1998; 18:87–92.
52. Chen WC, Lin HS, Tsai FJ, Li CW. Effects of Tamm-Horsfall protein and albumin on the inhibition of free radicals. Urol Int 2001; 67:305–309.
53. Chen WC, Lin HS, Chen HY, Shih CH, Li CW. Effects of Tamm-Horsfall protein and albumin on calcium oxalate crystallization and importance of sialic acids. Mol Urol 2001; 5:1–5.
54. http://smart.embl-heidelberg.de/.

55. Bleyer AJ, Hart TC, Shihabi Z, Robins V, Hiyer JR. Mutations in the uromodulin gene decrease urinary excretion of Tamm-Horsfall protein. Kiney Int 2004; 66:974–977.
56. Horton JK, Davis M, Topley N, Thomas D, Williams JD. Activation of the inflammatory response of neutrophils by Tamm-Horsfall glycoprotein. Kidney Int 1990; 37:717–726.
57. Thomas DB, Davies M, Peters JR, Williams JD. Tamm Horsfall protein binds to a single class of carbohydrate specific receptors on human neutrophils. Kidney Int 1993; 44:423–429.
58. Cavallone D, Malagolini N, Serafini-Cessi F. Binding of human neutrophils to cell-surface anchored Tamm-Horsfall glycoprotein in tubulointerstitial nephritis. Kidney.
59. Thomas DB, Davies M, Williams JD. Release of gelatinase and superoxide from human mononuclear phagocytes in response to particulate Tamm-Horsfall protein. Am J Pathol 1993; 142:249–260.
60. Su S-J, Chang K-L, Lin T-M, Huang YH, Yeh TM. Uromodulin and Tamm Horsfall protein induce human monocytes to secrete TNF and express tissue factor. J Immunol 1997; 158:3449–3456.
61. Kumar S. Tamm-Horsfall protein-uromodulin (1950–1990). Kidney Int 1990; 37:1395–1401.
62. Huan Y, Van Adelsburg J. Polycistin-1, the PKD1 gene product, is in a complex containing E-cadherin and the catenins. J Clin Invest 1999; 104:1459–1468.
63. Nurnberger J, Bacallao RL, Phillips CL. Inversin forms a complex with catenins and N-cadherin in polarized epithelial cells. Mol Biol Cell 2002; 13:3096–3106.
64. Vos HL, Devarayalu S, deVries Y, Bornstein P. Thrombospondin 3, a new member of the thrombospondin gene famile. J Biol Chem 1992; 267:12192–12196.
65. Hugo C. The thrombospondin 1-TGF beta axis in fibrotic renal disease. Nephrol Dial Transplant 2003; 18:1241–1245.
66. Ohno I, Ichida K, Okabe H, et al. Familial juvenile gouty nephropathy: exclusion of 16p12 from the candidate locus. Nephron 2002; 92:573–575.
67. Ichida K, Hosoyamada M, Kimura H, et al. Urate transport via human PAH transporter hOAT1 and its gene structure. Kidney Int 2003; 63:143–155.
68. Enomoto A, Kimura H, Chairoungdua A, et al. Molecular identification of a renal urate-anion exchanger that regulates blood urate levels. Nature 2002; 417:447–452.
69. Tanaka M, Itoh K, Matsushita K, et al. Two male siblings with hereditary renal hypouricemia and exercise-induced ARF. Am J Kidney Dis 2003; 42:1287–1292.
70. Tureci O, Schmitt H, Fadle N, Pfreundschuh M, Sahin U. Molecular definition of a novel human galectin which is immunogenic in patients with Hodgkin's disease. J Biol Chem 1997; 272:6416–6422.
71. Lipkowitz MS, Leal-Ointo E, Rappoport JZ, Najfeld V, Abramson RG. Functional reconstruction, membrane targeting, genomic structure and chromosomal localization of a human urate transporter. J Clin Invest 2001; 107:1103–1115.
72. Bingham C, Ellard S, van't Hoff WG, et al. Atypical familial juvenile hyperuricemic nephropathy associated with a hepatocyte nuclear factor -1β gene mutation. Kidney Int 2003; 63:1645–1651.

73. Mendel DB, Hansen LP, Graves MK, Conley PB, Crabtree GR. HNF-1alpha and HNF-1beta (vHNF-1) share dimerization and homeodomains, but not activation domains, and form heterodimers in vitro. Genes Dev 1991; 5:1042–1056.
74. Lazzaro D, de Simone V, de Magistris L, Lehtonen E, Cortese R. LFB1 and LFB3 homeoproteins are sequentially expressed during kidney development. Development 1992; 114:469–479.
75. Fairbanks LD, Cameron JS, Venkat-Raman G, et al. Early treatment with allopurinol in familial juvenile hyperuricemic nephropathy (FJHN) ameliorates the long-term progression of renal disease. Q J Med 2002; 95:597–607.
76. Cheng LS-C, Chiang S-L, Tu H-P, et al. Genome-wide scan for gout in Taiwanese aborigines reveals linkage to chromosome 4q25. Am J Hum Genet 2004; 75:498–503.
77. Wang WH, Chang SJ, Wang TN, et al. Complex segregation and linkage analysis of familial gout in Taiwanese aborigines. Arthritis Rheum 2004; 50:242–246.
78. Puca AA, Daly MJ, Brewster SJ, et al. A genome wide scan for linkage to human exceptional longevity identifies a locus on chromosome 4. Proc Natl Acad Sci USA 2001; 98:10505–10508.
79. Cutler RG. Urate and ascorbate: their possible roles as antioxidants in determining longevity of mammalian species. Arch Gerontol Geriatr 1984; 3:321–348.
80. Zitnan D, Sitaj S. Mnohopocentna familiarna kalcifikacin articularnych chrupiek. Bratisl Lek Listy 1958; 38:217–228.
81. Zitnan D, Sitaj S. Chondrocalcinosis articularis. I. Clinical and radiologic study. Ann Rheum Dis 1963; 22:142–169.
82. McCarty DJ, Hollander JL. Identification of urate crystals in gouty synovial fluid. Ann Intern Med 1961; 54:452–460.
83. Moskowitz RW, Katz D. Chondrocalcinosis (pseudogout syndrome): a family study. JAMA 1964; 188:867–871.
84. Louyot P, Peterschmitt J, Barthelme P. Chondrocalcinose articulaire diffuse familiale. Rev Rhum 1964; 31:659–663.
85. Aschoff H, Boehm P, Schoen EJ, Schurholz K. Hereditaere chondrocalcinosis articularis. Untersuchung einer familie. Humangenetik 1966; 3:98–103.
86. Reginato AJ, Valenzuela F, Martinez VA, Passano G, Doza S. Polyarticular and familial chondrocalcinosis. Arthritis Rheum 1970; 13:197–213.
87. van der Korst JK, Geerards J, Driessens FCM. A hereditary type of idiopathic articular chondrocalcinosis. Am J Med 1974; 56:307–314.
88. Reginato AJ, Hollander JL, Martinez V, et al. Familial chondrocalcinosis in the Chiloe Islands, Chile. Ann Rheum Dis 1975; 34:260–268.
89. Gaucher A, Faure G, Netter P, et al. Hereditary diffuse articular chondrocalcinosis. Dominant manifestation without close linkage with the HLA system in a large pedigree. Scand J Rheumatol 1977; 6:217–221.
90. Gaudreau A, Camerlain M, Piborot ML, Beauregard G, Lebrun A, Petitclerc C. Familial articular chondrocalcinosis in Quebec. Arthritis Rheum 1981; 24:611–615.
91. Bjelle AO. Pyrophosphate arthropathy in two Swedish families. Arthritis Rheum 1982; 25:66–74.
92. Sakaguchi M, Ishikawa K, Mizuta H, Kitagawa T. Familial pseudogout with destructive arthropathy. Ryumachi 1982; 22:4–13.

93. Richardson BC, Chafetz NI, Ferrell LD, Zulman JI, Genant HK. Hereditary chondrocalcinosis in a Mexican-American family. Arthritis Rheum 1983; 26:1387–1396.
94. Fernandez-Dapica MP, Gomez-Reino J. Familial chondrocalcinosis in the Spanish population. J Rheumatol 1986; 13:631–633.
95. Rodriguez-Valverde V, Zuniga M, Casanueva B, Sanchez S, Merino J. Herditary articular chondrocalcinosis: clinical and genetic features in 13 pedigrees. Am J Med 1988; 84:101–106.
96. Balsa A, Martin-Mola E, Gonzalez T, Cruz A, Ojeda S, Gijon-Banos J. Familial articular chondrocalcinosis in Spain. Ann Rheum Dis 1990; 49:531–535.
97. Eshel G, Gulik A, Halperin N, et al. Hereditary chondrocalcinosis in an Ashkenazi Jewish family. Ann Rheum Dis 1990; 49:528–530.
98. Doherty M, Hamilton E, Henderson J, Misra H, Dixey J. Familial chondrocalcinosis due to calcium pyrophosphate dihydrate crystal deposition in English families. Br J Rheumatol 1991; 30:10–15.
99. Hamza M, Meddeb N, Bardin T. Hereditary chondrocalcinosis in a Tunisian family. Clin Exp Rheumatol 1992; 10:43–49.
100. Andrew LJ, Brancolini V, de al Pena LS, et al. Refinement of the chromosome 5p locus for familial calcium pyrophosphate dihydrate deposition disease. Am J Hum Genet 1999; 64:136–145.
101. Williams CJ, Zhang Y, Timms A, et al. Autosomal dominant familial calcium pyrophosphate dihydrate deposition disease is caused by mutation in the transmembrane protein ANKH. Am J Hum Genet 2002; 71:985–991.
102. Riestra JL, Sanchez A, Rodriquez-Valverde V, Alonso JL, de la Hera M, Merino J. Radiographic features of hereditary articular chondrocalcinosis: a comparative study with the sporadic type. Clin Exp Rheumatol 1988; 6:369–372.
103. Ryan LM, McCarty DJ. Calcium pyrophosphate crystal deposition disease; pseudogout; articular chondrocalcinosis. In: McCarty DJ, Koopman WJ, eds. Arthritis and Allied Conditions. Philadelphia: Lea & Febiger, 1993:1835–1855.
104. Bjelle AO. Morphological study of articular cartilage in pyrophosphate arthropathy (chondrocalcinosis articularis or calcium pyrophosphate dehydrate crystal deposition disease). Ann Rheum Dis 1972; 31:449–456.
105. Bjelle AO. Cartilage matrix in hereditary pyrophosphate arthropathy. J Rheumatol 1981; 8:959–964.
106. Williams CJ, Considine EL, Knowlton RG, et al. Spondyloepiphyseal dysplasia and precocious osteoarthritis in a family with an Arg75→Cys mutation in the procollagen type II gene (COL2A1). Hum Genet 1993; 92:499–505.
107. Reginato AJ, Passano GM, Neumann G, et al. Familial spondyloepiphyseal dysplasia tarda, and precocious osteoarthritis associated with an arginine75 to cysteine mutation in the procollagen type II gene in a kindred of Chiloe Islanders. I. Clinical, radiographic, and pathologic findings. Arthritis Rheum 1994; 37:1078–1086.
108. Muniz O, Pelletier J-P, Martel-Pelletier J, Morales S, Howell DS. NTP pyrophosphohydrolase in human chondrocalcinotic and osteoarthritic cartilage. I. Some biochemical characteristics. Arthritis Rheum 1984; 27:186–192.
109. Howell DS, Martel-Pelletier J, Pelletier J-P, Morales S, Muniz O. NTP pyrophosphohydrolase in human chondrocalcinotic and osteoarthritic cartilage. II. Further studies on histologic and subcellular distribution. Arthritis Rheum 1984; 27:193–196.

110. Ryan LM, Wortmann RL, Karas B, McCarty DJ. Pyrophosphohydrolase activity and inorganic pyrophosphate content of cultured human skin fibroblasts: elevated levels in some patients with calcium pyrophosphate dihydrate deposition disease. J Clin Invest 1986; 77:1689–1696.
111. Lust G, Faure G, Netter P, Gaucher A, Seegmiller JE. Evidence of a generalized metabolic defect in patients with hereditary chondrocalcinosis: increased inorganic phosphate in cultured fibroblasts and lymphoblasts. Arthritis Rheum 1981; 24:1517–1522.
112. Lust G, Faure G, Netter P, Gaucher A, Seegmiller JE. Increased pyrophosphate in fibroblasts and lymphoblasts from patients with hereditary diffuse articular chondrocalcinosis. Science 1981; 214:809–810.
113. Baldwin CT, Farrer LA, Adair R, Dharmavaram R, Jimenez S, Anderson L. Linkage of early-onset osteoarthritis and chondrocalcinosis to human chromosome 8q. Am J Hum Genet 1995; 56:692–697.
114. Hughes AE, McGibbon D, Woodward E, Dixey J, Doherty M. Localisation of a gene for chondrocalcinosis to chromosome 5p. Hum Mol Genet 1995; 4:1225–1228.
115. Ho A, Johnson M, Kingsley DM. Role of the mouse ank gene in tissue calcification and arthritis. Science 2000; 289:265–270.
116. Sweet HO, Green MC. Progressive ankylosis, a new skeletal mutation in the mouse. J Hered 1981; 72:87–93.
117. Hakim FT, Cranley R, Brown KS, Eanes ED, Harne L, Oppenheim JJ. Hereditary joint disorder in progressive ankylosis (ank/ank) mice. I. Association of calcium hydroxyapatite deposition with inflammatory arthropathy. Arthritis Rheum 1984; 27:1411–1420.
118. Hakim FT, Brown KS, Oppenheim JJ. Hereditary joint disorder in progressive ankylosis (Ank/Ank) mice. II. Effect of high dose hydrocaortisone treatment on inflammation and intraarticular calcium hydroxyapatite deposits. Arthritis Rheum 1986; 29:114–123.
119. Sampson HW, Davis JS. Histopathology of the intervertebral disc of progressive ankylosis mice. Spine 1988; 13:650–654.
120. Mahowald ML, Krug H, Halverson J. Progressive ankylosis (Ank/Ank in mice: An animal model of spondyloarthropathy. II. Light and electron microscopic findings. J Rheumatol 1989; 16:60–66.
121. Pendleton A, Johnson MD, Hughes A, et al. Mutations in ANKH cause chondrocalcinosis. Am J Hum Genet 2002; 71:933–940.
122. Williams CJ, Pendleton A, Bonavita G, et al. Mutations in the amino terminus of ANKH in two US families with calcium pyrophosphate dihydrate crystal deposition disease. Arthritis Rheum 2003; 48:2627–2631.
123. Von Heijne G. Membrane protein structure prediction: hydrophobicity analysis and the positive inside rule. J Mol Biol 1992; 225:487–494.
124. Cannon RB, Schmid FR. Calcific periarthritis involving multiple sites in identical twins. Arthritis Rheum 1973; 16:393–396.
125. Zaphiropoulos G, Grahame R. Recurrent calcific periarthritis involving multiple sites. Proc R Soc Med 1973; 66:351–353.
126. Marcos JC, DeBenyacar MA, Garcia-Morteo O, et al. Idiopathic familial chondrocalcinosis due to apatite crystal deposition. Am J Med 1981; 71:557–564.

127. Caspi D, Rosenbach TO, Yaron M, McCarty DJ, Graff E. Pariarthritis associated with basic calcium phosphate crystal deposition and low levels of serum alkaline phosphatase-report of three cases from one family. J Rheumatol 1988; 15:823–827.
128. McCarty DJ, Halverson PB, Carrera GF, Brewer BJ, Kozin F. "Milwaukee shoulder"—association of microspheroids containing hydroxyapatite crystals, active collagenase, and neutral protease, with rotator cuff defects. I. Clinical aspects. Arthritis Rheum 1981; 24:464–474.
129. Hajiroussou VJ, Webley M. Familial calcific periarthritis. Ann Rheum Dis 1983; 42:469–470.
130. Pons-Estel BA, Gimenez C, Sacnun M, et al. Familial osteoarthritis and Milwaukee shoulder associated with calcium pyrophosphate and apatite crystal deposition. J Rheumatol 2000; 27:471–480.

4

Gout: Presentation, Natural History, and Associated Conditions

N. Lawrence Edwards

Section of Rheumatology, Department of Medicine, University of Florida and VA Medical Center, Gainesville, Florida, U.S.A.

INTRODUCTION

Gout is a disease caused by the deposition of monosodium urate monohydrate crystals in joints and surrounding tissues. Symptomatic crystal deposition includes attacks of, typically, acute monoarticular arthritis; tophi, which elicit a chronic inflammatory response causing a destructive arthritis; and urolithiasis. The natural course of classic gout passes through three stages: asymptomatic hyperuricemia, acute intermittent gout, and chronic tophaceous or advanced gout (Fig. 1). The rate of progression from asymptomatic hyperuricemia to chronic tophaceous gout varies considerably from one person to another and is dependent on numerous endogenous and exogenous factors. The clinical manifestations of urate crystal deposition and the natural history of gout are reviewed in this chapter.

STAGES OF CLASSIC GOUT

Asymptomatic Hyperuricemia

Hyperuricemia is a very common biochemical abnormality and can be defined in terms of physiology, epidemiology, or disease risk. In extracellular fluids at pH 7.4, 98% of uric acid exists in the form of monosodium urate. The solubility of monosodium urate (MSU) in human serum (or plasma) reaches saturation at concentrations of approximately 6.8 mg/d. Serum concentrations greater than this

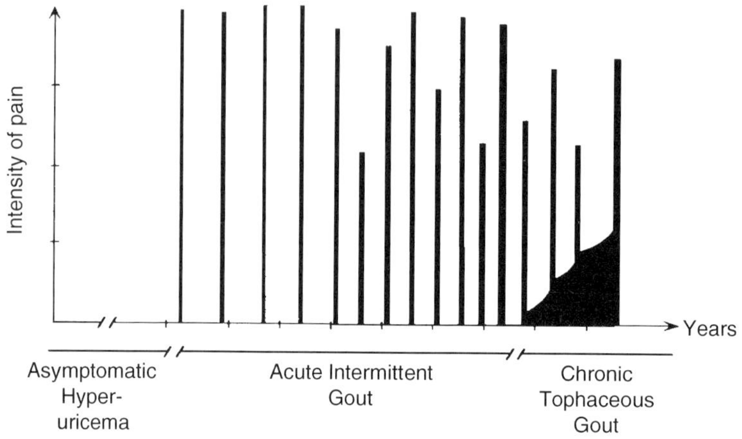

Figure 1 The three stages of disease progression in classic gout. The period of asymptomatic hyperuricemia lasts decades, followed by acute intermittent gout with painless intercritical periods, which finally leads to chronic tophaceous gout with progressive and persistent pain and joint destruction.

are therefore supersaturated and considered to be physiologic hyperuricemia (1). However, it is common for clinical laboratories to define hyperuricemia as a serum urate level that is greater than two standard deviations above the mean value in a gender- and age-matched healthy population. This method may provide normal ranges above 8.1 mg/dL in adult men or 7.2 mg/dL in adult women. This method, though statistically accurate, is inappropriate for serum urate levels, because individuals with urates above 6.8 mg/dL (i.e., but within the "normal range") are at risk for gout. In fact, gout is exceedingly rare in individuals with urate levels below 6.8 mg/dL, and the risk of developing gout increases the higher the serum urate level is above that level (2). The term asymptomatic hyperuricemia is applied to the state in which the serum urate concentration is abnormally high but symptoms have not occurred.

In males, adult urate levels are reached during puberty. Serum urate levels for women run approximately 1 to 2 mg/dL lower than those for men but rise to a similar level after menopause.

Accordingly, in men, primary hyperuricemia frequently begins at puberty, whereas in women, it is usually delayed until menopause. Once established, asymptomatic hyperuricemia frequently lasts a lifetime, but gout may develop in hyperuricemic individuals at any point. The prevalence of asymptomatic hyperuricemia among adult American males has been estimated at 5% to 8%, but even higher prevalence rates have been reported in Asian-Pacific populations (3,4). Management of hypertension and congestive heart failure with diuretics and the epidemic of obesity in this country have expanded an already large population of individuals with asymptomatic hyperuricemia, particularly among elderly women.

Few studies have assessed the risks of asymptomatic hyperuricemia. In a cohort of 2046 initially healthy men followed for 15 years with serial measurements of serum urate concentrations, the annual incidence of gout was 4.9% for a serum urate of 9 mg/dL or more (2). In contrast, the incidence rate was only 0.5% for values between 7.0 and 8.9 mg/dL, and 0.1% for values below 7.0 mg/dL. Throughout this prospective study, no evidence existed of renal deterioration attributable to hyperuricemia. This finding was confirmed by a study of 4693 subjects enrolled in a hypertension detection and follow-up program (5). Therapy with thiazide-type diuretics increased both serum urate and creatinine concentrations. However, lowering urate values with drug therapy did not influence creatinine values. In addition, the incidence of gouty attacks in subjects at risk was only 2.7% over a 5-year period. One study concluded that hyperuricemia is of no clinical importance with respect to renal outcomes until serum urate levels reach at least 13 mg/dL in men and 10 mg/dL in women, limits beyond which little information is available (6). Urolithiasis was rare among previously asymptomatic hyperuricemic individuals, with an annualized incidence rate of 0.4% compared with 0.9% in gouty patients. In the Framingham study, gout developed in only 12% of patients with urate levels between 7.0 and 7.9 mg/dL over a period of 14 years (7). Values greater than 9.0 mg/dL had a sixfold greater predictive value but represented only 20% of the gouty population.

Acute and Intermittent Gout

The initial episode of acute gout usually follows decades of asymptomatic hyperuricemia (Fig. 1). Thomas Sydenham, the famous 17th century physician writing of his personal experiences with gout, eloquently described the initial hours of an acute attack in the following way:

"He goes to bed and sleeps well, but about Two a Clock in the Morning, is waked by the Pain, seizing either his great Toe, the Heel, the Calf of the Leg, or the Ankle; this Pain is like that of dislocated Bones, with the Sense as it were of Water almost cold, poured upon the Membranes of the part affected, presently shivering and shaking follow with a feverish Disposition; the Pain is first gentle, but increased by degrees—till dash towards Night it comes to its height, accompanying itself neatly according to the Variety of the bones of the Tarsus and Metatarsus, whose Ligaments it seizes, sometimes resembling a violent stretching or tearing of those ligaments, sometimes gnawing of a dog, and sometimes a weight; more over, the Part affected has such a quick and exquisite Pain, that it is not able to bear the weight of the cloths upon it, nor hard walking in the Chamber" (8). This classic description captures the exquisite pain frequently associated with acute gouty arthritis, and it is this clinical picture most commonly evoked by the term gout.

In men, the first attacks usually occur between the fourth and sixth decades of life. In women, age at onset is older and varies with several factors,

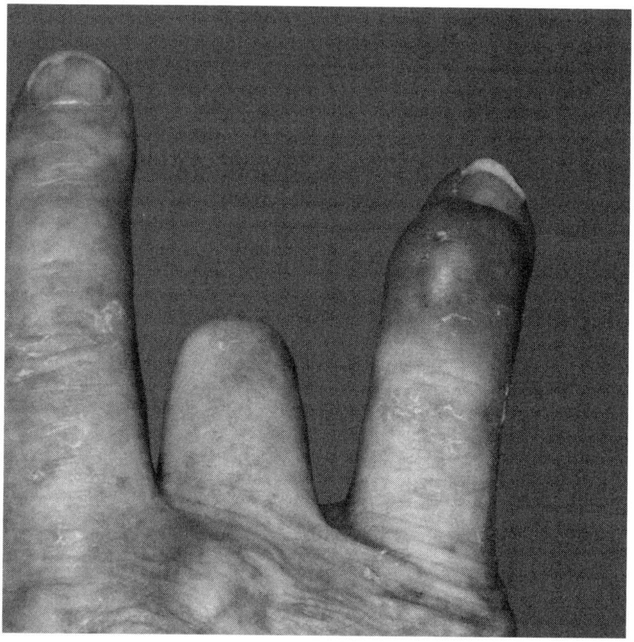

Figure 2 Acute, erythematous swelling of the distal interphalangeal joint suggestive of acute gouty arthritis.

the most important of which is age at menopause. The onset of a gouty attack is usually heralded by the rapid development of warmth, swelling, erythema, and exquisite pain in the affected joint (Fig. 2). Pain escalates from its faintest twinges to its most intense level over an 8- to 12-hour period. The initial attack is usually monoarticular and in one-half of patients involves the first metatarsophalangeal joint. Eventually this joint is affected in 90% of individuals with gout. Other joints that are frequently involved in this early stage are the midfoot, ankles, heels, and knees and less commonly the wrists, fingers, and elbows. The intensity of pain is characteristically very severe, but may vary among subjects. Classically, patients cannot stand even the weight of a bed sheet, and most find walking difficult or impossible when lower extremity joints are involved.

Systemic symptoms such as fever, chills, and malaise may accompany acute gout. Although most patients are afebrile during the acute episode, body temperatures over 38.5°C can occur. The cutaneous erythema associated with the gouty attack may extend beyond the involved joint and resemble bacterial cellulitis. Early in the acute intermittent stage, episodes of acute arthritis are infrequent and intervals between attacks sometimes last for years.

Trivial episodes of pain ("petite attacks") lasting only hours and sometimes recurrent over several years may precede the first dramatic gouty attack.

The initial attack of gout often occurs with explosive suddenness, typically awakening the patient or becoming apparent as a foot is placed on the floor upon arising. The skin over the affected joint soon becomes reddened and warm; extreme tenderness of the affected joint and periarticular tissues is noted. The slightest pressure produces exquisite pain. Leukocytosis and elevation of the erythrocyte sedimentation rate often occur. Without treatment, the signs of inflammation will spontaneously resolve over a period of 10 to 14 days, and the skin over the involved joint may desquamate as the episode subsides.

Factors capable of provoking episodes of acute gouty arthritis are those that cause fluctuation in serum urate levels and include trauma, surgery, alcohol ingestion, starvation, overindulgence in foods with high purine content, and ingestion of certain drugs. Interestingly, factors that cause sudden lowering of serum urate levels are more likely to trigger attacks than those that raise levels. The precise relationship of these factors to the attacks remains speculative.

On recovery, the patient reenters an asymptomatic phase termed the *intercritical period*. Even though the attack may have been incapacitating, with excruciating pain and swelling, resolution is usually complete, and the patient is once again well. This freedom from symptoms during the intercritical period is an important feature of gout in the differential diagnosis of acute monoarticular arthritis. The course of untreated acute gout is variable. Mild attacks may subside in several hours or may persist for only a few days and not reach the intensity described by Sydenham.

A clear and detailed history of an acute arthritic attack followed by a completely asymptomatic intercritical period before a recurrence is valuable in pointing toward the diagnosis of gout. During this period, aspiration of a previously inflamed joint can frequently corroborate the diagnosis of gout (9). For example, in an untreated gouty population, 36 of 37 synovial fluid aspirates obtained during intercritical periods yielded urate crystals if the knee aspirated had been subject to past gouty attacks (10). By comparison, the yield was only 22% if there was no history of prior acute involvement in the aspirated knee and was 50% in previously inflamed knees in patients on urate-lowering medication. Without therapy, most gouty patients will experience a second episode within two years. In one large series, 62% of patients had recurrences within the first year, and 78% within 2 years, with only 7% free of recurrences for 10 years or more (2).

As the disease progresses in the untreated patient, acute attacks occur with increasing frequency and are often polyarticular, more severe, longer-lasting, and occasionally associated with a fever (Fig. 1). Although affected joints may continue to recovery completely, bony erosions may develop. As many as one-third of patients with late polyarticular attacks reported that their initial attack was also polyarticular (11). Joints may flare in sequence, in a migratory pattern, or, as in pseudogout, several neighboring joints may be involved simultaneously in a cluster attack. Frequently, periarticular sites such as bursae and tendons are also involved.

Advanced Gout or Chronic Gouty Arthritis

Eventually, the untreated patient will progress to chronic polyarticular gout where the pain-free intercritical periods have disappeared This stage of gouty arthritis usually develops after 10 or more years of acute intermittent gout, although patients have been reported with tophi as their initial clinical manifestation (12). The transition from acute intermittent gout to chronic tophaceous gout occurs when the intercritical periods are no longer free of pain (Fig. 1). The involved joints are now persistently uncomfortable and swollen, although the intensity of these symptoms is much less than during acute flares. Gouty attacks can continue to occur against this painful background, and without therapy they may recur as often as every few weeks. The amount of background pain also steadily increases with time if appropriate intervention is not started. Clinically evident tophi may or may not be detected on physical examination during the first few years of this stage of gout. However, periarticular or boney tophi detected by magnetic resonance imaging and synovial "microtophi" discovered through the arthroscope are often present early in this stage of gout (13). Polyarticular involvement becomes much more frequent during this time. With diffuse and symmetric involvement of small joints in the hand and feet, chronic tophaceous gout can occasionally be confused with the nodal osteoarthritis of the hand (Fig. 3) or the symmetric polyarthritis of rheumatoid arthritis.

The subcutaneous tophus is the most characteristic lesion of chronic gouty arthritis (Fig. 4). Similar appearing nodules are clinically observed in other rheumatic disorders such as rheumatoid arthritis and multicentric reticulohistiocytosis and may lead to diagnostic confusion (14,15). Parallels can be drawn between nodule formation in rheumatoid arthritis and tophus formation in gout. The nodular aspects of both diseases are generally observed in the most chronic and severe cases but are not a universal consequence of the disease process and may appear in patients with clinically unapparent joint

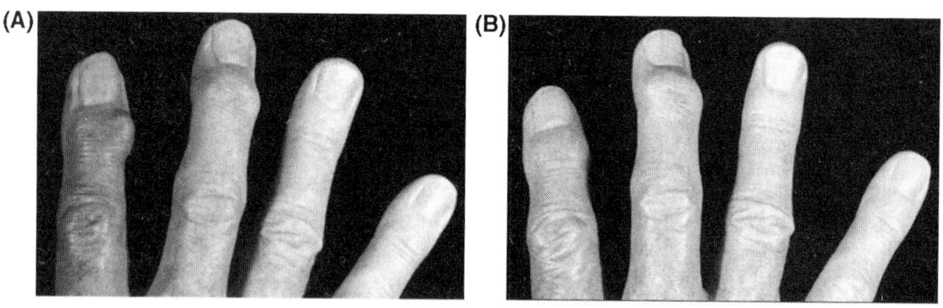

Figure 3 (**A**) Hard nodules over the distal interphalangeal joints of the second and third digits give the appearance of osteoarthritic Heberden's nodes. (**B**) After a year of allopurinol therapy the second distal interphalangeal is much smaller, suggesting that the nodules on that finger were actually gouty tophi.

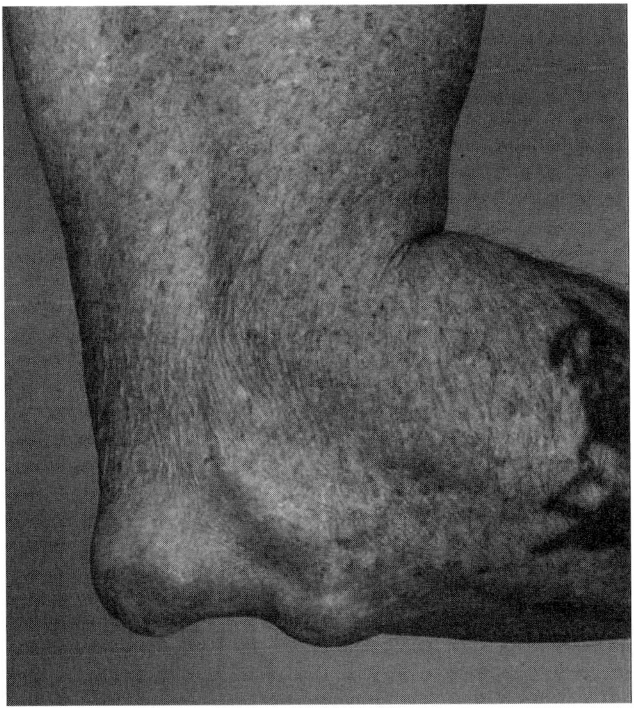

Figure 4 Typical location of gouty tophi over the olecranon process and along the ulnar surface of the forearm.

disease. However, the subcutaneous collection of monosodium urate crystals is pathognomonic for gout. Like the chronic destructive arthritis that they are frequently associated with, tophi may lead to physical disability and pain in their own right.

Tophaceous gout is often associated with an early age of onset, a long duration of active (but untreated) disease, frequent attacks, high serum urate values, and a predilection for upper extremity and polyarticular episodes. Characteristics of the arthritis include asymmetric, ascending joint involvement in which chronic inflammation is typical (16). Although ethanol consumption and diuretic use are frequently associated with gout in this population, suboptimal management and patient compliance are considered to be major factors in the progression from monoarticular gout to chronic polyarticular status.

The development of tophaceous deposits of monosodium urate is a function of the duration and severity of hyperuricemia (17). The identification of tophi with or before the initial gouty attack, once considered rare in primary gout, has been documented more frequently in recent years (18–20). In patients without tophi, the mean serum urate concentration was 9.2 mg/dL. Values of 10 to 11 mg/dL were found in subjects with minimal to moderate deposits, and patients with extensive tophaceous deposits had urate concentrations in excess of 11 mg/dL. In untreated patients, the interval from the first gouty attack to the beginning of chronic arthritis or visible tophi is highly variable, ranging from 3 to 42 years, with an average of 11.6 years (21).

Subcutaneous gouty tophi may be found anywhere over the body but occur most commonly in the fingers, wrists, ears, knees, olecranon bursa, and pressure points such as the ulnar aspect of the forearm (Fig. 4) and the Achilles' tendon (22,23). In patients with nodal osteoarthritis, tophi have a propensity for forming in Heberden's nodes (Fig. 3) (24). Tophi may also occur in connective tissues at other sites, such as renal pyramids, heart valves, and sclerae (25). Before antihyperuricemic agents were available, as many as 50% of patients with gout eventually developed clinical or radiographic evidence of tophi. Since the introduction of allopurinol and the uricosuric agents, the incidence of tophaceous gout has declined.

Gout at this stage may be confused with rheumatoid arthritis, especially if tophaceous nodules are mistaken for rheumatoid nodules. On occasion, the disease may progress from initial podagra to a rheumatoid arthritis-like chronic deforming arthritis without remissions but with synovial thickening and the early development of tophi (Fig. 5). Eventually, the untreated patient will progress to chronic polyarticular gout where the pain-free intercritical periods have disappeared. Unlike rheumatoid arthritis, in which polyarticular inflammation is most often synchronous and symmetric, inflamed gouty joints are frequently out of phase with each other. Another sign of gout is the involvement of the distal interphalangeal joints of the hands, joints not affected by rheumatoid arthritis (Fig. 6). Conversely, subcutaneous nodules in patients with "rheumatoid nodulosis" are easily confused with tophi (26). Coexistence of gout and rheumatoid arthritis is rare, however, and the appropriate diagnosis is best established by demonstrating the presence or absence of urate crystals by aspiration of affected joints or tophaceous deposits.

LESS CLASSIC PRESENTATIONS OF GOUT

Early-Onset Gout

Between 3% and 6% of patients with gout have symptom onset before the age of 25. Early-onset gout represents a special subset of patients who generally have a genetic component, a more accelerated clinical course, and require more aggressive antihyperuricemic therapy. In large epidemiologic studies of classic gout, a family history of gout and/or nephrolithiasis is present in 25% to 30% of cases. In early-onset gout, the incidence of family history of gout is about 80%. In this younger group, detailed questioning about the kindred over several generations may yield enough information to suggest a mode of inheritance (X-linked or autosomal dominant or recessive).

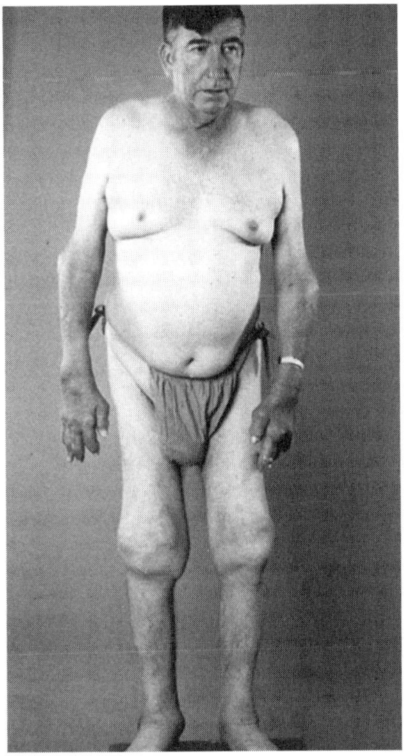

Figure 5 Advanced gout involving virtually every peripheral joint. This man was misdiagnosed as having rheumatoid arthritis for nearly 20 years because of the symmetric destruction of multiple joints.

Like classic gout, early-onset gout may be due to either overproduction of urate or reduced renal clearance of uric acid. Diseases associated with overproduction of urate in children and young adults include enzymatic defects in the purine pathway, glycogen storage diseases, and hematologic disorders such as hemoglobinopathies and leukemias. The complete deficiency of hypoxanthine-guanine phosphoribosyl transferase is an X-linked inherited inborn error or purine metabolism with a characteristic clinical presentation known as the Lesch-Nyhan syndrome (27,28). In addition to severe neurologic abnormalities and self-mutilative behavior, these boys develop gout and kidney stones in their first decade of life if they are not treated early with allopurinol. The partial deficiency of HGPRT (the Kelley-Seegmiller syndrome) results in early-onset gout or uric acid nephrolithiasis and is also X-linked in its inheritance (29). Patients with this syndrome have minor or no neurologic problems, and the onset of gouty symptoms may not occur until they are in their second or third decade of life. Similarly, early-onset gout maybe seen in the

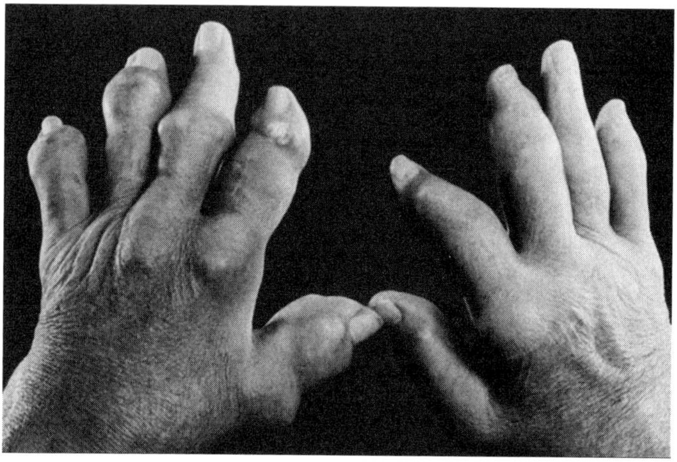

Figure 6 The hands of the patient in Figure 5. The extensive involvement of distal interphalangeal (DIP) joints, especially on the left hand, is evidence against rheumatoid arthritis in this patient. The left second DIP lesion was draining chalky urate crystals.

X-linked disorder phosphribosylpyrophosphate synthase overactivity (30). Glycogen storage disease types I, III, V, and VII are associated with early-onset gout and are inherited as autosomal recessive diseases (31,32). Sickle cell disease, beta-thalassemia, and nonlymphocytic leukemias may all be complicated by gouty arthritis in the young adult years. These disorders are described in further detail in Chapter 12.

Conditions associated with uric acid underexcretion in young patients include a specific renal tubular disorder known as familial urate nephropathy (33). This autosomal dominant disorder causes hyperuricemia from a very young age, before any evidence of renal insufficiency. The condition may lead to progressive renal failure and end-stage kidney disease by age 40. Other nephropathies associated with early-onset gout include polycystic kidney disease, chronic lead intoxication, medullary cystic disease, and focal tubulointerstitial disease.

Gout and Organ Transplants

Hyperuricemia reportedly develops in 75% to 80% of heart transplant recipients who routinely take cyclosporine for preventing allograft rejection (34). A slightly lower frequency (approximately 50%) of kidney and liver transplant recipients develop hyperuricemia, presumably because lower doses of cyclosporine are used in these individuals. Whereas in the general population asymptomatic hyperuricemia progresses to clinical gout in approximately one out of 30 subjects, cyclosporine-induced hyperuricemia leads to gout in one of six patients (35). Other differences between primary and cyclosporine-induced gout include the marked shortening of the asymptomatic hyperuricemia and acute intermittent gout stages with the rapid appearance of tophi. The stage of asymptomatic hyperuricemia lasts for 20 to 30 years in classic gout but is present for only 6 months to 4 years in cyclosporine-induced disease. Similarly, the duration of the acute intermittent stage is only 1 to 4 years in transplant recipients, whereas it may last 8 to 15 years in classic gout. Because other medications such as systemic corticosteroids and azathioprine are being used by organ transplant patients, their gouty symptoms are frequently less dramatic than those of classic gouty subjects. There is also the suggestion that corticosteroids may potentiate urate crystal deposition (36).

Gout in Women

Unlike most other rheumatic conditions, gout is less common in women. In most large reviews, women account for no more than 5% of all gouty subjects (37). Ninety percent of women are postmenopausal at the time of their initial attack. Postmenopausal gout is clinically similar in presentation and course to classic gout except that the age of onset is later in women than in men (mean age 60 years in women vs. 49 years in men). Several associated conditions are much more common in postmenopausal women with gout than in men. Diuretic use (95%), hypertension (73%), and renal insufficiency (50%) have strong associations with postmenopausal gout, as does preexisting joint disease such as osteoarthritis (38). Women who develop gout before menopause have hypertension and renal insufficiency or are using thiazide diuretics. Similar to early-onset gout in men, gout in premenopausal women has a strong hereditary component. The rare woman with premenopausal gout and normal renal function should be evaluated for the autosomally inherited familial hyperuricemia nephropathy or the even more rare non-X-linked inborn errors of purine metabolism (33,38).

Normouricemic Gout

Gout attacks not infrequently occur in individuals with serum urate levels less than 6.8 mg/dL. In one study this was observed in half of the attacks (39). The two most frequent explanations for gout in such individuals are: (1) the patient doesn't have gout, or (2) the serum urate is normal at the time measured, but the patient is actually chronically hyperuricemic. Accordingly, crystal identification is essential before diagnosing "normouricemic gout."

Several articular conditions can closely mimic gout, including other arthropathies caused by other crystals, such as calcium pyrophosphate dihydrate, basic calcium (apatite), and liquid lipid (40). Other causes of acute monoarthropathies such as infection, sarcoidosis, and trauma should also be considered (41) (and see Chapter 12).

A misunderstanding about the definition of hyperuricemia may also contribute to the misdiagnosis of "normouricemic" gout. Any sustained serum urate level above 6.8 mg/dL provides a permissive environment for urate crystal formation. For various reasons, patients with acute and chronic gout occasionally have urate values below this biochemical definition of hyperuricemia. It is, in fact, rather common for a patient presenting with acute gout to have a normal serum urate during the episode of severe pain. This finding probably results from the uricosuric effect of IL-6 released during the acute flare and the increased glomerular filtration associated with the stress of the painful process (39). Normalization of serum urate values during acute gouty flares may be more common in alcoholics than in nondrinkers. Aside from the standard urate-lowering agents (allopurinol, probenecid, and sulfinpyrazone), other drugs such as high-dose salicylates (greater than 2 g per 24 hours), corticosteroids, losartan, fenofibrate, dicumarol, glycerol guaiacholate, and X-ray contrast agents may also lower serum urate values and lead to the false impression of normouricemic gout.

In a large study, 1.6% of 2145 gouty patients were found to have sustained normouricemia even after not taking allopurinol or uricosuric agents for months (42). In most of these cases, hyperuricemia eventually was observed, although several patients with very mild gouty symptoms remained normouricemic over a prolonged period.

Neurologic Complications of Gout

Carpal tunnel syndrome resulting from tophi in the wrists is recognized as a complication of gout (43). However, other neurologic symptoms attributed to this disease are rare. Nevertheless, tophi can develop in the axial skeleton, and when they do, cause dramatic clinical consequences. These include presentations of acute-onset back pain with fever mimicking an epidural infection, progressive myelopathy with six weeks of progressive leg weakness later accompanied by urinary incontinence, and acute paraplegia (44–46). Computed tomography or magnetic resonance imaging is useful in identifying focal abnormalities in these settings, but emergent surgical intervention followed by appropriate medical management is necessary for good outcomes.

CLINICAL ASSOCIATES OF GOUT

Urolithiasis

Uric acid stones account for 5% to 10% of all renal stones in the United States and Europe, and 40% of renal stones in Israel (47). The overall prevalence of uric acid stones in adults in the United States is estimated to be 0.01%. However, in a series of 1258 patients with primary gout and 59 patients with secondary gout, the prevalence of renal lithiasis was 22% and 42%, respectively (48). More than 80% of calculi in these gouty patients consisted entirely of uric acid, with the remainder composed of calcium oxalate or calcium phosphate, often with a central nidus of uric acid. The several-hundred-fold higher incidence of uric acid stones in gout patients is accompanied by a 10- to 30-fold increased incidence of calcium oxalate stones (49). In studies of gouty individuals, higher prevalence rates of uric acid urolithiasis are associated with increased uric acid excretion. In gouty patients with daily excretion of more than 1100 mg of uric acid, the prevalence of stones was 50%, or 4.5 times greater than in patients excreting less than 300 mg/d (48). Many clinical circumstances result in hyperuricosuria, including inherited enzymatic defects and hematologic disorders that lead to accelerated purine biosynthesis, diets high in purine, and administration of uricosuric drugs (50).

Kidney Disease

Apart from arthritis and tophus formation, renal disease is the most frequently reported clinical association of hyperuricemia. In addition to promoting urolithiasis, hyperuricemia may affect the kidney through the deposition of urate crystals in the renal interstitium, referred to as urate nephropathy, or by the concentration of uric acid crystals in the collecting tubules, an entity referred to as uric acid nephropathy. Acute uric acid nephropathy with accompanying acute renal tubular damage and an obstructive uropathic clinical picture is very uncommon except in patients with malignancy and hyperuricemia treated by radiation or chemotherapy, or with inherited enzyme defects resulting in markedly increased uric acid excretion. In addition to these direct effects of hyperuricemia, other causes of renal dysfunction, such as hypertension, diabetes mellitus, alcohol abuse, nephrotoxic drug therapy, and lead nephropathy are also prevalent in the gouty population. The isolation of hyperuricemia or gout as primary risk factors for progressive renal disease is thus exceedingly difficult (2,6,51–53).

Significant impairment of renal function in up to 40% of patients with gout was reported in two older series of patients, and renal failure was the eventual cause of death in 18% to 25% of patients (51,53). Recent evaluations, however, have de-emphasized a primary causal relationship between hyperuricemia/gout and renal disease and suggest that the incidence of renal disease among gouty individuals is probably no greater than that in subjects of comparable age with similar degrees of hypertension, obesity, and primary renal disease (6,52).

Hypertension and Cardiovascular Disease

Interestingly, recent studies support a direct causal effect of hyperuricemia on endothelial dysfunction in renal arterioles (54,55). This may explain why 25% to 50% of gouty patients are hypertensive and why 2% to 14% of hypertensive subjects have gout (56). Since serum urate concentration correlates directly with peripheral and renal vascular resistance, reduced renal blood flow may account for the association between hypertension and hyperuricemia. Factors such as obesity and male gender also link hypertension and hyperuricemia.

Several recent studies in humans have found that hyperuricemia is an independent risk factor for cardiovascular disease when controlling for other associated risk factors using multivariate analysis (57–59). To date, however, the data are inconclusive with in regards to this issue. This issue is debated further in Chapter 12.

Obesity, Hyperlipidemia, and the Metabolic Syndrome

Hyperuricemia and gout are highly correlated with body weight for both men and women, and individuals with gout are commonly overweight compared to the general population. Obesity may be a common factor linking hyperuricemia, hypertension, hyperlipidemia, and atherosclerosis. Serum triglycerides are elevated in 80% of patients with gout. The association between hyperuricemia and serum cholesterol is controversial, although serum levels of high-density lipoprotein are generally decreased in patients with gout.

The metabolic syndrome is a constellation of disorders characterized by insulin-resistant hyperglycemia, hypertriglyceridemia, and obesity. It is estimated that 23% of the population in the United States meets criteria for the metabolic syndrome (60). One study found that 86% of gout patients met the criteria for this syndrome (61). Insulin resistance in the metabolic syndrome leads to increased circulating level of insulin which leads to increased sodium and urate reabsorption in the proximal convoluted tubule. This promotes both hypertension and gout (62). Obesity is another link between the metabolic syndrome and hyperuricemia. The elevated serum leptin levels in patients with metabolic syndrome impair urate excretion by the kidney (63).

Gout and Alcohol Consumption

Alcohol is both a predisposing and provocative factor in gout. These relationships have long been recognized. Over a century ago Garrod wrote, "There is no truth in medicine better established than the fact that the use of fermented liquors is the most powerful of all the predisposing causes of gout; nay, so powerful, that it may be a question whether gout would ever have been known to mankind had such beverages not been indulged in" (64). Although consumption of all forms of alcohol is recognized as inducing hyperuricemia, beer appears to be the most significant contributor among these (65,66). In one a study of 354 patients with gout, 37% consumed a minimum average daily intake of two pints of beer or two double whiskies (67). In contrast, in Saudi Arabia, where alcohol consumption is quite rare, a survey of 487 adults demonstrated the prevalence of hyperuricemia to be 8.42%, but no cases of gout were found (68).

The chronic use of alcohol promotes hyperuricemia by stimulating de novo purine biosynthesis (69). In addition "binge drinking" may cause lactic acidosis which causes sudden increases in the serum urate concentration by blocking the urinary excretion of uric acid. The changes in serum urate concentrations that occur related to alcohol can be dramatic. The administration of alcohol, orally or intravenously, to normal subjects causes increases in serum urate levels ranging between 1.0 and 3.0 mg/dL, and the change occurs within three hours. Conversely, decreases in serum urate levels ranging from 4.0 to 6.5 mg/dL were observed over 11 days in hospitalized patients who were intoxicated at the time of admission (70).

Although the increase in serum urate could provoke an acute bout of arthritis, attacks more commonly accompany the rapid fall in serum urate concentration that occurs with resolution of the acidosis and restoration of normal renal uric acid clearance. This practical clinical observation was confirmed by a study in which alcoholic individuals with a history of gout were hospitalized and given alcohol until inebriated. This was associated with increased serum urate concentrations. However, acute gouty arthritis did not develop until hours after they stopped drinking alcohol and the urate levels returned to or below baseline levels (71). Curiously, the finding of "normouricemic gout" is more common in alcoholics (72).

Saturnine Gout

Hyperuricemia and gout are well-recognized complications of chronic lead intoxication. A poorly defined renal defect appears to be responsible for the hyperuricemia (73,74). The earliest implication of lead being involved with gout involved the epidemic of gout that occurred in England in the late 17th century (75). At that time gout was quite common among the English upper class compared to Ireland and Scotland. In the latter two countries the diets contained little meat and the preferred alcoholic beverage was whiskey. In England the upper class ate copious amounts of meat and organic foods and consumed beer and port. It is estimated that it was common for the members of this society to imbibe 200 or more grams of alcohol in the course of an evening. Port had become a major source of alcohol after 1659 when the parliament passed the Navigation Act which forbid all imports other than those carried either on English ships or ships from the product's country of origin. The Act thereby prevented the importation of French wine on Dutch ships. As a result, wine in the diet was replaced by port produced in Portugal and Spain. The port was implicated as a contribution to gout, not only because of its higher alcohol content (estimated at 19%), but also because of its high lead content, which is acquired from sitting in lead-contaminated containers.

The prevalence of lead-intoxicated adults having documented gout, termed saturnine gout, ranges from 6% to in excess of 50% (76,77). Some patients with primary gout have increased blood lead levels, compared with age- and sex-matched controls, despite the absence of a history of overt lead exposure. These findings suggest that occult chronic lead intoxication may play an etiologic role in some cases of primary gout.

REFERENCES

1. Loeb J. The influence of temperature on the solubility of monosodium urate. Arthritis Rheum 1972; 15:189–192.
2. Campion EW, Glynn RJ, DeLabry LO. Asymptomatic hyperuricemia: risks and consequences in the normative aging study. Am J Med 1987; 82:421–426.
3. Gibson T, Waterworth R, Hatfield P, et al. Hyperuricemia, gout and kidney function in New Zealand Maori men. Br J Rheumatol 1984; 23:276–282.
4. Darmawan J, Valkenburg HA, Muirden KD, et al. The epidemiology of gout and hyperuricemia in a rural population of Java. J Rheumatol 1992; 19:1595–1599.
5. Langford HG, Blaufox MD, Borhani NO, et al. Is thiazide-produced uric acid elevation harmful? Analysis of data from the hypertension detection and follow-up program Arch Intern Med 1987; 147:645–649.
6. Fessel JW. Renal outcomes of gout and hyperuricemia. Am J Med 1979; 67:74–82.
7. Hall AP, Barry PE, Dawber TR, et al. Epidemiology of gout and hyperuricemia: a long-term population study. Am J Med 1967; 42:27–37.
8. Sydenham T. The whole works of that excellent practical physician, Dr. Thomas Sydenham. 7th ed. translated by John Pechey. London, Feals, 1717.
9. Agudelo CA, Weinberger A, Schumacher HR, et al. Definite diangonosi of gout by identification of urate crystals in asymptomatic metatarsophalangeal joints. Arthritis Rheum 1979; 22:559–560.
10. Pascual E. Persistence of monosodium urate crystals and low-grade inflammation in the synovial fluid of patients with untreated gout. Arthritis Rheum 1991; 34:141–145.
11. Raddatz DA, Mahowald ML, Bilka PJ. Acute polyarticular gout. Ann Rheum Dis 1983; 42:117–122.
12. Wernick R, Winkler C, Campbell S. Tophi as the initial manifestation of gout: report of six cases and review of the literature. Arch Intern Med 1992; 152:873–876.
13. Popp JD, Bidgood WD, Edwards NL. Magnetic resonance imaging of tophaceous gout in the hands and wrists. Semin Arthritis Rheum 1996; 25:282–289.
14. Ziff M. The rheumatoid nodule. Arthritis Rheum 1990; 33:761–767.
15. Campbell DA, Edwards NL. Multicentric reticulohistiocytosis: systemic macrophage disorder. Clin Rheumatol 1991; 5:301–319.
16. Nakayama DA, Barthelemy C, Carrera G, et al. Tophaceous gout: a clinical and radiographic assessment. Arthritis Rheum 1984; 27:468–471.
17. Popp JD, Bidgood WD, Edwards NL. The gouty tophus. Rheumatol Rev 1993; 2:163–168.
18. Wernick R, Winkler C, Campbell S. Tophi as the initial manifestation of gout: report of six cases and review of the literature. Arch Intern Med 1992; 152:873–876.
19. Iglesias A, Londono JC, saaibi DL, et al. Gouty nodulosis: widespread subcutaneous deposits without gout. Arthritis Care Res 1996; 9:74–77.
20. Liu K, Moffatt EJ, Hudson ER, et al. Gouty tophus presenting as a soft-tissue mass diagnosed by fine needle aspiration: a case report. Diagn Cytopathol 1996; 15:246–249.
21. McGill NW, Dieppe PA. The role of serum and synovial fluid components in the promotion of urate crystal formation. J Rheumatol 1991; 18:1042–1045.
22. Holland NW, Jost D, Beutler A, et al. Finger pad tophi in gout. J Rheumatol 1996; 23:690–692.
23. Fam AG, Assad D. Intradermal urate tophi. J Rheumatol 1997; 24:1126–1131.

24. Good AE, Rapp R. Bony ankylosis: a rare manifestation of gout. J Rheumatol 1978; 5:335–337.
25. Lichtenstein L, Scott HW, Levin MH. Pathologic changes in gout: survey of 11 necropsied cases. Am J Pathol 1956; 32:871–895.
26. Ginsberg MH, Genant HK, Yu T-F, et al. Rheumatoid nodulosis: an unusual variant of rheumatoid disease. Arthritis Rheum 1975; 18:49–58.
27. Lesch M, Nyhan WL. A familial disorder of uric acid metabolism and central nervous system function. Am J Med 1964; 36:561–569.
28. Seegmiller JE, Rosenbloom EM, Kelley WN. An enzyme defect associated with a sex-linked human neurological disorder and excessive purine synthesis. Science 1967; 155:1682–1685.
29. Kelley WN, Rosenbloom EM, Henderson JF, et al. A specific enzyme defect associated with overproduction of uric acid. Proc Natl Acad Sci USA 1967; 57:1735–1739.
30. Becker MA, Losman MJ, Itkin P, et al. Gout and superactive phosphoribosyl-pyrophosphate synthetase due to increased enzyme catalytic rate. J Lab Clin Med 1982; 99:495–502.
31. Mineo I, Kono N, Hara N, et al. Myogenic hyperuricemia. A common pathophysiologic feature of glycogenosis types III, V, and VII. N Engl J Med 1987; 317:75–80.
32. Cohen JL, Vinik A, Faller A, Fox IH. Hyperuricemia in glycogen storage disease type I: contributions by hypoglycemia and hyper glucagonemia to increased urate production. J Clin Invest 1985; 75:25–259.
33. Stibrkova B, HMajewski J, Sebesta I, et al. Familial juvenile hyperuricemic nephropathy: localization of the gene on chromosome 16p11.2-and evidence for genetic heterogeneity. Am J Hum Genet 2000; 66:1989–1994.
34. Burack DA, Griffith BP, Thompson ME, et al. Hyperuricemia and gout among heart transplant recipients receiving cyclosporine. Am J Med 1992; 92:141–146.
35. Howe S, Edwards NL. Controlling hyperuricemia and gout in cardiac transplant recipients. J Musculoskel Med 1995; 12:15–24.
36. Vazquez-Mellado J, Cuan A, Magana M, et al. Intradermal tophi in gout: a case-control study. J Rheumatol 1999; 26:136–140.
37. Lally EV, Ho G, Kaplan SR. The clinical spectrum of gouty arthritis in women. Arch Intern Med 1986; 146:2221–2225.
38. Puig JG, Michan AD, Jimenez ML, et al. Female gout: clinical spectrum and uric acid metabolism. Arch Intern Med 1991; 151:726–732.
39. Urano W, Yamanaka H, Tsytani H, et al. The inflammatory process in the mechanism of decreased serum uric acid concentration during acute gouty arthritis. J Rheumatol 2002; 29:1950–1953.
40. Reginato AJ, Schumacher HR, Allan DA, Rabinowitz JL. Acute monoarthritis associated with lipid liquid crystals. Ann Rheum Dis 1985; 44:537–543.
41. Baker DG, Schumacher HR. Acute monoarthritis. N Engl J Med 1993; 329:1013–1020.
42. Yu T-F. Diversity of clinical features in gouty arthritis. Semin Arthritis Rheum 1984; 13:360–368.
43. Weinzweiig J, Gletcher JW, Lindburg RM. Flexor tendonitis and median nerve compression caused by gout in a patient with rheumatoid arthritis. Plast Reconstr Surg 2000; 106:1570–1572.

44. Barrett K, Miller M, Wilson JT. Tophaceous gout of the spine mimicing epidural infection: case report and review of the literature. Neurosurgery 2001; 48:1170–1173.
45. St. George E, Liller CEM, Hatfield R. Spinal cord compression: an unusual neurologic complication of gout. Rheumatology 2001; 40:711–712.
46. Wang L-C, Hung Y-C, Lee E-J, et al. Acute paraplegia in a patient with spinal tophi: a case report. J Formos Med Assoc 2001; 100:205–208.
47. Yu T-F. Uric acid nephrolithiasis. In: Weiner IM, Kelley WN, eds. In: Uric Acid: Handbook of Experimental Pharmacology, Vol. 51. New York: Springer-Verlag, 1978:397–422.
48. Yu T-F, Gutman AB. Uric acid nephrolithiasis in gout: predisposing factors. Ann Intern Med 1967; 67:1133–1148.
49. Coe FL, Kavalach AG. Hypercalciuria and hyperuricosuria in patients with calcium nephrolithiasis. N Engl J Med 1974; 291:1344–1350.
50. Zollner N, Griebsch A. Diet and gout. Adv Exp Med Biol 1974; 41B:435–442.
51. Berger L, Yu T-F. Renal function in gout: 4. An analysis of 524 gouty subjects including long-term follow-up studies. Am J Med 1975; 59:605–613.
52. Reif MC, Constantiner A, Levitt MF. Chronic gouty nephropathy: a vanishing syndrome? N Engl J Med 1981; 304:535–536.
53. Talbott JH, Terplan KL. The kidney in gout. Medicine 1960; 39:405–468.
54. Mazali M, Hughes J, Kim Y-G, et al. Elevated uric acid increases blood pressure in the rat by a novel crystal-independent mechanism. Hypertension 2001; 38:1101–1115.
55. Sanchez-Lozada LG, Tapia E, Avila-Casado C, et al. Mild hyperuricemia induces glomerular hypertension in normal rats. Am J Physiol Renal Physiol 2002; 283:F1105–F1110.
56. Cannon PJ, Stason WB, Demartini FE, et al. Hyperuricemia in primary and renal hypertension. N Engl J Med 1966; 275:457–464.
57. Selby JV, Friedman GD, Quesenberry CP. Precursors of essential hypertension: pulmonary function, heart rate, uric acid, serum cholesterol and other serum chemistries. Am J Epidemiol 1990; 131:1017–1027.
58. Jossa F, Farinaro E, Panico S, et al. Serum uric acid and hypertension: the Olivetti heart study. J Hum Hypertens 1994; 8:677–681.
59. Fang J, Alderman MH. Serum uric acid and cardiovascular mortality: the NHANESI Epidemiologic follow-up study. 1971–1992. JAMA 2000; 283:2404–2410.
60. Grundy SM, Hanson B, Smith SC, et al. Clinical management of the metabolic syndrome. Circulation 2004; 109:551–556.
61. Vazquez-Mellado J, Garcia CG, Vazquez SG, et al. Metabolic syndrome and ischemic heart disease in gout. J Clin Rheum 2004; 10:105–109.
62. Beiber JD, Terbeltaub RA. Gout: on the brink of novel therapeutic options for an ancient disease. Arthritis Rheum 2004; 50:2400–2414.
63. Fruehwald-Schultes B, Peters A, Kern W, et al. Serum leptin is associated with serum uric acid concentrations in humans. Metabolism 1999; 48:677–680.
64. Garrod AB. In: A Treatise on Gout and Rheumatic Gout. London: Longmans, 1876:218–245.
65. Choi HK, Karlson EW, Willett W, Curhan G. Alcohol intake and risk of incident gout in men: a prospective study. Lancet 2004; 363:1277–1281.

66. Yamamoto T, Moriwaki Y, Takahashi S, et al. Effect of sauna bathing and beer ingestion on plasma concentrations of purine bases. Metabolism 2004; 53:772–776.
67. Lin KC, Lin HY, Chou P. The interaction between uric acid level and other risk factors on the development of gout among asymptomatic men. I. a prospective study. J Rheumatol 2000; 27:1501–1505.
68. Al-Arfaj AS. Hyperuricemia in Saudi Arabia. Rheumatol Int 2001; 20:61–64.
69. Faller J, Fox IH. Ethanol-induced hyperuricemia: evidence for increased urate production by activation of adenine nucleotide turnover. N Engl J Med 1982; 307:1598–1602.
70. Wyngaarden JD, Kelley WN. Gout and Hyperuricemia. New York: Grune and Stratton, 1976.
71. Rodnan GP. The pathogenesis of aldermanic gout: procatarctic role of fluctuations in serum concentration in gouty arthritis provoked by feast and alcohol. Clin Res 1980; 28:359A.
72. Vandenberg MK, Moxley G, Breitbach SA, Roberts WN. Gout attacks in chronic alcoholics occur at lower serum urate levels than in nonalcoholics. J Rheumatol 1994; 21:700–704.
73. Marsden PA. Increased body lead burden—cause or consequence of chronic renal insufficiency? N Engl J Med 2003; 248:345–347.
74. Lin JL, Tan DT, Ho HH, Yu CC. Environmental lead exposure and urate excretion in the general population. Am J Med 2003; 113:563–568.
75. Healey LA. Port wine and the gout. Arthritis Rheum 1975; 18:659–662.
76. Emmerson BT. Chronic lead nephropathy: the diagnostic use of calcium EDTA and the association with gout. Australas Ann Med 1963; 12:310–324.
77. Batuman V, Maesaka JK, Haddad B, Tepper E, Landy E, Wedeen RP. The role of lead in gout nephropathy. N Engl J Med 1981; 304:520–523.

5

Asymptomatic Hyperuricemia

John Kanellis

Department of Nephrology, Monash Medical Centre, Clayton, Melbourne, Victoria, Australia

Duk-Hee Kang

Division of Nephrology, College of Medicine, Ewha Women's University and Ewha Research Center, Seoul, Korea

Daniel I. Feig

Renal Section, Department of Pediatrics, Baylor College of Medicine, Houston, Texas, U.S.A.

Richard J. Johnson

Section of Nephrology, Hypertension, and Transplantation, University of Florida, Gainesville, Florida, U.S.A.

INTRODUCTION

This chapter discusses the significance of asymptomatic hyperuricemia and the current views regarding the need to treat this entity. Various controversies regarding the possible effects of uric acid are reviewed with reference to epidemiological, experimental animal, and in vitro studies. Although the traditional and historical view has been to avoid treating asymptomatic hyperuricemia, recent studies and a reappraisal of the historical allows one to question this approach (1). In particular, there is significant experimental evidence that hyperuricemia may contribute to the development of hypertension, vascular disease, and to renal disease progression. As a result, there is now a critical need to reassess the impact of urate-lowering therapy on various disease processes in humans.

URIC ACID: BIOCHEMISTRY

Uric acid is a metabolic breakdown product of purines in humans and exists in blood and synovial fluid in the form of monosodium urate. Urate is produced from hypoxanthine and xanthine via the action of the enzyme xanthine dehydrogenase or its isoform, xanthine oxidase (Fig. 1). Oxidants in the form of superoxide (O_2^-) are also generated in the xanthine oxidase-mediated reaction. See Chapter 12 for additional information.

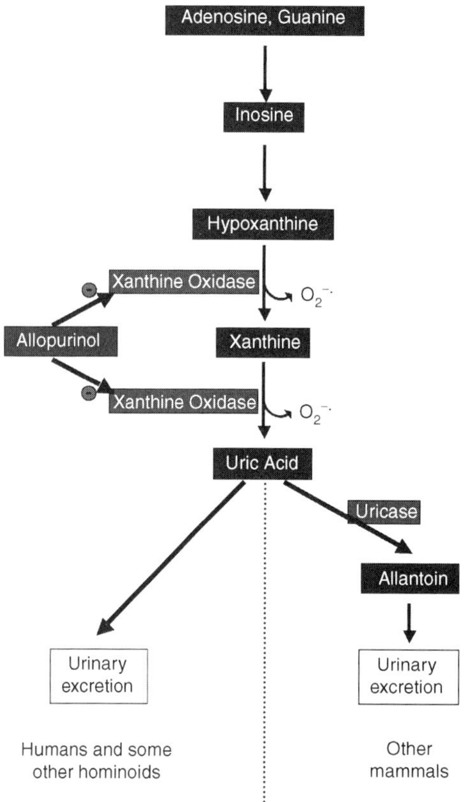

Figure 1 Purine metabolism and the production of uric acid in mammals. Purines (adenosine and guanine) are broken down via hypoxanthine to xanthine and then uric acid via the enzyme xanthine oxidase. Superoxide (O_2^-) is generated in the process. The action of xanthine oxidase can be directly blocked using allopurinol. In most mammals, urate is further degraded to allantoin via the enzyme uricase (urate oxidase). This step is not possible in humans and in other higher hominoid species due to mutation of the uricase gene.

THE URICASE GENE IS MUTATED IN HUMANS AND IN OTHER HOMINOIDS

In most mammals, urate is further degraded by the hepatic enzyme urate oxidase (or uricase) to allantoin, which is then freely excreted in the urine (Fig. 1). In humans, however, urate is generally not further metabolized, and soluble urate must therefore be excreted by the kidneys or the gastrointestinal tract in the form of uric acid. This difference between humans and most other mammals has arisen due to several parallel but distinct mutations that occurred in the uricase gene in hominoid species during the Miocene Epoch, 5 to 20 million years ago (2). Consequently, humans, the great apes, and some New World monkeys have serum urate levels three- to six-fold higher than other mammals, in which values are less than 2 mg/dL (0.12 mmol/L). In humans, some allantoin is made by the oxidative degradation of urate, but the amount is not particularly significant (3).

Much speculation exists concerning the likely survival advantage these mutations might have provided during the Miocene and their possible maladaptive effect in modern times (2). Since uric acid is an anti-oxidant, it has been suggested that the mutation in uricase may have occurred to replace the loss of vitamin C synthesis that had occurred previously (4). Indeed, some have speculated that the higher levels of urate may account for why primates live longer than most other mammals. It has also been proposed that these mutations allowed blood pressure levels to be adequately maintained in evolving hominoids when climatic conditions became drier, and salt and water were lacking in prehistoric diets (5). Under this hypothesis, the beneficial effect that hyperuricemia exerted on blood pressure during the Miocene has become a maladaptive adaptation in modern times where salt and water intake are no longer limited (5).

HYPERURICEMIA IN HUMANS: A DEFINITION

In humans, hyperuricemia is typically defined as a serum urate level greater than 6.8 mg/dL (0.4 mmol/L), because, above this concentration, body fluids are supersaturated with urate. In general, levels are higher in men and in post-menopausal women, partly because estrogen is uricosuric (6). These values were originally derived from epidemiological studies whereby 95% of healthy age and sex matched subjects fell below these limits (7). However, given the gradual rise in mean serum urates over the last 50 years, a larger percentage of individuals now qualify as hyperuricemic when statistical analysis is applied.

Studies examining urate solubility in plasma or serum show that saturation occurs at a concentration of above 6.8 mg/dL at 37°C. Substantially higher concentrations can be achieved in supersaturated solutions from which crystals can easily precipitate. Increased temperature and a higher pH are two well-known factors that increase urate and uric acid solubility (8). In urine at pH 5, saturation occurs at 15 mg/dL. At a urinary pH of 7, uric acid can remain soluble up to a concentration as high as 200 mg/dL (9). Less well-defined factors in both serum and urine also appear to increase solubility. In urine it appears that urea, various proteins, and mucopolysaccharides can all help increase solubility substantially (10).

Serum urate levels can vary significantly based on diet, exercise, and many other factors (11). Therefore, the percentage of individuals with hyperuricemia varies based on whether a single or multiple measurements are made. For example, based on a single determination in the Framingham study, 22% of males had serum urate levels above 6.0 mg/dL while 4.8% had levels above 7.0 mg/dL. Using repeated measurements over 14 years, this increased to 44% and 9.3%, respectively (12). There is evidence that mean serum urate levels have been rising over the last century, as has the frequency of gout (13,14). This may relate to the increased intake of fatty meats and fructose-containing sweets and beverages, as both are known to increase serum urate levels (15).

HYPERURICEMIA AND THE RISK OF GOUTY ARTHRITIS, CALCULI, AND NEPHROPATHY

Prior to the 1980s, urate-lowering agents were often prescribed for patients with asymptomatic hyperuricemia, particularly when the serum urate levels were greater than 9.0 mg/dL. This was because early data from the Framingham study indicated that hyperuricemia was an independent risk factor for coronary artery disease (1). In addition, prior to the advent of uricosuric agents and allopurinol, a high percentage of individuals with gout died of renal failure, a complication attributed to hyperuricemia. It was, therefore, logical to lower the serum urate in order to prevent heart and kidney disease. Subsequently the Framingham data was reanalysed and it was concluded that hyperuricemia alone was not an independent risk factor for coronary heart disease (2) and analyses of large cohorts of gout patients followed over a long period of time revealed that their renal failure resulted from uncontrolled hypertension and not hyperuricemia (3). Consequently, the value of treating asymptomatic hyperuricemia appeared to be minimal, and the recommendation has been to not use specific urate-lowering agents based on serum urate levels alone in the absence of clinical gout or calculi (16). It has never been recommended that asymptomatic hyperuricemia be ignored, however. Its cause should be determined and any association such as hypertension, obesity, hyperlipidemia, and alcohol consumption should be addressed. The approach of not using specific urate-lowering agents in the face of asymptomatic hyperuricemia has recently been strongly challenged, with various epidemiological, experimental animal, and in vitro studies suggesting a role for hyperuricemia in the pathogenesis of hypertension, cardiovascular disease, and renal disease progression (1).

If one disregards the controversial issues surrounding hyperuricemia and its association with vascular disease, renal disease, and hypertension, what then is the risk of developing gout at certain serum urate levels? Not too surprisingly, as serum urate levels rise, so does the risk of developing gouty arthritis. In a large French study from the 1970s, the prevalence of gouty arthritis in males with serum levels between 7.0 and 7.9 mg/dL was 4.7% (17). This rose to 47.6% in subjects with serum levels greater than 10 mg/dL. Higher rates were found in the Framingham study with a prevalence of 14.2% in males with serum urate levels between 7.0 and 7.9 mg/dL, 18.7% for levels between 8.0 and 8.9 mg/dL, and an impressive 83.3% for urate levels over 9.0 mg/dL (18).

In a similar fashion, the risk of developing renal calculi increases as serum urate levels rise. With serum urate levels between 7.0 and 7.9 mg/dL, the prevalence of calculi was 12.7% in males and 7.1% in females. For males, this rose to 22% and 40% for uric acid levels of between 8.0 and 8.9 mg/dL or greater than 9.0 mg/dL, respectively (18). In another study, the risk of developing calculi was about 50% when serum uric acid levels were greater than12 mg/dL (19).

In the absence of stones, the risk of renal injury from asymptomatic hyperuricemia alone (i.e.,"gouty nephropathy") has generally been considered to be low (20). In earlier studies on this topic, it was found that subjects with asymptomatic hyperuricemia frequently developed renal insufficiency, but this was often in association with hypertension, aging, renal vascular disease, or renal calculi with pyelonephritis. When these subjects were eliminated from the analysis, the presence of asymptomatic hyperuricemia was only occasionally associated with renal disease progression, and this was most frequent when the serum urate levels were above 10 mg/dL in women or 12 mg/dL in men (20,21). However, a problem with this type of analysis is that it assumes that hyperuricemia must act independently of hypertension or renal vascular disease in order to be nephrotoxic (22). If urate causes renal disease in part by causing hypertension and/or renal vascular disease, then urate would be considered a major risk factor for renal disease progression. Indeed, more recent studies do in fact suggest this very thing—namely that hyperuricemia is a powerful predictor for the development of hypertension, renal vascular disease, and renal disease progression.

DIETARY AND PHYSIOLOGICAL FACTORS THAT CAN INFLUENCE SERUM URATE LEVELS

Serum urate levels vary significantly within humans due to factors that alter its production and excretion. Increased production of urate may result from a high purine or protein diet and/or from alcohol consumption; from high cell turnover (i.e., myeloproliferative disease or polycythemia); or from enzymatic defects (i.e., increased phosphoribosylpyrophosphate synthetase or deficiency in hypoxanthine-guanine phosphoribosyltransferase) (Table 1).

Recently there has been renewed attention on the role of fructose-containing foods in the causation of hyperuricemia. Fructose is rapidly taken up into hepatocytes where it is phosphorylated to fructose 1-phosphate by fructokinase. The consequences of the reaction include depletion of ATP and a

Table 1 Factors and Medical Conditions Associated with Hyperuricemia

Associated factor/condition	Mechanism
High purine diet	Increased urate intake
Cell breakdown, tumor lysis (hematological disorders, chemotherapy)	Increased urate production
Alcohol ingestion	Increases urate generation and decreases urate excretion (23)
Males/postmenopausal females	Estrogen is uricosuric (6)
Diuretic use	Volume contraction promotes urate reabsorption (24)
Renal disease	Decreased GFR increases urate levels
Metabolic syndrome, obesity, insulin resistance (25)	Insulin increases sodium reabsorption and is linked to urate reabsorption (26)
Hypertension, vascular disease (27)	Increased renal vascular resistance increases urate reabsorption. Microvascular disease predisposes to tissue ischemia, leading to increased urate generation and reduced excretion (lactate competes with urate transporter in the proximal tubule) (28)

Abbreviation: GFR, glomerular filtration rate.

rapid increase in urate production. Serum urate levels increase within 30 minutes of fructose ingestion, and may be sustained if the fructose intake is high (29). The marked increase in fructose ingestion in recent years is a consequence of the use of high fructose corn syrup as a major sweetener in sodas and pastries.

Hyperuricemia may also result from decreased renal excretion of uric acid. A reduction in glomerular filtration rate will increase serum urate levels, in spite of the significant compensatory increase in gastrointestinal excretion that occurs under this circumstance (30). More commonly hyperuricemia results from increased net tubular absorption. Following filtration uric acid undergoes both reabsorption and secretion in the proximal tubule, a process which is mediated by a urate/anion exchanger and a voltage-sensitive urate channel. The urate transporter has been recently identified and is called URAT-1 (31,32). Several anions, such as lactate and β-hydroxybutyrate, decrease urate secretion by competitive inhibition of the organic anion exchanger, whereas other substances, including probenecid and benziodarone, have opposite effects (33).

HYPERURICEMIA IS ASSOCIATED WITH HYPERTENSION, VASCULAR DISEASE, AND THE "METABOLIC SYNDROME"

Some of the medical factors associated with hyperuricemia are outlined in Table 1. Hyperuricemia is frequently observed in subjects at increased cardiovascular risk (34,35). Obesity, insulin resistance, and dyslipidemia ("the metabolic syndrome") are all associated with hyperuricemia. This has been attributed to the ability of insulin to stimulate sodium reabsorption in the proximal tubule, an action that is tightly linked to urate reabsorption. Thiazide diuretics increase serum urate levels by inducing volume contraction, which stimulates both sodium and urate reabsorption in the proximal tubule. Thiazides may also compete with urate via the organic anion transport system. Alcohol intake results in elevated serum urate levels due to both increased generation (from increased adenine nucleotide turnover) and decreased excretion (due to lactate blocking tubular transport of urate) (23).

Hyperuricemia is commonly associated with hypertension, and is present in 25% of untreated hypertensive subjects, in 50% of subjects on diuretics, and in over 75% of subjects with malignant hypertension (1). The increase in serum urate levels in these subjects may be due to several mechanisms. Subjects with hypertension frequently have elevated renal vascular resistance, which is strongly associated with hyperuricemia in both normotensive and hypertensive individuals (28). The administration of agents that cause renal vasoconstriction (such as angiotensin II and norepinephrine) results in an immediate fall in urinary uric acid excretion (36). The mechanism may be due to increased sodium reabsorption in the proximal tubule that is linked with increased urate reabsorption (26). Hypertension can also result in microvascular disease. This can lead to local tissue ischemia, which in turn results in increased urate levels. In addition to the release of lactate, which stimulates urate reabsorption in the proximal tubule, ischemia also results in increased urate synthesis.

Under ischemic conditions, ATP is degraded to adenine and xanthine and xanthine oxidase activity is induced. The increased availability of substrate (xanthine) and enzyme (xanthine oxidase) results in increased urate generation as well as oxidant ($O_2\cdot$) formation. The finding that ischemia results in an increase in serum urate levels may account for the hyperuricemia that develops in patients with pre-eclampsia (34,37), systemic hypertension (with microvascular disease) (27), and congestive heart failure (36,38). The association of hyperuricemia and vascular injury may explain why serum urate levels are elevated in subjects with microalbuminuria (39). Other factors may also contribute to why hyperuricemia is associated with hypertension, including alcohol abuse (23), lead intoxication (38,40), obesity (25), and diuretic use (24). In contrast, the association of urate with obesity, insulin resistance, microalbuminuria, and hypertension may also be epiphenomena sustained by (or associated with) decreased insulin sensitivity.

THE PROGNOSTIC SIGNIFICANCE OF SERUM URATE LEVELS

In humans, serum urate levels have been found to powerfully and independently predict the development of hypertension (41) and in some studies to have significant independent prognostic value in cardiovascular disease, cardiac failure (42,43), stroke (44), and renal disease (45–47). These various studies would suggest that urate may have a direct role in the pathogenesis of these disorders. Data from animal and in vitro studies support the hypothesis that elevated urate levels are more than simply an "epiphenomenon," and that hyperuricemia itself may have harmful effects.

In other epidemiological studies, however, hyperuricemia has not been clearly shown to be an independent risk factor for cardiovascular and renal disease after controlling for other risk factors (1). As a consequence, the issue of whether hyperuricemia is somehow a causal factor in these disease processes has become extremely controversial.

URIC ACID: BENEFICIAL OR HARMFUL?

Soluble urate appears capable of promoting both antioxidant and pro-oxidant actions depending on the biochemical environment. Although some believe urate acts purely as an antioxidant and is therefore vasculoprotective, data exist that can refute this possibly limited opinion.

Among the antioxidant actions, soluble urate can scavenge superoxide ($O_2\cdot$), singlet oxygen, hydroxyl radical ($OH\cdot$), and peroxynitrite ($OONO\cdot$) as well as chelate transitional metals (4,48). Urate can also prevent extracellular superoxide dismutase (SOD3) degradation thereby increasing $O_2\cdot$ dismutation to hydrogen peroxide (H_2O_2). This decreases the availability of $O_2\cdot$, preventing its harmful interaction with nitric oxide (NO) (49).

Pro-oxidant effects of urate include an ability to generate aminocarbonyl radicals that are capable of amplifying the oxidation of liposomes and low-density lipoprotein (LDL) cholesterol (50,51). These pro-oxidant effects appear to be more pronounced in the setting of relative deficiency of other water-soluble antioxidants, such as ascorbic acid (52–54).

Various studies indicate that urate may have direct harmful effects on endothelium and on vascular smooth muscle cells (55,56). Data from experimental animal models also suggest that mild elevations in serum urate levels can contribute to the development of hypertension, vascular disease, and renal disease progression (5,55,57–60).

URATE MAY BE A USEFUL BIOMARKER

The reluctance to treat asymptomatic hyperuricemia stems partly from the view that it is simply associated with other disease processes and is of otherwise little significance (61,62). Cumulative evidence, however, suggests that hyperuricemia may either in itself be harmful, or that it can act as a "biomarker," which may be somehow targeted to allow fine tuning of other disease-modifying treatments (1,63,64). The "biomarker" effect of hyperuricemia is strongly suggested in studies which demonstrated that serum urate levels (divided into quartiles) provide useful prognostic information in subjects with heart failure (43).

When combined with a very comprehensive seven-parameter heart failure severity score, uric acid levels independently and powerfully predicted cardiovascular outcome.

Strong indirect evidence for harmful cardiovascular effects linked to elevated serum urate levels comes from the LIFE study. Data from this study indicate that the beneficial effect of losartan (which has uricosuric effects) over atenolol in terms of cardiovascular outcome was partly related to lower urate levels in the losartan group (63). Interestingly, a preceding reanalysis of the Systolic Hypertension in the Elderly Program (SHEP trial) also found that urate levels helped determine outcome independent of other parameters such as blood pressure (65). In these studies, patients treated successfully for hypertension with diuretics, who also had an increase in serum urate levels to greater than 10.0 mg/dL (600 μmol/L) while on treatment, failed to show any benefit in cardiovascular event rates when compared to placebo.

Despite suggestive data, there are very few studies directly looking at the effect of treating asymptomatic hyperuricemia in humans. Of note are recent findings in adolescents with essential hypertension, indicating that mild hyperuricemia is surprisingly common (64,66). Lowering urate levels with allopurinol improved blood pressure control in these individuals, strongly supporting a direct role for the urate metabolic pathway in the pathogenesis of essential hypertension. Similar studies will be required in hypertensive adults and in subjects with ischemic heart disease, cardiac failure, and cerebrovascular disease.

URATE AND ENDOTHELIAL DYSFUNCTION

Cardiovascular disease is commonly associated with endothelial dysfunction, oxidant generation, and a pro-inflammatory state (37). Oxidants generated via xanthine oxidase can potentially cause endothelial dysfunction through effects on NO synthesis and availability. Xanthine oxidase also produces urate, which may explain why hyperuricemia, oxidant generation, and endothelial dysfunction are all associated.

The exact role of urate in this setting has been a matter of debate. Some view urate as being protective due to the anti-oxidant effects described above (4). Various studies, however, suggest that urate may have directly harmful effects. While the oxidants produced (superoxide) in the generation of urate by xanthine oxidase could be harmful to the vasculature, there is also suggestive evidence that urate itself can have direct adverse effects unrelated to this (57,58,67).

The effect of allopurinol does not allow this issue to be resolved as it blocks xanthine oxidase-mediated generation of both urate and oxidants. Thus, the beneficial effects of allopurinol have usually been attributed to "anti-oxidant" properties rather than to any effect on urate levels per se. These beneficial effects include a reduction in cardiovascular complications following coronary artery bypass, and in patients with dilated cardiomyopathy (68–70). Allopurinol has also been found to correct impaired NO production in patients with hypertension, diabetes, and heart failure (67,71,72). Of course, allopurinol also lowers urate levels, and in some studies, the degree of lowering correlated very strongly with the improvement in endothelial function (67). Allantoin levels, a measure of oxygen free radical generation, did not correlate with these improvements or with the degree of lowering of serum uric acid levels, suggesting a direct role for urate itself. Similarly, in the animal studies, urate seems to have been the important factor leading to decreased NO production, vascular changes in the kidney, and hypertension (57,58).

Despite the studies mentioned above, very recent work does not support a direct role for urate in causing endothelial dysfunction (73). Urate infused into the forearms of resting healthy human subjects had no effect and was not associated with impaired acetylcholine-induced vasodilation or altered endothelial NO release. Subjects with pre-existing increased oxidative stress (i.e., heart failure or vascular disease) were not examined. This may be relevant because urate may have different effects in this setting. Certainly there is evidence that urate has different biochemical effects in different cellular environments. In addition to the increased pro-oxidant activity of urate when ascorbate is low (52), there is also evidence that bicarbonate concentrations can greatly influence the effect of urate on peroxynitrite-mediated nitration reactions (74).

EFFECTS OF URATE ON VASCULAR SMOOTH MUSCLE

Soluble urate has been shown to induce vascular smooth muscle cell proliferation in vitro via a pathway involving increased platelet-derived growth factor-A (PDGF-A) expression (75). Other studies have confirmed this and also show that urate-induced vascular smooth muscle cell proliferation is mediated by the activation or induction of extracellular signal-regulated kinase (ERK), mitogen-activated protein kinases (MAPK), and cyclooxygenase-2 (COX-2) (5,55). These various pro-inflammatory effects appear to require entry of urate via an organic anion transporter (OAT) expressed by the vascular smooth muscle cell (Fig. 2) (1). Drugs such as probenecid and benzbromarone interfere with entry of the urate into vascular smooth muscle cells.

Adding further to this pathway and to the potential harmful vascular effects, physiologic concentrations of crystal-free urate have been found to increase vascular smooth muscle cell expression of the chemokine monocyte chemoattractant protein-1 (MCP-1) in vitro (56). Various nuclear transcription factors, COX-2, MAP kinases, and redox alterations were all associated with this effect. Of note, MCP-1 has been implicated in several studies as a major contributor to the process of atherogenesis (76–80), raising the possibility that asymptomatic hyperuricemia could influence vascular disease through this pro-inflammatory pathway.

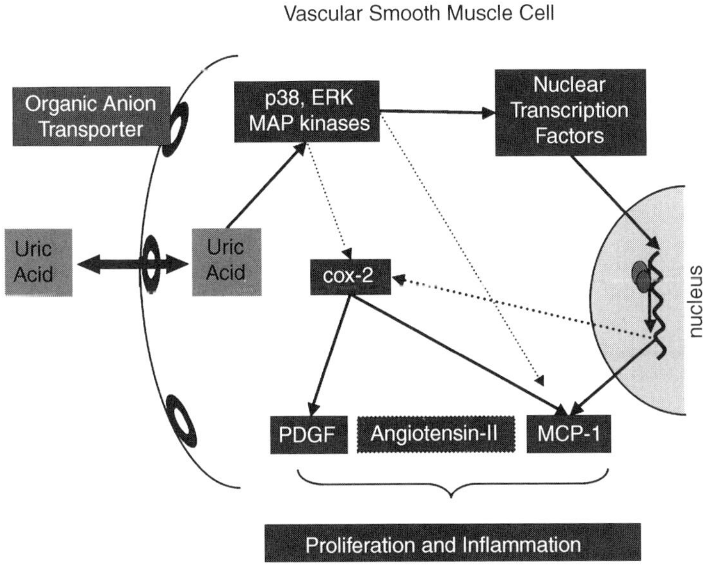

Figure 2 Urate-mediated pro-inflammatory and proliferative effects on vascular smooth muscle cells. Urate enters vascular smooth muscle cells via an anion exchanger/transporter where it appears to alter intracellular redox, activate mitogen activated protein kinases (ERK1/2 and p38 MAPK), increase cyclooxygenase-2 (COX-2) expression, and activate nuclear transcription factors (1,55,56). Downstream of these pathways there is a resulting increase in the production of platelet-derived growth factor (PDGF) and monocyte chemoattractant protein-1 (MCP-1). Studies have also demonstrated a role for the renin–angiotensin system and angiotensin II.

ANIMAL MODELS OF HYPERURICEMIA

Additional evidence suggesting that urate is a mediator of endothelial dysfunction, vascular disease, and inflammation is derived from various animal experiments (5,55,57–59,81). Animal models with increased serum urate levels (increased above the normal level for the animal, but below the physiochemical saturation level of 6.8 mg/dL) have been generated by feeding rats the uricase inhibitor oxonic acid (Fig. 3). Intrarenal vascular disease and salt-sensitive hypertension, in the absence of intrarenal urate crystal deposition, have been observed in these models (5,55,57–59).

In these models, activation of the renin-angiotensin system is evident, as is mild inflammation, and there is an associated decrease in NO synthase expression (57,58). Lowering serum urate levels with allopurinol or benziodarone reverses these findings, as does treatment with an angiotensin converting enzyme inhibitor (57,58). In contrast, treatment with a thiazide diuretic lowers blood pressure but does not improve urate levels or reverse the intrarenal vascular changes (57,58).

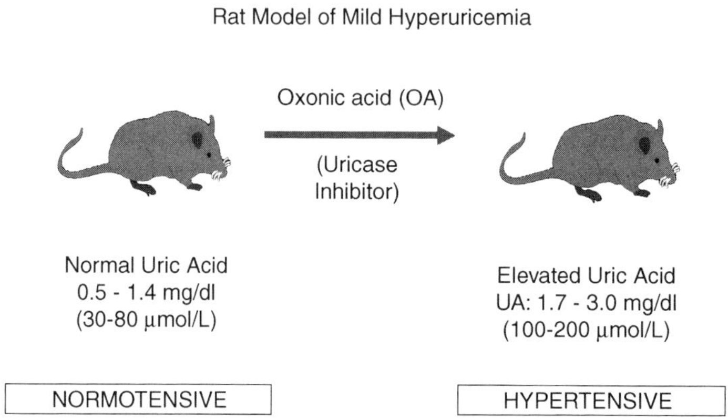

Figure 3 Rat model of mild hyperuricemia associated with hypertension. Sprague-Dawley rats that are fed oxonic acid (a uricase inhibitor) develop mild hyperuricemia and hypertension (57). A characteristic intrarenal vascular lesion develops (afferent arteriolopathy), which is associated with salt sensitive hypertension (5).

Also of note, in a cyclosporine toxicity model, mild hyperuricaemia exacerbated the nephrotoxicity (59), whereas in a hyperuricemic remnant kidney model, lowering the serum urate was markedly renoprotective (55).

SHOULD ASYMPTOMATIC HYPERURICEMIA BE TREATED?

Recent pilot studies in adolescent hypertensive children with otherwise asymptomatic hyperuricemia suggest a beneficial effect of allopurinol on the control of blood pressure (64,66). There is also evidence from various epidemiological, animal, and in vitro studies that lowering serum urate levels in subjects with increased cardiovascular disease risk, cardiac failure, established vascular disease, or known renal disease may be of some benefit. Regardless of these possibilities, it is apparent that serum urate levels serve as a powerful "biomarker" or independent predictor of prognosis and outcome in renal, cardiovascular, and cerebrovascular diseases. Whether these outcomes can be improved by specifically treating the hyperuricemia remains inadequately resolved and controversial.

For these reasons, the longstanding view that hyperuricemia should not be treated unless associated with gout or kidney stones remains the current recommendation (16). It is hoped that well-designed clinical studies will help resolve this issue in the future and clarify what the approach should be in various situations associated with asymptomatic hyperuricemia. These studies will need to determine both the impact on disease outcome of specific treatment aimed at lowering urate levels, as well as the value of using urate as a "biomarker" to help guide other disease-modifying therapies.

FURTHER READING

Berger L, Yu TF. Renal function in gout. IV. An analysis of 524subjects including long-term follow-up. Am J Med 1975; 59:605–613.

Hall APL. Correlations among hyperuricemia, hypercholesterolemia, coronary artery disease and hypertension. Arthritis Rheum 1965; 8:846–852.

Myers A, Epsstein FH, Dodge JH, et al. The relationship of serum uric acid to risk factors in coronary heart disease. Am J Med 1968; 45:520–528.

REFERENCES

1. Johnson RJ, Kang DH, Feig D, et al. Is there a pathogenetic role for uric acid in hypertension and cardiovascular and renal disease? Hypertension 2003; 41:1183–1190.
2. Wu XW, Muzny DM, Lee CC, Caskey CT. Two independent mutational events in the loss of urate oxidase during hominoid evolution. J Mol Evol 1992; 34:78–84.
3. Lagendijk J, Ubbink JB, Vermaak WJ. The determination of allantoin, a possible indicator of oxidant status, in human plasma. J Chromatogr Sci 1995; 33:186–193.
4. Ames BN, Cathcart R, Schwiers E, Hochstein P. Uric acid provides an antioxidant defense in humans against oxidant- and radical-caused aging and cancer: a hypothesis. Proc Natl Acad Sci USA 1981; 78:6858–6862.
5. Watanabe S, Kang DH, Feng L, et al. Uric Acid, hominoid evolution, and the pathogenesis of salt-sensitivity. Hypertension 2002; 40:355–360.
6. Nicholls A, Snaith ML, Scott JT. Effect of oestrogen therapy on plasma and urinary levels of uric acid. BMJ 1973; 1:449–451.
7. Mikkelsen WM, Dodge HJ, Valkenburg H. The distribution of serum uric acid values in a population unselected as to gout or hyperuricemia: Tecumseh, Michigan 1959–1960. Am J Med 1965; 39:242–251.
8. Seegmiller JE. The acute attack of gouty arthritis. Arthritis Rheum 1965; 8:714–725.
9. Goldfinger S, Klinenberg JR, Seegmiller JE. The renal excretion of oxypurines. J Clin Invest 1965; 44:623–628.
10. Sperling O, De Vries A, Kedem O. Studies on the etiology of uric acid lithiasis. IV. Urinary non-dialyzable substances in idiopathic uric acid lithiasis. J Urol 1965; 94:286–292.
11. Maclachlan MJ, Rodnan GP. Effect of food, fast and alcohol on serum uric acid and acute attacks of gout. Am J Med 1967; 42:38–57.
12. Abbott RD, Brand FN, Kannel WB, Castelli WP. Gout and coronary heart disease: the Framingham Study. J Clin Epidemiol 1988; 41:237–242.
13. Gresser U, Gathof B, Zollner N. Uric acid levels in southern Germany in 1989. A comparison with studies from 1962, 1971, and 1984. Klin Wochenschr 1990; 68:1222–1228.

14. Pascual E, Pedraz T. Gout. Curr Opin Rheumatol 2004; 16:282–286.
15. Johnson RJ, Rideout BA. Uric acid and diet—insights into the epidemic of cardiovascular disease. N Engl J Med 2004; 350:1071–1073.
16. Duffy WB, Senekjian HO, Knight TF, Weinman EJ. Management of asymptomatic hyperuricemia. JAMA 1981; 246:2215–2216.
17. Zalokar J, Lellouch J, Claude JR, Kuntz D. Serum uric acid in 23,923 men and gout in a subsample of 4257 men in France. J Chronic Dis 1972; 25:305–312.
18. Hall AP, Barry PE, Dawber TR, McNamara PM. Epidemiology of gout and hyperuricemia. A long-term population study. Am J Med 1967; 42:27–37.
19. Yu T, Gutman AB. Uric acid nephrolithiasis in gout. Predisposing factors. Ann Intern Med 1967; 67:1133–1148.
20. Berger L, Yu TF. Renal function in gout. IV. An analysis of 524 gouty subjects including long-term follow-up studies. Am J Med 1975; 59:605–613.
21. Fessel WJ, Siegelaub AB, Johnson ES. Correlates and consequences of asymptomatic hyperuricemia. Arch Intern Med 1973; 132:44–54.
22. Johnson RJ, Kivlighn SD, Kim YG, Suga S, Fogo AB. Reappraisal of the pathogenesis and consequences of hyperuricemia in hypertension, cardiovascular disease, and renal disease. Am J Kidney Dis 1999; 33:225–234.
23. Ramsay LE. Hyperuricaemia in hypertension: role of alcohol. BMJ 1979; 1:653–654.
24. Steele TH, Oppenheimer S. Factors affecting urate excretion following diuretic administration in man. Am J Med 1969; 47:564–574.
25. Lee J, Sparrow D, Vokonas PS, Landsberg L, Weiss ST. Uric acid and coronary heart disease risk: evidence for a role of uric acid in the obesity-insulin resistance syndrome. The Normative Aging Study. Am J Epidemiol 1995; 142:288–294.
26. Cappuccio FP, Iacone R, Strazzullo P. Serum uric acid and proximal sodium excretion: an independent association in man (the Olivetti Study). J Hypertens Suppl 1991; 9:S280–S281.
27. Cannon PJ, Stason WB, Demartini FE, Sommers SC, Laragh JH. Hyperuricemia in primary and renal hypertension. N Engl J Med 1966; 275:457–464.
28. Messerli FH, Frohlich ED, Dreslinski GR, Suarez DH, Aristimuno GG. Serum uric acid in essential hypertension: an indicator of renal vascular involvement. Ann Intern Med 1980; 93:817–821.
29. Davies PM, Simmonds HA, Singer B, et al. Plasma uridine as well as uric acid is elevated following fructose loading. Adv Exp Med Biol 1998; 431:31–35.
30. Sorensen LB. Role of the intestinal tract in the elimination of uric acid. Arthritis Rheum 1965; 8:694–706.
31. Enomoto A, Kimura H, Chairoungdua A, et al. Molecular identification of a renal urate anion exchanger that regulates blood urate levels. Nature 2002; 417:447–452.
32. Leal-Pinto E, Cohen BE, Abramson RG. Functional analysis and molecular modeling of a cloned urate transporter/channel. J Membr Biol 1999; 169:13–27.
33. Roch-Ramel F, Guisan B, Diezi J. Effects of uricosuric and antiuricosuric agents on urate transport in human brush-border membrane vesicles. J Pharmacol Exp Ther 1997; 280:839–845.
34. Moriarity JT, Folsom AR, Iribarren C, Nieto FJ, Rosamond WD. Serum uric acid and risk of coronary heart disease: atherosclerosis risk in communities (ARIC) study. Ann Epidemiol 2000; 10:136–143.

35. Brand FN, McGee DL, Kannel WB, Stokes J, 3rd, Castelli WP. Hyperuricemia as a risk factor of coronary heart disease: The Framingham study. Am J Epidemiol 1985; 121:11–18.
36. Ferris TF, Gorden P. Effect of angiotensin and norepinephrine upon urate clearance in man. Am J Med 1968; 44:359–365.
37. Many A, Hubel CA, Roberts JM. Hyperuricemia and xanthine oxidase in preeclampsia, revisited. Am J Obstet Gynecol 1996; 174:288–291.
38. Leyva F, Anker S, Swan JW, et al. Serum uric acid as an index of impaired oxidative metabolism in chronic heart failure. Eur Heart J 1997; 18:858–865.
39. Nishijo M, Nakagawa H, Morikawa Y, Miura K, Tabata M, Ishizaki M. Microalbuminuria and hypertension in nondiabetic Japanese men. Am J Hypertens 1999; 12:16–20.
40. Sanchez-Fructuoso AI, Torralbo A, Arroyo M, et al. Occult lead intoxication as a cause of hypertension and renal failure. Nephrol Dial Transplant 1996; 11:1775–1780.
41. Jossa F, Farinaro E, Panico S, et al. Serum uric acid and hypertension: the Olivetti heart study. J Hum Hypertens 1994; 8:677–681.
42. Verdecchia P, Schillaci G, Reboldi G, Santeusanio F, Porcellati C, Brunetti P. Relation between serum uric acid and risk of cardiovascular disease in essential hypertension. The PIUMA study. Hypertension 2000; 36:1072–1078.
43. Anker SD, Doehner W, Rauchhaus M, et al. Uric acid and survival in chronic heart failure: validation and application in metabolic, functional, and hemodynamic staging. Circulation 2003; 107:1991–1997.
44. Weir CJ, Muir SW, Walters MR, Lees KR. Serum urate as an independent predictor of poor outcome and future vascular events after acute stroke. Stroke 2003; 34:1951–1956.
45. Syrjanen J, Mustonen J, Pasternack A. Hypertriglyceridaemia and hyperuricaemia are risk factors for progression of IgA nephropathy. Nephrol Dial Transplant 2000; 15:34–42.
46. Ohno I, Hosoya T, Gomi H, Ichida K, Okabe H, Hikita M. Serum uric acid and renal prognosis in patients with IgA nephropathy. Nephron 2001; 87:333–339.
47. Iseki K, Oshiro S, Tozawa M, Iseki C, Ikemiya Y, Takishita S. Significance of hyperuricemia on the early detection of renal failure in a cohort of screened subjects. Hypertens Res 2001; 24:691–697.
48. Squadrito GL, Cueto R, Splenser AE, et al. Reaction of uric acid with peroxynitrite and implications for the mechanism of neuroprotection by uric acid. Arch Biochem Biophys 2000; 376:333–337.
49. Hicks M, Wong LS, Day RO. Identification of products from oxidation of uric acid induced by hydroxyl radicals. Free Radic Res Commun 1993; 18:337–351.
50. Maples KR, Mason RP. Free radical metabolite of uric acid. J Biol Chem 1988; 263:1709–1712.
51. Santos CX, Anjos EI, Augusto O. Uric acid oxidation by peroxynitrite: multiple reactions, free radical formation, and amplification of lipid oxidation. Arch Biochem Biophys 1999; 372:285–294.
52. Abuja PM. Ascorbate prevents prooxidant effects of urate in oxidation of human low density lipoprotein. FEBS Lett 1999; 446:305–308.
53. Bagnati M, Perugini C, Cau C, Bordone R, Albano E, Bellomo G. When and why a water-soluble antioxidant becomes pro-oxidant during copper-induced low-density lipoprotein oxidation: a study using uric acid. Biochem J 1999; 340:143–152.

54. Patterson RA, Horsley ET, Leake DS. Prooxidant and antioxidant properties of human serum ultrafiltrates toward LDL: important role of uric acid. J Lipid Res 2003; 44:512–521.
55. Kang DH, Nakagawa T, Feng L, et al. A role for uric acid in the progression of renal disease. J Am Soc Nephrol 2002; 13:2888–2897.
56. Kanellis J, Watanabe S, Li JH, et al. Uric acid stimulates monocyte chemoattractant protein-1 production in vascular smooth muscle cells via mitogen-activated protein kinase and cyclooxygenase-2. Hypertension 2003; 41:1287–1293.
57. Mazzali M, Hughes J, Kim YG, et al. Elevated uric acid increases blood pressure in the rat by a novel crystal-independent mechanism. Hypertension 2001; 38:1101–1106.
58. Mazzali M, Kanellis J, Han L, et al. Hyperuricemia induces a primary renal arteriolopathy in rats by a blood pressure-independent mechanism. Am J Physiol Renal Physiol 2002; 282:F991–F997.
59. Mazzali M, Kim YG, Suga S, et al. Hyperuricemia exacerbates chronic cyclosporine nephropathy. Transplantation 2001; 71:900–905.
60. Nakagawa T, Mazzali M, Kang DH, et al. Hyperuricemia causes glomerular hypertrophy in the rat. Am J Nephrol 2002; 23:2–7.
61. Culleton BF, Larson MG, Kannel WB, Levy D. Serum uric acid and risk for cardiovascular disease and death: the Framingham heart study. Ann Intern Med 1999; 131:7–13.
62. Alderman MH. Serum uric acid as a cardiovascular risk factor for heart disease. Curr Hypertens Rep 2001; 3:184–189.
63. Hoieggen A, Alderman MH, Kjeldsen SE, et al. The impact of serum uric acid on cardiovascular outcomes in the LIFE study. Kidney Int 2004; 65:1041–1049.
64. Feig DI, Nakagawa T, Karumanchi SA, et al. Hypothesis: uric acid, nephron number, and the pathogenesis of essential hypertension. Kidney Int 2004; 66:281–287.
65. Franse LV, Pahor M, Di Bari M, et al. Serum uric acid, diuretic treatment and risk of cardiovascular events in the systolic hypertension in the elderly program (SHEP). J Hypertens 2000; 18:1149–1154.
66. Feig DI, Johnson RJ. Hyperuricemia in childhood primary hypertension. Hypertension 2003; 42:247–252.
67. Doehner W, Schoene N, Rauchhaus M, et al. Effects of xanthine oxidase inhibition with allopurinol on endothelial function and peripheral blood flow in hyperuricemic patients with chronic heart failure: results from 2 placebo-controlled studies. Circulation 2002; 105:2619–2624.
68. Cappola TP, Kass DA, Nelson GS, et al. Allopurinol improves myocardial efficiency in patients with idiopathic dilated cardiomyopathy. Circulation 2001; 104:2407–2411.
69. Coghlan JG, Flitter WD, Clutton SM, et al. Allopurinol pretreatment improves postoperative recovery and reduces lipid peroxidation in patients undergoing coronary artery bypass grafting. J Thorac Cardiovasc Surg 1994; 107:248–256.
70. Johnson WD, Kayser KL, Brenowitz JB, Saedi SF. A randomized controlled trial of allopurinol in coronary bypass surgery. Am Heart J 1991; 121:20–24.
71. Butler R, Morris AD, Belch JJ, Hill A, Struthers AD. Allopurinol normalizes endothelial dysfunction in type 2 diabetics with mild hypertension. Hypertension 2000; 35:746–751.

72. Farquharson CA, Butler R, Hill A, Belch JJ, Struthers AD. Allopurinol improves endothelial dysfunction in chronic heart failure. Circulation 2002; 106:221–226.
73. Waring WS, Adwani SH, Breukels O, Webb DJ, Maxwell SR. Hyperuricaemia does not impair cardiovascular function in healthy adults. Heart 2004; 90:155–159.
74. Whiteman M, Ketsawatsakul U, Halliwell B. A reassessment of the peroxynitrite scavenging activity of uric acid. Ann N Y Acad Sci 2002; 962:242–259.
75. Rao GN, Corson MA, Berk BC. Uric acid stimulates vascular smooth muscle cell proliferation by increasing platelet-derived growth factor A-chain expression. J Biol Chem 1991; 266:8604–8608.
76. Nelken NA, Coughlin SR, Gordon D, Wilcox JN. Monocyte chemoattractant protein-1 in human atheromatous plaques. J Clin Invest 1991; 88:1121–1127.
77. Reape TJ, Groot PH. Chemokines and atherosclerosis. Atherosclerosis 1999; 147:213–225.
78. Boring L, Gosling J, Cleary M, Charo IF. Decreased lesion formation in CCR2-/- mice reveals a role for chemokines in the initiation of atherosclerosis. Nature 1998; 394:894–897.
79. Furukawa Y, Matsumori A, Ohashi N, et al. Anti-monocyte chemoattractant protein-1/monocyte chemotactic and activating factor antibody inhibits neointimal hyperplasia in injured rat carotid arteries. Circ Res 1999; 84:306–314.
80. Yla-Herttuala S, Lipton BA, Rosenfeld ME, et al. Expression of monocyte chemoattractant protein 1 in macrophage-rich areas of human and rabbit atherosclerotic lesions. Proc Natl Acad Sci USA 1991; 88:5252–5256.
81. Sanchez-Lozada LG, Tapia E, Avila-Casado C, et al. Mild hyperuricemia induces glomerular hypertension in normal rats. Am J Physiol Renal Physiol 2002; 283:F1105–F1110.

6

Pseudogout: Presentation, Natural History, and Associated Conditions

Ann K. Rosenthal
Division of Rheumatology, Department of Medicine, Medical College of Wisconsin, Milwaukee, Wisconsin, U.S.A.

INTRODUCTION

Arthritis associated with articular calcium pyrophosphate dihydrate (CPPD) crystals was first described in the early 1960s with the discovery of uricase-resistant crystals in patients with an acute gout-like arthritis (1). Simultaneous studies describing an unusual form of familial oligoarticular arthritis associated with articular calcium crystals rapidly confirmed the clinical importance of this finding (2). The careful work of these astute physician-scientists led to the description of a whole new disease, now commonly called CPPD crystal deposition disease. Subsequent work showed that CPPD crystals were found in a variety of clinical settings and were not exclusive to patients with an acute monoarticular arthritis. Studies demonstrating the inflammatory nature of these crystals and their destructive effects on articular tissues provided further support for their clinical importance (3).

Forty years after its initial clinical description, CPPD deposition disease remains an underdiagnosed and incompletely understood entity. The heterogeneity of the clinical presentations of CPPD deposition disease as well as the propensity of this arthritis to mimic other conditions is partly responsible for this phenomenon. In addition, the ability of the average clinical laboratory to identify CPPD crystals in articular fluids and tissues is often lacking (4,5). Careful clinical studies of CPPD deposition disease lag far behind the sophisticated laboratory studies currently used to approach disease pathogenesis. Yet a review of what is known about the clinical presentation, natural history, and conditions associated with CPPD deposition may help direct future work on this disease.

EPIDEMIOLOGY

The incidence and prevalence rates of CPPD deposition are currently unknown. Cited prevalence rates of 0.9 per 1000 for clinical CPPD deposition disease are based on data from retrospective single-center hospital-based studies and may significantly underestimate the true prevalence (6). Most population-based studies of CPPD crystal deposition rely on radiographic or autopsy diagnoses and do not consider clinically significant joint disease (7). These studies reveal prevalence rates between 6% and 34%. Many studies use radiographic chondrocalcinosis to identify articular CPPD crystals. Chondrocalcinosis is defined as a finely stippled calcification most typically seen in the articular or fibrocartilage of the knee, the triangular cartilage of the wrist, or the pubic symphysis (Fig. 1). The frequency of radiographic chondrocalcinosis in population-based studies varies from 10% to 27% (7,8). The prevalence of pathologic chondrocalcinosis in patients over sixty years of age is about 20% at autopsy (9).

Aging is the major epidemiologic risk factor for CPPD deposition disease. Rates of radiographic and clinical CPPD disease dramatically increase with age.

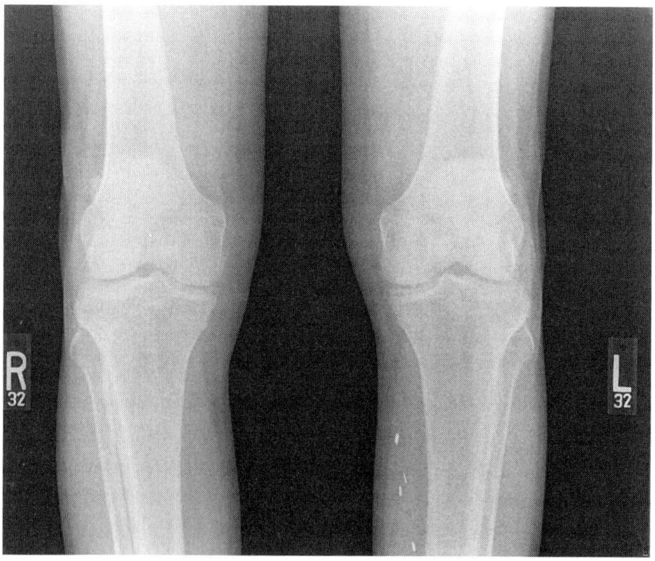

Figure 1 Chondrocalcinosis of the knee joints: abundant chondrocalcinosis of the articular hyaline and fibrocartilage is visible in the joint space in this patient.

CPPD deposition disease is rare under the age of 60. For example, one study demonstrated a 7% prevalence of radiographic chondrocalcinosis in subjects aged 60 to 69 years. Rates rose to 43% in subjects over the age of 80 years (7).

The literature is unclear whether more women (6,7,10–12) or more men (6,13) have clinically apparent CPPD deposition. The pattern of disease, however, may, influenced by sex. Acute pseudogout may be more common in men, while a polyarticular presentation is more common in women (13).

Racial and ethnic predilections for CPPD deposition disease are not well understood. Several small studies suggest an increased prevalence in one ethnic group (8,14). However, in general, differences in susceptibility among various racial groups have not been proven.

CLINICAL PRESENTATION

Overview

Although initially described in the setting of an acute monoarthritis clinically indistinguishable from gout, articular CPPD crystals are associated with variable clinical presentations (1). At least five clinical presentations have subsequently been associated with articular CPPD crystals (Table 1) (10). In addition, CPPD crystals are recognized in other situations as well. For example, crowned dens syndrome and tophaceous CPPD crystal deposits presenting as nerve compression syndromes are rare, but clinically well described (15,16).

The frequency of various clinical patterns of CPPD deposition remains poorly studied. It has been suggested that 50% of patients with CPPD deposition disease presented with a pseudo-osteoarthritis–like picture (10). These patients display a chronic degenerative type of arthritis, affecting joints not typically involved in primary osteoarthritis and with or without superimposed acute inflammatory attacks. Approximately a quarter of patients have an oligo- or mono-articular inflammatory presentation consistent with pseudogout. Others present with less common patterns including a polyarticular inflammatory arthritis similar to rheumatoid arthritis in about 5%. A neuropathic joint-like pattern is seen considerably less frequently. The frequency of asymptomatic (lanthanic) articular CPPD crystals remains unstudied, but is probably the most

Table 1 Clinical Presentations of Calcium Pyrophosphate Dihydrate Crystal Deposition

Acute monoarticular arthritis (pseudogout or pseudoseptic arthritis)
Polyarticular noninflammatory arthritis (pseudo-osteoarthritis with or without acute inflammatory flares)
Polyarticular inflammatory arthritis (pseudo-rheumatoid arthritis)
Neuropathic-like joint destruction (pseudo-Charcot joint)
Lanthanic (asymptomatic)

prevalent form. A recent case collection of 50 patients from Portugal showed a similar distribution of clinical presentations. Fifty-eight percent of these patients had an osteoarthritis-like picture, while 16% had monarticular arthritis, and 8% had a pseudo- rheumatoid presentation (17).

Pseudogout

CPPD crystals were originally described in patients with acute monoarticular arthritis clinically indistinguishable from gout. This remains perhaps the most widely clinically recognized presentation of CPPD crystals. Patients with acute pseudogout typically present with sudden onset of symptoms usually affecting a single joint. In many cases, several joints are involved (12). Like gout, pseudogout is an inflammatory process manifest by joint effusions and signs and symptoms of articular inflammation. Patients typically experience pain, stiffness, and swelling in the affected joint. Signs include swelling with variable erythema and warmth. Compared to true gout, pseudogout attacks may take longer to reach peak intensity, and are often considerably longer lasting than gout attacks. Symptoms can last 3 to 120 days despite therapy (12). Lightening or fleeting attacks with brief episodes of pain have been described in affected joints, as have been described in gout (10). Pseudogout is more common in large than in small joints. The knee is the most commonly involved joint, followed by the wrist, ankle, elbow, toe, shoulder, and hip (12).

Pseudo-Osteoarthritis

Most patients with clinically apparent CPPD crystal deposition have an unusually severe, oddly distributed, degenerative arthritis resembling osteoarthritis. They present with the gradual onset of joint pain and stiffness, typically involving knees, shoulders, wrists, spine, elbows, and ankles. Involvement is usually asymmetric. Half of these patients will have acute attacks superimposed on their chronic symptoms, and half do not describe any such attacks (10). Symptoms are rarely self-limiting. The natural history of polyarticular CPPD crystal deposition is not well described. However, joint involvement is often severe and aggressive compared to typical osteoarthritis (18).

This type of presentation can be difficult to differentiate from osteoarthritis and consequently may be significantly under-recognized. In one series, 30% of patients diagnosed with osteoarthritis had CPPD crystals in their affected joints at the time of knee replacement (19). Although radiographic findings, including chondrocalcinosis, may support a diagnosis of CPPD deposition disease, synovial analysis remains necessary to confirm the diagnosis.

Pseudo-Rheumatoid Arthritis

In a minority of patients, CPPD deposition disease presents as a chronic, polyarticular inflammatory arthritis. These patients experience subacute attacks of inflammation which last from one to several months. Involvement of both small and large joints is common. A generally symmetric pattern may be observed. Although onset is often subacute, an acute presentation can occur. In the elderly, this acute polyarticular presentation can be quite dramatic, presenting with fever, chills, and mental status changes. Often systemic infection is suspected (20). Elevated levels of circulating interleukin-6, a potent pyrogen, may be responsible for the systemic manifestations in these patients (21). These attacks can be self-limited. The natural history of disease in patients with this type of presentation is not well described.

The polyarticular inflammatory form of CPPD deposition disease can easily be confused with true rheumatoid arthritis. Further confusion may result from the observation that about 10% of patients with articular CPPD crystals have a positive rheumatoid factor (22). Thus, differentiating between CPPD deposition disease and rheumatoid arthritis can be particularly challenging. By chance alone, 1% of patients with CPPD deposition disease would have rheumatoid arthritis. Patients with primary CPPD deposition have joint inflammation in multiple joints, but episodes tend not to begin and end simultaneously. This contrasts with the symmetric polyarticular episodes typical of rheumatoid arthritis. Beyond finding CPPD crystals in affected joints, radiographic clues such as abundant osteophytes, bony sclerosis, and of course, chondrocalcinosis, all support a diagnosis of primary CPPD crystal deposition. The absence of osteopenia and classic erosions also make a diagnosis of rheumatoid arthritis less likely.

Pseudo-Neuropathic Joint

Some patients with CPPD deposition disease have a severe destructive monarthritis similar to that seen in neuropathic joints. This is perhaps the most controversial of the clinical presentations of CPPD crystal deposition. It was originally described by McCarty and Hoskins in a study characterizing radiographic changes in patients with CPPD deposition (23). A case collection of patients with severe monarticular destructive arthropathy followed (24). These patients had no neurologic abnormalities, and yet presented with a painful monoarthritis, associated with dramatic destructive radiographic changes. The distribution of involvement was quite atypical for osteoarthritis. These patients may just represent end-stage pseudogout-like CPPD deposition disease, and may not have a unique entity. The natural history of patients with this type of CPPD deposition disease is not well described.

Lanthanic

There are clearly some people with radiographic or pathologic evidence of articular chondrocalcinosis who have no clinically apparent arthritis. This finding was termed "lanthanic" CPPD deposition by McCarty and is of uncertain significance (10). These patients have not been rigorously studied to see if they develop signs and symptoms of clinical arthritis with a greater frequency than the unaffected population.

Other Presentations

Unlike monosodium urate crystals, CPPD crystals are not commonly found in tissues other than cartilage. Even in synovium, CPPD crystals typically form in areas of chondrometaplasia (25). In rare instances, CPPD crystals occur in the sclera of the eye (26). Deposits near the mandible or clavicles can mimic gouty tophi (27). Because of their ability to erode adjacent bones, they can also be mistaken for neoplastic lesions (28). CPPD crystals in periarticular tissues occur rarely and can present as a nerve compression syndrome, such a carpal or cubital tunnel syndrome (16). Spinal ligaments seem peculiarly prone to CPPD crystal deposition. Affected patients often present with myleopathy (29). Almost one-fourth of patients undergoing decompressive laminectomy for lumbar spinal stenosis had CPPD crystal deposits in their ligamenta flava. Clinically, patients with CPPD crystals had more acute onset of symptoms than those without crystals (30).

DIAGNOSIS

The diagnosis of CPPD deposition disease is most commonly and accurately made by identifying CPPD crystals in the synovial fluids of affected joints using polarizing light microscopy. The identification of CPPD crystals with polarizing light microscopy requires expertise. Clinical laboratories often miss CPPD crystals in clinical specimens (4,5). The weak birefringence of CPPD crystals render them much more difficult to discern than urate crystals. In addition they can also be quite sparse in number and very small in size. Methods for definitive crystal identification, such as X-ray diffraction or Fourier transform infrared spectroscopy, are cumbersome, expensive, and often require extensive specimen preparation (31). These methods are not commonly used in clinical practice. Synovial fluid characteristics can vary from inflammatory to non-inflammatory in CPPD deposition disease and are most useful in ruling out other diagnoses. In pseudogout patients, synovial fluid may be turbid, watery, or hemorrhagic. Average white cell counts are approximately 12,000 cells/mm^3 in pseudogout fluids, but may be in the non-inflammatory range in other clinical presentations (12).

Histologic examination of cartilage or synovial biopsies can also be helpful, as long as the methods used to prepare the specimens preserve crystals (31). The presence of chondrocalcinosis on X-rays is certainly supportive of the diagnosis, but should not be relied on as definitive evidence of CPPD deposition disease. Rarely, chondrocalcinosis is caused by crystals other than CPPD, such as dicalcium phosphate dihydrate. Vascular calcification can also be mistaken for chondrocalcinosis (32). In cases of acute monoarticular arthritis, all patients should undergo arthrocentesis. This is necessary to rule out infection or gout, conditions which are clinically indistinguishable from pseudogout.

Drs. Ryan and McCarty set out diagnostic criteria for CPPD deposition disease (Table 2) (33). In the absence of CPPD crystals in tissue or fluid samples, these criteria rely heavily on clinical presentation, and should be used with caution. For example, the presence of acute or chronic arthritis in joints not typically involved in osteoarthritis may suggest CPPD deposition disease. Unusual radiographic features, such as superior cortical erosions on the patella, large or extensive subchondral cysts, severe radiographic destruction, osteophytes, tendon calcifications (Achilles, triceps, obturator), and axial skeletal involvement, can also be used to identify patients that have possible CPPD arthritis. Although these findings can be suggestive, a definitive diagnosis should only be made when CPPD crystals can be identified in affected joints.

Precipitating Factors

Flares of CPPD deposition disease have been noted in certain clinical settings. These include the post-operative period, the days after parathyroidectomy, the period after a medical illness, and after exposure to certain drugs. Most patients with CPPD deposition disease have no clear precipitating factors.

Postoperative Pseudogout

Pseudogout is well described in the postoperative period. Almost 10% of patients with pseudogout have at least one attack in the postoperative period. These findings are very similar to the statistics with true gout (22). Among hospitalized patients, 23 of the 31 patients with pseudogout had attacks during the post-operative period in one study (6). Although it is unlikely that the type of surgery affects the development of pseudogout, some have noted a high frequency of orthopedic procedures preceding pseudogout attacks (6). This may simply reflect the high frequency of orthopedic surgery in the susceptible population.

Pseudogout After Parathyroidectomy

Attacks of acute pseudogout often occur after parathyroidectomy, presumably related to fluxes of serum calcium levels (6,34). Most reported cases occurred in the setting of iatrogenic post-operative hypoparathyroidism. This observation spawned theories about crystal shedding precipitating inflammation when

Table 2 Proposed Criteria for the Diagnosis of Calcium Pyrophosphate Dihydrate Crystal Deposition Disease

Definite: CPPD crystals are demonstrated in tissues or synovial fluid by definitive means, such as X-ray diffraction, or if crystals compatible with CPPD are demonstrated by compensated light microscopy and typical calcifications are seen on roentgenograms
Probable: Only one of the above criteria is met

Abbreviation: CPPD, calcium pyrophosphate dihydrate.
Source: From Ref. 33.

circulating calcium levels were suddenly lowered (6). This is similar to the way in which sudden changes in serum urate levels could precipitate attacks of true gout. However, pseudogout attacks often continued to occur as calcium levels return to normal. Furthermore, radiographic chondrocalcinosis was not improved by resolution of hypercalcemia (6).

Pseudogout After Medical Illness

Pseudogout can also be precipitated by serious medical illness. Vascular diseases such as cerebrovascular accidents and myocardial infarctions seem particularly common. Because these are such common major illnesses in the elderly population, causation would be difficult to prove.

Drug-Induced Pseudogout

Several case reports suggest the possibility that intra-articular sodium hyaluronate preparations can cause acute attacks of pseudogout (35,36). Pamidronate and GM-CSF have also been reported to precipitate pseudogout flares (37,38).

CLASSIFICATION OF CPPD DEPOSITION DISEASE

McCarty originally divided clinical CPPD disease patients into three catagories, loosely based on etiology (Table 3) (10). These included hereditary (familial) CPPD deposition disease, sporadic (or idiopathic) CPPD deposition disease, and CPPD deposition disease associated with metabolic conditions. Others have proposed similar schema (39). Most cases of CPPD deposition disease are sporadic, and the pathogenesis in these cases remains unknown.

Hereditary CPPD Deposition Disease

The true frequency of familial CPPD deposition disease among CPPD deposition disease cases is difficult to determine. The late onset phenotype of this condition, in combination with its high rate of clinical mimics, renders familial CPPD deposition disease particularly challenging to study (40). Despite this, the literature describes numerous kindreds with multiple family members affected by CPPD deposition disease. Among others, families of French-Canadian, Swedish, English, and Dutch descent have been characterized (40). Most of the reported families display autosomal dominant inheritance with no sex-linkage, but phenotypes can vary widely (32). Some families show evidence of CPPD crystal

Table 3 Etiologic Classification of Calcium Pyrophosphate Dihydrate Crystal Deposition Disease

Sporadic
Hereditary
Associated with another condition

formation which clearly predates the clinical appearance of arthritis (41). Some have associated neurologic findings such as febrile seizures (42). Others have basic calcium phosphate crystals as well as CPPD crystals in affected joints (43). This clinical heterogeneity suggests the presence of a variety of genetic abnormalities in these kindreds. Indeed, several different chromosomal loci have been implicated in familial CPPD deposition disease. The CCAL1 locus on chromosome 8q was the first locus to be described (44). Identification of the CCAL2 locus on chromosome 5p and abnormalities of the type II procollagen gene quickly followed (45). The identity of the involved genes on chromosome 8q remains unknown. However, the 5p locus has recently been reported to be the site of the ANK gene (46). ANKH is a transmembrane protein responsible for transporting inorganic pyrophosphate to the extracellular space (46). Pyrophosphate is the anionic component of CPPD crystals and high extracellular levels promote CPPD crystal formation (47). Mutations in the ANKH gene are felt to alter pyrophosphate metabolism and to favor CPPD crystal formation in some affected families (40). Further discussion of the genetics of CPPD deposition is in Chapter 3 and CPPD biochemistry is in Chapter 13.

Associated Conditions

Articular CPPD crystal deposition is linked to a heterogeneous group of metabolic conditions (Table 4). Some of these associations are well established, but many are poorly supported by clinical data (48). Ideally, for an association to be important, an increased prevalence of severe and premature CPPD deposition disease should occur in affected patients. A plausible explanation as to causality makes a true association even more attractive. Fairly good clinical evidence supports an association of CPPD crystal deposition with aging, osteoarthritis, prior injury, hyperparathyroidism, hemochromatosis, gout, hypophosphatasia, and hypomagnesemia. Rare metabolic conditions, such as ochronosis, Wilson's disease, and acromegaly, may be associated with a higher rate of CPPD deposition, but lack good clinical data to support a true association. Weaker associations exist with common conditions including diabetes and hypothyroidism. Case reports of CPPD deposition in the setting of very rare conditions warrant further study. In general, patients with newly diagnosed CPPD deposition disease should be screened for associated conditions with a serum calcium, magnesium and phosphorus, alkaline phosphatase, ferritin, iron, and total iron binding capacity.

Age

Age is the strongest known risk factor for CPPD deposition disease (9). This disease is rare in patients under the age of 60, and rates double with each decade thereafter (7). Important changes in aging articular cartilage may predispose to CPPD deposition (49). Repeated minor injuries that accumulate with age may also cause damage to cartilage and permit CPPD crystal formation.

Table 4 Conditions Associated with Calcium Pyrophosphate Dihydrate Crystal Deposition Disease

Conditions
Strongly associated
Age
Osteoarthritis
Injury
Gout
Hyperparathyroidism
Hemochromatosis
Hypophosphatasia
Hypomagnesemia
Weakly associated
Hypothyroidism
Not associated
Diabetes
Potentially associated
Wilson's disease
Acromegaly
Hyaluronidase deficiency
X-linked hypophosphatemic rickets
Familial hypocalciuric hypercalcemia
Ochronosis

Osteoarthritis

Osteoarthritis frequently coexists with CPPD crystal deposition, occurring in 40% to 70% of patients (48,50). Osteoarthritis has a complex relationship with CPPD deposition. It remains unclear whether CPPD deposition disease is a clinical variant of osteoarthritis, a marker of severe disease, or a separate entity altogether (51). However, there is good evidence to suggest that radiographic chondrocalcinosis is a risk factor for osteoarthritis (52). A recent population-based study from Nottingham reinforced this association (53). Because CPPD crystals can initiate or perpetuate cartilage damage, it is unlikely that they are innocent bystanders in osteoarthritis (54). Moreover, because CPPD crystals are associated with an uniquely distributed arthritis, they are probably not simply markers of cartilage damaged by osteoarthritis.

Injury

Local joint damage, particularly meniscal injury in the knee, often antedates clinically apparent CPPD deposition disease (55–57). This association is strengthened by the premature appearance of CPPD crystals in these individuals and the localization of the crystals to previously damaged areas. The concept that cartilage damage leads to or permits CPPD crystal formation in otherwise unmineralized cartilage matrix is an attractive one. It links CPPD crystal formation to inflammatory and non-inflammatory conditions causing damage as well as to the repetitive minor injuries that accumulate with age.

Gout

CPPD crystal deposition disease has been linked with both gout and hyperuricemia through small case collections (48). One controlled study confirmed a small but significant increase in the risk for chondrocalcinosis among patients with hyperuricemia and acute arthritis compared to controls (58). It is possible that one type of crystal can serve to nucleate another. Equally plausible, however, is the theory that joint damage from repeated gout attacks can promote CPPD crystal formation.

Hyperparathyroidism

Hyperparathyroidism was one of the first syndromes to be associated with CPPD crystal deposition. This association has withstood the test of time, despite a lack of good studies. It also has the advantage of a plausible causative link, as high calcium levels in hyperparathyroid patients may directly or indirectly participate in CPPD crystal formation. In addition, parathyroid hormone has important effects in cartilage which may facilitate crystal formation (59). Although most data suggesting a connection is in a case report format, a few controlled studies confirm an increase in premature and severe chondrocalcinosis in the setting of hyperparathyroidism (60,61). Importantly, an increased risk for pseudogout was also observed in this population (61). A simple connection between high parathyroid hormone levels or high calcium levels and CPPD crystal deposition disease is refuted by the clinical course of hyperparathyroid patients. They typically continue to have clinical evidence of articular CPPD crystal deposition for years after resolution of their clinical hyperparathyroidism.

Hemochromatosis

Hemochromatosis is another of the better-established metabolic conditions associated with CPPD deposition disease. It is estimated that as many as 50% of patients with hemochromatosis have clinical CPPD deposition disease (62,63). These patients tend to be younger at age of presentation than those with sporadic CPPD disease. Arthritis may be the presenting feature of hemochromatosis (64). Intriguing studies suggested a role for iron in CPPD crystal deposition (65). Recent reports of increased levels of circulating PTH in patients with hemochromatosis support an additional theory of pathogenesis (66). Interestingly, the course of arthritis does not appear to be improved by correcting iron overload with phlebotomy (62).

Hypophophatasia

Hypophosphatasia is a rare group of syndromes resulting from congenital alkaline phosphatase deficiency (67). These have clearly been associated with premature and severe CPPD deposition disease (68). There is also some evidence to suggest an increased prevalence of clinical CPPD deposition disease in heterozygotes with this condition (69). A clear causal connection stems from the ability of alkaline phosphatase to act as a pyrophosphatase and to degrade CPPD crystals (70,71).

Hypomagnesemia

Hypomagnesemia is strongly associated with an increased risk of CPPD crystal deposition (48). In this setting the disease has a premature onset and is severe. Magnesium is a cofactor for many pyrophosphatases (72,73). Therefore, a deficiency of magnesium might limit the activities of these enzymes and result in pyrophosphate accumulation and subsequent CPPD crystal formation. Bartter's syndrome has been associated with chondrocalcinosis (74,75). Recent data suggest that the Gitelman's variant of Barrter's syndrome is the variant most frequently associated with low serum magnesium levels. Most cases of chondrocalcinosis reported in Bartter's syndrome patients likely had the Gittelman's variant (76). Other causes of chronic hypomagnesemia have also been associated with chondrocalcinosis. For example, renal magnesium wasting can occur in familial forms (77,78). In many cases, magnesium supplementation seems to improve the arthritis in patients with hypomagnesemia, but this has not been rigorously studied (79). Diuretic use might predispose to chondrocalcinosis through a shared association with hypomagnesemia (48). Nevertheless, there is little additional evidence that hypomagnesemia contributes significantly to the pathogenesis of sporadic CPPD (80,81).

Hypothyroidism

A link between hypothyroidism and chondrocalcinosis persists in our clinical consciousness despite the lack of good evidence to support a true association between these conditions. For example, three studies looking for an increased rate of chondrocalcinosis in patients with hypothyroidism compared to appropriate controls showed no statistically significant association between chondrocalcinosis and hypothyroidism (82–84). However, when these smaller studies were combined and a meta-analysis done, the relative risk for chondrocalcinosis in hypothyroidism was 1.94 (CI 1.06–9.72) (48). Thus a significant but small link between the two conditions is possible but of uncertain clinical significance. An etiologic connection remains unclear.

Diabetes Mellitus

Diabetes is often cited as a risk factor for CPPD deposition disease. However, there is no evidence suggesting a true association between these common age-related conditions (48).

Wilson's Disease

The association between Wilson's disease and CPPD deposition disease remains speculative. One series of 22 patients found three with radiographic chondrocalcinosis (85). The association is based on case reports which lack even morphologic identification of crystals. Further studies are necessary to confirm any association with this relatively rare condition.

Acromegaly

An association between acromegaly and CPPD deposition disease is often cited, but remains poorly supported. A handful of case reports and case series comment on the presence of chondrocalcinosis in acromegalic patients (86,87). However, only two out of 314 patients had documented chondrocalcinosis in one combined study (48). Whether this is a true association remains unclear.

Other Associated Conditions

There are numerous case reports of CPPD deposition disease occurring in the setting of a variety of rare conditions. These conditions, including hylauronidase deficiency (88), X-linked hypophosphatemic rickets (89), and familial hypocalciuric hypercalcemia (90), are so rare that it is impossible to determine if true associations exist. Pseudogout has been reported in peripheral joints in patients with ochronosis (50). However, other changes in cartilage in ochronotic patients can make chondrocalcinosis difficult to identify, and good evidence for a true association is lacking.

CONCLUSIONS

It has been forty years since the original descriptions of arthritis associated with CPPD crystals. Although we have learned a great deal about the clinical manifestations of these crystals, major clinical questions remain. The heterogeneous clinical presentation of articular CPPD crystals and the multitude of seemingly unrelated metabolic conditions associated with their presence suggest that many factors are involved in their pathogenesis. Additional careful clinical studies of CPPD deposition disease may contribute to the development of specific therapies for this common condition.

REFERENCES

1. McCarty D, Kohn N, Faires J. The significance of calcium pyrophosphate crystals in the synovial fluid of arthritic patients. 1. Clinical aspects. Ann Intern Med 1962; 56:711–737.
2. Zitnan D, Sitaj S. Chondrocalcinosis articularis: section I. Clinical and radiological study. Ann Rheum Dis 1963; 22:142–152.
3. Landis R, Haskard D. Pathogenesis of crystal-induced inflammation. Curr Rheum Rep 2001; 3:36–41.
4. Hasselbacher P. Variation in synovial fluid analysis by hospital laboratories. Arthritis Rheum 1987; 30:637–642.
5. McGill N, York H. Reproducibility of synovial fluid examination for crystals. Aust NZ J Med 1991; 21:710–713.
6. O'Duffy J. Clinical studies of acute pseudogout attacks. Comments on prevalence, predisposition and treatment. Arthritis Rheum 1976; 19:349–352.
7. Sanmarti R, Kanterewicz E, Pladevall M, et al. Analysis of the association between chondrocalcinosis and osteoarthritis: a community based study. Ann Rheum Dis 1996; 55:30–33.
8. Ellman M, Levin B. Chondrocalcinosis in elderly persons. Arthritis Rheum 1975; 18:43–47.
9. Mitrovic D, Stankovic A, Iriarte-Borda O, et al. The prevalence of chondrocalcinosis in the human knee joint. An autopsy survey. J Rheumatol 1988; 15:633–641.
10. McCarty D. Calcium pyrophosphate dihydrate crystal deposition disease-1975. Arthritis Rheum 1975; 19:275–286.
11. Doherty M, Dieppe P. Clinical aspects of calcium pyrophosphate dihydrate crystal deposition. Rheum Dis Clin North Am 1988; 14:395–414.
12. Masuda I, Ishikawa K. Clinical features of pseudogout attack: a survey of 50 cases. Clin Orthop Relat Res 1987; 229:173–181.
13. McCarty DJ. Pseudogout: articular chondrocalcinosis; calcium pyrophosphate crystal deposition disease. In: Hollander J, McCarty D, Jr., eds. Arthritis and Allied Conditions. 8th ed. Philadelphia: Lea and Febiger, 1972:1140–1160.
14. Hamza M, Elleach M, Sellami S, et al. Frequence de la chondrocalcinose articulaire dans deux groupes ethniques. Press Med 1989; 18:493–494.
15. Bouvet J, le Parc J-M, Michalski B, et al. Acute neck pain due to calcification surrounding the odontoid process: the crowned dens syndrome. Arthritis Rheum 1985; 28:1417–1420.
16. Taniguchi Y, Yoshida M, Tamaki T. Cubital tunnel syndrome associated with calcium pyrophosphate dihydrate crystal deposition disease. J Hand Surg 1996; 21A:870–874.
17. Canhao H, Fonseca J, Leandro M, et al. Cross-sectional study of 50 patients with calcium pyrophosphate dihydrate crystal arthropathy. Clin Rheumatol 2001; 20:119–122.
18. Menkes C, Simon F, Delrieu F, et al. Destructive arthropathy in chondrocalcinosis articularis. Arthritis Rheum 1985; 19:329–348.
19. Derfus B, Kurian J, Butler J, et al. The high prevalence of pathologic calcium crystals in pre-operative knees. J Rheumatol 2002; 29:570–574.
20. Bong D, Bennett R. Pseudogout mimicking systemic disease. JAMA 1981; 246:1438–1440.

21. Guerne P, Terkeltaub R, Zuraw B, et al. Inflammatory microcrystals stimulate interleukin-6 production and secretion by human monocytesand synoviocytes. Arthritis Rheum 1989; 32:1443–1452.
22. McCarty DJ. Diagnostic mimicry in arthritis: patterns of joint involvement associated with calcium pyrophosphate dihydrate crystal deposits. Ann Rheum Dis 1975; 25:804–809.
23. McCarty DJ, Haskin M. The roentgenologic aspects of pseudogout (articular chondrocalcinosis). An analysis of 20 cases. Am J Roentgenol 1963; 90:1248–1257.
24. Menkes C, Simon F, Delrieu F, et al. Destructive arthropathy in chondrocalcinosis articularis. Arthritis Rheum 1976; 19:329–348.
25. Beutler A, Rothfuss S, Clayburne G, et al. Calcium pyrophosphate dihydrate crystal deposition in synovium. Arthritis Rheum 1993; 36:704–715.
26. Daiker B. Tophus-like, conglomerated, crystalline calcification of the sclera. Opthalmoligica 1996; 210:223–228.
27. Li-Yu J, Schumacher HR, Gratwick G. Invasive tophaceous pseudogout in temporalmandibular joint: misdiagnosis as tumor. J Clin Rheumatol 2000; 6:272–277.
28. Allen E, Ali S, Erozan Y. Tumoral calcium pyrophosphate dihydrate deposition disease: ctyopathologic findings on fine-needle aspiration. Diagn Cytopathol 1996; 15:349–351.
29. Zunkeler B, Schelper R, Menezes A. Periodontoid calcium pyrophosphate dihydrate deposition disease: “pseudogout” mass lesions of the craniocervical junction. J Neurosurg 1996; 85:803–809.
30. Markiewitz A, Boumphrey F, Bauer T, et al. Calcium pyrophosphate dihydrate crystal deposition disease as a cause of lumbar canal stenosis. Spine 1996; 21:506–511.
31. Rosenthal A, Mandel N. Identification of crystals in synovial fluids and joint tissues. Curr Rheumatol Rep 2001; 3:11–16.
32. Rosenthal A, Ryan L. Calcium pyrophosphate crystal deposition disease, pseudogout, and articular chondrocalcinosis. In: Koopman W, ed. Arthritis and Allied Conditions, Vol. 2. Philadelphia: Williams and Wilkens, 2000:2348–2371.
33. Ryan L, McCarty D. Calcium pyrophosphate crystal deposition disease; pseudogout; articular chondrocalcinosis. In: McCarty D, ed. Arthritis and Allied Conditions. Philadelphia: Lea & Febiger, 1985:1515–1546.
34. Bilezikian J, Aurbach G, Connor T, et al. Pseudogout after parathyroidectomy. Lancet 1973; 1:445–449.
35. Luzar M, Altawil B. Pseudogout following intraarticular injection of sodium hyaluronate. Arthritis Rheum 1998; 41:939–940.
36. Kroesen S, Schmid W, Theiler R. Induction of an acute attack of calcium pyrophosphate dihydrate arthritis by intra-articular injection of Hylan G-F 20 (Synvisc). Clin Rheumatol 2000; 19:147–149.
37. Malnick S, Ariel-Ronen S, Evron E, et al. Acute pseudogout as a complication of pamidronate. Ann Pharmacother 1997; 31:499–500.
38. Sandor V, Hassan R, Kohn E. Exacerbation of pseudogout by granulocyte colony-stimulating factor. Ann Intern Med 1996; 125:781.
39. Agudelo C, Wise C. Crystal-associated arthritis. Clin Geriatr Med 1998; 14:495–513.

40. Williams C. Familial calcium pyrophosphate dihydrate deposition disease and the ANKH gene. Curr Opin Rheumatol 2003; 15:326–331.
41. Bjelle A. Pyrophosphate arthropathy in two Swedish families. Arthritis Rheum 1982; 25:66–74.
42. Hughes A, McGibbon D, Woodward E, et al. Localisation of a gene for chondrocalcinosis to chromosome 5p. Hum Mol Genet 1995; 4:1225–1228.
43. Pons-Estel B, Giminez C, Sacnun M, et al. Familial osteoarthritis and Milwaukee shoulder associated with calcium pyrophosphate and apatite crystal deposition. J Rheumatol 2000; 27:471–480.
44. Baldwin C, Farrer L, Adair R, et al. Linkage of early onset osteoarthritis and chondrocalcinosis to human chromosome 8q. Am J Hum Genet 1995; 56:692–697.
45. Williams C, Considine E, Knowlton R, et al. Spondyloepiphyseal dysplasia and precocious osteoarthritis in a family with an Arg75 to Cys mutation in the procollagen type II gene (COL2A1). Hum Genet 1993; 92:499–505.
46. Ho A, Johnson M, Kingsley D. Role of the mouse ank gene in tissue calcification and arthritis. Science 2000; 289:265–270.
47. Costello J, Ryan L. Modulation of chondrocyte production of extracellular inorganic pyrophosphate. Curr Opin Rheum 2004; 16:268–272.
48. Jones AC, Chuck AJ, Arie EA, Green DJ, Doherty M. Diseases associated with calcium pyrophosphate deposition disease. Semin Arthritis Rheum 1992; 22:188–202.
49. Rosenthal AK, Ryan LM. Ageing increases growth factor-induced inorganic pyrophosphate elaboration by articular cartilage. Mech Ageing Dev 1994; 75:35–44.
50. Hamilton E. Diseases associated with CPPD deposition disease. Arthritis Rheum 1976; 19:353–357.
51. Jaovisidha K, Rosenthal A. Calcium crystals in osteoarthritis. Curr Opin Rheumatol 2002; 14:298–302.
52. Felson D, Anderson J, Naimark A, et al. The prevalence of chondrocalcinosis in the elderly and its association with knee osteoarthritis: the Framingham study. J Rheumatol 1989; 16:1241–1245.
53. Neame R, Carr A, Muir K, et al. UK community prevalence of knee chondrocalcinosis: evidence that correlation with osteoarthritis is through a shared association with osteophyte. Ann Rheum Dis 2003; 42:513–518.
54. Fam A, Morava-Protzner I, Purcell C, et al. Acceleration of experimental lapine osteoarthritis by calcium pyrophosphate microcrystalline synovitis. Arthritis Rheum 1995; 38:201–210.
55. Doherty M, Watt I, Dieppe P. Localised chondrocalcinosis in post-meniscetomy knees. Lancet 1982; 1:1207–1210.
56. DeLange E, Keats T. Localized chondrocalcinosis in traumatized joints. Skeletal Radiol 1985; 14:249–256.
57. Linden B, Nilssen B. Chondrocalcinosis following osteochondritis desicans in the femur condyles. Clin Orthop 1978; 130:223–227.
58. Stockman A, Darlington L, Scott J. Frequency of chondrocalcinosis of the knee and avascular necrosis of the femoral heads in gout. A controlled study. Ann Rheum Dis 1980; 39:7–11.

59. Schwartz Z, Semba S, Graves D, et al. Rapid and long-term effects of PTH(1-34) on growth plate chondrocytes are mediated through two different pathways in a cell-maturation -dependent manner. Bone 1997; 21:249–259.
60. Pritchard M, Jessop J. Chondrocalcinosis in primary hyperparathyroidism. Ann Rheum Dis 1977; 36:146–151.
61. Rynes R, Merzig E. Calcium pyrophosphate crystal deposition disease and hyperparathryoidism: a controlled prospective study. J Rheumatol 1978; 5:460–468.
62. Hamilton E, Willimans R, Barlow K, et al. The arthropathy of idiopathic hemochromatosis. Q J Med 1968; 37:171–182.
63. Dymock I, Hamilton E, Laws J, et al. Arthropathy of haemochromatosis. Ann Rheum Dis 1970; 29:469–476.
64. Gordon D, Little H. The arthropathy of hemochromatosis without hemochromatosis. Arthritis Rheum 1973; 16:305–312.
65. Hearn P, Russell R, Elliott J, et al. Formation product f calcium pyrophosphate crystals in vitro and the effect of iron salts. Clin Sci 1978; 54:29P.
66. Pawlotsky Y, Dantec PL, Moirand R, et al. Elevated parathryoid hormone 44-68 and osteoarticular changes in patients with genetic hemochromatosis. Arthritis Rheum 1999; 42:799–806.
67. Whyte M. Hypophosphatasia. In: Scriver C, Beaudet A, Sly W, al E, eds. The Metabolic Basis of Inherited Disease. Vol. 2. New York: McGraw-Hill, 1989:22843–22856.
68. Chuck A, Pattrick M, Hamilton E, et al. Crystal deposition in hypophosphatasia: a reappraisal. Ann Rheum Dis 1989; 48:571–576.
69. Macfarlane J, Kroon H, Cats A. Ectopic calcification in hypophosphatasia. Eur J Radiol 1986; 6:228–230.
70. Russell R. Excretion of inorganic pyrophosphate in hypophosphatasia. Lancet 1965; 2:461–464.
71. Xu Y, Cruz T, Pritzker K. Alkaline phosphatase dissolves calcium pyrophosphate dihydrate crystals. J Rheumatol 1991; 18:1606–1610.
72. Rachow J, Ryan L. Inorganic pyrophosphatase metabolism in arthritis. Rheum Dis Clin North Am 1988; 14:289–302.
73. Doherty M, Chuck A, Hosking D, et al. Inorganic pyrophosphatase in metabolic diseases predisposing to calcium pyrophosphate dihydrate crystal deposition. Arthritis Rheum 1991; 34:1297–1303.
74. Bauer F, Glasson P, Vallatton M, et al. Syndrome de Bartter, chonrocalcinose and hypomagnesemia. Schwitz Med Wschr 1979; 34:1251–1256.
75. Resnick D, Rausch J. Hypomagnesia with chondrocalcinosis. J Assoc Can Radiol 1984; 35:214–216.
76. Punzi L, Calo L, Schiavon F, et al. Chondrocalcinosis is a feature of Gitelman's variant of Bartter's syndrome: a new look at the hypomagnesemia associated with calcium pyrophosphate dihydrate crystal deposition diseae. Rev Rheum [Engl Ed] 1998; 65:571–574.
77. Runeberg L, Collan Y, Jokinen E, et al. Hypomagnesemia due to renal disease of unknown etiology. Am J Med 1975; 59:873–881.
78. Milazzo S, Ahern M, Cleland L, et al. Calcium pyrophosphate dihydrate deposition disease and familial hypomagnesemia. J Rheumatol 1981; 8:767–771.

79. Smilde T, Haverman J, Schipper P, et al. Familial hypokalemia/hypomagnesemia and chondrocalcinosis. J Rheumatol 1994; 21:1515–1519.
80. McCarty DJ, Silcox D, Coe F, et al. Diseases associated with calcium pyrophosphate dihydrate crystal deposition. A controlled study. Am J Med 1974; 56:704–714.
81. Ellman M, Brown N, Porat A. Laboratory investigation in pseudogout patients and controls. J Rheumatol 1980; 7:77–81.
82. Gordon T, Smith M, Ebert B, et al. Articular chondrocalcinosis in a hospital population: an Australian experience. Aust NZ J Med 1984; 14:655–659.
83. Komatireddy G, Ellman M, Brown N. Lack of association between hypothyroidism and chondrocalcinosis. J Rheumatol 1989; 16:807–808.
84. Job-DesLandre C, Menkes C, Guinot M, et al. Does hypothyroidism increase the prevalence of chondrocalcinosis? Hung Rheumatol 1991; 32:5–55.
85. Menerey KA, Eider W, Brewer GJ, et al. The arthropathy of Wilson's disease. J Rheumaol 1988; 15:331–337.
86. Lamotte M, Segrestaa J-M, Krassinine G. Arthrite microcristalline calcique (pseudo-goutte) chez un acromegale. Semin Hop Paris 1966; 41:2420–2424.
87. Podorski M, Robinson B, Weissberger A, et al. Articular manifestations of acromegaly. Aust NZ J Med 1988; 18:28–35.
88. Natowicz M, Short P, Wang Y, et al. Clinical and biochemical manifestations of hyaluronidase deficiency. NEJM 1996; 335:1029–1033.
89. Hardy D, Murphy W, Siegel B, et al. X-linked hypophosphatemia in adults: prevalence of skeletal radiographic and scintigraphic features. Radiology 1989; 171:403–414.
90. Marx S, Attie M, Levine M, et al. The hypocalciuric or benign variant of familial hypercalcemia: clinical and biochemical features in fifteen kindreds. Medicine 1981; 60:397–412.

7

Clinical Manifestations of Basic Calcium Phosphate (Apatite) Deposition Disease

Kanyakorn Jaovisidha

Division of Rheumatology, Department of Medicine, Bangkok Hospital, Bangkok, Thailand

Lawrence M. Ryan

Division of Rheumatology, Department of Medicine, Medical College of Wisconsin, Milwaukee, Wisconsin, U.S.A.

INTRODUCTION

Basic calcium phosphate (BCP) deposition disease encompasses clinical syndromes caused by pathologic deposits of a variety of crystalline mineral including octacalcium phosphate, tricalcium phosphate, and most often carbonate-substituted apatite. If sufficient mineral deposits are present they can be detected radiographically, but not specifically identified. Methods for specific identification are detailed in Chapter 10, and include X-ray diffraction, Fourier transform infrared spectroscopy, transmission and scanning electron microscopy with energy dispersive analysis, and atomic force microscopy. These methods have variable degrees of specificity and require varying quantities of mineral for precise characterization.

Clinical manifestations of BCP deposition disease can be acute as in acute calcific tendinitis or periarthritis or can be chronic as in Milwaukee shoulder syndrome. Pathologic deposition of these crystals leads to multiple clinical manifestations that can be categorized into four groups: sporadic or aging, hereditary, disease-associated, and drug-associated deposition diseases.

SPORADIC OR IDIOPATHIC BCP CRYSTAL DEPOSITION DISEASE

Sporadic or idiopathic BCP deposition diseases include Milwaukee shoulder syndrome, calcific periarthritis, osteoarthritis, mixed crystal deposition disease, diffuse idiopathic skeletal hyperostosis (DISH), and calcification of common posterior cervical ligament (1).

Non-Inflammatory Arthropathy

Perhaps the best analyzed clinical expression of BCP deposition is a non-inflammatory arthropathy. The term Milwaukee shoulder syndrome was given to this condition involving the shoulder and was first described in a group of patients exhibiting large effusions in unstable shoulders (2). This clinical presentation was identical to that previously described as cuff tear arthropathy (3). Analysis of patients, synovial fluids, radiographs, and surgical specimens offers insights into pathogenesis of a basically non-inflammatory yet destructive arthropathy. Subsequently it was recognized that the destructive effects related to BCP crystal deposition were not limited to the shoulder, but could occur in any peripheral joint. For example, "Philadelphia fingers" is used to describe erosive destructive arthropathy due to BCP crystals in the finger joints.

The original cohort of patients with Milwaukee shoulder syndrome were recognized by their large non-inflammatory joint effusions and remarkable glenohumeral instability (4). The unifying feature of these patients was the presence of synovial fluid BCP crystals as assessed by (^{14}C) ethane-1-hydroxy-1, 1-diphosphonate (EHDP) binding. Repetitive joint aspirate specimens consistently contained BCP. Coexistent calcium pyrophosphate dihydrate (CPPD) crystals were found in one-half of fluids. Similar non-inflammatory but destructive arthritis affected the knees of many patients with Milwaukee shoulder syndrome. As in the shoulders, BCP and often CPPD crystals were seen in knee fluids. At the time of shoulder arthrotomy, dissolution of articular cartilage, rotator cuff, and long head of the biceps tendon was apparent. Realizing that proteases would be necessary to digest the thick collagenous articular cartilage and tendons, investigators measured protease activity in fluids. Collagenolytic and proteolytic activities were measurable in most instances (5,6). Subsequent studies, reviewed in Chapter 17, detail mechanisms by which calcium-containing crystals can produce synovial lining proliferation seen in Milwaukee shoulder syndrome as well as synthesis and release of collagenases and neutral proteases.

The syndrome has a predilection for elderly women. Women outnumber men with a ratio of approximately four to one. Symptoms include chronic pain worsened by activity and nocturnal pain, especially when lying on the affected side. The pain can be severe enough to occur at rest. Painless swelling, however, is also encountered (7). As expected with lysis of the rotator cuff and the long head of biceps tendon, active range of motion is severely limited. Often, both shoulders are affected. However, passive motion is preserved and instability is often apparent. Effusions vary in size with aspirates yielding 5 to 200 mL. Crepitus can be obvious. Intra-articular bleeding can result in joint rupture and dissection of bloody synovial fluid into the anterior chest wall and upper arm resulting in the quarter panel sign (8). Rarely, Milwaukee shoulder syndrome is complicated by the development of a draining sinus from the severely swollen joints (7). Predisposing factors include trauma and overuse, such as with use of crutches.

Synovial fluids are non-inflammatory with white cell count usually less than 1,000 per mm^3. Fluids predictably contain only BCP crystals, while some fluids also contain CPPD crystals.

Radiographic features reveal upward subluxation of the humeral head, degeneration of the glenohumeral joint, and soft tissue calcification (Fig. 1). Osteophyte formation may not be prominent despite severe degenerative and destructive changes. Pseudoarticulation between humeral head and coracoacromial vault caused by the displaced humeral head may result in acromial stress fracture and severe erosion of the anterior portion of acromion, distal end of clavicle, and coracoid process. Collapse of the humeral head completes the syndrome (3). In the knee, narrowing of the lateral femorotibial space is typical, followed by collapse of articular surfaces, fragmentation, and valgus deformity.

Acute Inflammatory Arthritis

Acute arthritis induced by BCP crystals in the absence of osteoarthritis manifests similarly to an acute gout or pseudogout attack but is a much less common

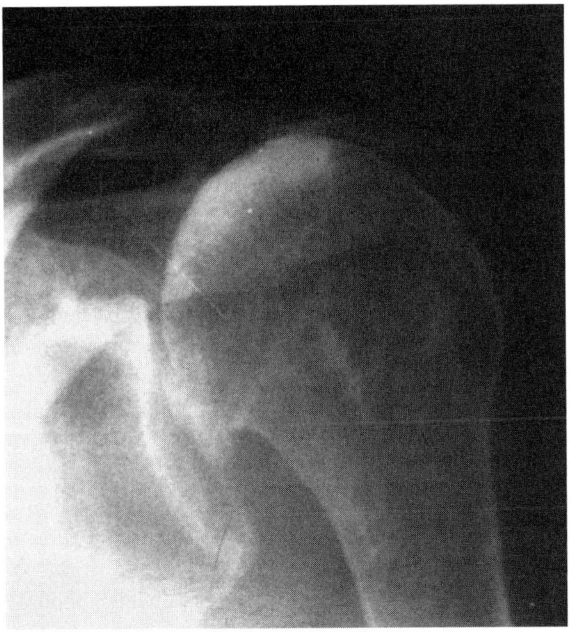

Figure 1 AP view of the left shoulder shows cephalad migration of the humeral head, remodeling of the superior humeral head and overlying acromion and clavicle, osteophyte formation, subchondral sclerosis, and minor cystic formation in a patient with Milwaukee shoulder syndrome.

condition. Symptoms begin with pain, swelling, and erythema in metacarpophalangeal, metatarsophalangeal, proximal, and distal interphalangeal joints in relatively young persons (9). Synovial fluids from these joints may contain high white cell counts as well as BCP crystals. Radiographs of joints are normal during initial attacks, but BCP crystal-induced acute arthritis predicts later development of erosive osteoarthritis (10). Acute arthritis in the costovertebral joint has also been reported and presumably is due to the release of crystals deposited adjacent to intervertebral disk (11). BCP release is also occasionally responsible for an acute flare in osteoarthritic joint. Acute arthritis and periarthritis infrequently occur in individuals with tumoral calcinosis, chronic renal failure, heterotopic calcification due to neurologic catastrophes, connective tissue diseases, synovial osteochondromatosis, and epiphyseal dysplasia (1).

Acute Calcific Periarthritis

Acute calcific periarthritis is an acute inflammatory process in periarticular tendons, ligaments, and bursae as a result of deposition of BCP crystals, mainly carbonate-substituted apatite (12). Women are affected three to four times more commonly than men. Acute calcific periarthritis presents with warmth, erythema, swelling, and pain in a localized area which lasts from a few days to a few weeks. Occasionally, it is accompanied by low-grade fever (usually below 38°C), elevated acute phase reactants, and low-grade leukocytosis (13). The most common sites to be involved are around the shoulders and hips. Less common sites include fingers, toes, wrists, elbows, and ankles (13,14). Rarely the temporomandibular joint is affected (15). When arising in the first metatarsophalangeal joint, this entity resembles acute gouty arthritis, hence the term "hydroxyapatite pseudopodagra" (16–18). Careful physical examination usually reveals relative preservation of normal passive range of motion unless the process results in rupture of tendons (19) or adhesive periarthritis.

Most patients with calcific periarthritis are middle-aged to elderly, with the exception of hydroxyapatite pseudopodagra that mostly affects young women (20). Recurrent periarthritis or simultaneous involvement in multiple sites suggests an associated systemic disease such as hypoparathyroidism, surgically treated primary hyperparathyroidism, connective tissue diseases, or others as described below. These presentations may be seen in one-third to two-thirds of individuals (21).

Periarticular calcification, often asymptomatic, is common in the fifth to seventh decades of life (21). Deposits vary in size, shape, and location. Radiographically, the initial calcifications appear cloud-like, but later become denser, homogeneous, and better-delineated. Use of special views and bright light may be necessary to visualize small deposits. The size of deposits does not predict or correlate with symptoms. Symptoms occur when deposits interfere with motion or expand into adjacent soft tissue. Deposits may differ in appearance depending on their phase. For example, in the asymptomatic phase in the shoulder, calcific deposits are commonly confined to the supraspinatus tendon. When symptoms such as pain or restricted motion are present, the calcifications may remain unchanged or have enlarged and raise the floor of the subdeltoid bursa. However, calcification may not be observed radiographically at the time of symptoms. After an acute attack, the deposit may remain, fade, or totally disappear, then recur at a later date. Dissolution of extracellular crystals is due to increased blood flow and intracellularly results after they are phagocytosed into the acidic phagolysosome. Even large calcification can completely disappear within 7 days (13).

Deposits may spread under or into the bursa. In some instances, the deposit may involve bone and be seen as an intraosseous calcified cyst. BCP crystals can deposit almost anywhere in the body. Frequent sites of calcification identified radiographically include the insertion of the supraspinatus on the promontory of the greater tuberosity, the attachment of the infraspinatus and teres minor on the greater tuberosity, the attachment of the subscapularis on the lesser tuberosity, the long head of the bicipital tendon in the bicipital grove and along the humeral shaft, the short head of the biceps near the coracoid process, within the flexor carpi ulnaris tendon, the insertions of the gluteus into the greater trochanter, and near the first metatarsophalangeal joint (21). Calcification of the longus colli muscle is usually located anterior to C1 and C2 vertebral bodies. Cortical erosion may accompany mineral deposits adjacent to the bone diaphysis (22).

The differential diagnoses of acute periarthritis includes infection of soft tissue and joints, acute gouty attack, and pseudogout. Rarely, peri- and intra-articular inflammation may coexist with septic arthritis (23). In rare instances of deposits in the longus colli muscle, patients may present with odynophagia and mimic a retropharyngeal abscess (24,25). Within the carpal tunnel, the deposits result in inflammation and median nerve compression causing carpal tunnel syndrome (26,27). CPPD deposition can also occur in tendons, but that tends to cause more elongated appearing calcifications as compared to the tumor-like or cloud-like densities in BCP deposition. Chondrocalcinosis is unusual in periarticular BCP deposition disease.

Osteoarthritis and BCP Crystal Deposition

BCP crystals are present in synovial fluids in a large subset of patients with osteoarthritis. Half of articular cartilages with advanced osteoarthritis contained hydroxyapatite-type crystals (28). Studies of synovial fluids from osteoarthritic knee joints reveal apatite crystals in approximately 30% to 60%, and such fluids more often contain both BCP and CPPD crystals than either species alone (29–32). The presence of BCP correlates with more severe radiographic joint degeneration and at times is associated with neuropathic-like arthropathy on X-ray (21). Moreover, the progression of degenerative arthritis in BCP-containing joints can be very rapid. For example, protrusio acetabuli or lysis of the femoral head can develop within one year. However, BCP crystals are often overlooked in synovial fluids because they are small and lack birefringence. Degeneration in BCP-containing osteoarthritic knees typically involves the lateral and patellofemoral compartments, while primary osteoarthritis unassociated with crystals usually involves the medial and patellofemoral compartments (21). The existence of BCP crystals in small joints of the hands is a possible predictor of erosive osteoarthritis (10).

Diffuse Idiopathic Skeletal Hyperostosis

DISH, or Forrestier's disease, is an ossifying skeletal disorder involving spinal and extraspinal sites. DISH predominates in men and the elderly. Depending on the criteria used, the prevalence ranges between 2.6% and 28% in individuals over age 39 years (33). In older age groups men and women are equally affected. DISH is more common in Caucasians than in Asians. It is generally diagnosed by the presence of flowing ossification along the anterolateral aspect of at least four consecutive vertebral bodies, due to ossification of the anterior longitudinal ligament, and large bridging osteophytes. This is most commonly seen between the seventh to the eleventh thoracic vertebrae and between the first and the third lumbar vertebrae (34). Clinically, DISH is often asymptomatic or presents as spinal stiffness and moderate degree of limitation of motion (35). Back pain is mild or absent despite the significant calcium deposition. In the cervical spine, large ossification can result in dysphagia, hoarseness, dyspnea, stridor, and difficult intubation (36). DISH accounts for up to 10.5% of individuals with dysphagia over the age of 59 years. Ossification of the posterior longitudinal ligament, which occurs in high percentage of patients, can be severe enough to cause spinal stenosis. Ossification of a long segment of the spine increases the risk of spinal fracture from hyperextension even after minor trauma (37,38). Cervical myelopathy can also result from pseudoarthrosis between the first and second cervical vertebrae and from anterior atlantoaxial subluxation (36).

Compared to osteoarthritis of the spine, in DISH the intervertebral discs are normal or only slightly decreased in height, and neither vacuum phenomenon nor marginal sclerosis of the vertebra are observed. Radiolucent lines, which correspond to anterolateral disc extension sandwiched between ossified mass superiorly and inferiorly, can be observed anterior to the vertebrae on lateral films. Radiolucent lines may also be seen on lateral films in the unossified areas between the anterior borders of the vertebrae and the deposited bone (34). DISH usually evolves over a period of several years (39).

In extraspinal sites, large enthesophytes, whiskering bone proliferation, and ligament calcification are observed. Enthesophytes usually develop at sites of ligament or tendon attachments such as the calcaneus, the olecranon process, and the patella. Sacrotuberous and iliolumbar ligament calcification are found. Calcaneal involvement may be associated with heel pain and Achilles tendinitis. Thoracic outlet syndrome is a rare complication of DISH. In keeping with the ossifying nature of DISH, affected patients have a five-fold increase in risk of developing heterotopic ossification after total hip arthroplasty (40).

The cause of DISH is unknown. An association between DISH and hyperglycemia is controversial. The prevalence in patients with diabetes is higher than healthy subjects, but the association is lost when adjusted to body mass index (35,41,42). Patients treated with synthetic retinoic acid also develop skeletal disorder similar to DISH. Rarely, hypoparathyroidism causes flowing ossification anterior to the vertebral bodies similar to that seen in DISH (43).

Calcification of the Spine and Intervertebral Disks

Idiopathic calcification of the spinal ligaments and disks is common in the elderly. It can be asymptomatic or can present with signs and symptoms of cord compression, especially in the cervical region. Ossification of the posterior longitudinal ligaments, a condition common in the Japanese, and calcification of the ligamentum flavum can cause cervical myelopathy (44). Less severe manifestations are radiculopathy and neck pain. Both BCP and CPPD crystals may be found in such deposits (45,46). The lesions are easily visualized on plain radiographs of the spine and are demonstrated clearly with CT scanning. A murine disease model, which exhibits a phenotype similar to human ossification of posterior longitudinal ligaments, has been analyzed and found to result from deficiency of an ectoenzyme that generates inorganic pyrophosphate, an inhibitor of BCP formation. These so-called tiptoe-walking mice suffer from myelopathy (47).

Calcification in the disks is usually localized to one or two disks and involves the anulus fibrosus, nucleus pulposus, and cartilaginous end plates. The clusters of BCP crystals appear globular in shape, are usually seen in the mid-thoracic and upper lumbar levels, and are commonly seen in association with degenerative disease of the spine.

Mixed Crystal Deposition Disease

Synovial fluids often contain both BCP and CPPD crystals. This indicates mixed crystal deposition disease, which is probably more common than deposition disease arising from either CPPD or BCP crystals alone. Mixed crystal deposition disease can be recognized radiographically when chondrocalcinosis is present in multiple sites in conjunction with extensive calcification in joint capsules or dense homogeneous deposits in tendons (21). Mixed crystal deposition disease is associated with severe degenerative arthritis (30,48).

HEREDITARY BCP CRYSTAL DISEASE

Hereditary BCP deposition disease has been reported in multiple forms of manifestations from many countries around the world. The manifestations include calcific bursitis, tendinitis, and arthritis; enthesopathy in X-linked hypophosphatemia; idiopathic tumoral calcinosis; Milwaukee shoulder syndrome and other forms of destructive shoulder arthropathy; fibrodysplasia ossificans progressiva; and idiopathic infantile arterial calcification (1).

Idiopathic Tumoral Calcinosis

Idiopathic tumoral calcinosis, also termed lipocalcinosis granulomatosis, is a rare syndrome characterized by the presence of irregular calcifying masses in periarticular soft tissue. The condition usually affects young patients of African descent, although it has occurred in other ethnic groups as well. Patients who present at an older age may represent a form fruste of the disease. Although these tumor-like masses are observed around the shoulders, hips, and elbows, they do not limit motion (49,50). These masses can be unifocal or multifocal. Complications include skin ulceration with secondary infection, draining sinus, cachexia, and amyloidosis (49). Compression of nerve roots, spinal cord, and peripheral nerves is not uncommon (51,52).

A proportion of patients have high serum phosphate levels as well as metabolic derangements involving calcium, alkaline phosphatase, 25-hydroxy-vitamin D, and parathyroid hormone. Some patients have affected siblings, suggesting this is a hereditary disease (53). The hyperphosphatemic subset of tumoral calcinosis is transmitted by autosomal recessive inheritance and is the result of mutation in the gene GALNT3, which encodes a glycosyl transferase (54). This gene has been mapped to chromosome 2q24-q31. Genetic abnormalities in the normophosphatemic subset have not been identified.

Fibrodysplasia Ossificans Progressiva

Fibrodysplasia ossificans progressiva, or myositis ossificans progressiva, is a rare hereditary disorder manifesting in childhood. It is characterized by extensive ectopic calcification in striated muscles, fascia, aponeuroses, and fibrous structures related to muscles, especially paraspinal muscles (49). This condition is transmitted as an autosomal dominant trait with incomplete penetrance. The course of disease is one of exacerbations and remissions. The onset begins at 4 to 5 years of age (range 1 to 16 years) with inflammation followed by calcification over weeks. At times the calcification follows local trauma, surgery, injection, venipuncture, and dental treatment (55–57). Acute lesions may or may not be associated with inflammation and do not always progress to ossification. During remission, visible and palpable soft tissue masses, especially on the back of head and neck, may develop and are associated with progressive stiffness (58). Remission can last many years.

Smooth muscle, heart, diaphragm, tongue, and sphincters are spared (56). Massive periarticular ossification can lead to severe disability by limiting joint motion and causing joint contractures in the lower extremities. About one-fourth of patients have a synostosis between the humerus and chest wall which leads to superior subluxation of the humeral head (59). Entire muscles may be replaced by new bone formation causing marked limitations of movement. Movement of the cervical spine may be abolished entirely by ankylosis of the cervical spine and pseudoexostoses arising from the occiput. Pain may be caused by pseudoexostoses on the long bones and calcaneus. Diagnostically helpful features found in the majority of individuals include bilateral microdactyly of the first metatarsal bones and proximal phalanges as well as hallux valgus. Deafness is common. Complications include nerve compression, limited chest wall capacity, dependence on diaphragmatic breathing, and respiratory tract infection (60,61). A fall can cause serious injury and worsen functional limitation. Sixty-seven percent of falls lead to exacerbation of calcification (62). Fatal outcomes result from respiratory failure and inanition from calcification in muscles of mastication. Despite the possible debilitating and fatal course of the disorder, prolonged survival is not rare and patients can live into their eighth decade (61–63). Laboratory findings include elevated serum alkaline phosphatase levels, but no abnormalities in calcium or phosphorus metabolism have been identified. The differential diagnosis includes ankylosing spondylitis, idiopathic tumoral calcinosis, and causes of metastatic calcification due to disorders of calcium and phosphorus metabolism.

Idiopathic Infantile Arterial Calcification

Idiopathic infantile arterial calcification is a rare and fatal disorder characterized by pathologic calcification and intimal proliferation of medium-sized and large arteries in infants. Calcium deposits, mainly calcium hydroxyapatite, are found near the internal elastic lamina and in the tunica media. The disease is associated with mutations in the gene ENPP1 (ectonucleotide pyrophosphatase/phosphodiesterase1) which encodes for the enzyme plasma cell membrane glycoprotein-1 (an important inhibitor of bone mineralization) (64,65). This results in low levels of pyrophosphate, an inhibitor of calcification, in plasma and urine (66,67). The disease manifests with cardiovascular compromise, cardiac failure, and systemic hypertension occurring in utero, at birth, or shortly thereafter. Calcification in abdominal viscera, brain, thyroid gland, periarticular tissues, and soft tissues may be present (68–70). Calcified vessels may not be apparent radiographically when cardiac symptoms develop (66). Normal values of serum calcium, phosphorus, parathyroid hormone, and vitamin D are expected. Affected infants usually die in the first 6 months of life of severe cardiac failure and myocardial infarction. However, a rare case of spontaneous disappearance of calcification with long-term survival and a case of late presentation at 33 months of age have been reported (69–71).

Other Hereditary Hydroxyapatie Deposition Diseases

Reports of familial cases of BCP deposition disease suggest that genetic risks may play a pathogenetic role. The phenotype found in these families is heterogeneous.

In one family, five members were affected with different manifestations, namely multiple intervertebral disk calcification, arthritis, and degenerative changes of small joints of the hands, shoulders periarthritis, and periarticular calcific deposits (72). BCP crystals in the deposits were confirmed. A relationship with HLA antigen was not found. In another report of Italo-Argentinian kindred with 75 affected members from five generations, osteoarthritis, chondrocalcinosis, and Milwaukee shoulder syndrome were observed and were probably transmitted as an autosomal dominant inheritance (73). Incomplete Milwaukee shoulder syndrome was strikingly detected radiographically in seven members aged less than 53 years. Both BCP and CPPD crystals were identified in synovial fluids from two cases. Again, none of the genetic risks tested showed a positive correlation. Recurrent calcific periarthritis in multiple sites has been reported in identical twins in the United States (74). In another family, recurrent calcific periarthritis was diagnosed in a 47-year-old proband who had two relatives with asymptomatic periarticular calcific deposits (75). Low serum levels of alkaline phosphatase has been observed in some patients with familial calcific periarthritis (76–79). Multiple crystal deposition disease, manifesting with calcific periarthritis, gout and chondrocalcinosis, has been reported in four members of a single family (80).

SYSTEMIC DISEASES ASSOCIATED WITH BCP CRYSTAL DEPOSITION

BCP crystal deposition disease frequently arises in patients with comorbidities such as renal failure, connective tissue diseases, hypercalcemia, trauma, and neurologic injuries. Occasionally, it is the presenting manifestation of the underlying disorder.

End Stage Renal Disease

In patients with chronic renal failure, calcification may be observed in multiple sites including soft tissue, subcutaneous tissue and periarticular tissue as well as in blood vessels, viscera, cornea, and conjunctiva. Infrequently, crystal deposits are found in the intervertebral disks and in articular tissues (1). Release of these crystals may lead to periarthritis or acute arthritis (15). The term "tumoral calcinosis" has been used widely to describe large periarticular calcific deposits associated with chronic renal failure and other conditions. After hemodialysis and peritoneal dialysis, calcification typically continues to progress, although resolution of calcification can occur (43). A positive calcium balance induced by the use of calcium-containing phosphate binders and high calcium dialysate may worsen calcification (81). Calcification is less frequent with better control of calcium x phosphate product by means of phosphate binders, increasing dialysis frequency, and renal transplantation. Sometimes calcific deposits resolve after parathyroidectomy (82). Vitamin D should be used cautiously to prevent hypervitaminosis D, which aggravates calcification (83).

Connective Tissue Diseases

BCP crystals are found deposited in the subcutaneous tissues in patients with a variety of connective tissue diseases with no evidence of abnormal calcium or phosphorus metabolism. The most common example is in patients with juvenile dermatomyositis. Risk factors for calcification in dermatomyositis are delayed treatment, suboptimal steroid therapy, and unresponsiveness to steroid therapy (84). In limited or late-stage diffuse systemic sclerosis, calcification is observed in 36% of patients (85) and is typically present in the skin or subcutaneous tissue on the flexor side of terminal phalanges, in the digital pads and periarticular tissues of the hands, the extensor surface of the forearms, the olecranon bursae, prepatellar areas, buttocks, cervical synovial articulations, and thoracic and lumbar spine (85,86). Acute calcific periarthritis may follow subcutaneous or bursal deposits (20,87). Resolution of the deposit after an acute attack is incomplete and less frequent than is the norm for idiopathic calcific periarthritis. Secondary complications include skin ulcers, drainage of paste-like material, and infection. Calcinosis and periarticular and intra-articular calcification has also been reported in systemic lupus erythematosus (88,89), mixed connective tissue disease (90), and rheumatoid arthritis (91). In these diseases, calcification in the cervical area can be extensive, involving multiple levels and resulting in osteolysis and erosion of adjacent bone and joints (92).

Hypercalcemia

Hypercalcemic metastatic calcification arises in patients with hyperparathyroidism, hypervitaminosis D, sarcoidosis, metastatic cancer, plasma cell myeloma, and leukemia (93). Calcification is noted in various organs including stomach, lung, arterial walls, skin, and eyes. It may improve after treatment of the hypercalcemia. Occasionally, calcific deposits enlarge, forming a subcutaneous mass or tumoral calcinosis. If large, these deposits may erode bones (94). Calcifications in primary hyperparathyroidism can be composed of CPPD crystals as well as BCP crystals.

Myositis Ossificans Traumatica

This condition is characterized by localized soft tissue ossification (myositis ossificans circumscripta) typically in soft tissues and large muscles in the upper arms and thighs (95). Trauma precedes this type of heterotopic ossification in 60% to 75% of patients, who are usually young adults (93). In the remainder the trauma was probably quite minor or simply not remembered. Patients present with mass-like lesions that can mimic soft tissue tumor, sometimes in conjunction with limitation of motion. Signs of local inflammation and low-grade fever may be noted. If the lesions are around the joint, they may mimic acute gout (96). Lesions in the head and neck are rare (97). Myositis ossificans is also an uncommon complication of neurologic catastrophes such as prolonged coma, head trauma, anoxic brain injury, paraplegia and hemiplegia from stroke and spinal cord injury

(1,98,99). Sixteen percent to 53% of patients developed this condition one to four months after spinal cord injury (100). In this particular situation, the hip joints are most frequently involved. Other sites include knees, shoulders, elbows, and spine. The condition is seldom reported in lumbosacral and conus-cauda areas lesions which do not limit ambulation. In 2% to 30% of patients, decreased range of motion is present, while only about 3% of ossification results in severe limitation of movement and ankylosis (101). When myositis ossificans develops in the absence of trauma, it is named pseudomalignant osseous tumor of soft tissue.

Serum alkaline phosphatase is elevated in some patients during the early phase of bone formation (101). Two major radiographic findings in myositis ossificans are a peripheral rim of calcification and ossification surrounding a lucent center, and a radiolucent band separating myositis ossificans from its adjacent bone, both of which correlate the pathological findings and are clearly demonstrated by CT scans (93).

DRUG-RELATED BCP CRYSTAL DEPOSITION

A number of medications have been associated with BCP crystal deposition. Intravenous calcium gluconate injection causes calcinosis cutis in neonates at site of extravasation (102,103). Intra-articular injection of corticosteroid infrequently causes calcification in soft tissue (104,105). Rarely, calcification arises locally in the area of long-term subcutaneous injection such as insulin injection in insulin-dependent diabetes (106,107). In these latter cases, calcification is restricted to the skin. Synthetic retinoid therapy, such as etretinate and isotretinoin at low and high doses, has also been implicated in extraspinal tendon and ligament calcification, spinal hyperostosis, and DISH (108,109). Milk-alkali syndrome also may cause soft tissue calcification (110).

CONCLUSION

BCP crystal deposition leads to a variety of clinical manifestations in the musculoskeletal system with acute or insidious onset, local or systemic presentation, and variable prognosis. Treatment of symptomatic BCP crystal deposition is mainly symptomatic. Formulation of successful prophylaxis or treatments will require a better understanding of the processes involved in BCP deposition.

REFERENCES

1. Reginato AJ, Reginato AM. Diseases associated with deposition of calcium pyrophosphate or hydroxyapatite. In: Ruddy S, Harris ED, Jr., Sledge C, eds. Kelley's Textbook of Rheumatology. 6th ed. Philadelphia: W.B. Saunders, 2001:1377–1390.

2. Adams R. Illustration of the Effect of Rheumatic Joint in Chronic Rheumatic Arthritis of All the Articulations; with Descriptive and Explanatory Statements. London: John Churchill, 1857.
3. Neer CS, II, Craig EV, Fukuda H. Cuff tear arthropathy. J Bone Joint Surg Am 1983; 65:1232–1244.
4. McCarty DJ, Halverson PB, Carrera GF, Brewer BJ, Kozin F. "Milwaukee shoulder"—association of micro spheroids containing hydroxyapatite crystals, active collagenase, and neutral protease with rotator cuff defects. I. Clinical aspects. Arthritis Rheum 1981; 24:464–473.
5. Halverson PB, Cheung HS, McCarty DJ. 'Milwaukee shoulder': association of micro spheroids containing hydroxyapatite crystals, active collagenase and neutral protease with rotator cuff defects: II. Synovial fluid studies. Arthritis Rheum 1981; 24:474–483.
6. Cheung HS, Halverson PB, McCarty DJ. Release of collagenase, neutral protease, and prostaglandins from cultured mammalian synovial cells by hydroxyapatite and calcium pyrophosphate dihydrate crystals. Arthritis Rheum 1981; 24:1338–1344.
7. Klimaitis A, Carroll G, Owen E. Rapidly progressive destructive arthropathy of the shoulder—a viewpoint on pathogenesis. J Rheumatol 1988; 15:1859–1862.
8. McCarty DJ, Swanson AB, Ehrhart RH. Hemorrhagic rupture of the shoulder. J Rheumatol 1994; 21:1134–1137.
9. Schumacher HR, Jr., Smolyo AP, Tse RL, Maurer K. Arthritis associated with apatite crystals. Ann Intern Med 1977; 87:411–416.
10. Gerster JC. Intraarticular apatite crystal deposition as a predictor of erosive osteoarthritis of the fingers. J Rheumatol 1994; 21:2164–2165.
11. Mutschler C, Le Hir PX, Laredo JD, Arriv L. Hydroxyapatite-associated arthritis of a thoracic costovertebral joint. AJR 1999; 173:1711–1712.
12. Hamada JI, Ono W, Tarnai K, Saotome K, Hoshino T. Analysis of calcium deposits in calcific periarthritis. J Rheumatol 2001; 28:809–813.
13. Yosipovitch G, Yosipovitch Z. Acute calcific periarthritis of the hand and elbows in women. A study and review of the literature. J Rheumatol 1993; 20:1533–1538.
14. Claudepierre P, Rahmouni A, Bergamasco P, Montazel J-L, Larget-Piet B, Chevalier X. Misleading clinical aspects of hydroxyapatite deposits: a series of 15 cases. J Rheumatol 1997; 24:531–535.
15. Best JA, Shapiro RD, Kalmar J, Westesson P-L. Hydroxyapatite deposition disease of the temporomandibular joint in a patient with renal failure. J Oral Maxillofac Surg 1997; 55:1316–1322.
16. Fam AG, Rubinstein J. Hydroxyapatite pseudopodagra. A syndrome of young women. Arthritis Rheum 1989; 32:741–747.
17. Fam AG, Stein J. Hydroxyapatite pseudopodagra in young women. J Rheumatol 1992; 19:662–664.
18. Mines D, Abbuhl SB. Hydroxyapatite pseudopodagra in a young man: acute calcific periarthritis of the first metatarsophalangeal joint. Am J Emerg Med 1996; 14:180–182.
19. De Smet L, Baeten Y. Closed rupture of both flexor tendons of the fifth finger due to a calcium hydroxyapatite deposit in the carpal tunnel. Acta Orthop Belg 1998; 64:336–338.

20. Fam AG, Pritzker KP. Acute calcific periarthritis in scleroderma. J Rheumatol 1992; 19:1580–1585.
21. Resnick D. Calcium hydroxyapatite crystal deposition disease. In: Resnick D, ed. Diagnosis of Bone and Joint Disorders. 4th ed. Philadelphia: WB Saunders, 2002:1619–1657.
22. Fritz P, Bardin T, Laredo JD, et al. Paradiaphyseal calcific tendinitis with cortical bone erosion. Arthritis Rheum 1994; 37:718–723.
23. Razzaq A, Kokko K, Agudelo CA. Case report: coexistence of acute calcific periarthritis and infection. Am J Med Sci 1996; 312:140–141.
24. De Maeseneer M, Vreugde S, Laureys S, Sartoris DJ, De Ridder F, Osteaux M. Calcific tendinitis of the longus colli muscle. Head Neck 1997; 19:545–548.
25. Figler T. Radiologic case study. Calcific tendonitis of the longissimus colli muscle. Orthopedics 1993; 16:1365.
26. Verfaillie S, De Smet L, Leemans A, Van Damme B, Fabry G. Acute carpal tunnel syndrome caused by hydroxyapatite crystals: a case report. J Hand Surg Am 1996; 21:360–362.
27. el Maghraoui A, Lecoules S, Lechevalier D, Magnin J, Eulry F. Acute carpal tunnel syndrome caused by calcific periarthritis of the wrist (letter). Clin Exp Rheumatol 2001; 19:107.
28. Doyle DV. Tissue calcification and inflammation in osteoarthritis. J Pathol 1982; 136:199–216.
29. Derfus BA, Kurian JB, Butler JJ. The high prevalence of pathologic calcium crystals in preoperative knees. J Rheumatol 2002; 29:570–574.
30. Gibilisco PA, Schumacher HR, Jr., Hollander JL, Soper KA. Synovial fluid crystals in osteoarthritis. Arthritis Rheum 1985; 28:511–515.
31. Swan A, Chapman B, Heap P, Seward H, Dieppe P. Submicroscopic crystals in osteoarthritic synovial fluids. Ann Rheum Dis 1994; 53:467–470.
32. Halverson PB, McCarty DJ. Patterns of radiographic abnormalities associated with basic calcium phosphate and calcium pyrophosphate dihydrate crystal deposition in the knee. Ann Rheum Dis 1986; 45:603–605.
33. Kim SK, Choi BR, Kim CG, et al. The prevalence of diffuse idiopathic skeletal hyperostosis in Korea. J Rheumatol 2004; 31:2032–2035.
34. Resnick D. Diffuse idiopathic skeletal hyperostosis. In: Resnick D, ed. Bone and Joint Imaging. 2nd ed. Philadelphia: W.B. Saunders, 1996:378–387.
35. Moskowitz RW, Holderbaum D. Clinical and laboratory findings in osteoarthritis. In: Koopman WJ, ed. Arthritis and Allied Conditions. 14th ed. Philadelphia: Lippincott Williams & Wilkins, 2001:2216–2245.
36. Mader R. Clinical manifestations of diffuse idiopathic skeletal hyperostosis of the cervical spine. Semin Arthritis Rheum 2002; 32:130–135.
37. Israel Z, Mosheiff R, Gross E, Muggia-Sullam M, Floman Y. Hyperextension fracture-dislocation of the thoracic spine with paraplegia in a patient with diffuse idiopathic skeletal hyperostosis. J Spinal Disord 1994; 7:455–457.
38. Burkus JK, Denis F. Hyperextension injuries of the thoracic spine in diffuse idiopathic skeletal hyperostosis. Report of four cases. J Bone Joint Surg Am 1994; 76:237–243.
39. Mader R. Diffuse idiopathic skeletal hyperostosis: isolated involvement of cervical spine in a young patient. J Rheumatol 2004; 31:620–621.

40. Guillemin F, Mainard D, Rolland H, Delagoutte JP. Antivitamin K prevents heterotopic ossification after hip arthroplasty in diffuse idiopathic skeletal hyperostosis. A retrospective study in 67 patients. Acta Orthop Scand 1995; 66:123–126.
41. Kiss C, Szilagyi M, Paksy A, Poor G. Risk factors for diffuse idiopathic skeletal hyperostosis: a case-control study. Rheumatology (Oxford) 2002; 41:27–30.
42. Daragon A, Mejjad O, Czernichow P, Louvel JP, Vittecoq O, Durr A, et al. Vertebral hyperostosis and diabetes mellitus: a case-control study. Ann Rheum Dis 1995; 54:375–378.
43. Resnick D. Parathyroid disorders and renal osteodystrophy. In: Resnick D, ed. Bone and Joint Imaging. 2nd ed. Philadelphia: W.B. Saunders, 1996:552–571.
44. Pascal-Moussellard H, Cabre P, Smadja D, Kaidomar S, Catonne Y. Myelopathy due to calcification of the cervical ligamenta flava: a report of two cases in West Indian patients. Eur Spine J 1999; 8:238–240.
45. Okada G, Hosoi S, Kato K, et al. Case report 779. Carbonate apatite calcification of ligamentum flavum. Skelet Radiol 1993; 22:211–213.
46. Muthukumar N, Karuppaswamy U. Tumoral calcium pyrophosphate dihydrate deposition disease of the ligamentum flavum. Neurosurgery 2003; 53:103–108.
47. Okawa A, Nakamura I, Goto S, Moriya H, Nakamura Y, Ikegawa S. Mutation in Npps in a mouse model of ossification of the posterior longitudinal ligament of the spine. Nat Genet 1998; 19:271–273.
48. Halverson PB, Cheung HS, Johnson R, Struve J. Simultaneous occurrence of calcium pyrophosphate dihydrate and basic calcium phosphate (hydroxyapatite) crystals in a knee. Clin Orthop Relat Res 1990; 257:162–165.
49. Halverson PB. Basic calcium phosphate (apatite, octacalcium phosphate, tricalcium phosphate) crystal deposition diseases and calcinosis. In: Koopman WJ, ed. Arthritis and Allied Conditions. 14th ed. Philadelphia: Lippincott Williams & Wilkins, 2001:2372–2392.
50. Harwood CA, Cook MG, Mortimer PS. Tumoral calcinosis: an unusual cause of cutaneous calcification. Clin Exp Dermatol 1996; 21:163–166.
51. Flores J, Munoz J, Gallego S, Bujan A, Ferreiro I, Gonzalez A. Spinal cord compression due to tumoral idiopathic calcinosis. Spinal Cord 2003; 41:413–416.
52. Sanchez-Martin A, Proubasta-Renart I. Acute carpal tunnel syndrome caused by idiopathic tumoral calcinosis. J S Orthop Assoc 2001; 10:92–94.
53. Slavin RE, Wen J, Kumar D, Evans EB. Familial tumoral calcinosis. A clinical, histopathologic, and ultrastructural study with an analysis of its calcifying process and pathogenesis. Am J Surg Pathol 1993; 17:788–802.
54. Topaz O, Shurman DL, Bergman R, et al. Mutations in GALNT3, encoding a protein involved in a-linked glycosylation, cause familial tumoral calcinosis. Nat Genet 2004; 36:579–581.
55. Brantus JF, Meunier PJ. Effects of intravenous etidronate and oral corticosteroids in fibrodysplasia ossificans progressiva. Clin Orthop 1998; 346:117–120.
56. Goldman AB. Collagen diseases, epiphyseal dysplasias, and related conditions. In: Resnick D, ed. Bone and Joint Imaging. 2nd ed. Philadelphia: W.B. Saunders, 1996:1109–1127.
57. Chichareon V, Arpornmaeklong P, Donsakul N. Fibrodysplasia ossificans progressiva and associated osteochondroma of the coronoid process in a child. Plast Reconstr Surg 1999; 103:1238–1243.

58. Smith R, Russell RG, Woods CG. Myositis ossificans progressiva. Clinical features of eight patients and their response to treatment. J Bone Joint Surg Br 1976; 58:48–57.
59. Sawyer JR, Klimkiewicz JJ, Iannotti JP, Rocke DM. Mechanism for superior subluxation of the glenohumeral joint in fibrodysplasia ossificans progressiva. Clin Orthop 1998; 346:130–133.
60. Druce M, Morris VH, Stamp TC. A case report of myositis ossificans progressiva complicated by femoral nerve compression treated with radiotherapy. Rheumatolgy (Oxford) 2002; 41:947–948.
61. Kussmaul WG, Esmail AN, Sagar Y, Ross J, Gregory S, Kaplan FS. Pulmonary and cardiac function in advanced fibrodysplasia ossificans progressiva. Clin Orthop 1998; 346:104–149.
62. Glaser DL, Rocke DM, Kaplan FS. Catastrophic falls in patients who have fibrodysplasia ossificans progressiva. Clin Orthop 1998; 346:110–116.
63. Dua T, Kabra M, Kalra V. Familial fibrodysplasia ossificans progressiva: trial with etidronate disodium. Indian Pediatr 2001; 38:1305–1309.
64. Rutsch F, Ruf N, Vaingankar S, et al. Mutations in ENPP1 are associated with 'idiopathic' infantile arterial calcification. Nat Genet 2003; 34:379–381.
65. Rutsch F, Vaingankar S, Johnson K, et al. PC-1 nucleoside triphosphate pyrophosphohydrolase deficiency in idiopathic infantile arterial calcification. Am J Pathol 2001; 158:543–554.
66. Rutsch F, Schauerte P, Kalhoff H, Petrarulo M, August C, Diekmann L. Low levels of urinary inorganic pyrophosphate indicating systemic pyrophosphate deficiency in a boy with idiopathic infantile arterial calcification. Acta Paediatr 2000; 89:1265–1269.
67. Stuart AG. Idiopathic arterial calcification of infancy and pyrophosphate deficiency. J Pediatr 1993; 123:170–171.
68. Van Dyck M, Proesmans W, Van Hollebeke E, Marchal G, Moerman P. Idiopathic infantile arterial calcification with cardiac, renal and central nervous system involvement. Eur J Pediatr 1989; 148:374–377.
69. Patel M, Andronikou S, Solomon R, Sinclair P, McCulloch M. Idiopathic arterial calcification in childhood. Pediatr Radiol 2004; 34:652–655.
70. Eronen M, Pohjavuori M, Heikkila P. Fatal outcome of two siblings with idiopathic arterial calcification of infancy diagnosed in utero. Pediatr Cardiol 2001; 22:167–169.
71. Sholler GF, Yu JS, Bale PM, Hawker RE, Celermajer JM, Kozlowski K. Generalized arterial calcification of infancy: three case reports, including spontaneous regression with long-term survival. J Pediatr 1984; 105:257–260.
72. Marcos JC, De Benyacar MA, Garcia-Morteo O, et al. Idiopathic familial chondrocalcinosis due to apatite crystal deposition. Am J Med 1981; 71:557–564.
73. Pons-Estel BA, Gimenez C, Sacnun M, et al. In: Familial Osteoarthritis and Milwaukee Shoulder Associated with Calcium Pyrophosphate and Apatite Crystal Deposition. J Rheumatol 2000; 27:471–480.
74. Cannon RB, Schmid FR. Calcific periarthritis involving multiple sites in identical twins. Arthritis Rheum 1973; 16:393–396.
75. Zaphiropoulos G. Recurrent calcific perarthritis involving multiple sites. Proc R Soc Med 1973; 66:351–352.

76. Caspi D, Rosenbach TO, Varon M, McCarty DJ, Graff E. Periarthritis associated with basic calcium phosphate crystal deposition and low levels of serum alkaline phosphatase report of three cases from one family. J Rheumatol 1988; 15:823–827.
77. Chuck AJ, Pattrick MG, Hamilton E, Wilson R, Doherty M. Crystal deposition in hypophosphatasia: a reappraisal. Ann Rheum Dis 1989; 48:571–576.
78. Hajiroussou VJ, Webley M. Familial calcific periarthritis. Ann Rheum Dis 1983; 42:469–470.
79. Lassere MN, Jones JG. Recurrent calcific periarthritis, erosive osteoarthritis and hypophosphatasia: a family study. J Rheumatol 1990; 17:1244–1248.
80. Doherty M, Dieppe PA. Multiple microcrystal deposition within a family. Ann Rheum Dis 1985; 44:544–548.
81. Jones G, Kingdon E, Sweny P, Davenport A. Tumoral calcinosis and calciphylaxis presenting in a dialysis patient. Nephrol Dial Transplant 2003; 18:2668–2670.
82. Sabeel A, Al-Homrany M. Complete resorption of massive soft tissue calcification in a hemodialysis patient after parathyroidectomy. Am J Nephrol 2000; 20:421–424.
83. Kay J, Bardin T. Osteoarticular disorders of renal origin: disease-related and iatrogenic. Baillieres Best Pract Res Clin Rheumatol 2000; 14:285–305.
84. Miller FW. Inflammatory myopathies: polymyositis, dermatomyositis, and related conditions. In: Koopman WJ, ed. Arthritis and Allied Conditions. 14th ed. Philadelphia: Lippincott Williams & Wilkins, 2001:1562–1590.
85. Walden CA, Gilbert P, Rogers LF, Hendrix RW. Case report 620. Progressive systemic sclerosis (PSS) with paraspinous and intraspinous calcifications. Skeletal Radiol 1990; 19:377–378.
86. Medsger TA. Systemic sclerosis (Scleroderma): clinical aspects. In: Koopman WJ, ed. Arthritis and Allied Conditions. 14th ed. Philadelphia: Lippincott Williams & Wilkins, 2001:1590–1624.
87. Rashad SM, Abdelaty EM, Rooney J, Schumacher HR, Jr. Acute inflammation at the site of calcinosis in limited cutaneous scieroderma. J Rheumatol 2002; 29:402–403.
88. Quismorio FP, Dubois EL, Chandor SB. Soft-tissue calcification in systemic lupus erythematosus. Arch Dermatol 1975; 111:352–356.
89. Weinberger A, Kaplan JG, Myers AR. Extensive soft tissue calcification (calcinosis universal is) in systemic lupus erythematosus. Ann Rheum Dis 1979; 38:384–386.
90. Hutton CW, Maddison PJ, Collins AJ, Berriman JA. Intra-articular apatite deposition in mixed connective tissue disease: crystallographic and technetium scanning characteristics. Ann Rheum Dis 1988; 47:1027–1030.
91. Dossick PH, Bansal M, Figgie MP, Boskey AL. Intramedullary deposits of hydroxyapatite crystals in a patient with rheumatoid arthritis. Clin Orthop 1994; 298:240–245.
92. Schweitzer ME, Cervilla V, Manaster BJ, et al. Cervical paraspinal calcification in collagen vascular diseases. AJR 1991; 157:523–525.
93. Resnick D. Soft tissues. In: Resnick D, ed. Bone and Joint Imaging. 2nd ed. Philadelphia: W.B. Saunders, 1996:1240–1272.
94. Grant GA, Wener MH, Yaziji H, et al. Destructive tophaceous calcium hydroxyapatite tumor of the infratemporal fossa. J Neurosurg 1999; 90:148–152.

95. Sirvanci M, Ganiyusufoglu AK, Karaman K, Tezer M, Hamzaoglu A. Myositis ossificans of psoas muscle: magnetic resonance imaging findings. Acta Radiol 2004; 45:523–525.
96. Siegert JJ, Wortmann RL. Myositis ossificans simulating acute monoarticular arthritis. J Rheumatol 1986; 13:652–654.
97. Hynes B, Lubynski RA. Perimandibular myositis ossificans. J Otolaryngol 2003; 32:205–206.
98. Chua KS, Kong KH. Acquired heterotopic ossification in the settings of cerebral anoxia and alternative therapy: two cases. Brain Inj 2003; 17:535–544.
99. Goldberg MA, Schumacher HR. Heteroropic ossification mimicking acute arthritis after neurologic catastrophes. Arch Int Med 1977; 137:619–621.
100. Stover SL, Niemann KM, Miller JM, III. Disodium etidronate in the prevention of postoperative recurrence of heterotopic ossification in spinal-cord injury patients. J Bone Joint Surg Am 1976; 58:683–688.
101. van Kuijk AA, Geurts AC, van Kuppevelt HJ. Neurogenic heterotopic ossification in spinal cord injury. Spinal Cord 2002; 40:313–326.
102. Mu SC, Lin CH, Sung TC. Calcinosis cutis following extravasation of calcium gluconate in neonates. Acta Paediatr Taiwan 1999; 40:34–35.
103. Speer ME, Rudolph AJ. Calcification of superficial scalp veins secondary to intravenous infusion of sodium bicarbonate and calcium chloride. Cutis 1983; 32:65–66.
104. Gerster JC, Fallet GH. Periarticular hand hydroxyapatite deposition after corticosteroid injections. J Rheumatol 1987; 14:1156–1159.
105. Ohira T, Ishikawa K. Hydroxyapatite deposition in articular cartilage by intra-articular injections of methylprednisolone. A histological, ultrastructural, and x-ray-microprobe analysis in rabbits. J Bone Joint Surg Am 1986; 68:509–520.
106. Ullman HR, Dasgupta A, Recht M, Cash JM. CT of dystrophic calcification in subcutaneous soft tissues secondary to chronic insulin injection. J Comput Assist Tomogr 1995; 19:657–659.
107. Skidmore RA, Davis DA, Woosley JT, McCauliffe DP. Massive dystrophic calcinosis cutis secondary to chronic needle trauma. Cutis 1997; 60:259–262.
108. DiGiovanna JJ, Helfgott RK, Gerber LH, Peck GL. Extraspinal tendon and ligament calcification associated with long-term therapy with etretinate. N Engl J Med 1986; 315:1177–1182.
109. DiGiovanna JJ. Isotretinoin effects on bone. J Am Acad Dermatol 2001; 45:S176–S182.
110. Duthie JS, Solanki HP, Krishnamurthy M, Chectow BS. Milk-alkali syndrome with metastatic calcification. Am J Med 1995; 99:102–103.

8

Differential Diagnosis of Monarthritis

Kevin D. Deane and Sterling G. West

Division of Rheumatology, University of Colorado Health Sciences Center, Denver, Colorado, U.S.A.

INTRODUCTION

Pain in one joint area may occur due to a problem with the joint (arthritis, internal derangement), from adjacent bone (fracture, tumor, osteomyelitis), or from surrounding soft tissues (ligament, bursa, tendon, muscle, or nerve). Arthritis generally causes diffuse joint pain which is aggravated by movement. The presence of an effusion and limitation of active and passive range of motion in all planes strongly supports an intra-articular process, although these findings may also result from a problem in the adjacent bone. Alternatively, a juxta-articular bone or soft tissue problem usually has localized pain and limitation of active range of motion in only one plane with preserved passive motion.

The purpose of this chapter is to discuss the diagnostic approach and differential diagnosis of acute and chronic monoarticular arthritis. Although almost any cause of arthritis including those that are traditionally polyarticular (e.g., rheumatoid arthritis) may begin as a monarthritis, there are a relatively limited number that commonly present as arthritis of a single joint (Table 1).

The causes of monarthritis can be divided into two groups: inflammatory and noninflammatory disorders. Of the various causes, infectious arthritis, crystal-induced arthritis, and traumatic arthritis are the most important for the evaluating physician to rule out initially since these conditions require an urgent diagnosis with differing and aggressive therapies (1,2).

DIAGNOSTIC APPROACH

History

The history and physical examination are helpful in narrowing the differential diagnosis in a patient presenting with monarthritis. The initial evaluation should

Table 1 Causes of Monarthritis

Acute (<4 wk)	Chronic (>4 wk)
Inflammatory	**Inflammatory**
Infection	Infection
Bacterial	Fungi
Viral	Mycobacteria
Brucella	Lyme disease[a]
Lyme disease[a]	Whipple's disease[a]
Fungi (candida)[a]	Osteomyelitis
Whipple's disease[a]	Parasites/spirochetes (syphilis)
Crystalline	Autoimmune
Gout	Rheumatoid arthritis[a] (adult, juvenile)
Pseudogout[a]	Seronegative spondyloarthritis[a]
Basic calcium phosphate	Behcet's disease
Calcium oxalate	Other
Autoimmune	Sarcoidosis[a]
Rheumatoid arthritis (adult, juvenile)	Foreign body (plant thorn, sea urchin spine)
Systemic lupus erythmatosis	
Seronegative spondyloarthropathies[a]	**Non-inflammatory**
Palindromic rheumatism	Tumors
Still's disease	Pigmented villonodular synovitis[b]
Rheumatic fever	Metastatic tumors
Relapsing polychondritis	Osteogenic sarcoma
Intestinal disease[a]	Synovioma
Crohn's disease	Osteoid osteoma
Ulcerative colitis	Osteochondroma
Intestinal bypass	Paraneoplastic syndromes
Pancreatic fat necrosis	Amyloidosis
Other	Metabolic conditions
Sarcoidosis[a]	Hemachromatosis
Hereditary periodic fever syndromes	Wilson's disease
Non-inflammatory	Gaucher's disease
Trauma	Other
Internal derangement[a,b]	Osteoarthritis
Fracture[b]	Hypertrophic osteoarthropathy
Prosthetic loosening[a]	Legg-Calve-Perthes disease
Hemoglobinopathies[a,b]	Slipped capital femoral epiphysis
Transient osteoporosis	Neuropathic arthropathy
Hemarthrosis	
Osteonecrosis[a]	

[a]May be acute or chronic.
[b]Frequently hemorrhagic.

focus on the time course of the joint symptoms and whether or not inflammatory signs are present. Diffuse pain at rest and with normal use, prolonged stiffness which is worse in the morning or after inactivity (gelling), and the presence of swelling with an effusion, warmth, erythema, and limited range of motion are all characteristics of an inflammatory arthritis.

The acute onset of inflammatory symptoms and signs which rapidly reach peak intensity within hours to a few days always requires immediate evaluation to rule out an infectious or crystalline arthritis. If symptoms acutely occur following an injury then traumatic arthritis, internal derangement (meniscal tear or ligamentous injury), or intraarticular fracture with hemarthrosis should be considered. In patients with a known polyarticular arthritis (i.e., rheumatoid arthritis) who develop an acutely inflamed joint out of proportion to their other joint disease, an infection (and rarely crystal-induced arthritis) must be urgently excluded (3,4). Likewise, infection and hardware loosening should be considered in patients with pain and swelling in a prosthetic joint.

A history of previous episodes of an intensely painful inflammatory monoarticular arthritis that resolves spontaneously in a few days suggests a non-infectious cause such as crystalline arthritis or palindromic rheumatism. If the skin overlying the inflamed joint desquamates following the attack, a crystal-induced arthritis is the most likely diagnosis (5).

Patients with more prolonged symptoms (greater than 4 weeks) can be a diagnostic challenge. Chronic inflammatory monoarticular arthritic symptoms are seen in patients with an infectious arthritis due to slow-growing organisms (fungal, mycobacterial), foreign body synovitis due to penetrating trauma, or an autoimmune process such as a seronegative spondyloarthropathy or pauciarticular juvenile idiopathic arthritis (1,2). As noted above, virtually any cause of a polyarticular inflammatory arthritis may start as a monarthritis.

Chronic monarthritis lacking characteristic signs of inflammation is typical of osteoarthritis and internal derangements where symptoms wax and wane depending on joint use. Notably, knee osteoarthritis may on occasion present with a tense and warm effusion that does not wane. Locking of the joint is common with an internal derangement (torn meniscus, loose bodies). Important but less common causes of locking such as synovial or bony tumors should also be considered.

The sex, age, and ethnicity of the patient may help to narrow the differential in a patient with monarthritis. Pauciarticular juvenile idiopathic arthritis can present as a monarthritis, frequently associated with a chronic uveitis, most commonly in a young girl under the age of 5 (6). In slightly older children, slipped capital femoral epiphysis or Legg-Calve-Perthes disease are common causes of hip pain. Caucasian males under the age of 40 are more likely to develop a seronegative spondyloarthropathy. Young, sexually active individuals are most at risk to develop gonococcal septic arthritis. Males over the age of 25 to 30 of any ethnicity, but particularly South Pacific Islanders and Asians, are the most likely to develop gout, whereas premenopausal females rarely develop this disorder unless they have an underlying metabolic disorder (5,7). Individuals older than 55 to 60 years are the most common group to develop chondrocalcinosis and pseudogout (8). Family history may be important especially if the monarthritis occurs in a patient with a family history of gout, psoriasis, or a seronegative spondyloarthropathy.

The joint affected by the monarthritis may also be helpful in identifying the cause. The knee more than other weight-bearing joints is most commonly involved in an acute or chronic infectious arthritis. Acute infections of fibrocartilaginous joints (sternoclavicular, sacroiliac, symphysis pubis, and spinal disc) are seen more commonly in intravenous drug users, while chronic infections of the sacroiliac joint or spine are seen in mycobacterial, brucella, and Blastomyces infections (9–12). In gout, the first metatarsophalangeal joint is most commonly involved, but any joint can be affected (5). In contrast, with pseudogout, the knee and the wrist are more commonly involved (8). Seronegative spondyloarthropathies such as reactive arthritis preferentially involve lower extremity joints, while osteoarthritis and osteonecrosis preferentially affect the hip and knee (13).

The presence of past or current extra-articular manifestations may provide important clues to the etiology of acute monoarticular symptoms. Fever suggests infection, although it can be seen with crystal-induced arthritis, Still's disease, and familial periodic fever syndromes. A history of a rash such as psoriasis, erythema chronicum migrans (Lyme disease), or erythema nodusum (inflammatory bowel disease, sarcoid arthritis) is helpful. Recurrent painful oral and genital ulcers may indicate Behcet's disease or inflammatory bowel disease. Other important associated symptoms include a history of diarrhea or abdominal pain, urethral discharge, low back pain, and uveitis which may indicate a reactive arthritis or other seronegative spondyloarthropathy.

A review of the patient's concomitant medical conditions is extremely important. The use of anticoagulants or a history of a bleeding disorder predisposes a person to a hemarthrosis. Certain disorders like renal insufficiency, obesity, and alcoholism or use of medications such as diuretics and cyclosporine among others are associated with gouty arthritis, while hyperparathyroidism and hemochromatosis are associated with chondrocalcinosis and pseudogout. Sexual history should be elicited to help exclude gonococcal arthritis and human immunodeficiency virus (HIV) exposures. A history of blood transfusions or intravenous drug use puts a patient at risk for hepatitis C, HIV, or septic arthritis. Patients with immunodeficiency, a history of splenectomy, or on immunosuppressive medications are predisposed to infectious arthritis from any organism. High dose corticosteroid use may cause osteonecrosis. Finally, pregnancy has been associated with transient osteoporosis of the hip which can present with acute symptoms mimicking a septic joint or osteonecrosis. A similar disorder, termed transient osteoporosis of the knee, has also been seen in other conditions including runners and middle-aged obese females (14).

Travel history or a history of a tick bite in an endemic area may indicate Lyme disease. Travel history can also be instrumental in determining if a fungal infection such as coccidioidomycosis or histoplasmosis should be considered. Certain avocations may lead to exposures that might predispose to unusual causes of monarthritis such as gardening (plant thorn synovitis), water and fish exposures (atypical mycobacterial infection, sea urchin spine synovitis), or ingestion of unpasteurized dairy products (brucellosis).

Physical Examination

The physical examination in a patient with monoarticular symptoms should be used to verify the presence of historical features as well as additional findings that the patient may not report. Vital signs can help determine the severity of illness, with fever the most important. Rashes reported by the patient should be examined, keeping in mind that the findings may be subtle and not noticed by the patient. For example, psoriatic skin lesions may only be present behind the ears or in the anal crease, while patients with reactive arthritis may not have noted the keratoderma blennorrhagicum lesions on the soles of their feet. Likewise, gouty tophi should be looked for on the ears, elbows, and other peripheral sites. Ocular inflammation, mouth sores, and heme-positive stools should be sought. The presence of a cardiac murmur (suggesting endocarditis), pneumonia, cellulitis, or throat infection may indicate the source for a patient's infectious arthritis.

In addition to the symptomatic joint, other joints should be examined to make sure the arthritis is truly monoarticular. Particular attention should be given to the spine examination to rule out an underlying spondyloarthropathy. Upon examination of the symptomatic joint, the presence of warmth, erythema, tenderness, effusion, stability, and range of motion should all be documented. Care must be taken to ensure that the joint is truly involved and not symptomatic due to an adjacent process in the bone or soft tissue. Likewise, if the joint appears normal, referred pain from another site such as from the hip to the knee should be considered.

Synovial Fluid Analysis

Although the history and physical examination can provide important clinical clues, a definite diagnosis frequently requires an arthrocentesis with synovial fluid analysis. It is mandatory to perform an arthrocentesis if an infected joint is possible. Synovial fluid analysis will also confirm if the fluid is inflammatory and if a hemarthrosis or crystals are present. Arthrocentesis can be performed in almost any patient, including those on anticoagulants provided the INR is less than 5.0 (15).

Studies that can be performed on synovial fluid analysis include a gross examination, total white blood cell (WBC) count with differential, culture, gram stain, and examination of wet preparation for crystals, fat, and other microscopic abnormalities (16,17). All these studies can be performed on as little as 1 milliliter of fluid. When only a few drops are available, one drop can provide an estimated leukocyte count (each WBC seen per high-powered field at 40X magnification equals 500 cells/mm^3). Another drop can be used for crystal examination and gram stain. A third drop can be sent for routine culture.

Normal synovial fluid is clear, viscous, and does not clot. Inflammatory synovial fluid is cloudy (due to an elevated WBC count), watery, and may clot spontaneously. Hemarthrosis can be seen with traumatic arthritis, fracture, pigmented villonodular synovitis (PVNS), synovial hemangiomas, Charcot joints, and bleeding due to a coagulopathy or complication of anticoagulation therapy. Fat floating on top of a bloody joint aspirate suggests an intraarticular fracture with release of bone marrow elements into the synovial fluid.

Normal synovial fluid contains less than 200 WBCs/mm^3 with a mononuclear cell predominance. A noninflammatory fluid usually contains less than 1000 WBCs/mm^3. Synovial fluid with over 2000 WBCs/mm^3 indicates an inflammatory cause for the monarthritis. The higher the leukocyte count and the higher the percentage of neutrophils, the more likely an infection is present. Synovial fluids with greater than 100,000 WBCs/mm^3 and a predominance of polymorphonuclear leukocytes in the differential should be concerning for infection, although many cases of septic arthritis have lower WBC counts (18). Alternatively, some noninfectious causes of monoarticular inflammation, including crystal-induced arthritis, can have very high synovial fluid WBC counts. However, the presence of crystals in synovial fluids with high WBC counts does not rule out infection, because the two conditions can occur simultaneously in the same joint (19).

An inflammatory synovial fluid should be sent for gram stain and bacterial culture. The frequency of a positive gram stain differs depending on the infecting organism. In culture-positive specimens, gram-positive bacteria appear on gram stain over 80% of the time, and gram-negative organisms are seen only 50% of the time (20). In selected patients who are immunosuppressed or with an undiagnosed chronic inflammatory monarthritis, special stains and cultures for fungi and mycobacterial organisms should be obtained. Polymerase chain reaction (PCR) of synovial fluid may be used to identify DNA from organisms that are notoriously difficult to culture with standard techniques. Such agents include Borrelia burgdorferi (Lyme disease), Neisseria organisms, mycobacterial organisms, and Tropheryma whipplei (responsible for Whipple's disease).

The synovial fluid should be examined for crystals and other microscopic abnormalities (see Chapter 9 for more detailed information). Monosodium urate (MSU) crystals are needle-shaped, easily seen on polarized light microscopy, and negatively birefringent. Calcium pyrophosphate dihydrate (CPPD) crystals are rhomboid or block-shaped, smaller, and less bright with polarized light microscopy than MSU crystals, and positively birefringent. Basic calcium phosphate or apatite crystals are the hardest to identify. With light and polarized microscopy these crystals look like nondescript shiny debris (shiny coins) and with Wright's staining, they may appear as purple clumps inside of neutrophils or mononuclear cells. While the crystalline structure of basic calcium phosphate cannot be seen with standard microscopy, it can be determined with electron microscopy (21). Special preparation of synovial fluid with Alizarin red S stain can confirm that these are calcium-containing crystals. Rarely, calcium oxalate crystals which have a bipyramidal appearance are seen, especially in patients with chronic renal failure (17). Another important microscopic abnormality includes fat droplets which suggest an intraarticular fracture into the marrow space, osteonecrosis, or pancreatic fat necrosis due to elevations in circulating lipase from a diseased pancreas. Stains such as Oil red O can confirm the presence of fat droplets (21). Synovial fluid protein, lactate dehydrogenase (LDH), and glucose determinations add little information. Low synovial fluid glucose levels 40 mg% less than a corresponding fasting serum glucose suggest an infection. Urate concentration, rheumatoid factor (RF), antinuclear antibodies (ANA), and complement levels should not be obtained on a synovial fluid analysis.

Laboratory Tests

A limited number of laboratory tests are helpful in the evaluation of monarthritis. A complete blood count showing an elevated leukocyte level and an elevated erythrocyte sedimentation rate or C-reactive protein are not specific but should be present in a patient with an infectious arthritis (22). In cases of suspected crystal-induced arthritis, an elevated serum urate level does not confirm gout as the cause of the patient's monarthritis. Conversely, the serum urate level may be in the normal range during an acute gout flare (5). Measurement of the serum creatinine and liver-associated enzymes may be indicated if a systemic disease is suspected or the use of a nonsteroidal anti-inflammatory drug is anticipated. Elevated serum lipase or amylase may be present in cases of arthritis due to pancreatic fat necrosis. A protime (PT), partial thromboplastin time (PTT), platelet count, and bleeding time should be obtained on a patient with an unexplained hemarthrosis. Serologic testing for syphilis, HIV, Lyme disease, and other more unusual infections such as brucellosis or fungal infections may be helpful in selected cases since synovial fluid cultures are often negative in patients with monarthritis due to these diseases. In Whipple's disease, PCR analysis of peripheral blood may rarely identify the organism. In a patient with suspected reactive arthritis, genital-urethral swabs for evidence of Chlamydial infection can be useful. Also in cases of reactive arthritis, stool cultures for pathogenic organisms (Yersinia, Campylobacter, Shigella, and Salmonella species) may be helpful in making a diagnosis and guiding therapy with antimicrobial agents. Rarely, in cases of arthritis associated with occult inflammatory bowel disease or Whipple's disease, intestinal biopsy may need to be performed in order to confirm a diagnosis.

In a patient with suspected infectious arthritis, blood, urine, and synovial fluid cultures should be obtained with the caveat that these cultures are not always positive, particularly in patients who have a gonococcal septic arthritis (25–50% positive) (23). These patients should also have oropharyngeal, cervical-urethral, and rectal cultures performed using Thayer-Martin medium. Cultures for gonococcus from normally sterile sites including synovial or tenosynovial fluid and skin lesions should be placed on chocolate agar without impregnated antibiotics. In appropriate individuals with a chronic inflammatory monarthritis, synovial fluid stains and cultures for fungi and mycobacteria, as well as tuberculosis skin testing, can be helpful. Serologies such as RF and ANA are usually not indicated, although an occasional rheumatoid arthritis patient may initially present with a monarthritis (24). A young child with monarthritis (usually knee) due to juvenile idiopathic arthritis frequently has a positive ANA.

Radiography

Except for soft tissue swelling and the identification of intra-articular fluid, plain radiography is unremarkable in most cases of acute monarthrits. However, in the appropriate clinical setting, radiographs may be helpful in establishing a diagnosis. The findings of chondrocalcinosis or osteoarthritic changes suggest these diagnoses, although these findings on radiography do not prove the etiology without corresponding synovial fluid analysis. Other potentially important radiographic findings include tumors, fractures, osteomyelitis, loose bodies, osteonecrosis, or Paget's disease, all of which may not be readily suspected on history and physical examination.

Radionuclide bone scans are sensitive but not specific for bone and joint abnormalities. These scans may be particularly useful to confirm abnormalities in deep joints such as the spine, sacroiliac joints, or hips. Computerized tomography (CT) scanning can detect fractures and other bony abnormalities. However, in most cases, magnetic resonance imaging (MRI) is superior to CT scanning in detecting bony abnormalities such as osteonecrosis, tumors, fractures, and osteomyelitis. MRI is also superior to other modalities for detecting soft tissue abnormalities including meniscal or ligamentous injuries, loose bodies, and PVNS (25). More recently, MRI has been shown to be a powerful tool in detecting early erosive changes in rheumatoid arthritis and other inflammatory conditions, but the clinical usefulness of this aspect of MR imaging in the evaluation of an acute monarthritis has yet to be determined (26). Ultrasound has limited value in the evaluation of an acute monarthritis, but may be better than other imaging modalities at identifying foreign bodies in patients with foreign body synovitis (27,28).

Synovial Biopsy

A synovial biopsy obtained by closed needle technique or during arthroscopy should be obtained in patients with an unexplained chronic monarthritis (1,29). Patients with chronic arthritis due to fungal, mycobacterial, or spirochete infections often have negative synovial fluid cultures. These infections can be confirmed in nearly all cases with culture and special staining of synovial tissue. Synovial biopsy is also useful to diagnose infiltrative diseases such as PVNS, tumors, amyloidosis, and sarcoidosis.

Closed needle biopsy has the advantage of being less traumatic and less expensive, while arthroscopic biopsy can observe the joint pathology directly as well as obtain a larger synovial biopsy for more extensive testing. Due to the difficulty in removing foreign bodies, an open surgical biopsy is indicated in patients with foreign body synovitis. In patients with suspected infections of fibrocartilaginous joints, open surgical biopsy is also necessary if radiographically-guided needle biopsy is non-diagnostic.

SPECIFIC DISEASES THAT CAUSE MONARTHRITIS

The preceding discussion describes the appropriate diagnostic approach when evaluating a patient presenting with a monarthritis, including historical features, examination findings, laboratory testing, synovial analysis, and radiographic imaging. What follows is a more detailed discussion of the specific etiologies of both acute and chronic monoarticular arthritis that should be considered in the differential diagnosis of crystal-associated diseases.

Infections

Bacterial. As the most destructive and life-threatening of the causes of an acute monarthritis, bacterial infection must be considered whenever a patient presents with acute joint symptoms. Typically patients with septic arthritis present with a rapidly worsening, painful, swollen joint of a few days duration, although multiple joints can be involved. Systemic findings such as fevers or other organ system involvement are often present and can lead to an early suspicion for infection (30). In general, large joints are more often affected than small joints, with the knee and the hip being most commonly involved (31).

The age of the patient can have significant bearing on the organism responsible for the arthritis (32). In sexually active adults, gonococcal infections are the most common cause of septic arthritis, and can often present with concomitant tenosynovitis and a characteristic pustular rash (33). Usually, the monarthritis seen with disseminated gonococcal infections develops after a prodrome of polyarthralgia and polyarthritis. In many patients, an antecedent history of symptoms of a sexually-transmitted disease is absent (33). Synovial fluid from patients with gonococcal arthritis typically has an elevated leukocyte count, although levels below 10,000 cells/mm^3 have been reported (23). Other diagnostic strategies for determining if a gonoccocal infection is present have been discussed earlier.

Non-gonococcal organisms comprise the next group of pathogens leading to septic arthritis. In this category, Staphylococcus aureus is most commonly implicated in septic arthritis in adults, with other pathogens such as Streptococcal species and gram-negative organisms playing lesser roles. Polymicrobial joint infections are rare but have been reported (34).

Prosthetic joint infections are typically caused by gram-positive organisms, with coagulase-negative organisms predominating in early post-surgical infections and *Staphylococcus aureus* being more common in later infections. Gram-negative prosthetic joint infections are possible, and in one series accounted for 14% of total prosthetic hip infections (35). Anaerobic prosthetic joint infections are more unusual but have been identified in up to 8% of infections (35).

Encapsulated organisms such as *Streptococcus pneumoniae* and *Neisseria* species are seen less commonly in septic arthritis, but can lead to disease in immunocompromised hosts such as surgically splenectomized patients or those with functional asplenia from diseases such as sickle-cell anemia or systemic lupus erythematosus (30).

Viral Arthritis. Viral pathogens can lead to an acute arthritis, although the usual presentation is polyarticular and symmetric with signs of systemic illness varying depending on the type of viral infection (36–39). HIV is associated with an acute monoarticular arthritis, typically presenting as an acutely painful joint with features of a seronegative spondyloarthropathy (40,41). Varicella zoster dermatomal involvement may mimic a septic joint, but is likely due to nerve root involvement rather than true joint inflammation. Also, initial infection with the varicella zoster virus (chickenpox) may lead to an acute monarthritis (42). The discovery of new viruses such as human retrovirus-5 (HRV-5) and human T-cell leukemia virus-1 (HTLV-1), which have been associated with synovitis in several arthritis syndromes, may imply that some cases of unexplained monarthritis may be viral in origin (40,43).

Lyme Arthritis. Lyme disease is caused by the spirochete, *Borrelia burgdorferi*, and occurs after an individual has been bitten by a tick harboring the organism, usually in the spring or summer months. The disease has been reported in nearly all of the 50 United States as well as in Europe and Russia, but the majority of cases in the U.S. are from the Northeast and upper Midwest regions. The illness is characterized by a rash (erythema migrans) and multiple organ system involvement. Articular involvement in Lyme disease includes migratory arthralgias within the first weeks after infection, monoarticular or polyarticular arthritis usually developing within days or weeks of initial infection and often involving the knee, and a chronic form of arthritis diagnosed if symptoms persist longer than 1 year (44). Lyme disease as a cause of acute monoarticular arthritis should be considered in any individuals with a history of appropriate geographic exposure. Serologies are usually performed to establish the diagnosis as the *Borrelia* organism is difficult to culture from body tissue samples, although PCR techniques can be used on synovial samples to establish the diagnosis.

Brucellosis. Although an uncommon cause of arthritis in the United States, brucellosis is an important cause of acute infectious mono- or polyarticular arthritis in much of the rest of the world (12). In humans, the disease is caused by several species of Brucella. Humans acquire the infection generally through ingestion of contaminated food, usually dairy products. In the United States, cases of brucellosis are most commonly linked to the consumption of unpasteurized dairy products often found in foods of Latin American origin.

The acute systemic illness is characterized by fever, hepatosplenomegaly, and cytopenias. Multiple musculoskeletal manifestations of brucellosis can occur including sacroiliitis, peripheral arthritis, osteomyelitis, and spinal infection. The peripheral arthritis is usually monoarticular and in the lower extremity, with the knee being the most common joint involved, although upper extremity involvement with the elbow and shoulder is also seen. A self-limited form of arthritis may occur and likely represents a sterile, reactive-type arthritis. True joint infections with brucella organisms require antibiotic therapy and often drainage (12). The diagnosis can be made either from direct culture or serologic analysis.

Mycobacterial Arthritis. Mycobacterium tuberculosis can lead to peripheral monoarticular arthritis, although typically the clinical course is indolent and rarely presents as an acute monarthritis (45). Most of these patients will have a positive tuberculosis skin test (PPD) (>90%); however, only 30% of patients will have evidence of pulmonary tuberculosis (46). The pathogenesis of the disease usually involves hematogenous spread of the mycobacterial organisms from the site of primary infection, although local extension from osteomyelitis or superficial infections may occur (46). Acid-fast staining of synovial fluid is positive in only 10–20%. Cultures of synovial fluid improve yield to approximately 80%, with synovial tissue culture yields of up to 94% (47). PCR analysis has even higher yield and is becoming more commonly available, although cultures still need to be performed for assessment of drug sensitivities (48).

Infections with atypical mycobacterial organisms including *M. marinum, M. kansasii*, and *M. avium-intracellulare* have also been reported (49). Again, these infections are usually indolent, and can be difficult to diagnose as tuberculosis skin testing is often negative and chest radiography is usually normal. Patients are often immunosuppressed, but these organisms have been implicated in infections in normal hosts (49).

Poncet's disease, an acute mono- or polyarticular sterile arthritis in the setting of an active mycobacterial infection elsewhere in the body, has also been described. The arthritis is usually seen in the lower extremities and is thought to be a form of reactive arthritis (50).

Fungal Arthritis. Multiple fungal species can lead to articular syndromes, but in developed countries, *Sporothrix* species are the most common cause of fungal joint infections. Sporotrichosis can lead to an acute monarthritis by direct joint invasion from nearby cutaneous lesions or hematogenous seeding, but can also result in a diffuse arthritis if the infection becomes systemic (51).

Infection with *Histoplasmosis capsulatum* can lead to polyarthralgia and at times a mono- or oligoarticular arthritis (52). In the United States, histoplasmosis can present with hilar adenopathy and erythema nodosum, mimicking acute sarcoidosis (52). The articular manifestations are usually self-limiting, although true septic joints have been reported, especially in Africa where the organism *H. capsulatum var. duboisii* has a tendency to cause osteomyelitis with extension of infection into adjacent joints.

Infection with *Coccidioides immitis*, the etiologic agent of Valley Fever, can also lead to acute mono- or polyarticular arthritis, and can be seen in up to 8% of primary infections (53). This acute arthritis is usually self-limiting and thought to be part of a reactive process rather than true infection (54). However, in disseminated coccidioidomycosis, a chronic infectious arthritis can occur.

Other fungal infections including blastomycosis, paracoccidioides, cryptococcus, aspergillus, and candida can also present with chronic monoarticular arthritis in an immunocompromised host. Both candida and blastomycosis can also cause acute monoarticular arthritis (51).

Other Infections. Rare infectious causes of monoarticular arthritis include parasitic infections with protozoans, nematodes, or trematodes. Arthritis caused by these organisms is usually chronic in nature, and affected individuals have a history of travel to endemic areas or immunosuppression (55). Other rare forms of monarthritis include syphilitic arthritis and leprosy, which typically cause chronic symptoms.

Crystalline Arthritis

Crystal deposition is one of the most common causes of rapid-onset monoarticular arthritis, especially in men over 40. However, as this text is dedicated to the discussion of crystalline arthropathies, we will only briefly discuss these here.

Monosodium urate (MSU) and calcium pyrophosphate dihydrate (CPPD) crystals are the most common etiologies of crystalline arthropathy, leading to the clinical syndromes of gout and pseudogout respectively. Calcium hydroxyapatite is also a cause of acute arthropathy, but more often is associated with tendonitis or periarthritis, although true arthritis can develop. Other forms of crystalline arthropathy such as calcium oxalate-induced arthritis in renal failure patients and lipid crystals are more rare.

Gout. In most cases, gouty attacks present as acute pain, swelling, warmth, and redness in a joint. The pain felt during a flare of gout is often severe and reaches a maximum intensity at times within hours of the initial onset, unlike septic arthritis which often has a more gradual onset of pain. The overlying erythema can have a similar appearance to a cellulitis, especially if the flare is in the midfoot region. Fever can be present, although it rarely exceeds 102 degrees Fahrenheit. Gouty attacks are typically self-limiting, usually lasting from days to weeks, but in some cases inflammation can persist leading to chronic inflammatory arthritis. The joints most commonly involved in order of decreasing frequency include the first metatarsophalangeal (MTP) joint, the midfoot, the ankle, and the knee. Less commonly involved are the wrists, fingers, and elbows. Over time, greater than 90% of patients with gout will experience first MTP joint involvement, and eliciting this history can be helpful in making a diagnosis. Gouty flares are usually monarticular, although polyarticular flares can be seen, especially in patients with conditions that predispose to high serum levels of uric acid including diuretic use, renal insufficiency, or renal transplant. Gout is more common in men than women, with a ratio of approximately 5:1. This difference is thought to be due to a protective effect of estrogen on uric acid metabolism (7). Factors associated with gout include family history, renal insufficiency, alcohol intake, high purine intake, and the use of medications that can elevate uric acid levels including diuretics, cyclosporine, ethambutol, and pyrazinamide. The synovial fluid from an acute gouty attack is typically inflammatory with leukocyte counts ranging from 20,000 to over 100,000 WBCs/mm^3. As mentioned earlier, the presence of crystals does not eliminate the possibility of infection and synovial fluid should always be cultured (19). In early disease, radiographs are often normal, or show only acute changes such as soft tissue swelling or effusions. However, late in disease, erosive changes with characteristic sclerotic rims can be seen (56).

Pseudogout: The clinical presentation of pseudogout arthropathy can be quite similar to that of gout with acute onset of pain, swelling, redness, and warmth in a joint. However, with pseudogout, the peak onset of pain is generally slower than that seen with gout, and maximal pain may be somewhat less (8). Similar to gouty flares, most patients will have self-limited attacks lasting from days to weeks, but in a small percentage of individuals, a persistent inflammatory arthritis may develop. Systemic findings in pseudogout flares may be more common than in their gouty counterparts. Fevers can range up to 103°F, and in the elderly mental status changes can be present (8). Pseudogout flares are often precipitated by physical stress such as a concomitant illness or surgery, often leading to flares several days after hospitaltization for other illnesses. The pattern of joint involvement seen with pseudogout flares differs slightly from joints involved with gout. In pseudogout, the knees are most commonly affected, followed by wrists, fingers, hips, shoulders, elbows, and ankles. Shoulder involvement with gout is rare, and correspondingly, first MTP involvement with pseudogout is unusual.

During acute flares, peripheral leukocytosis may be present. Synovial fluid is generally inflammatory with crystals present. MSU and CPPD crystals can be present in the same joint, as can infection, so these diagnoses must be considered (56). Radiographs show chondrocalcinosis in the majority of cases; however, its absence does not eliminate CPPD as the cause of an acute monarthritis.

Basic Calcium Phosphate: Calcium hydroxyapatite crystals are part of a larger group of basic calcium phosphate (BCP) crystals that can lead to arthritic syndromes. BCP crystal deposition can lead to calcific tendinitis, calcific periarthritis, and joint arthropathy, specifically the Milwaukee shoulder syndrome (56, 58). While the inflammation engendered is often in periarticular structures, the proximity to the joint can mimic acute monarthritis, and in the case of the Milwaukee shoulder syndrome, can involve the true joint. Attacks of acute calcific periarthritis can occur in multiple regions of the body. In young women, attacks can occur at the first MTP joint, mimicking a gouty flare (59). However, on joint aspiration, no gout crystals will be seen, and occasionally tendon calcification will be seen on radiography. Attacks elsewhere in the body can occur after trauma, or occasionally spontaneously. The Milwaukee shoulder can present as an acute monoarthritis or as a more indolent process, usually in women above the age of 70 (58). Synovial fluid is usually non-inflammatory although it may be bloody, and radiographs typically show severe degenerative changes of the shoulder. A similar syndrome due to BCP crystals has also been described in finger joints. The appropriate clinical setting with non-inflammatory synovial fluid, absence of MSU or CPPD crystals, and radiographs showing calcified tendinous structures can help make the diagnosis of BCP-associated arthropathy. The identification of basic calcium phosphate crystals by microscopy was described earlier in this chapter.

Traumatic Arthritis

Trauma is perhaps the most straightforward of the causes of an acute monarthritis to identify. Typically, the patient will describe joint pain and swelling occurring within seconds to minutes after the injury. Features of the patient's description of the injury can help to isolate the particular injury. Falls onto an outstretched wrist may result in fracture or ligamentous injury. Lateral knee injuries may indicate meniscal or ligamentous injury, while abrupt stopping or twisting injuries may indicate cruciate tears. An acutely injured joint may be warm, swollen, and tender, mimicking an inflammatory process. In patients who are poor historians, careful attention needs to be made to ensure an inflammatory process did not precede the perceived joint injury (57). Hemorrhagic synovial fluid containing fat droplets in the setting of trauma should lead to consideration of a fracture.

Osteoarthritis

Osteoarthritis is a common disease and can present with an acute or chronic monoarticular arthritis. Typically the patient has a history of pain in the joint that may have worsened with increased activity or minor trauma. If loose bodies are present, the patient may describe joint locking or intermittent pain. On examination, an effusion can be present, as can mild warmth. Examination findings of other joints with features typical of OA such as Bouchard's or Heberden's nodes may help narrow the differential. Erosive osteoarthritis may more commonly present with inflammatory symptoms.

Autoimmune Disease

Autoimmune diseases that affect the joints typically involve multiple sites in a symmetric fashion. However, these diseases uncommonly can present with an acute-onset monoarticular arthritis which may persist and become a chronic monarthritis.

Rheumatoid arthritis can present with monoarticular symptoms, both as an initial manifestation in an undiagnosed patient and in a patient with established disease (24). Special care must be taken not to miss a septic joint in a patient with established rheumatoid arthritis who flares in just one joint. Pseudoseptic arthritis can also be present in patients with rheumatoid arthritis, presenting as an acute monarthritis with synovial leukocyte counts exceeding 100,000 WBCs/mm^3 (61). Pseudosepsis usually occurs when there has been a change in therapy in a patient with known RA, but infection must always be ruled out. Crystal-induced arthropathies can occur in patients with rheumatoid arthritis or systemic lupus erythematosus, but they are rare. Nevertheless, they should also be considered in the differential diagnosis (4).

Palindromic rheumatism, a possible variant of rheumatoid arthritis, can cause dramatic acute monoarticular arthritis. A history of previous episodes of similar joint pain in the presence or absence of a positive rheumatoid factor (RF) may help clarify this diagnosis (62). Patients will often present with a rapid onset of symptoms that can mimic crystal-induced or infectious arthritis. However, symptoms typically abate after several hours to a few days in the case of palindromic rheumatism.

Still's disease should also be considered in a patient with a monarthritis, rash, or systemic symptoms (60–62). Monoarticular arthritis is rare in systemic lupus erythematosus (SLE) and if it develops in a patient with that diagnosis, other causes should be considered (63).

Seronegative spondyloarthropathies often presents with an acute monoarticular arthritis that can mimic septic arthritis (13). The joints involved are usually in the lower extremities, although upper extremity involvement is common in psoriatic arthritis (66). Often the arthritis has a rapid onset, but symptoms can persist for prolonged periods of time, helping to differentiate these cases from crystal-induced arthropathies. The patient may have a history of urethritis or diarrhea, inflammatory eye disease, or associated symptoms such as a psoriaform rash or abdominal complaints consistent with inflammatory bowel disease. Celiac disease can also present with monoarticular symptoms (67).

Acute rheumatic fever (ARF) following infection with Group A streptococcal organisms can also lead to a monoarticular arthritis (68). Arthritis develops in nearly 70% of cases, usually appears early in the course of the disease, and is classically manifested by rapid migration of the joint pain with each joint being involved for only a few days. Large joints are more commonly involved and the arthritis rarely exceeds 4 wk duration. Other features of disease may be present including fever, rash, carditis, chorea, and nodules, helping to confirm the diagnosis. A history of antecedent sore throat may also be present. The diagnosis can be confirmed by the presence of elevated and rising titers of specific antibodies including antistreptolysin-O antibodies, antideoxyribonuclease-B (DNAase B) antibodies, and anti-hyaluronidase antibodies (68). A similar arthritis can be seen after streptococcal infection in the absence of a full ARF picture that may be related to a reactive process (69). This arthritic presentation is most common in adults.

Sarcoidosis

Acute sarcoidosis causes symmetric, painful, warm joints, usually in the lower extremity. Monoarticular arthritis has also been reported (70). Associated findings may include fever, hilar adenopathy on chest radiography, and erythema nodosum. Elevated serum levels of angiotensin converting enzyme may be present, but normal levels should not exclude the diagnosis. Chronic sarcoidosis may also present with a monarthritis, but the time course is usually prolonged, and inflammatory findings are minimal (70). Synovial biopsy is often required to confirm the diagnosis. Hyperuricemia is not uncommon in patients with sarcoidosis, and symptomatic gout may coexist with this disease.

Bleeding Diatheses

Disorders of coagulation such as hemophilia or therapeutic anticoagulation can lead to acute monarthritis due to hemarthrosis (71). A history of bleeding or the use of anticoagulants should be present, and synovial fluid aspiration should be hemorrhagic. There are reported cases of hemarthrosis from acquired hemophilia due to anti-factor VIII antibodies. In these rare cases, a family or personal history of hemophilia may not be present (72).

Sickle Cell Disease

Acutely painful joints are often seen in sickle cell disease. The causes of joint pain in this setting include acute osteonecrosis due to sickle crisis, as well as septic arthritis with salmonella predominating as the causative organism (73). In addition to osteonecrosis and sepsis, patients with sickle cell disease can develop non-inflammatory effusions or synovitis and a rapidly progressive destructive arthritis of unclear etiology (74). Patients with sickle cell disease have hyperuricemia, but the incidence of gouty arthritis is low (75).

Rare Causes of Monarthritis

Rare causes of acute or chronic monoarthritis include Whipple's disease in which articular symptoms may precede gastrointestinal symptoms by years (76), foreign bodies (77), and metastatic or joint-based tumors including PVNS (78). PVNS should be considered in a painful, swollen joint with hemorrhagic synovial fluid upon aspiration. Joint involvement with PVNS is usually chronic, although acute worsening of symptoms mimicking a process such as infection or crystal-induced arthropathy can occur with intra-articular hemorrhage from the tumor.

Osteonecrosis can also present with acute or chronic monoarticular joint pain. Factors putting an individual at risk for this include corticosteroid use, trauma, excessive alcohol use, deep-sea diving, sickle-cell disease, and thrombotic disorders (79).

Neuropathic arthropathy (Charcot joint) is usually a more chronic process, but acute fracture can cause monoarthritis of the ankle or knee (80). Amyloidosis can also present with monarthritis, although typically the course is more indolent (81).

Pancreatic disease can lead to a mono- or polyarticular arthritis (82). The most common underlying pancreatic disease is cancer, although alcohol-induced pancreatic disease and traumatic pancreatic disease have also been described. The most common joints involved are the knee and ankle, and joint findings are

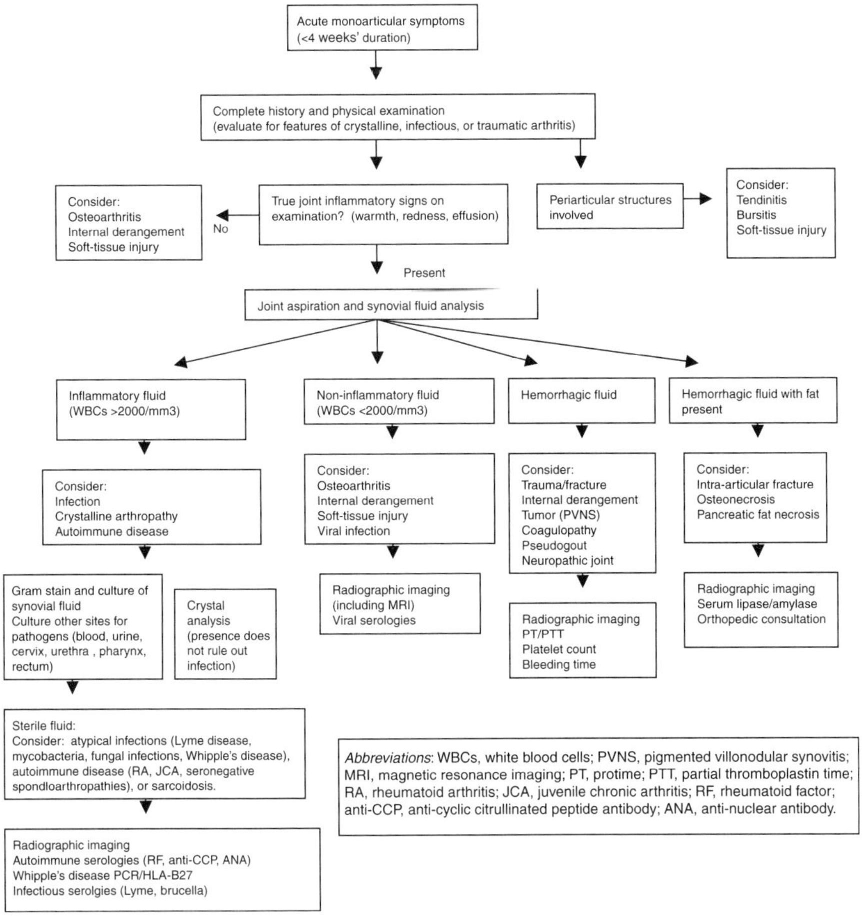

Figure 1 Evaluation of acute monoarticular symptoms (<4 weeks' duration). *Source*: Adapted from Ref. 84.

usually accompanied by a characteristic subcutaneous panniculitis. Interestingly, abdominal symptoms are absent in a minority of cases, but serum pancreatic enzymes (amylase and lipase) are usually markedly elevated (82,83). Synovial fluid is usually cloudy due to lipid droplets from necrosis of fat in the synovial membrane caused by circulating pancreatic enzymes (83). Other rare causes of monoarthritis are included in Table 1.

Mimics of Monarthritis

Several periarticular conditions can mimic acute or rarely chronic monarthritis. Tendonitis, bursitis, or overlying soft-tissue inflammation can appear to involve the true joint. In particular, olecranon bursitis or prepatellar bursitis can simulate

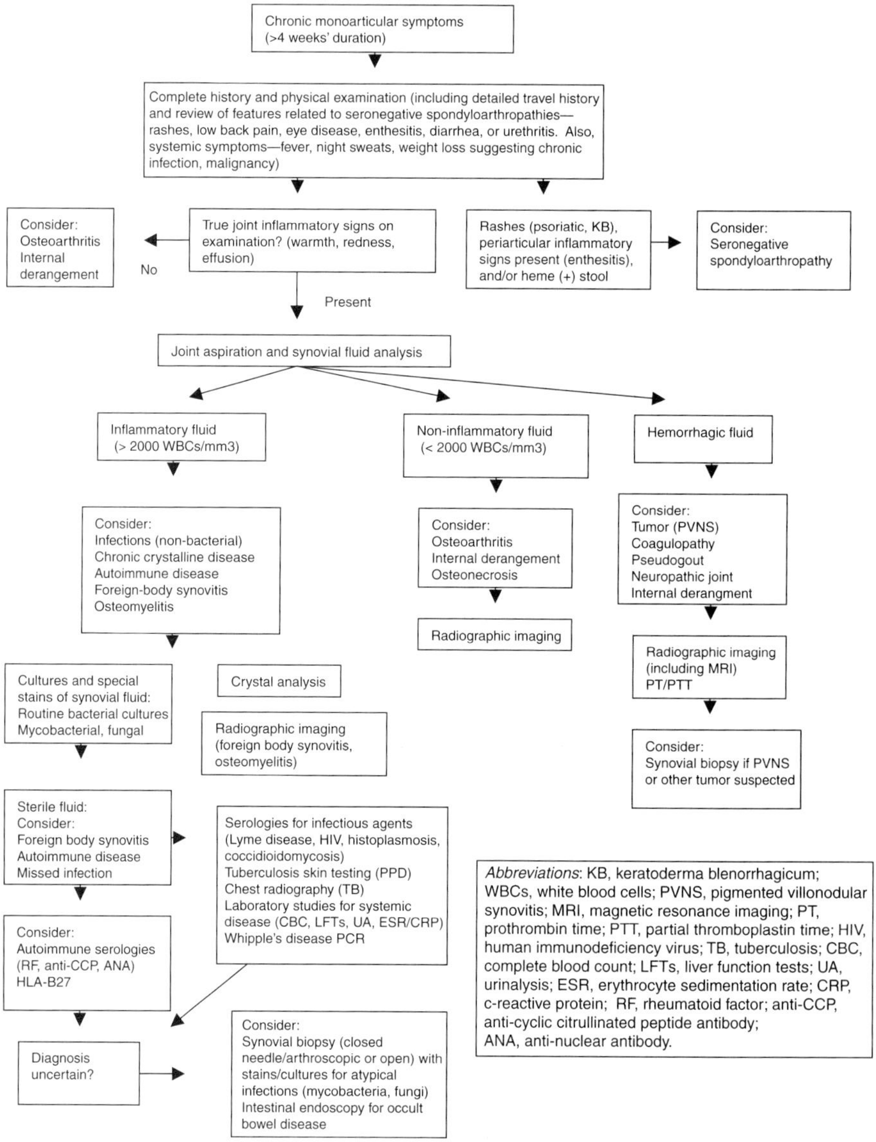

Figure 2 Evaluation of chronic monoarticular symptoms (>4 weeks' duration).

true joint involvement, and careful consideration must be taken to differentiate these processes. As mentioned, neuropathic processes such as herpes zoster can also mimic an acute arthritis, as can referred pain such as spinal radiculopathy mimicking hip disease or pain referred from the hip to the knee.

SUMMARY

There are multiple etiologies for monoarticular symptoms ranging from trauma to life-threatening infection. Historical factors, physical examination findings, laboratory testing, synovial fluid analysis, and radiographic imaging can lead to the appropriate diagnosis in the majority of cases, with synovial biopsies being reserved for more difficult diagnoses. Evaluation must be timely and complete to arrive at the correct diagnosis and initiate appropriate treatment (Figs. 1 and 2).

REFERENCES

1. Baker DG, Schumacher HR. Acute monoarthritis. NEJM 1993; 329:1013–1020.
2. Sack K. Monoarthritis: differential diagnosis. Am J Med 1997; 102:1A30S–1A34S.
3. Gardner GG, Weisman MH. Pyarthrosis in patients with rheumatoid arthritis: a report of 13 cases and a review of the literature from the past 40 years. Am J Med 1990; 88:503–511.
4. Rizzoli AJ, Trujeque L, Bankhurst AD. The coexistence of gout and rheumatoid arthritis: case reports and a review of the literature. J Rheumatol 1980; 7:316–324.
5. Agudelo CA, Wise CM. Gout: diagnosis, pathogenesis, and clinical manifestations. Curr Opin Rheumatol 2001; 13:234–239.
6. Al-Matar MJ, Petty RE, Tucker LB, et al. The early pattern of joint involvement predicts disease progression in children with oligoarticular juvenile rheumatoid arthritis. Arthritis Rheum 2002; 46:2708–2715.
7. Puig JG, Michan AD, Jimenez ML, et al. Female gout: clinical spectrum and uric acid metabolism. Arch Int Med 1991; 151:726–732.
8. Rosenthal AK, Ryan LM. Calcium pyrophosphate dehydrate crystal deposition disease: pseudogout; articular chondrocalcinosis. In: Koopman WJ, ed. Arthritis and Allied Conditions, 14th ed. Philadelphia: Lippincott, Williams, and Wilkins, 2001:2348–2371.
9. Ross JJ, Shamsuddin H. Sternoclavicular septic arthritis: review of 180 cases. Medicine (Baltimore) 2004; 83:139–148.
10. Ferraro K, Cohen MA. Acute septic sacroilitis in an injection drug user. Am J Emerg Med 2004; 22:60–61.
11. Ross JJ, Hu LT. Septic arthritis of the pubic symphysis: review of 100 cases. Medicine (Baltimore) 2003; 82:340–345.
12. Gotuzzo E, Alarcon GS, Bocanegra TS, et al. Articular involvment in human brucellosis: a retrospective analysis of 304 cases. Sem Arthritis Rheum 1982; 12:245–255.
13. Kvien T, Glennas A, Melby K, et al. Reactive arthritis: incidence, trigger agents, and clinical presentation. J Rheumatol 1994; 21:115–122.
14. Glockner JF, Sundaram M, Pierron RL. Radiologic case study: transient migratory osteoporosis of the hip and knee. Orthopedics 1998; 21:594–596.
15. Dunn AS, Turpie AG. Perioperative management of patients receiving oral anticoagulants: a systematic review. Arch Intern Med 2003; 163:901–908.
16. Shmerling RH, Delbanco TL, Tosteson ANA, Trentham DE. Synovial fluid tests: what should be ordered? JAMA 1990; 264:1009–1014.
17. Gatter RA, Schumacher HR. Joint aspiration: indications and technique. In: Gatter RA, Schumacher HR, eds. A Practical Handbook of Synovial Fluid Analysis. Philadelphia: Lea & Febiger, 1991:14.

18. McCutchan HJ, Fisher RC. Synovial leukocytosis in infectious arthritis. Clin Orthop 1990; 257:226–230.
19. Yu KH, Luo SF, Liou LB, et al. Concomitant septic and gouty arthritis: an analysis of 30 cases. Rheumatology (Oxford) 2003; 42:1062–1066.
20. Freed JF, Nies KM, Boyer RS, Louie JS. Acute monoarticular arthritis: a diagnostic approach. JAMA 1980; 243:2314–2316.
21. Gatter RA. A practical handbook of joint fluid analysis. Philadelphia: Lea and Febiger 1984.
22. Li SF, Henderson J, Dickson E, et al. Laboratory tests in adults with monoarticular arthritis: can they rule out a septic joint? Acad Emer Med 2004; 11:276–280.
23. Goldenberger DL. Gonococcal arthritis and other neisserial infections. In: McArthy DJ, Koopman WS, eds. Arthritis and Allied Conditions. 12th ed. Philadelphia: Lea & Febiger, 1993.
24. Masi HT. Articular patterns in the early course of rheumatoid arthritis. Am J Med 1983; 75:16–26.
25. Masih S, Antebi A. Imaging of pigmented villonodular synovitis. Semin Musculoskelet Radiol 2003; 7:205–216.
26. Hoving JL, Buchbinder R, Hall S, et al. A comparison of magnetic resonance imaging, sonography, and radiography of the hand in patients with early rheumatoid arthritis. J Rheumatol 2004; 31:663–675.
27. Stevens KJ, Theologis T, McNally EG. Imaging of plant thorn synovitis. Skelet Radiol 2000; 29:605–608.
28. Gibbon WW, Wakefield RJ. Ultrasound in inflammatory disease. Radiol Clin N Am 1999; 37:633–651.
29. Gibson T, Fagg N, Highton J, et al. The diagnostic value of synovial biopsy in patients with arthritis of unknown cause. Br J Rheumatol 1985; 24:232–241.
30. Mikhail IS, Alarcon GS. Nongonococcal bacterial arthritis. Rheum Dis Clin N Am 1993; 19:311–331.
31. Goldenberg DL, Reed JI. Bacterial arthritis. NEJM 1985; 312:764–771.
32. Adams WG, Deaver KA, Cochi SL, et al. Decline of childhood influenza type B(Hib) disease in the Hib vaccine era. JAMA 1993; 269:221–226.
33. Obrien JP, Goldenberg DL, Rice PA. Disseminated gonococcal infection: a prospective analysis of 49 patients and review of pathophysiology and immune mechanisms. Medicine 1983; 62:395–406.
34. Messieh M, Turner R, Bunch F, et al. Hip sepsis from retroperitoneal rupture of diverticular disease. Orthop Rev 1993; 22:597–599.
35. Tsukayama DT, Estrada R, Gustilo RB. Infection after total hip arthroplasty: a study of 106 infections. J Bone Joint Surg Am 1996; 78:512–523.
36. Rivera J, Garcia-Monforte A, Pineda A, et al. Arthritis in patients with chronic hepatitis C infection. J Rheum 1999; 26:420–424.
37. White DG, Woolf AD, Martinez DD, et al. Human parvovirus arthropathy. Lancet 1985; 1(8426):419–421.
38. Guilleven LL, Lhote F, Cohen P, et al. Polyarteritis nodosa-related hepatitis B virus: a prospective study with long term observation of 41 patients. Medicine 1995; 74:238–253.
39. Smith CA, Petty RE, Tingle AJ. Rubella virus and arthritis. Rheum Dis Clin N Am 1987; 13:265–274.
40. Espinoza LR. Retrovirus-associated rheumatic syndromes. In: McArthy DJ, Koopman WS, eds. Arthritis and Allied Conditions. 12th ed. Philadelphia: Lea and Farbinger, 1993.

41. Berman A, Cahn P, Perez H, et al. HIV infection associated arthritis: clinical characteristics. J Rheumatol 1999; 26:1158–1162.
42. Fierman AH. Varicella-associated arthritis occurring before the exanthema: a case report and literature review. Clin Pediatr (Phila) 1990; 29:188–190.
43. Griffiths DJ, Cooke SP, Herve C, et al. Detection of human retrovirus 5 in patients with arthritis and SLE. Arthritis Rheum 1999; 42:448–454.
44. Steer AC, Schoen RT, Taylor E. The clinical evolution of lyme arthritis. Ann Int Med 1987; 107:725–731.
45. Garrido G, Gomez-Reino JJ, Fernanoez-Dapka P, et al. A review of peripheral tuberculous arthritis. Semin Arthritis Rheum 1988; 18:142–149.
46. Haas DN. Mycobacteria tuberculosis. In: Mandell GL, Bennett J, Dolin R, eds. Principles and Practice of Infectious Disease. 5th ed. Edinburgh, Churchill, Livingston, 2000:2576–2607.
47. Wallace R, Cohen AS. Tuberculous arthritis: a report of two cases with review of biopsy and synovial fluid findings. Am J Med 1976; 61:277–282.
48. Van der Heijden IM, Wilbrink B, Schouls LM, et al. Detection of mycobacteria in joint samples from patients with arthritis using genus specific PCR and sequence analysis. Rheumatology 1999; 38:547–553.
49. Hirsch R, Miller SM, Kazi S, et al. HIV-associated atypical mycobacterial skeletal infections. Semin Arthritis Rheum 1996; 25:347–356.
50. Pugh MT, Southwod TR. Tuberculous rheumatism. Poncet's disease—a sterile controversy? (Editorial) Rev Rheum 1993; 60:735–740.
51. Cuellar ML, Silveira LH, Espinoza LR. Fungal arthritis. Ann Rheum Dis 1992; 51:690–697.
52. Rosenthal J, Brandt KD, Wheat LJ, Salama TG. Rheumatologic manifestations of histoplasmosis in the recent Indianapolis epidemic. Arthritis Rheum 1983; 26:1065–1070.
53. Stevens DA. Coccidioidomycosis. NEJM 1995; 332:1077–1082.
54. Koster FT, Galgian JN. Coccidioidal arthritis. In: Espinoza LR, Goldenberg DL, Arnett F, Alarcon GS, eds. Infections in the Rheumatic Diseases: A Comprehensive Review of Microbial Relations to Rheumatic Disorders. New York: Grune and Stratton, 1988:165–171.
55. Louie JS, Bocanegra TS. Mycobacterial, brucella, fungal, and parasitic arthritis. In: Hochberg MC, Silman AJ, Smolen JS, Weinblatt ME, Weisman MH, eds. Rheumatology 3rd ed. Elsevier, Ltd 2003:1077–1089.
56. Rosenthal AK. Calcium crystal-associated arthritis. Curr Opin Rheumatol 1998; 10:273–277.
57. Cline DM. Renal transplant-associated hyperuricernia and gout. J Am Soc Nephrol 2000; 11:974–979.
58. Halverson PB, Carrera GF, McCarty DJ. Milwaukee shoulder syndrome: fifteen additional cases and a description of contributory factors. Arch Int Med 1990; 150:677–682.
59. Fam AG, Stein J. Hydroxyapatite pseudopodagra in young women. J Rheumatol 1992; 19:662–664.
60. Doi K, Martell W. Monoarticular erosive arthritis: a possible source of confusion with infectious arthritis. J Clin Rheumatol 1995; 1:242.
61. Singleton JD, West SG, Nordstrom DM. Pseudoseptic arthritis complicating rheumatoid arthritis: a report of 6 cases. J Rheumatol 1991; 18:1319–1322.
62. Schumacher HR. Palindromic onset of rheumatoid arthritis: clinical, synovial fluid, and biopsy studies. Arthritis Rheum 1982; 25:366–369.

63. Cush JJ, Medsger TA, Christy WC, et al. Adult onset still's disease: clinical course and outcome. Arthritis Rheum 1987; 30:186–194.
64. Elkon KB, Hughes GR, Bywaters EGL, et al. Adult-onset still's disease: twenty year follow-up and further studies of patients with active disease. Arthritis Rheum 1982; 25:647–654.
65. Wong RC, Kong KO, Lin RU, Barkham T. Chronic monoarthritis of the knee in systemic lupus erythematosus. Lupus 2003; 12:324–326.
66. Kerr HE, Sturrock RD. Clinical aspects, outcome assessment, disease course, and extra-articular features of spondyloarthropathies. Curr Opin Rheum 1999; 11:235–237.
67. Falcini F, Ferruci R, Simonini G, Calabri GB, Pazzaglia A, Lionetti P. Recurent monoarthritis in an 11-year-old boy with occult celiac disease: successful and stable remission after gluten-free diet. Clin Exp Rheum 1999; 17:509–511.
68. Valtonen JM, Koskimies S, Miettinen A, Valtonen VV. Various rheumatic syndromes in adult patients associated with high ASO titers and their differential diagnosis with rheumatic fever. Ann Rheum Dis 1993; 52:527–530.
69. Grand rounds in rheumatology: acute rheumatic fever or post-streptococcal reactive arthritis: a clinical problem revisited. Br J Rheumatol 1998; 37:335–340.
70. Barnard J, Newman LS. Sarcoidosis: immunology, rheumatic involvement, and therapeutics. Curr Opin Rheumatol 2001; 13:84–91.
71. Hilgartner MW. Current treatment of hemophilic arthropathy. Curr Opin Pediatr 2002; 14:46–49.
72. Wendling D, Bertand MA. Hemarthrosis in aquired hemophilia: two case reports. Joint Bone Spine 2003; 70:532–534.
73. Bennett OM, Namnyak SS. Bone and joint manifestations of sickle cell anemia. J Bone Joint Surg Br 1990; 72:494–499.
74. Schumacher HR, Dorwart BB, Bond J, et al. Chronic synovitis with early cartilage destruction in sickle cell disease. Ann Rheum Dis 1977; 36:413–419.
75. Reynolds MD. Gout and hyperuricemia associated with sickle-cell anemia. Semin Arthritis Rheum 1983; 12:404–413.
76. Holden W, Orchard T, Wordsworth P. Enteropathic arthritis. Rheum Dis Clin North Am 2003; 29:513–530.
77. Miller EB, Gilad A, Schattner A. Cactus thorn arthritis and review of the literature. Clin Rheum 2000; 19:490–491.
78. Abraham JH, Canoso JJ. Tumors of soft tissue and bone. Curr Opin Rheumatol 1993; 5:193–198.
79. Vail TP, Covington DB. The incidence of osteonecrosis. In: Urbaniak JR, Jones JP, eds. Osteonecrosis: Etiology, Diagnosis, and Treatment 1st ed. American Academy of Orthopedic Surgeons 1st ed. 1997:43–49.
80. Schon LC, Easley ME, Weinfeld SB. Charcot neuropathy of the foot and ankle. Clinl Orthop 1998; 349:116–131.
81. Grateau G. Musculoskeletal disorders in secondary amyloidosis and hereditary fevers. Best Pract Res Clin Rheumatol 2003; 17:929–944.
82. Shbeeb MI, Duffy J, Bjornsson J, Ashby AM, Matteson EL. Subcutaneous fat necrosis and polyarthritis associated with pancreatic disease. Arthritis Rheum 1996; 39:1922–1925.
83. Francombe J, Kingsnorth AN, Tunn E. Panniculitis, arthritis, and pancreatitis. Br J Rheumatol 1995; 34:680–683.
84. Guidelines for the initial evaluation of the adult patient with acute musculoskeletal symptoms. American College of Rheumatology Ad Hoc Committee on Clinical Guidelines. Arthritis Rheum 1996; 39:1767–1768.

9

Synovial Fluid Analysis for Identification of Crystals

Lan X. Chen

Division of Rheumatology, Department of Medicine, University of Pennsylvania, Philadelphia, Pennsylvania, U.S.A.

H. Ralph Schumacher, Jr.

Division of Rheumatology, Department of Medicine, University of Pennsylvania and VA Medical Center, Philadelphia, Pennsylvania, U.S.A.

INTRODUCTION

Current concepts of gout and calcium pyrophosphate dihydrate (CPPD) deposition disease began with the microscopic identification of crystals in synovial fluid by Hollander and McCarty in 1961–1962 (1), and microscopic examination continues to be the principal method for crystal identification. Gout in fact is defined by the presence of monosodium urate (MSU) crystals. CPPD crystals can be seen in a variety of settings, may be a result of osteoarthritis or other joint diseases, and do not as clearly define a disease. Other crystals have now also been identified in joint fluids. These have a variety of implications.

Synovial fluid analysis for crystals is generally considered the gold standard. It can change clinically suspected diagnoses and can change treatment (2) but it does have limitations. Reliability of identification depends on training and experience of examiners and on the quality and proper maintenance of the microscope. Several studies have reported wide discrepancies of results on aliquots of fluid sent to different laboratories (3).

GROSS EXAMINATION

Evidence for the presence of crystals can begin to accumulate with the initial gross examination of the fluid aspirated (4). Some gouty fluids will have visible

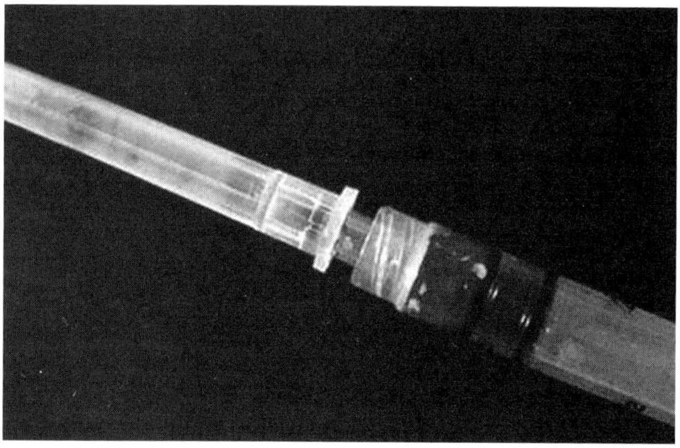

Figure 1 (*See color insert.*) White aggregates of tophaceous material in bloody synovial fluid.

white chunks (Fig. 1) that are virtually diagnostic and can be confirmed quickly on microscopic examination to be masses of MSU crystals from a tophaceous deposit in the joint. Less commonly, fluids aspirated from joints or bursas can be milky white liquids or pastes. These should raise suspicion for either gout or apatite disease. CPPD crystals rarely if ever produce such white effusions. Massive cholesterol crystal-laden fluids as occur in some chronically swollen shoulders or olecranon bursas may glisten with a gold paint appearance.

The gross appearance of the fluid may also give important information about the host response to crystals. Totally clear, almost colorless, viscous fluids may still contain MSU or CPPD crystals but suggest that there is little or no inflammatory response to the crystals. During acute attacks of gout or pseudogout effusions are cloudy because of the leukocyte response. Microscopic examination of a wet drop, differentials on a stained smear, and leukocyte counts are commonly used to further characterize the response. Effusions occasionally are bloody with any of the crystal induced diseases, but this may be especially common in the apatite associated destructive disease in the Milwaukee shoulder syndrome.

EXAMINATION OF A WET DROP PREPARATION

The standard approach to crystal identification still follows the preparation of a single wet drop of joint fluid as utilized by Hollander and McCarty (1). A single drop tends to have less distracting movement of the fluid. If few cells are present, effort may be needed to focus on the proper plane. Look with 10X or 40X objectives for cells, other debris, fat, etc. It may help to start at the margin of the cover slip where cells and crystals may clump.

The preparation should be examined using regular light before proceeding to the generally definitive use of compensated polarized light. This allows a quick impression about the cellular content of the fluid, identification of other possibly

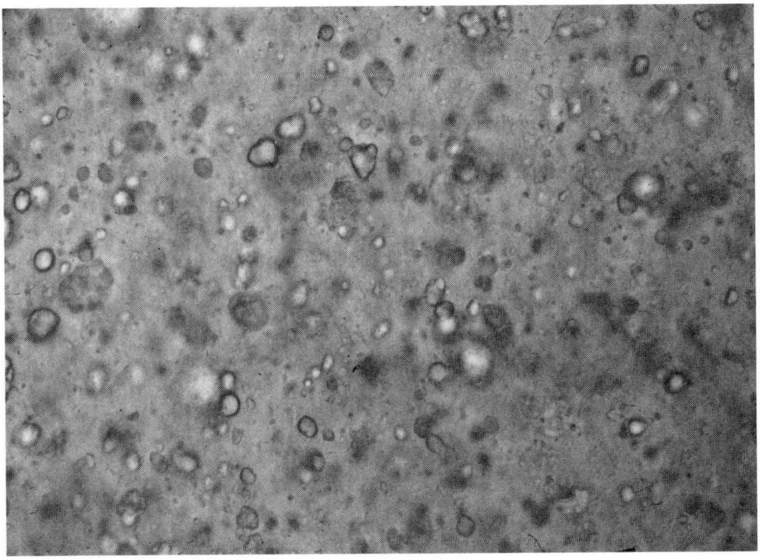

Figure 2 Shiny irregular clumps of apatite crystals.

important features such as fat droplets, fibrils, and cartilage or synovial fragments, and may provide the first clue to the presence of apatite, also called basic calcium phosphate (BCP) crystal clumps. These latter can appear as shiny, round or irregular 3 to 15 μ chunks (Fig. 2) (5). MSU and CPPD crystals can be seen and their nature suggested by their shapes and sizes. MSU crystals may be long needles up to 30 μ but also 3 to 10 μ rods. CPPD can also be rodlike but more characteristically are square, rhomboid, or more irregular and are mostly 3 to 7 μ. Since CPPD are often only weakly or virtually non-birefringent, they may actually be best seen on this regular light examination. Phase contrast or adjusting the condenser may produce a phase effect and can better delineate the CPPD crystals. Oil immersion may help identify small crystals. Especially when there are few cells, crystals may be best seen in clumps of tissue fibrils or tissue fragments.

Concentration of Specimens

If crystals are not seen on several minutes search, time can be saved and accuracy assured by also concentrating one aliquot of fluid by centrifugation or use of a cytocentrifuge (6). Crystals may be missed on initial examination of fluids for a variety of reasons beside paucity of crystals (7). Occasionally all crystals may be very small. The effusion aspirated may be from an adjacent sympathetic effusion not from the actual site of crystal induced inflammation.

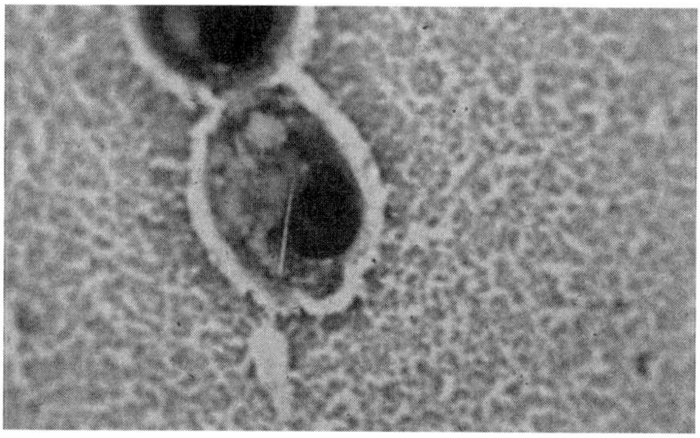

Figure 3 (*See color insert.*) Monosodium urate crystal in Wright's stained synovial fluid macrophage.

Examination of Stained Smears or Pellets

Dried smear preparations of inflammatory effusions can be stained and examined for crystals. Such specimens can be saved for later re-examination without concern for development of artifacts. Wright's stain or Diff Quick preparations have been reported to show either CPPD or MSU crystals which are especially easily characterized in cells (Fig. 3) (8,9). Gram stains prepared in microbiology laboratories have also shown crystals in specimens coexisting with or in the absence of bacteria.

Staining of Wet Preparations

The best studied but still not widely used technique for crystal identification is alizarin red S staining for apatites and other calcium containing crystals. This procedure, described by Paul et al. (10) stains apatite containing clumps as bright red, round, occasionally Chinese coin-like or irregular 3 to 15 μ bodies (Fig. 4). CPPD and oxalate (Fig. 5) will also stain red but retain their typical shapes and stain more slowly. Urate crystals have been stained with De Golantha silver stain (11) or methylene blue, but any clinical value of these has not been tested. A preparation called Testsimplets (Boehringer-Ingelheim), which has a dry stain on the slide and stains viable cells in fluid applied as a wet drop, defines cells well and does not dissolve crystals (12).

Compensated Polarized Light

Birefringent crystals such as MSU and CPPD can be highlighted and further characterized by use of polarized light which is best performed with commercial polarizing microscopes (13). In such microscopes a polarizing plate is placed above the light source. This orients the light into many parallel planes. A second similar polarizer (called the analyzer) above the specimen can be rotated 90° to these parallel planes of light. When this is done no light passes through and the field appears dark. If the specimen contains crystals, these will cause the direction of the

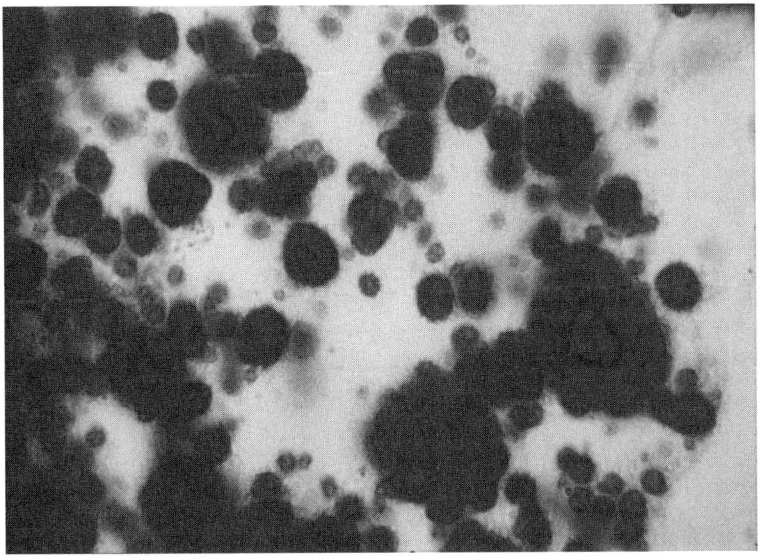

Figure 4 (*See color insert.*) Alizarin red stained clumps of apatite.

light planes to deviate so that bright white light will now pass through the analyzer and the examiner will see a white crystal shape against the dark background.

The technique now widely used to help distinguish MSU and CPPD crystals involves use of a first order red plate or compensator inserted between the polarizer and analyzer. This turns the background red or magenta. Crystals appear blue or yellow, and their orientation can be noted in relation to the axis of slow vibration of the compensator. This is usually marked by a line or arrow. The long axis of the crystal being examined is then aligned with the orienting arrow. If the crystal is blue in this position, it is said to have positive elongation (or positive birefringence). This is characteristic of most CPPD crystals (Fig. 6) (14). Crystals yellow parallel to the axis of slow vibration are termed to have negative elongation

Figure 5 Pyramidal-shaped oxalate crystal stained with alizarin red.

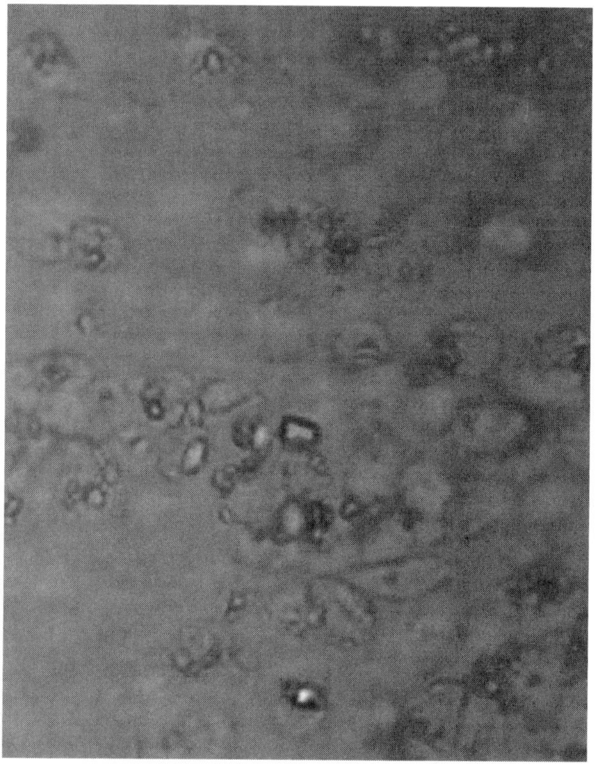

Figure 6 (*See color insert.*) Calcium pyrophosphate dihydrate (CPPD) crystals with compensated polarized light.

(negative birefringence) as is typical for MSU crystals (Fig. 7). If crystals are rotated or other crystals appear in the field, their color will be opposite when perpendicular to the line of orientation. That is, an MSU crystal will be blue when perpendicular to the axis of slow vibration.

Several other features can be noted. Blue or yellow birefringence will often disappear when rotated to midway between parallel and perpendicular to the orienting axis. This is termed extinction. MSU crystals are virtually always very bright. CPPD crystals can be bright but often are much less birefringent and occasionally show no birefringence with polarized light (15).

Less Common Crystals and Artifacts

Less common crystals can also be seen with compensated polarized light. These and a variety of artifacts need to be distinguished from the common pathogenetic crystals (16).

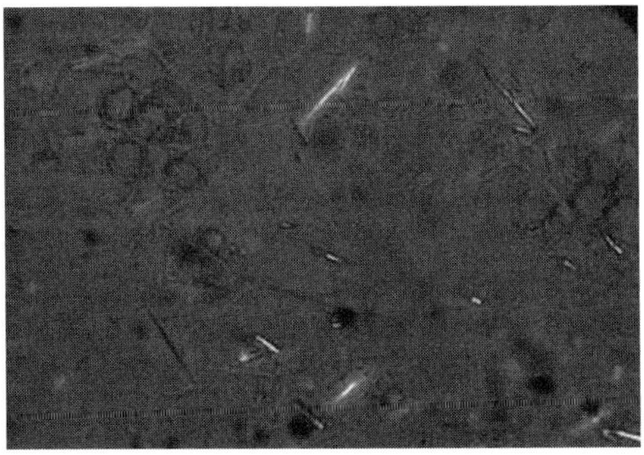

Figure 7 (*See color insert.*) Monosodium urate crystals with compensated polarized light.

Investigative Techniques

A variety of techniques not considered part of a practical synovial fluid analysis should also be mentioned as they may be used in research or called upon in rare situations to identify a puzzling finding in synovial fluid.

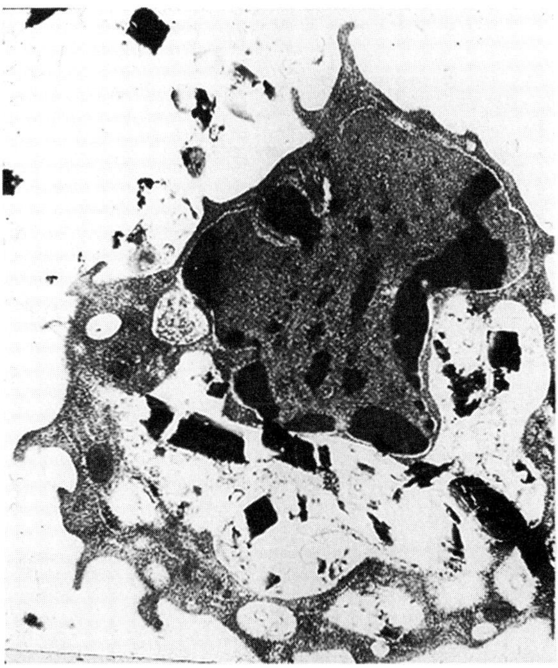

Figure 8 Tiny calcium pyrophosphate dihydrate (CPPD) crystals seen only by electron microscopy in vacuoles of a synovial fluid macrophage.

Electron microscopy can identify very small crystals by morphology (Fig. 8) (17) and can allow confirmation by electron diffraction elemental analysis (Fig. 9) (5). X-ray diffraction or Fourier transform infra red analysis are the most definitive methods for crystal identification but require more crystals than are often available. A technique using ^{14}Carbon labeled ethane-1-hydroxy-1 diphosphonate (EHDP) can detect small amounts of apatite but is not generally available (13,18). A recent report describes dissolution of urate crystals in synovial fluid with their measurement of soluble urate as a possible way to quantify urates (19).

Other Less Common Crystals and Artifacts

A rare example of suspected crystal associated arthritis will turn out to be related to or associated with a variety of less common crystals (16).

Oxalate crystals can complicate renal failure and appear as double pyramids or envelopes (20). Depot corticosteroids can vary in shape and size but are generally very brightly birefringent (21). These can cause an iatrogenic acute inflammation after injection in occasional patients (22). Liquid lipid crystals can appear like maltese crosses or beach balls and can be phagocytized and associated with acute inflammation (Fig. 10) (23). The broad notched plates typical of cholesterol crystals are generally not phagocytized or phlogistic. Proteins such

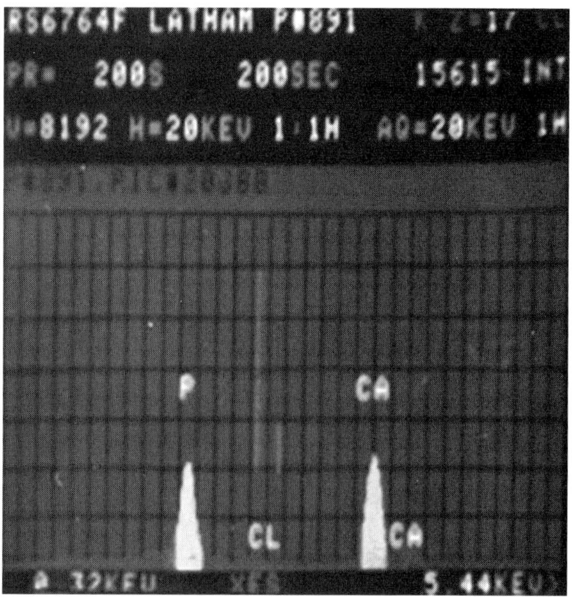

Figure 9 Elemental analysis showing equal amounts of calcium and phosphate in a calcium pyrophosphate dihydrate (CPPD) crystal.

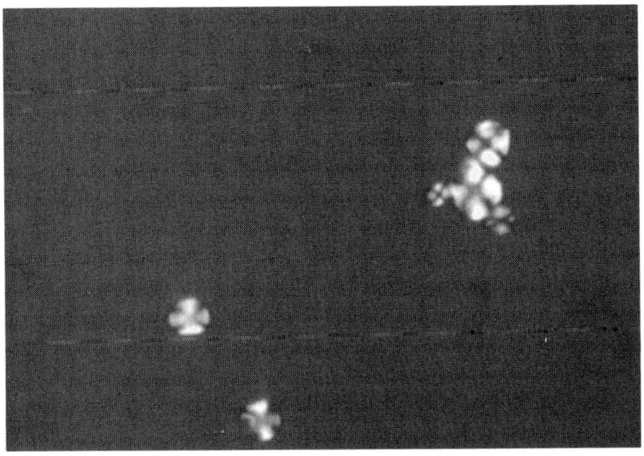

Figure 10 *(See color insert.)* Maltese cross-like lipid liquid crystals seen with compensated polarized light.

as cryoglobulins can form crystals; these and Charcot-Leyden crystals from eosinophilic exudates (Fig. 11) have been associated with arthritis (19).

Crystal-like artifacts include glass fragments, lipid crystals developing from cell breakdown, starch from gloves, oxalate, EDTA or lithium anticoagulants, hemoglobin breakdown products, drying artifacts, dust, and lens paper fibrils (24).

ARTHROCENTESIS

Identification of synovial fluid crystals assumes ability to successfully obtain synovial fluid. Patients may initially decline arthrocentesis but may be more willing if made aware that diagnosis can be wrong up to 20% of the time without proof of crystal presence and identity (2). Large bulging effusions at knees may be relatively easy to aspirate, but accurate and successful needle placement in knees may be achieved less often than many suspect. Confirmation by X-ray contrast injection has been used to study accuracy of injections (25,26).

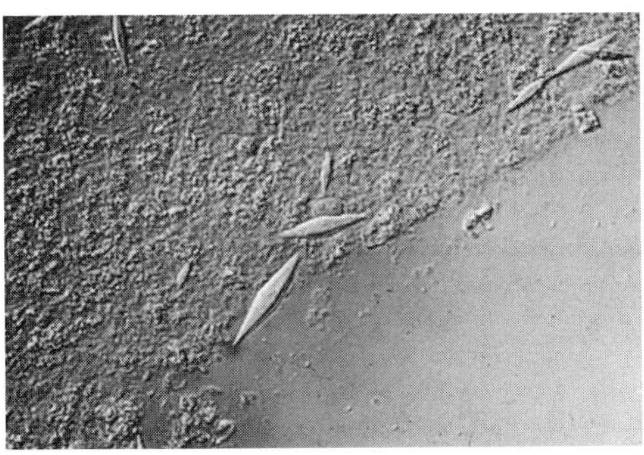

Figure 11 Charcot-Leyden crystals seen with regular light microscopy.

The superolateral route of entry into the suprapatellar pouch was most successful, medial retropatellar aspiration second best, and aspiration of the flexed knee medial or lateral to the patellar tendon least reliable. Shoulder arthrocentesis is less often successful. First metatarsophalangeal joints (and others) can be aspirated even without a detectable effusion (27), but no studies document rates of success. Ultrasound has been suggested to improve success with small effusions (28). Routes for aspiration of various other joints such as the shoulder have been described (29).

If no fluid is obtained on attempted aspiration, the plunger of the syringe should be withdrawn forcefully. Even if no fluid or material appears in the barrel of the syringe, there may still be some crystal-containing material in the needle. Therefore, in the case of an apparent "dry tap," the syringe should be removed from the needle, filled with air, and then reattached. Vigorously pushing in the plunger will often expel droplets or particles that can be examined by polarized light microscopy.

QUALITY CONTROL

No generally available system for quality control has been established for crystal identification. Ability to identify crystals in text books or lecture slides has not been confirmed to show ability to accurately detect the crystals in a given laboratory. A system to distribute embedded samples of crystals for use by individuals on their own microscopes has been proposed (30) but does not reproduce the clinical experience of the preparation techniques or totally reproduce the appearance of clinical specimens.

REFERENCES

1. McCarty DJ, Hollander JL. Identification of urate crystals in gouty synovial fluid. Ann Int Med 1961; 54:452–460.
2. Eisenberg JM, Schumacher HR, Davidson PK, Kauffman L. Usefulness of synovial fluid analysis in the evaluation of joint effusions. Use of threshold analysis and likelihood ratios to assess a diagnostic test. Arch Int Med 1984; 144:715–719.
3. Schumacher HR, Sieck MS, Rothfuss S, et al. Reproducibility of synovial fluid analyses: a study among four laboratories. Arthritis Rheum 1986; 29:770–774.
4. Schumacher HR, Reginato AJ. Atlas of Synovial Fluid Analysis and Crystal Identification. Philadelphia: Lea & Febiger, 1991.
5. Schumacher HR, Somlyo AP, Tse R, Maurer K. Apatite crystal associated arthritis. Ann Int Med 1977; 87:411–416.
6. Moreno MJ, Clayburne G, Schumacher HR. Processing of non-inflammatory synovial fluids with hyaluronidase for cytospin preparations impromes the accuracy of differential counts. Diagn Cytopathol 2000; 22:256–258.

7. Schumacher HR, Jimenez SA, Gibson T, et al. Acute gouty arthritis without urate crystals identified on initial examination of synovial fluid: report of 9 patients. Arthritis Rheum 1975; 18:603 612.
8. Petrocelli A, Wong AL, Swezey RI. Identification of pathologic synovial fluid crystals on gram stains. J Clin Rheum 1998; 4:103–105.
9. Selvi E, Manganelli S, Catenaccio M. Diff quik staining method for detection and identification of monosodium urate and calcium pyrophosphate crystals in synovial fluid. Ann Rheum Dis 2001; 60:194–198.
10. Paul H, Reginato AJ, Schumacher HR. Alizarin red S stainlng as a screening test to detect calcium compounds in synovial fluid. Arthritis Rheum 1983; 26:191–200.
11. de Galantha E. Techniques for preservation and microscopic demonstration of nodules in gout. Am J Clin Pathol 1935; 5:165–166.
12. Louthrenoo W, Sieck M, Clayburne G, et al. Supravital staining of cells in noninflammatory synovial fluids: analysis of the effect of crystals on cell populations. J Rheumatol 1991; 18:409–413.
13. Gatter RA, Schumacher HR. A Practical Handbook of Joint Fluid Analysis. 2nd ed. Philadelphia: Lea and Febiger, 1991 pp. 122.
14. Kohn NN, Hughes RE, McCarty DJ, Farres JS. The significance of calcium phosphate crystals in the synovial fluid of arthritic patients: the "pseudogout syndrome" II. Identification of crystals. Ann Int Med 1962; 56:711–737.
15. Ivorra J, Rosas J, Pascual E. Most calcium pyrophosphate crystals appear as non-birefrigent. Ann Rheum Dis 1999; 58:582–584.
16. Schumacher HR. Other crystals. In: Klippel JH, Dieppe PA, eds. Rheumatology. St. Louis: Mosby, 1994:7.15.1–7.15.4.
17. Cherlan V, Schumacher HR. Diagnostic potential of rapid electron microscopic analysis of joint effusions. Arth Rheum 1982; 25:98–100.
18. Halverson PB, McCarty DJ. Identification of hydroxyapatite crystals in synovial fluid. Arth Rheum 1979; 22:389–395.
19. Tiliakos AN, Tiliakos NA. Total joint fluid urate in gout. J Clin Rheum 2004; 10:250–251.
20. Hoffman GS, Schumacher HR, Paul H, et al. Calcium oxalate microcrystalline associated arthritis in end stage renal disease. Ann Intern Med 1982; 97:36–42.
21. Kahn CB, Hollander JL, Schumacher HR. Corticosteroid crystals in synovial fluid. JAMA 1970; 211:807–809.
22. Gordon GV, Schumacher HR. Electron microscopic study of depot corticosteroid crystals with clinical studies after intra-articular injections. J Rheumatol 1979; 6:7–14.
23. Reginato AJ, Schumacher HR, Allan DA, Rabinowitz JL. Acute monoarthritis associated with lipid liquid crystals. Ann Rheum Dis 1985; 44:537–543.
24. Chen LX, Clayburne G, Schumacher HR. Update on identification of pathogenic crystals in joint fluid. Current Rheum Rep 2004; 6:217–220.
25. Schumacher HR. Aspiration and injection therapies for joints. Arthritis Care Res 2003; 49:413–420.
26. Jackson DW, Evans NA, Thomas BM. Accuracy of needle placement into the intraarticular space of the knee. JBJS 2002; 84A:1522–1526.
27. Aqudelo CA, Weinberger A, Schumacher HR, Turner RA, Molina J. Definitive diagnosis of gout by identification of urate crystals in asymptomatic metatarsophalangeal joints. Arth Rheum 1979; 22:559–560.

28. Grassi E, Farina A, Fillippucci E, Cervini C. Sonographically guided procedures in rheumatology. Semin Arthritis Rheumatol 2001; 30:347–353.
29. Schumacher HR. Arthrocentesis of the shoulder. Hosp Med 1997; 33:57–60.
30. Schumacher HR, Sieck M, Clayburne G. Development and evaluation of a method for preservation of synovial fluid wet preparations for quality control testing of crystal identification. J Rheumatol 1990; 17:1369–1374.

10

Other Methods of Crystal Identification

Paul B. Halverson

Division of Rheumatology, Department of Medicine, Medical College of Wisconsin, Milwaukee, Wisconsin, U.S.A.

INTRODUCTION

Crystal-associated arthritis usually connotes either monosodium urate monohydrate (MSU) or calcium pyrophosphate dihydrate (CPPD) crystals. These two crystals are easily detected and identified by polarized light microscopy. Less common crystals, such as cholesterol and oxalate, may also be visualized by polarized light microscopy. Basic calcium phosphate (BCP) crystals, on the other hand, found in up to 60% of cases of knee osteoarthritis, usually can not be identified by this technique (1). The failure of polarized light microscopy to detect BCP crystals relates to the very small size of the crystals and the random orientation of crystals within a crystal mass. In rare cases, BCP crystals may be visualized with the light microscope as refractile "shiny coins" which represent laminations of crystals in a globular mass (2). Thus, other means have been necessary to identify BCP crystals.

Various other techniques that have been used to identify BCP crystal are listed in Table 1. These include light microscopy with alizarin red S staining, radio-labeled diphosphonate binding, electron microscopy, Fourier transform infrared spectroscopy, atomic force microscopy, and arsenazo III. These techniques vary considerably in their applicability, cost, ease of performance, sensitivity, and specificity. The advantages and disadvantages of each will be discussed.

ALIZARIN RED S STAINING

Alizarin red S is a calcium stain. It has been proposed that alizarin red S staining of joint fluid pellets is an acceptable method for detection of calcium-containing

Table 1 Techniques Used for the Detection of BCP Crystals

Method	Advantage/disadvantage	Comment
Alizarin red	Light microscopy, easy to perform	Very sensitive, lacks specificity
EHDP binding	EHDP not available	Semiquantitative
Electron microscopy		
Scanning (SEM)	Visualizes BCP microspheroids	Not as sensitive as TEM
Transmission (TEM)	Visualizes individual crystals	High specificity/sensitivity
Atomic force microscopy	Visualizes crystal lattice	High specificity/sensitivity
Fourier transform IR	Generally performs well	
X-ray diffraction	Requires relatively large specimen	Not recommended

Abbreviations: BCP, basic calcium phosphate; EHDP, ^{14}C-ethane-1-hydroxy-1, 1-disphonate; IR, infrared.

crystals (3,4). Other investigators, though, have found the method to lack specificity because of staining of non-calcium containing particles in joint fluids and/or precipitation of stain (5,6). Those who claim success with the method suggest that strong staining is reliable in detecting BCP crystals. It is likely that laboratories that frequently perform alizarin red S staining have greater confidence with the technique. The majority of clinical laboratories either do not perform alizarin red S staining or perform the test only infrequently. Therefore, alizarin red S staining can only be recommended as a screening technique for BCP crystals. An additional confirmatory test would be necessary for definite identification.

RADIONUCLIDE DIPHOSPHONATE BINDING

A technique utilizing ^{14}C-ethane-1-hydroxy-1,1-disphonate (EHDP) binding has been used to identify BCP crystals (7). In this method, EHDP is added to joint fluid and incubated to allow binding. The joint fluid is then centrifuged at high speed, and aliquots of the supernatant removed and compared to pre-centrifuge values. The amount bound is compared to a standard binding curve to determine an approximate amount of BCP mineral present in the fluid. The test is sensitive to approximately 2 milligrams hydroxyapatite standard per milliliter. This method is considered semi-quantitative. High levels of binding are very suggestive of the presence of BCP crystals. Low levels of binding should be confirmed by another more specific technique. Unfortunately, despite the relative ease of performing the test, radiolabelled EHDP is not commercially available.

ELECTRON MICROSCOPY

Electron microscopy, either scanning or transmission, is useful in detecting BCP crystals. Under scanning electron microscopy, BCP crystals appear as microspheroids (8). Identification of BCP crystals is dependent on X-ray energy dispersive analysis which yields calcium to phosphorus molar ratios of 1.3 to 1.7, suggesting mixtures of hydroxyapatite and octacalcium phosphate. Under transmission electron microscopy, individual crystals of hydroxyapatite may be visualized as tiny rods which are often found in large aggregates (9). Plate-like crystals are more suggestive of octacalcium phosphate. X-ray energy dispersive analysis confirms similar calcium to phosphorus ratios as described above. Electron microprobe is an alternative to X-ray energy dispersive analysis.

ATOMIC FORCE MICROSCOPY

Atomic force microscopy visualizes crystal surfaces at a molecular level (10). Crystal lattice structure can be determined including intramolecular spacing and angle or orientation. Some crystals may be identified which can be missed by polarized light microscopy and even transmission electron microscopy.

FOURIER TRANSFORM INFRARED SPECTROSCOPY

Fourier transform infrared spectroscopy was important in confirming that pathologic calcium deposition contained calcium-containing materials in addition to hydroxapatite (11). With this technique, spectra from known crystals-containing substances are subtracted from the spectra of a clinical specimen to determine the constituents. These deposits often contained mixtures of partially carbonate substituted hydroxyapatite, octacalcium phosphate, and rarely tricalcium phosphate. Subsequently the term BCP was proposed as the more appropriate term for these crystals.

X-RAY DIFFRACTION

X-ray diffraction is not recommended for identification of BCP crystals in joint fluid. Typically, only small quantities of mineral are isolated. Poor crystallization of the mineral results in broad diffraction minima which are difficult to interpret.

ARSENAZO III

Arsenazo III has been used in a quantitative colorimetric assay to measure calcium containing crystals in joint fluids (12). Results were calculated using a standard hydroxyapatite calibration curve. This technique provided values of 23.99 mg/dL for rheumatoid arthritis, gout, and miscellaneous arthropathies, 40.81 mg/dL for osteoarthritis, 53.18 for CPPD arthritis, and similar values for fluids containing hydroxyapatite. No further clinical studies using this technique have been reported. This method probably is probably not sufficiently specific to be of much utility.

REFERENCES

1. Halverson PB, McCarty DJ. Patterns of radiographic abnormalities associated with basic calcium phosphate and calcium pyrophosphate dihydrate crystal deposition in the knee. Ann Rheum Dis 1986; 45:603–605.
2. Schumacher HR, Rothfuss S, Bertken R, et al. Unusual laminated birefringent arrays of apatite crystals in inflammatory arthritis. Arthritis Rheum 1987; 30:S1063.
3. Paul H, Reginato AJ, Schumacher HR. Alizarin red S staining as a screening test to detect calcium compounds in synovial fluid. Arthritis Rheum 1983; 26:191–200.
4. Lazcano O, Li CY, Pierre RV, et al. Clinical utility of the alizarin red S stain on permanent preparations to detect calcium-containing compounds in synovial fluid. Am J Clin Pathol 1993; 99:90–96.
5. Bardin T, Bucki B, Lansaman J, et al. Coloration par le rouge alizarine des liquides articulaires. Rev Rhuem Mal Osteoarthritis 1987; 54:149–154.
6. Gordon C, Swan A, Dieppe P. Detection of crystals in synovial fluids by light microscopy: sensitivity and reliability. Ann Rheum Dis 1989; 48:737–742.
7. Halverson PB, McCarty DJ. Identification of hydroxyapatite crystals in synovial fluid. Arthritis Rheum 1979; 22:389–395.
8. Halverson PB, Cheung HS, McCarty DJ. "Milwaukee shoulder": association of microspheroids containing hydroxyapatite crystals, active collagenase and neutral protease with rotator cuff defects: II. Synovial fluid studies. Arthritis Rheum 1981; 24:474–483.
9. Cherian PV, Schumacher HR. Diagnostic potential of rapid electron microscopic analysis of joint effusions. Arthritis Rheum 1982; 25:98–100.
10. Blair JM, Sorenson LB, Arnsdorf MF, et al. The application of atomic force microscopy for the detection of microcrystals in synovial fluid from patients with recurrent synovitis. Semin Arthritis Rheum 1995; 24:359–369.
11. McCarty DJ, Lehr JR, Halverson PB. Crystal populations in human synovial fluid. Identification of apatite, octacalcium phosphate, tricalcium phosphate. Arthritis Rheum 1983; 26:1220–1224.
12. Fernandez-Dupica MP, Reginato AJ, Ramachandrula A. Quantitative analysis of BCP crystals in synovial fluid using Arsenazo III. Arthritis Rheum 1994; 37:S41.

11

Radiographic Changes of Crystal-Induced Arthropathies

Lawrence M. Ryan
Division of Rheumatology, Department of Medicine, Medical College of Wisconsin, Milwaukee, Wisconsin, U.S.A.

Guillermo F. Carrera
Department of Radiology, Medical College of Wisconsin, Milwaukee, Wisconsin, U.S.A.

INTRODUCTION—GOUT

The radiographic features of gout are usually nonspecific early in the disease course. Plain films may reveal soft tissue swelling of the involved part during the acute attack and may be normal during the asymptomatic (intercritical) periods. Over time, and long before apparent on physical examination, the inflammatory reaction to microscopic tophi leads to degenerative changes in bone and cartilage. These abnormalities are usually asymmetric and are most common in the feet and hands; may be seen in wrists, elbows, and knees in more severe disease; and can occur in almost any joint in the body on rare occasions.

The boney erosions that develop in gout have a characteristic appearance in many cases. The erosions are usually slightly removed from the joint margin, have a sclerotic "overhanging edge," and are often associated with a soft tissue density cause by the tophus. This is attributed to the inflammatory process, which has both atrophic and hypertrophic elements. The gouty erosion is further distinguished by the absence of associated juxta-articular osteopenia, a finding

(Text continues on page 187.)

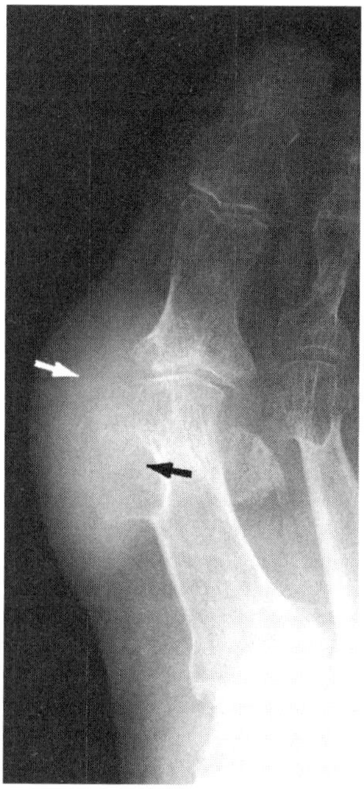

Figure 1 Tophaceous deposit with calcification (*white arrow*) and intraosseous lesions (*black arrow*) most prominent in the proximal phalanx of the great toe.

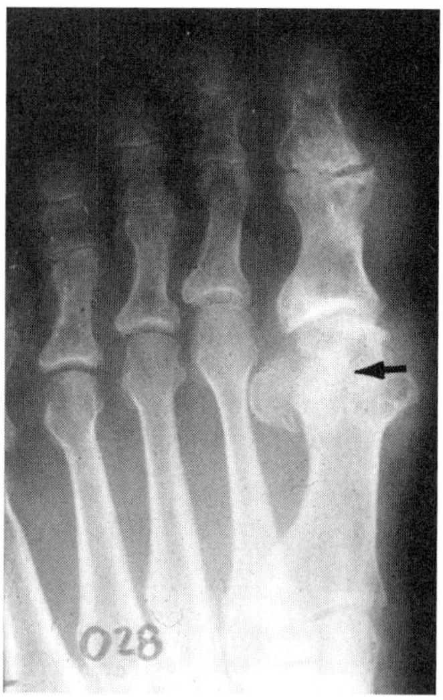

Figure 2 Tophi adjacent to medial aspect of interphalangeal and metatarsophalangeal joints of the great toe and erosions with overhanging edges (*arrow*). *Source*: From Ref. 1.

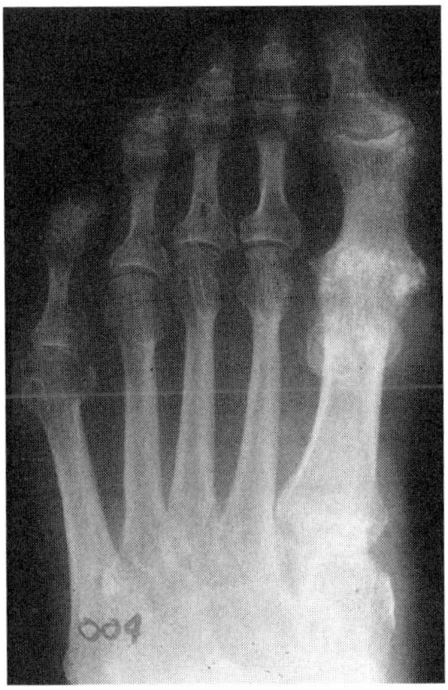

Figure 3 Tophus adjacent to medial aspect of metatarsophalangeal joint of the great toe. *Source*: From Ref. 1.

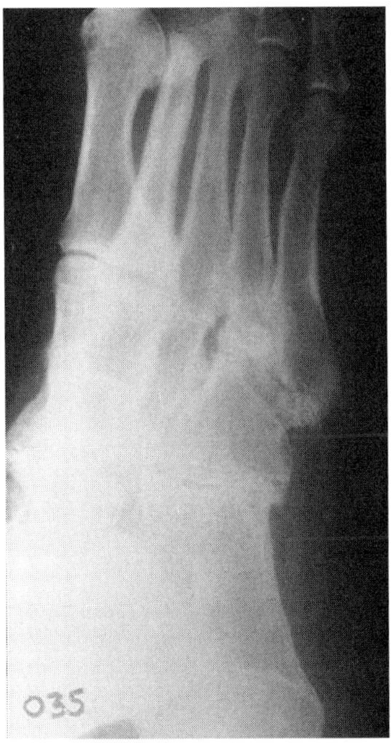

Figure 4 Erosions and sclerosis at the base of the fourth and fifth metatarsals in patient with gout. *Source*: From Ref. 1.

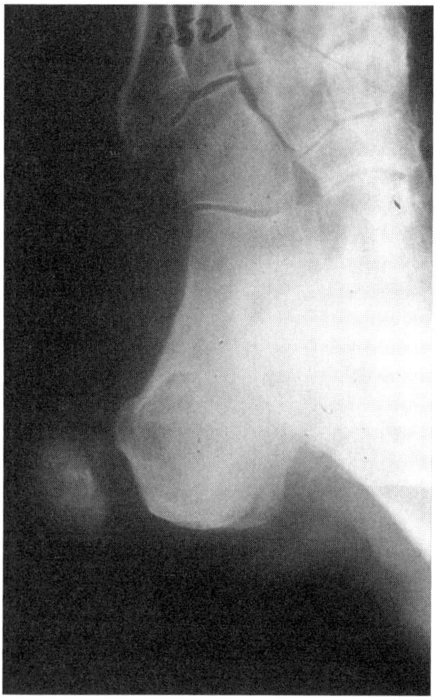

Figure 5 Calcified tophus in the heel. *Source*: From Ref. 1.

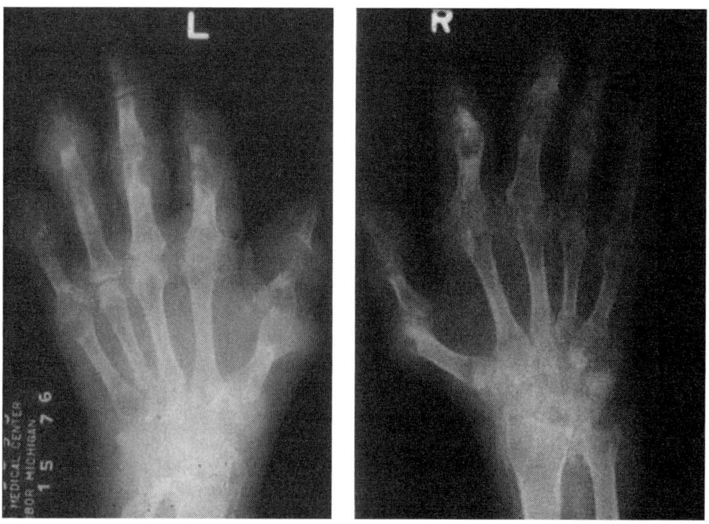

Figure 6 Tophi and destructive changes in multiple joints. *Source*: From Ref. 1.

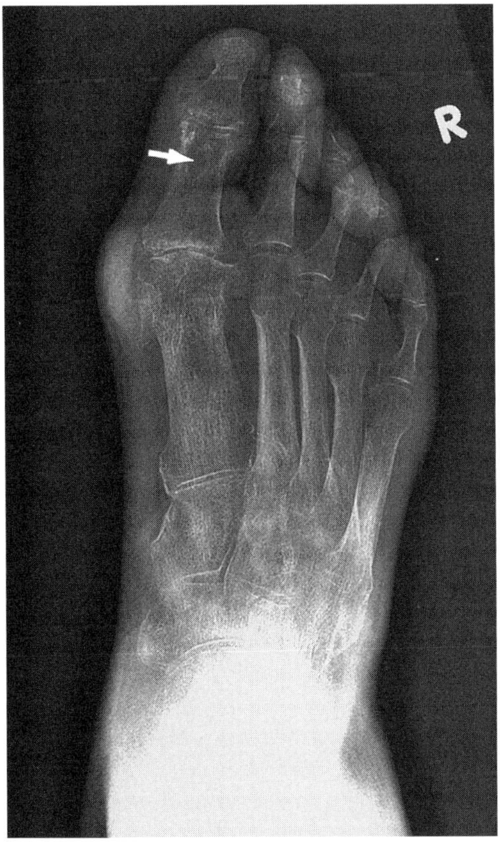

Figure 7 Tophaceous gout with soft-tissue mass (*arrow*) and bony lesions in the toes.

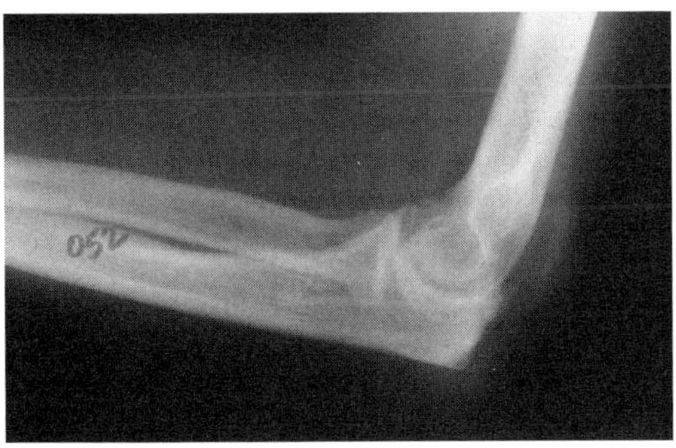

Figure 8 Elbow with soft-tissue swelling, calcifications, and erosions of the olecranon. *Source*: From Ref. 1.

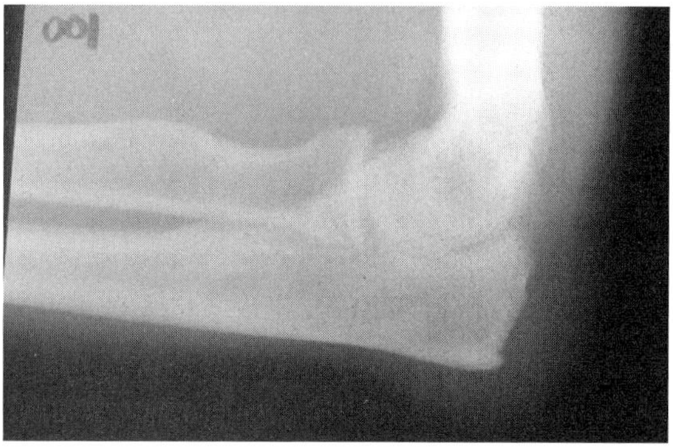

Figure 9 Elbow with soft-tissue swelling and calcifications. *Source*: From Ref. 1.

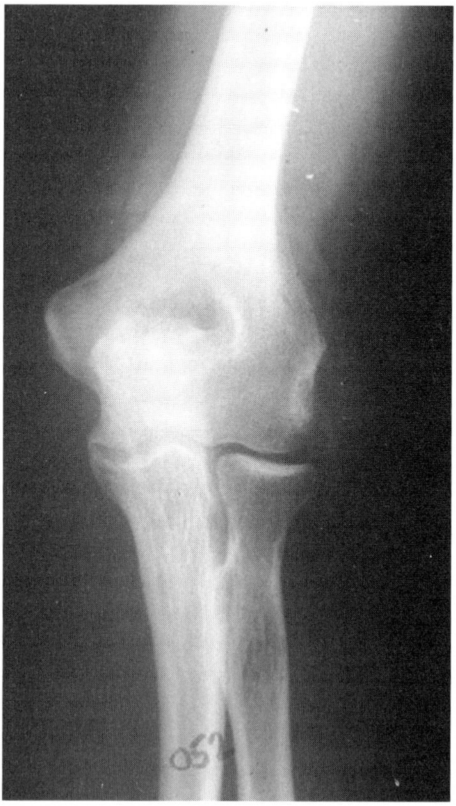

Figure 10 Elbow with erosion in lateral epicondyle adjacent to a tophus. *Source*: From Ref. 1.

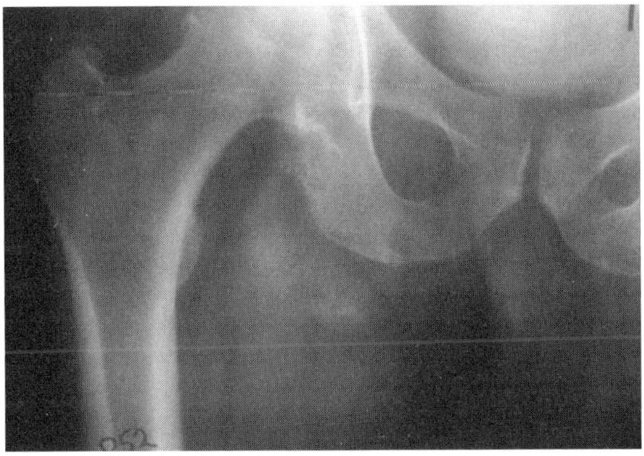

Figure 11 Large tophus near the ischial tuberosity and erosion at the ischial tuberosity. *Source*: From Ref. 1.

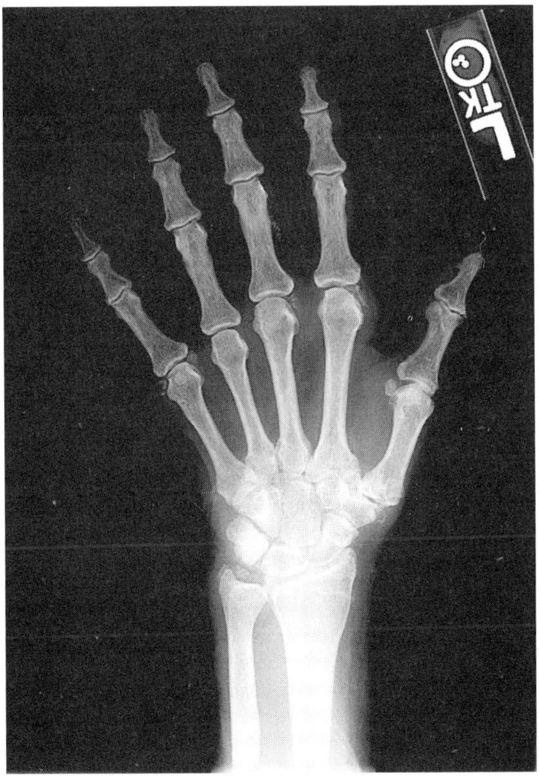

Figure 12 Calcium pyrophosphate dihydrate crystal deposition involving triangular fibrocartilage of the wrist, inter-carpal cartilages, and synovium/capsule of metacarpo-phalangeal joints.

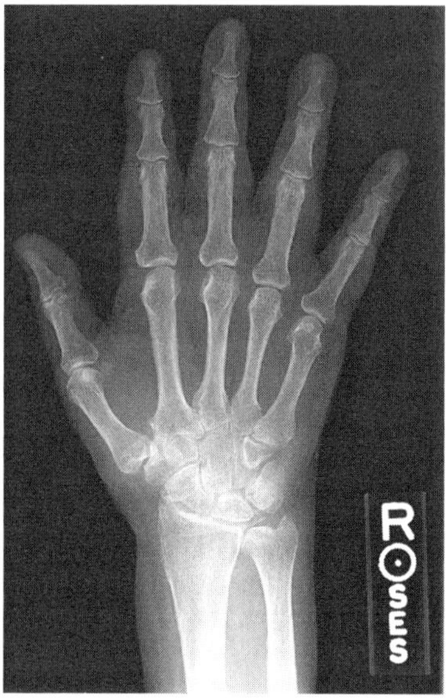

Figure 13 Chondrocalcinosis in the triangular fibrocartilage of the wrist, cartilage of triquetrum, and base of the proximal phalanx of the thumb.

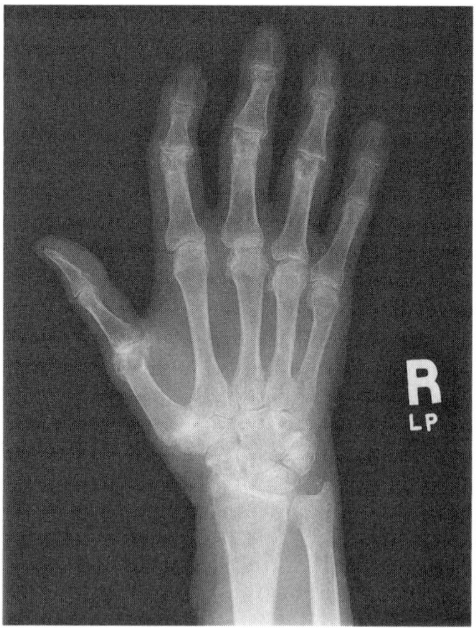

Figure 14 Hemochromatosis with chondrocalcinosis in the wrist and characteristic degenerative changes in metacarpophalangeal joints.

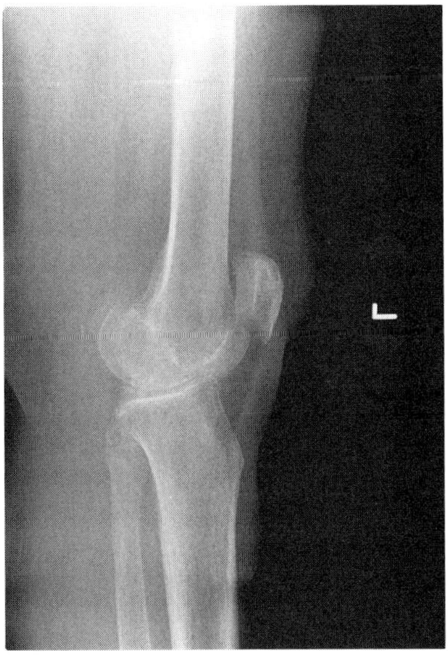

Figure 15 Chondrocalcinosis involving femoral condylar cartilage, patellar cartilage, and meniscus.

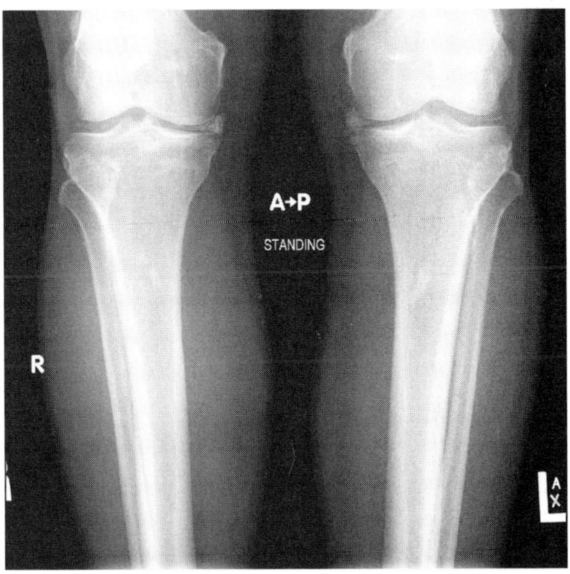

Figure 16 Medial and lateral meniscal calcification in both knees.

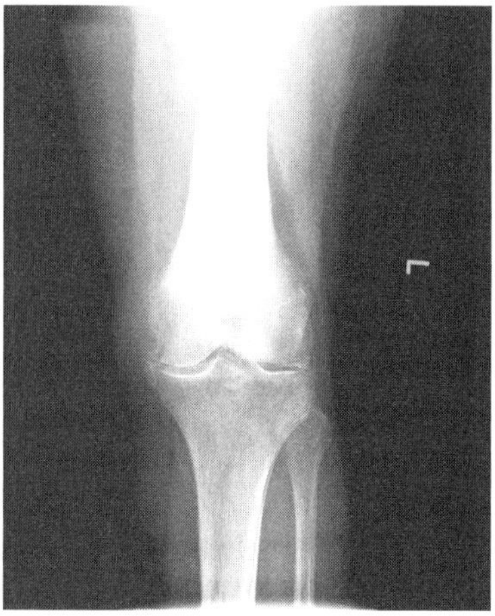

Figure 17 Chondrocalcinosis in lateral and medial menisci.

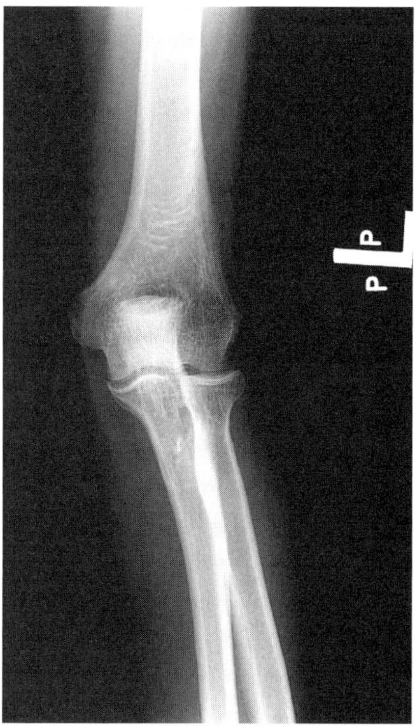

Figure 18 Chondrocalcinosis in cartilage of distal humerus.

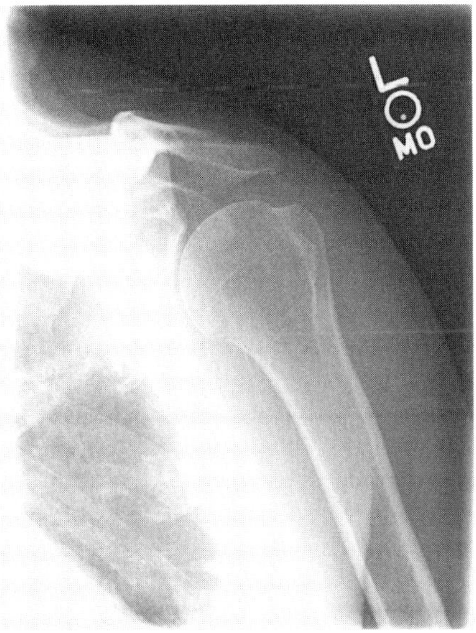

Figure 19 Chondrocalcinosis of the humeral head hyaline articular cartilage.

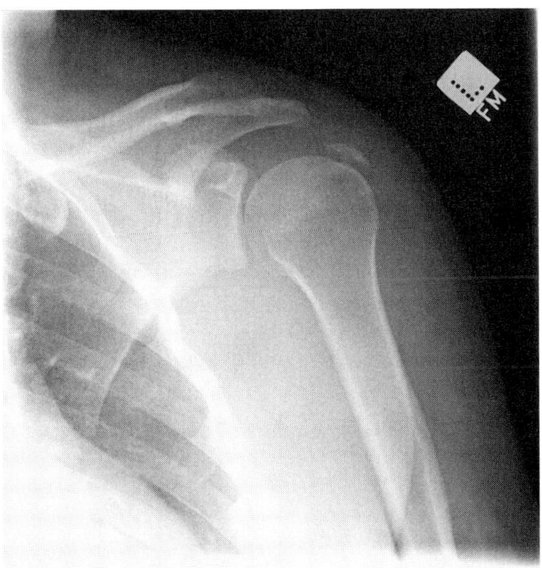

Figure 20 Subdeltoid/subacromial calcific bursitis.

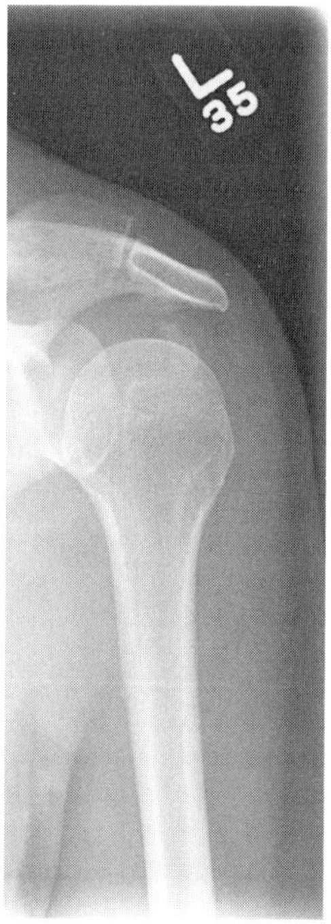

Figure 21 Calcific tendinitis of the supraspinatus tendon.

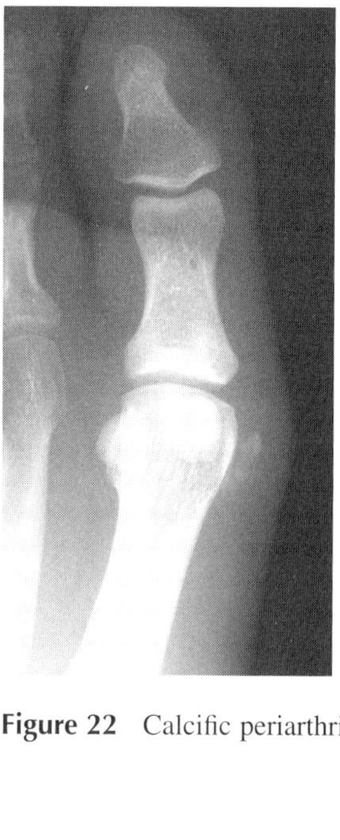

Figure 22 Calcific periarthritis of the toe.

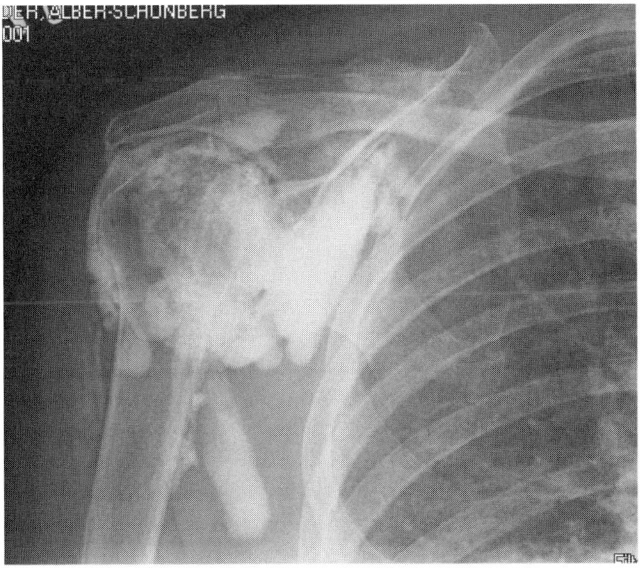

Figure 23 Tumoral calcinosis of the shoulder.

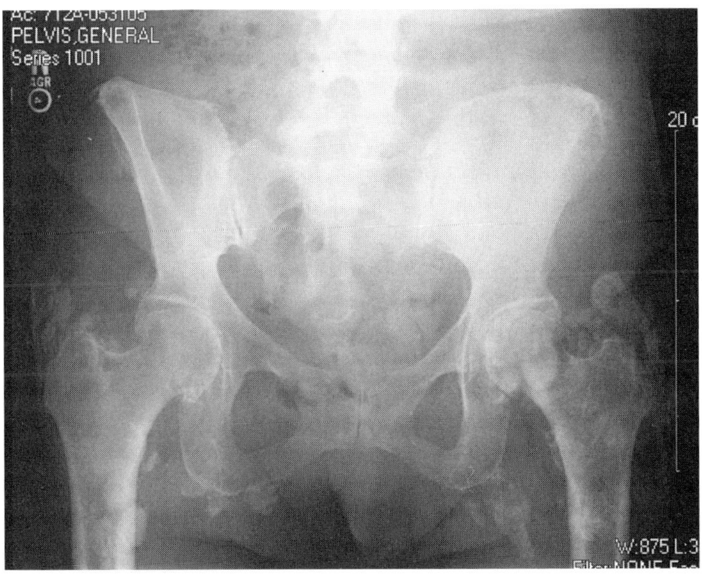

Figure 24 Tumoral calcinosis of the pelvis.

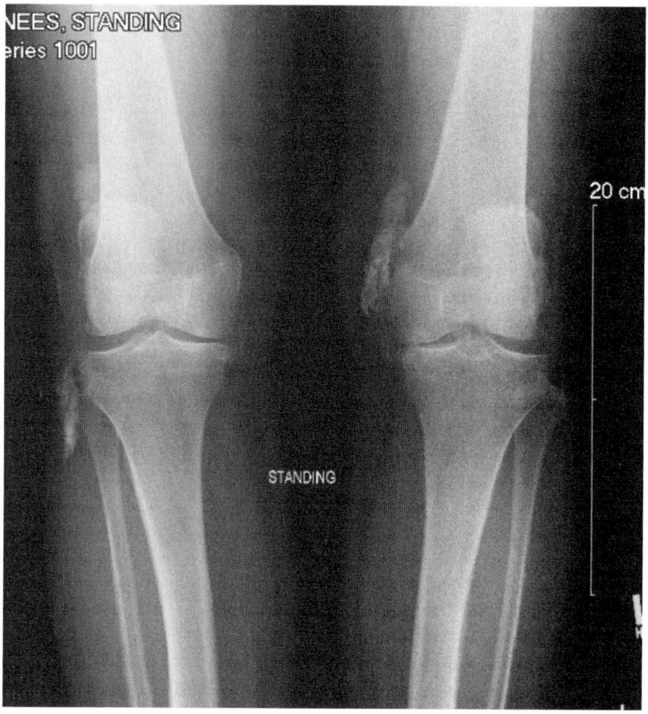

Figure 25 Tumoral calcinosis of the knees.

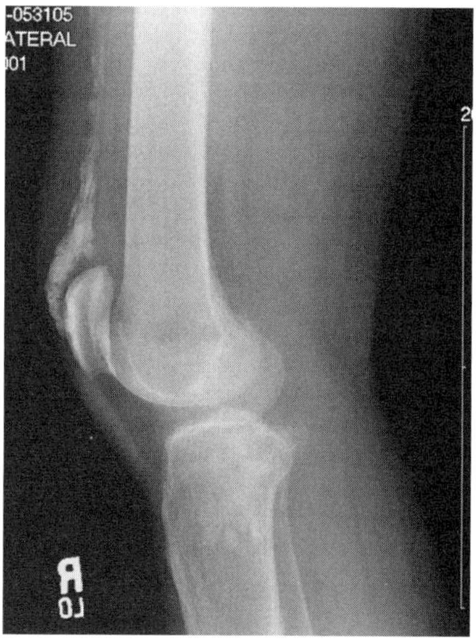

Figure 26 Tumoral calcinosis of the knee.

commonly associated with erosions seen in diseases such as rheumatoid arthritis or infections arthritis.

CALCIUM PYROPHOSPHATE DIHYDRATE CRYSTAL DEPOSITION DISEASE

The characteristic radiographic appearance of calcium pyrophosphate dihydrate (CPPD) deposition includes punctate and linear densities in articular hyaline and fibrocartilages. These changes are termed chondrocalcinosis. Calcific deposits may also appear in the articular capsule, ligaments, and tendons. When the deposits are typical and unequivocal, the radiographic appearance is nearly specific. The recognition and interpretation of faint deposits is, however, more difficult.

Although the earliest deposits occur in otherwise radiographically normal cartilage, degenerative changes often supervene. Chondrocalcinosis is not uncommonly seen in association with findings typical of osteoarthritis. The pattern of affected joints, however, tends to be different when CPPD deposition is present. For example, isolated patellofemoral join space narrowing, tricompartmental knee joint degeneration, and isolated wrist degeneration are typically related to CPPD deposition. Furthermore, degenerative changes in the metacarpophalangeal joints, such as squaring of the bone ends and hook-like osteophytes, may be seen with CPPD deposition alone. However, these changes are more commonly seen in patients with both hemochromatosis and CPPD deposition.

BASIC CALCIUM PHOSPHATE ARTHROPATHIES

Most soft tissue calcifications are due to the deposition of basic calcium phosphate (BCP) crystals. These calcifications are not uncommon at sites of injury and also represent the crystals seen in cases of calcific bursitis, tendinitis, and periarthritis. BCP crystals are believed to play a pathophysiologic role in the destructive degenerative arthropathy seen in advanced osteoarthritis, including the arthritis classified as Milwaukee shoulder. Finally, BCP crystals are the mineral in cases of tumoral calcinosis, which appears as conglomerate and globular calcifications in tendons, ligaments, joints, bursae, and juxta-articular soft tissues (Figs. 1–26).

REFERENCE

1. Barthelemy CR, Nakayama DA, Carrera GF, Lightfoot RW, Jr., Wortmann RL. Gouty arthritis: a prospective radiographic evaluation of sixty patients. Skel Radiol 1984; 11:1–8.

12

The Biochemistry of Gout

Michael A. Becker
Rheumatology Section, Department of Medicine, University of Chicago School of Medicine, Chicago, Illinois, U.S.A.

INTRODUCTION

The clinical manifestations of gout ultimately reflect consequences of urate/uric acid crystal deposition from biological fluids supersaturated for urate, the sparingly soluble end-product of purine metabolism in humans. Study of the biochemistry of gout, therefore, focuses on the processes determining urate levels in health and on alterations in these processes that result in states of urate supersaturation. Several definitions should expedite the aims of this discussion.

Uric acid (2, 6, 8-trioxypurine) is a weak organic acid derived in biological systems from sequential oxidation of the purine bases, hypoxanthine and xanthine. Ionization of uric acid at position 9 of the purine ring occurs with a pKa_1 of 5.75, so that dissociated urate predominates over undissociated uric acid in a ratio of about 50 to 1 at the pH of 7.4 in plasma and other extracellular fluids (Fig. 1). Nearly all dissociated urate ion functions as monosodium urate as a result of the high concentration of sodium ion in extracellular fluids. In acidic biological fluids (such as is usually the case for urine), however, undissociated uric acid predominates. These considerations explain why uric acid crystals are found in stones formed in the urinary tracts of some gouty individuals, in contrast to the monosodium urate monohydrate crystals that deposit in joints, tophi, renal interstitium, and other tissues in gouty patients.

Hyperuricemia is defined as a concentration of urate exceeding the solubility of this compound in serum or plasma and is a common biochemical

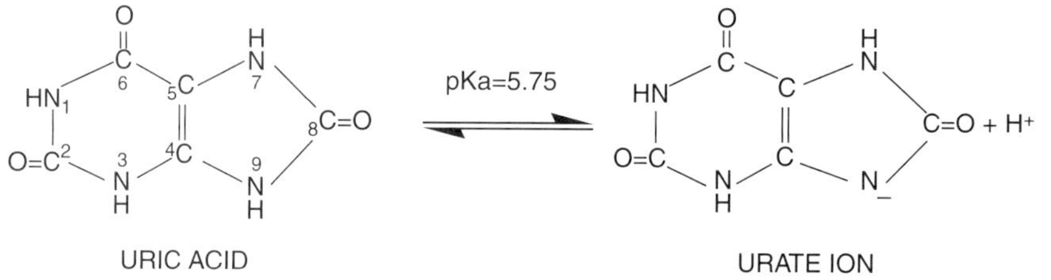

Figure 1 Uric acid and the urate ion.

abnormality. Estimates of the limit of solubility of urate in serum range from about 6.5 mg/dL to 7.0 mg/dL, but a value of 6.8 mg/dL is commonly stated, and values exceeding 7.0 mg/dL are clearly supersaturating. Under steady state conditions, persistent hyperuricemia reflects extracellular urate supersaturation predisposing to urate crystal formation and deposition in tissues. In fact, hyperuricemia of increasing magnitude is associated with a corresponding increase in risk for the clinical consequences of urate crystal deposition that define gout (1,2). Nevertheless, only a minority of chronically hyperuricemic individuals appear ever to express a manifestation of gout, such as a flare of gouty arthritis, renal colic, or, less commonly, the appearance of a tophaceous deposit. The majority of people with urate supersaturation thus remain in a state called asymptomatic hyperuricemia.

For several reasons, the physicochemical definition of hyperuricemia appears preferable to the population-based definition derived from measuring serum urate levels in putatively normal individuals. First, serum urate in the adult population is not normally distributed; rather, the distribution is skewed toward values in the higher range (Fig. 2) (3). Second, upper limits of "normal" serum urate values derived from studies of different populations often reach 7.5 or 8.0 mg/dL or greater, thereby including individuals whose sera are clearly supersaturated for urate. Finally, real differences in means and variances between adult men and women tend to obscure the facts that some women with serum urate levels exceeding two standard deviations above the mean for the sex may not have urate supersaturation or an increased risk for gout, and, conversely, that both men and women with urate levels exceeding saturation for similar durations are (it is believed) at similar risk for urate crystal deposition and gout.

Gout is the disease state manifesting clinical consequences of urate/uric acid crystal deposition from urate-supersaturated extracellular fluids. Because hyperuricemia most often does not eventuate in a disease state, careful distinction between hyperuricemia, a biochemical aberration, and the disease gout must be made. This has significance in consideration of therapeutic intervention, at least until the association of hyperuricemia and non-crystal-related degenerative diseases is clarified with regard to whether hyperuricemia plays a causal or an

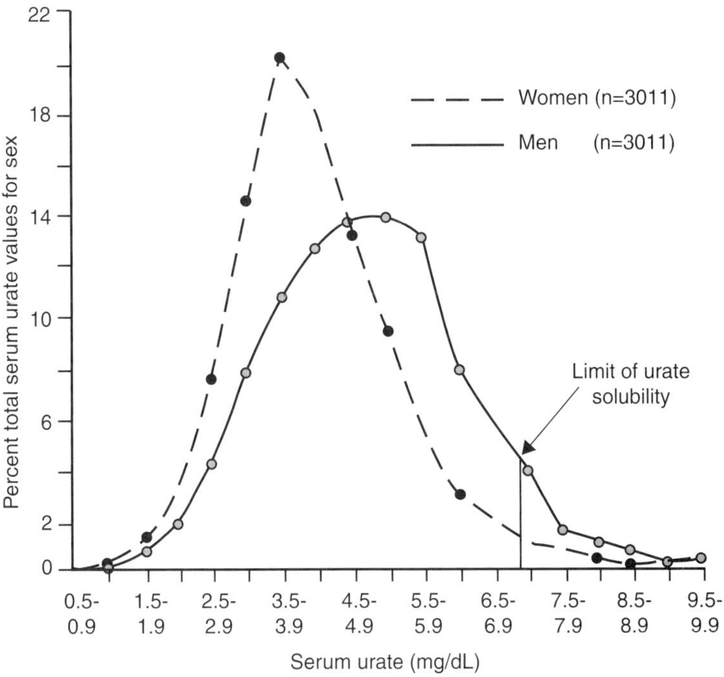

Figure 2 Frequency distribution of serum urate values in healthy men and women in Tecumseh, Michigan, U.S.A., 1959–1960. *Source*: Modified from Ref. 3.

epiphenomenologic role in the pathogenesis or progression of hypertension, chronic renal impairment, or cardiovascular disease (4).

This chapter will review normal purine production, interconversion, and catabolism and how these processes are regulated to support the multiple biological roles of purine compounds and, ultimately, provide substrate for urate production. Urate physiology and disposal are discussed elsewhere in this book (Chapter 16), but reference will be made here to the current understanding of the major pathogenetic mechanisms underlying hyperuricemia: urate overproduction and impaired renal excretion of uric acid. Finally, the phenotypic features accompanying inborn errors of human purine metabolism will be reviewed.

PURINE METABOLISM

Purine compounds are defined by the nine member purine nucleus, consisting of fused pyrimidine and imidazole rings (Fig. 1). Purines are essential components of all living cells. Purine nucleotides serve as building blocks for DNA and RNA, molecular energy sources, and high energy phosphate donors in many enzymatic reactions. Purines also function as neurotransmitters, intra- and extracellular signaling molecules, and, perhaps, as protectors against oxidant-induced tissue

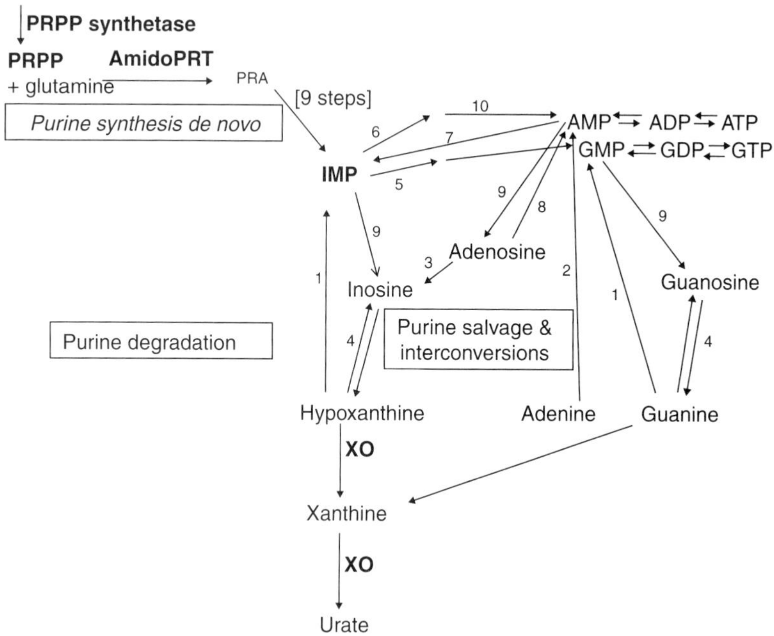

Figure 3 Schematic representation of the pathways of purine metabolism in humans. Purine compounds and certain key enzymes catalyzing reactions in the purine pathways are indicated in bold type or numbered as listed below. The component pathways are labeled in boxes. Numbered enzymes are: (1) hypoxanthine-guanine phosphoribosyltransferase (HPRT); (2) adenine phosphoribosyltransferase (APRT); (3) adenosine deaminase; (4) purine nucleoside phosphorylase; (5) inosinic acid dehydrogenase; (6) adenylosuccinate synthetase; (7) adenylate deaminase; (8), adenosine kinase; (9) specific 5′-nucleotidases and nonspecific phosphatases; and (10) adenylosuccinate lyase. In the absence of purine ingestion, all new purine compounds are ultimately derived from non-purine precursors contributing to the assembly of IMP through the 10-step pathway of purine synthesis de novo. Not shown are the pathways of deoxypurine synthesis and degradation. *Abbreviations*: PRPP, 5-phosphoribosyl 1-pyrophosphate; IMP, inosinic acid; AMP and GMP, ADP and GDP, ATP and GTP, the mono-, di- and triphosphate members of the adenylate and guanylate classes of purines, respectively; AmidoPRT, amidophosphoribosyltransferase; XO, xanthine oxidase.

damage (4) and neurodegenerative processes (5,6). The overall scheme of human purine metabolism (6) is customarily divided into four interfacing and, to some extent, overlapping compartments, which include purine nucleotide synthetic pathways; purine salvage reactions; purine nucleoside and nucleotide interconversions; and purine nucleotide degradation through purine nucleoside and base forms, culminating in irreversible oxidation of unreclaimed hypoxanthine and xanthine to urate (Figs. 3 and 4) (7).

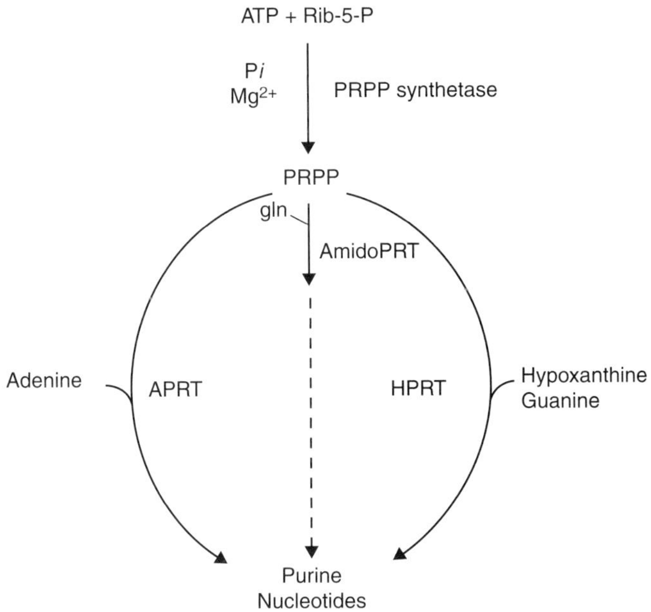

Figure 4 Schematic representation of the synthesis of purine nucleotides, emphasizing the role of 5-phosphoribosyl-1-pyrophosphate (PRPP) as a substrate common to the pathways of purine base salvage as well as purine synthesis de novo. Synthesis of PRPP from Mg-ATP and ribose-5-phosphate is catalyzed by PRPP synthetase in a reaction requiring magnesium ion (Mg^{2+}) and inorganic phosphate (Pi). *Abbreviations*: Amido-PRT, amidophosphoribosyltransferase; APRT, adenine phosphoribosyltransferase; ATP, adenosine triphosphate; HPRT, hypoxanthine-guanine phosphoribosyltransferase.

Purine Synthesis De Novo

Net contributions to body pools of purine compounds are provided only by dietary purine ingestion and endogenous synthesis of purine nucleotides in the process of purine synthesis de novo (Figs. 3 and 4) (7). The latter is a pathway of ten enzymatic reactions in which the purine ring of the parent purine nucleotide, inosinic acid (IMP), is sequentially constructed from non-purine small molecule donors on a ribose-5-phosphate backbone provided by the high energy sugar phosphate 5-phosphoribosyl-1-pyrophosphate (PRPP).

PRPP is a key substrate in and activator of purine synthesis de novo and is also utilized in purine base salvage reactions and in pyrimidine and pyridine nucleotide synthesis (8). PRPP is formed from Mg-ATP and ribose-5-phosphate in the PRPP synthetase reaction, catalyzed in humans by at least three independently active PRPP synthetase isoforms, designated PRS1, PRS2, and PRS3. Because the PRPP synthetase reaction is neither committed solely to nor rate-limiting for

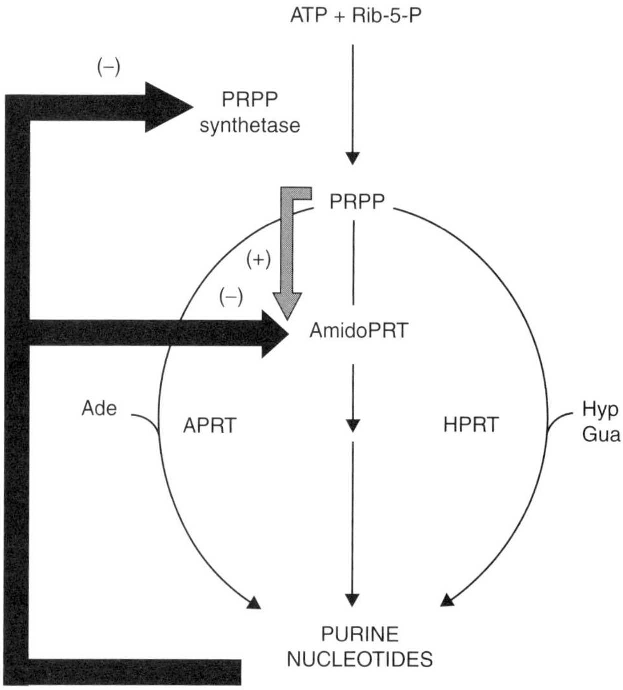

Figure 5 Schematic representation of the major sites and mechanisms of regulation of purine nucleotide synthesis. Both amidophosphoribosyltransferase (AmidoPRT) and 5-phosphoribosyl-1-pyrophosphate (PRPP) synthetase are allosteric enzymes inhibited by purine nucleotide products (*heavy black arrows*), with AmidoPRT being more sensitive to inhibition. PRPP is an activator (*heavy gray arrow*) as well as a substrate of AmidoPRT. The antagonistic interaction between PRPP and purine nucleotide inhibitors determines the activity of AmidoPRT and, consequently, the rate of the pathway of purine nucleotide synthesis de novo. *Abbreviations*: Ade, adenine; ATP, adenosine triphosphate; APRT, adenine phosphoribosyltransferase; Gua, guanine; Hyp, hypoxanthine; HPRT, hypoxanthine-guanine phosphoribosyltransferase.

purine synthesis de novo, it is not regarded as the first step in the pathway. This role is fulfilled by the succeeding reaction, catalyzed by amidophosphoribosyltransferase (amidoPRT), in which PRPP condenses irreversibly with L-glutamine to generate 5-phosphoribosyl-1-amine (PRA). As discussed below, the amidoPRT reaction is the primary site of control of purine nucleotide and, under ordinary circumstances, urate synthesis in humans (Figs. 5 and 6) (8,9). The structure and catalytic mechanisms of this critical enzyme have been studied in detail (largely in the Bacillus version of amidoPRT) (10,11), confirming that PRA synthesis is allosterically regulated and involves sequential steps at separate catalytic sites on the protein: first, hydrolysis of glutamine to glutamate and NH_3, and then inorganic

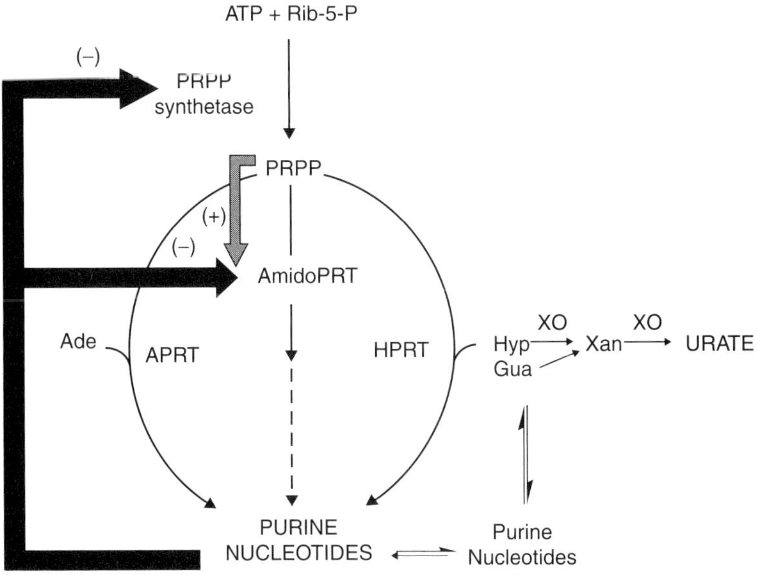

Figure 6 Schematic representation of purine nucleotide synthetic pathways and degradation to urate. The single-step salvage of hypoxanthine or guanine, catalyzed by hypoxanthine-guanine phosphoribosyltransferase (HPRT), both utilizes 5-phosphoribosyl-1-pyrophosphate (PRPP) and contributes to nucleotide pools, thus modulating rates of the pathway of purine synthesis de novo. Under baseline unfed conditions, activity of amidophosphoribosyltransferase (AmidoPRT), the rate-limiting reaction in purine synthesis de novo, is the major determinant of uric acid production. In HPRT deficiency, however, hypoxanthine and guanine reutilization in salvage synthesis of purine nucleotides is impaired, and these purine bases undergo oxidation to urate at higher rates. In addition, the reduced utilization of PRPP in salvage results in activation of AmidoPRT. This results in an acceleration of purine nucleotide synthesis de novo, which contributes further to urate production. In overactivity of PRPP synthetase, increased PRPP availability drives both purine synthesis de novo and urate production despite intact purine base salvage. *Abbreviations*: Ade, adenine, APRT, adeninc phosphoribosyltransferase; ATP, adenosine triphosphate; Hyp, hypoxanthine; Gua, guanine; Xan, xanthine; XO, xanthine oxidase.

pyrophosphate displacement from PRPP by NH_3. The additional nine enzyme-catalyzed reactions in the de novo pathway are directed at stepwise construction and closure of the purine ring (7).

Purine Base Salvage Synthesis of Nucleotides

Purine synthesis de novo is an energy-costly process, requiring six moles of ATP for each mole of IMP generated (7). Substantial cellular energy savings is achieved, however, by means of single-step salvage of preformed purine bases derived from endogenous purine catabolism, nucleic acid breakdown, and dietary purines. Purine base salvage involves the enzymes hypoxanthine-guanine phosphoribosyltransferase (HPRT) and adenine phosphoribosyltransferase (APRT), which catalyze phosphoribosylation of hypoxanthine and guanine and of adenine, respectively, to their corresponding mononucleotides (IMP, GMP, and AMP) by reaction with PRPP (7,8). HPRT and APRT, and amidoPRT are representatives of the PRPP-utilizing class of phosphoribosyltransferase enzymes required for the net synthesis of pyrimidine and pyridine as well as purine nucleotides (8). HPRT and APRT also accept alternative purine base and base analogue substrates and have thus served as important sites of chemotherapeutic and molecular genetic interest (8).

Purine Nucleotide Interconversions and Catabolism

All newly synthesized purines are ultimately derived from IMP, which serves as a branchpoint for the alternative biosynthetic pathways leading to production of the major classes of purine nucleotides (adenylates and guanylates) involved in RNA and DNA synthesis or to the purine catabolic pathway (Fig. 3). Two-step pathways are required for interconversion of IMP to AMP or to GMP, the respective precursors of ADP and ATP and of GDP and GTP (7).

The purine catabolic pathway in humans (Fig. 3) encompasses reactions through which purine nucleoside 5′-monophosphates (IMP, AMP, XMP, GMP) are converted to purine nucleosides and bases that ultimately undergo irreversible oxidation to urate (12). Dephosphorylation of these compounds to the respective ribonucleosides, with release of inorganic phospate, is catalyzed by nonspecific phosphatases and by specific purine 5′-nucleotidases (7). Purine nucleosides (other than adenosine) may be further catabolized to purine bases by phosphorolysis via the reversible purine nucleoside phosphorylase (PNP) reaction. In this reaction, inosine and guanosine (as well as their corresponding 2′deoxynucleosides) and, less effectively, xanthosine are cleaved to the respective purine bases, hypoxanthine, guanine, or xanthine, and ribose- (or deoxyribose-)1-phosphate (7). Adenosine, derived from both AMP and S-adenosylhomocysteine metabolism, is not a substrate for the human PNP. Rather, the catabolism of adenosine and a portion of AMP proceeds through deamination steps to inosine and IMP, respectively, in reactions catalyzed by adenosine deaminase and adenylate deaminase.

In contrast to adenosine, which can be salvaged by direct conversion to AMP, inosine and guanosine salvage to their respective nucleotides requires sequential PNP and HPRT reactions. In the course of this salvage sequence, the intermediate purine bases, hypoxanthine and guanine, can be alternatively directed into the final and irreversible catabolic steps resulting in urate formation (Fig. 3). In this process, guanine is converted to xanthine in a deamination reaction, and both of the oxidation steps converting hypoxanthine to xanthine and xanthine to urate are catalyzed by xanthine oxidase/dehydrogenase, a flavoenzyme containing Fe-S centers and molybdenum bound to a pterin cofactor (12).

Xanthine oxidase is found in greatest abundance in the human liver and proximal small intestine and, in trace amounts, in endothelial cells and muscle. In the course of catalyzing the oxidation reactions leading to production of urate, superoxide anion and H_2O_2 are generated, with further conversion of H_2O_2 to free hydroxyl radicals. Production of these mediators of inflammation and tissue injury during xanthine oxidase catalysis has led to a proposed role for xanthine oxidase in the events surrounding tissue injury after ischemia, circumstances that also promote adenine nucleotide catabolism and urate production (13,14).

Regulation of Purine Biosynthesis and Degradation

Purine nucleotide synthesis de novo and purine base salvage reactions provide alternative but concerted means for regulating production of purine nucleotides to fulfill cellular needs. The molecular mechanisms underlying this regulation largely involve control of rates of purine synthesis de novo determined in a regulatory domain encompassing the sequential allosteric enzymes, PRPP synthetase (15) and amidoPRT (Fig. 5) (16).

The allosteric regulatory and quaternary structural properties of amidoPRT are in accord with a functionally critical antagonistic interaction between PRPP and pathway end products on the activity of the enzyme (16–18). Binding of PRPP induces a conformational change favoring enzyme activation (17). Purine nucleotides (especially monophosphates) inhibit amidoPRT by binding at regulatory domains distinct from substrate binding sites (11,18). Purine nucleotides bearing different (amino and hydroxy) substituents at position 6 of the purine ring exert synergistic inhibition of amidoPRT activity, which, however, can be overcome by very high concentrations of PRPP (11,16,17). Because levels of PRPP in normal cells (8) are substantially less than the apparent affinity constant of amidoPRT for this compound (18), it is likely that PRPP availability provides the basis for rate limitation of the pathway at the amidoPRT reaction. In fact, with rare exception, increased intracellular PRPP concentration is associated with accelerated purine synthesis de novo, and depletion of PRPP slows the rate of the pathway (8).

Human amidoPRT can assume alternative and functionally significant quaternary conformations (16,17). An active smaller form is reversibly converted into an inactive larger form by addition of nucleotide inhibitors, and this effect is blocked by increasing concentrations of PRPP. This model provides a potential molecular mechanism for control of amidoPRT activity and has been confirmed in vivo as well as in purified preparations of the enzyme (16). The molecular cloning of vertebrate amidoPRT cDNAs (19) and the crystallographic and kinetic analyses of bacterial (Bacillus subtilis) amidoPRT have provided additional molecular insight into the amidotransferase and glutaminase functions of this important enzyme (10).

Purine nucleotide inhibition of PRPP synthetase activity provides a second level of inhibitory control of rates of purine synthesis de novo (Fig. 6) (15). Human

PRS1 is an allosteric and multimeric enzyme with a regulatory site defined by noncompetitive inhibition by the purine nucleotides ADP and GDP (8). The subunit of the erythrocyte enzyme has a molecular weight of 34.5 kDa and can undergo reversible enzyme concentration- and effector-mediated subunit association, with enzyme activity residing only in the two largest of many multimers (20,21). Recombinant human PRS1 and PRS2 isoforms have been characterized with respect to their kinetic and regulatory properties and confirm that PRPP synthetase is less sensitive to purine nucleotide inhibition than is the case for amidoPRT (15,22,23). PRPP synthetase activity may also be inhibited by pyrimidine and pyridine nucleotides, products of pathways which, like purine nucleotide synthesis, require PRPP (24). Regulation of purine synthesis de novo at successive early steps in the pathway appears well suited to maintaining of both fine and broad control over changes in endproduct availability. Fine control is effected by alterations in amidoPRT activity in response to small changes in purine concentrations (15–17,23), and broader control is maintained by changes in PRPP synthetase activity in response to larger variations in concentrations of nucleotide products of several biosynthetic pathways (15,23).

Several additional levels of control of purine metabolism have been proposed (Fig. 3). First, purine nucleotide interconversion reactions involved in the alternative conversion of IMP to either AMP or GMP are subject to endproduct inhibition directed at the first reaction in the respective sequence (25). In addition, GTP and ATP are required, respectively, for the synthesis of AMP and GMP from IMP, consistent with control over the balance of nucleotide classes produced by interconversion reactions. Second, ribonucleotide degradation is also a regulated process in which the critical reactions are catalyzed by AMP deaminase and 5′-nucleotidases. AMP deaminase is activated by ATP and ADP and is inhibited by GTP and inorganic phosphate. Release of this enzyme from inhibition, for example, in circumstances requiring rapid phosphorylation of substrates by ATP, results in accelerated nucleotide degradation to urate (26). Finally, although understanding of regulation at the level of dephosphorylation has been limited by the multiplicity of soluble 5′-nucleotidases, each with a different pattern of substrate preference and responsiveness to nucleotides and inorganic phosphate, it seems likely that nucleotides, especially ATP and ADP (as well as inorganic phosphate), are key modulators of nucleotide catabolism.

URATE HOMEOSTASIS AND MECHANISMS OF HYPERURICEMIA

Humans and certain primate species are unique among mammals in the requirement to excrete uric acid as the end product of purine metabolism. This is the result of a mutational silencing of the gene encoding the enzyme uricase, which catalyzes degradation of urate to the readily excreted compound allantoin (27,28). Lack of uricase is one of three circumstances conditioning all humans to the development of body fluids supersaturated for urate, with the attendant risks for urate crystal deposition and clinical sequelae. A second is the limited solubility of urate and uric acid. The theoretical limit of solubility of undissociated uric acid in aqueous solution is about 6.5 mg/dL. This form usually predominates in urine, where, at pH 5.0, saturation occurs at about 15 mg/dL (7). The solubility of the ionized urate form that constitutes 98% of the uric acid at the pH and sodium concentration of other extracellular fluids is comparably limited, only about 6.8 mg/dL. Thus, in many normal adult male populations at least, mean serum urate concentrations approach the limit of urate solubility in serum. The third predisposing circumstance is that 90% or more of urate filtered at the glomerulus is normally reabsorbed rather than excreted. Even though this process favors urate retention, most individuals excrete an acid urine with uric acid concentrations considerably in excess of saturation (7). Despite these conditioning circumstances, manifestations of urate deposition are relatively uncommon. The factors determining which persons will develop hyperuricemia and gout are diverse but can be more easily appreciated by considering the physiological mechanisms maintaining uric acid homeostasis in normal and hyperuricemic individuals.

Urate is synthesized mainly in the liver and is released into the circulation. Urate plasma protein binding is minimal (less than 4% under physiological conditions), and the vast majority of circulating urate filtered at the glomerulus is available for the subsequent mechanisms of renal uric acid handling. Both the overall contribution of renal excretion to uric acid disposal and the size and dynamics of the miscible pool of urate have been estimated at steady state in normal and gouty individuals by sequential measurements of isotopic enrichment of urinary uric acid following intravenous administration of [^{15}N] or [^{14}C] urate (7). Urinary uric acid excretion ordinarily accounts for two-thirds to three-fourths of daily uric acid disposal, and intestinal uricolysis, degradation by gut bacteria of uric acid secreted into the gut, accounts for nearly all urate disposed of by extrarenal routes (29). In normal men, the miscible urate pool averages about 1200 mg (range, about $\pm$300 mg), with a mean rate of turnover of about 700 mg/day (range, about 500 to 1100 mg/day) (7). Mean urate pool sizes of about 600 mg and turnover rates of 0.6 pool/day have been found in six normal women.

All untreated patients with gout have enlarged urate pools, usually ranging from 2000 to 4000 mg in the absence of evident tophi but estimated to reach 30,000 mg or more in tophaceous gout in which, however, measurements may be inaccurate when urate deposits are not in steady state with the soluble urate pool (7). Extrarenal urate disposal in hyperuricemic or gouty individuals is normal or increased to as much as 50% of total daily excretion, indicating that impaired intestinal uricolysis is not a mechanism of hyperuricemia (29). Many patients with gout have rates of turnover of the urate pool in the normal range. Increased rates of turnover have, however, invariably been found in patients with excessive rates of purine synthesis de novo and urate overproduction as reflected by increased incorporation of labeled precursor molecules into urinary uric acid and by daily urinary uric acid excretion clearly exceeding that of normal individuals (7,30).

Table 1 Classification of the Causes of Hyperuricemia and Gout

- Impaired renal uric acid excretion
  - Primary gout with decreased uric acid clearance
  - Secondary gout
    - Clinical disorders resulting in decreased uric acid clearance
      - Chronic renal failure
      - Polycystic kidney disease
      - Familial juvenile hyperuricemic nephropathy (UMOD mutations)
      - Medullary cystic kidney disease (UMOD mutations in type 2)
      - Hypertension
      - Dehydration
      - Salt restriction
      - Starvation
      - Diabetic ketoacidosis
      - Lactic acidosis
      - Obesity
      - Hyperparathyroidism
      - Hypothyroidism
      - Adrenal insufficiency
      - Nephrogenic diabetes insipidus
      - Sarcoidosis
      - Toxemia of pregnancy
      - Bartter syndrome
      - Chronic beryllium disease
      - Down syndrome
    - Drugs, toxins, or dietary habits
      - Ethanol
      - Lead nephropathy
      - Diuretics
      - Low dose salicylates ($\sim$0.3–3.0 grams/day)
      - Ethambutol
      - Pyrazinamide
      - Laxative abuse (alkalosis)
      - Levodopa
      - Methoxyflurane
      - Cyclosporine A
      - Tacrolimus
- Excessive urate production
  - Primary gout with accelerated urate synthesis
  - Secondary gout with purine nucleotide and/or uric acid overproduction
    - Inherited enzyme defects
      - HPRT deficiency
      - PRPP synthetase overactivity
      - Glucose-6-phosphatase deficiency (glycogenosis I)
      - Fructose-1-phosphate aldolase deficiency

(Continued)

Table 1 Classification of the Causes of Hyperuricemia and Gout *(Continued)*

Clinical disorders leading to urate overproduction
Polycythemia vera
Myeloproliferative disorders
Lymphoproliferative disorders
Malignancies
Hemolytic disorders
Psoriasis
Obesity
Tissue hypoxia
Glycogenoses III, V, VII
Drugs or dietary habits
Ethanol (beer > distilled spirits > red wine)
Meat- or fish-rich diet
Purine-rich diet
Pancreatic extract
Fructose
Nicotinic acid
Ethylamino-1,3,4-thiadiazole
4-Amino-5-imidazole carboxamide riboside
B_{12} (repletion in patients with pernicious anemia)
Cytotoxic drugs
Warfarin

Abbreviations: HPRT, hypoxanthine-guanine phosphoribosyltransferase; PRPP, 5-phosphoribosyl-1-pyrophosphate.

These findings provided evidence for heterogeneity in the mechanisms accounting for urate accumulation, hyperuricemia, and the consequent predisposition to urate crystal deposition among gouty patients (7). Additional study has confirmed that excessive urate production and impaired renal clearance of uric acid, operating singly or in combination, are the major abnormalities demonstrable among persistently hyperuricemic individuals with or without gout (31). Whether hyperuricemia results from an intrinsic metabolic disease (primary hyperuricemia), as the result of another disease, or as a consequence of drug use or exposure to a toxin (secondary hyperuricemia), one or both of these mechanisms underlie the development of hyperuricemia. The distinction between urate overproduction and impaired uric acid renal excretion provides the basis for a commonly employed classification of hyperuricemia and gout (Table 1).

CLASSIFICATION OF GOUT AND HYPERURICEMIA

Determination of the 24-hour urinary uric acid excretion usually allows discrimination between urate overproduction and impaired uric acid excretion (32). For adults ingesting a purine-free diet, uric acid excretion in excess of 600 mg per day is considered overproduction. Values in excess of 1000 mg per day with ingestion of a "regular" diet are also clearly abnormal and indicative of overproduction; values between 800 and 1000 mg/day are borderline. Lower values provide evidence that the hyperuricemia results from impaired renal uric acid excretion. These comments presume otherwise normal renal function. Within these two broad categories, the causes of hyperuricemia can be subclassified as primary or secondary (Table 1).

Primary Gout

Renal mechanisms, which may be under genetic control, are responsible for the hyperuricemia in over 90% of individuals with primary gout. Uric acid excretion rates and the capacity of the excretory mechanism for uric acid are the same for gouty subjects and non-gouty individuals, but the curve relating uric acid excretion to serum urate is shifted in the former group, so that gouty subjects require serum urate values 2 or 3 mg/dL higher than those of controls to achieve equivalent uric acid renal excretion rates (33). In both primary gout with impairment of renal uric acid excretion and primary gout resulting from urate overproduction, it is likely that several pathophysiological mechanisms underlie the development of hyperuricemia.

Secondary Gout

Numerous secondary causes of hyperuricemia and gout can be attributed to impaired renal excretion of uric acid. Decreased renal excretion of uric acid is thought to be an important mechanism for the hyperuricemia associated with hypothyroidism, adrenal insufficiency, nephrogenic diabetes insipidus, chronic lead intoxication, and disorders characterized by accumulation of organic acids (starvation, alcoholic ketosis, diabetic ketoacidosis, and lactic acidosis). Drugs that alter uric acid excretion also represent important causes of secondary hyperuricemia (34). These include diuretics, lower-dose aspirin, pyrazinamide, nicotinic acid, ethambutol, and cyclosporine A.

Secondary gout can also result from urate overproduction. This is the case with specific inborn metabolic defects, including HPRT deficiency (35,36), PRPP synthetase overactivity (37,38), glucose-6-phosphatase deficiency, and fructose-1-phosphate aldolase deficiency. Overproduction can also occur in patients with psoriasis, chronic hemolytic states, polycythemia, certain muscle glycogenoses, and lymphoproliferative and myeloproliferative disorders.

Hyperuricemia in patients with fructose-1-phosphate aldolase deficiency, glucose-6-phosphatase deficiency, or chronic alcoholism reflects a combination of mechanisms. In each of these conditions there is both accelerated purine nucleotide catabolism leading to urate overproduction and an acidemia that blocks renal excretion of uric acid. In the case of chronic alcohol use, nucleotide depletion activates de novo purine biosynthesis, with consequent urate overproduction (39). Acute excessive alcohol intake also provokes lactic acidosis, resulting in impaired uric acid excretion. In addition, some alcoholic beverages contain large quantities of purine precursors of urate (40).

Urate Overproduction

Excessive urinary uric acid excretion is demonstrable in 10% to 15% of patients with gout and primary hyperuricemia and in most patients in whom hyperuricemia reflects increased cell turnover (i.e., a lymphoproliferative or myeloproliferative disease or psoriasis) or a toxic state or pharmacologic intervention resulting in increased uric acid production (Table 1). Sustained urate overproduction in patients with gout and primary hyperuricemia indicates excessive rates of purine synthesis de novo, which in the framework of current understanding of the regulation of this pathway should reflect altered interaction between PRPP and purine nucleotides on amidoPRT activity (Fig. 6) (15,16). In fact, in several circumstances in which inherited or acquired hyperuricemia is associated with urate overproduction, alterations in the availability of these small molecule effectors have been demonstrated, with either increased PRPP availability or decreased purine nucleotide concentrations constituting the apparent basis for excessive purine nucleotide and urate synthesis.

Increased PRPP Availability

The role of PRPP as a critical component in the regulation of purine nucleotide, and urate production is supported by extensive biochemical, pharmacologic, and clinical investigation since first proposed by Wyngaarden and Kelley 30 years ago (7,15). Increased PRPP availability is the driving force for excessive rates of purine synthesis de novo in two X chromosome-linked inborn errors of purine metabolism, HPRT deficiency (35,36) and PRPP synthetase overactivity (37,38). Urate overproduction, hyperuricemia, and hyperuricosuria occur in each of these disorders in conjunction with increased intracellular PRPP concentrations but no apparent decreases in concentrations of purine nucleotides (7,15,35,37). In PRPP synthetase overactivity, increased PRPP levels result from overproduction of this regulatory substrate. In contrast, PRPP accumulates in excess in HPRT deficiency as a consequence of underutilization in this salvage reaction (8,41). Increased PRPP availability in both instances results in activation of amidoPRT and acceleration of purine nucleotide and urate synthesis, which readily explain the metabolic consequences of the disorders in most affected early adult-onset patients: gouty arthritis and urolithiasis. Unexplained, however, are the distinctive neurological syndromes encountered in infants or young children with more severe variants of HPRT deficiency (Lesch-Nyhan syndrome) or PRPP synthetase overactivity (sensorineural deafness, neurodevelopmental impairment) (42–44).

PRPP synthetase superactivity and HPRT deficiency account for only a small proportion of patients with primary uric acid overproduction, but represent the only states in which excessive PRPP availability clearly constitutes the sole basis of urate overproduction. A unique or contributory role for increased PRPP availability has been suggested, however, in several other proposed or established enzymatic defects or metabolic states in which there is evidence for urate overproduction, such as in patients with glucose-6-phosphatase deficiency (glycogen storage disease, type I), where multifactorial hyperuricemia may appear as early as infancy, and gout has been reported by the end of the first decade of life (7). Purine and urate overproduction in this disorder of carbohydrate metabolism is of particular interest as a potential model system for clarifying an apparent link between disordered carbohydrate metabolism and hyperuricemia in disorders like obesity and hypertriglyceridemia. A potential mechanism could be that in states of carbohydrate excess and accelerated lipogenesis, metabolic flux through the pentose phosphate shunt is increased with consequent increase in PRPP production.

Decreased Purine Nucleotide Concentrations

Despite impaired purine base salvage, normal intracellular purine nucleotide concentrations have been found in cells deficient in HPRT (41,45). Urate overproduction due to nucleotide depletion has, however, been identified in a number of circumstances in which net degradation of ATP results from either increased ATP consumption or impaired ATP regeneration (46). When the supply of inorganic phosphate, oxygen, glucose, or fatty acids is restricted, ATP synthesis may be impaired, and severe ATP depletion and accompanying hyperuricemia may ensue, particularly if the demands for ATP consumption are concomitantly increased. Net ATP degradation results in accumulation of ADP and AMP, which are rapidly converted to uric acid through the intermediates inosine, hypoxanthine, and xanthine (Fig. 3). Increases in any or all of these intermediates accompanying excessive urate levels in serum or uric acid in urine provide evidence in support of this mechanism of hyperuricemia. Among the unusual physiological and pathological states that can provoke net ATP degradation and consequent hyperuricemia are: strenuous exercise or prolonged training in otherwise normal individuals; glycogen storage diseases, types I, III, V, and VII; acute alcohol ingestion; and diseases with acute tissue hypoxia (14,46,47).

Impaired Uric Acid Excreton

Renal Handling Mechanisms

Renal excretion of uric acid is a complex physiological function currently undergoing significant clarification as a result of the cloning and characterization of human urate transporters. This topic is reviewed in Chapter 16. Suffice to say, prior concepts of how human renal uric acid handling results in net retention of about 90% of filtered urate emerged over several decades of pharmacological and physiological studies in experimental animals and in humans (48). The result was an operationally defined four-component model incorporating glomerular filtration, proximal tubular reabsorption, proximal tubular secretion, and post-secretory reabsorption. Because of the complicated phenomenology of metabolite and drug effects on renal uric acid excretion, however, validation of this model remained incomplete and awaited understanding at genetic and molecular levels of how renal uric acid excretion is regulated and, in turn, regulates serum urate levels in normal individuals (48). Such an understanding appears imminent and should serve to clarify mechanisms of impaired urate handling in gout patients as well.

Reduced urate clearance contributes to hyperuricemia in over 90% of patients with primary gout (7). Absolute amounts of uric acid in the daily urine are not reduced in most of these individuals compared with non-gouty persons. Most gouty subjects, however, have lower than normal fractional clearances of urate than do normal subjects, and for any plasma concentration of urate, gouty persons excrete on average 41% less uric acid than normal subjects (33). These patients show a greater increase in plasma urate concentrations in response to exogenously administered purines, presumably as a result of decreased urate clearances. Overall, gouty patients require plasma urate levels 2 to 3 mg/dL higher than non-gouty persons to achieve comparable uric acid excretion rates.

To date, efforts to identify precise mechanistic defects underlying impaired renal urate excretion in primary gout patients have had only marginal success. Reduced urate filtration as a result of increased urate binding to plasma proteins has been proposed, but not confirmed, as an explanation of the high rates of hyperuricemia and gout in the Maoris of New Zealand (49). In a few patients with no evident uric acid overproduction, diminished renal urate secretion per nephron was found, and some additional support for impaired tubular urate secretion has been presented (50). In contrast, evidence to support the idea of enhanced tubular reabsorption of uric acid as an explanation of primary hyperuricemia has, to date, not been compelling.

A better understanding of mechanisms of aberrant renal uric acid handling in gouty patients has arisen from several recent advances. The first is the identification and characterization of the autosomal dominantly transmitted disorders familial juvenile hyperuricemic nephropathy (FJHN) (51,52) and medullary cystic kidney disease 2 (MCKD2) (53), which are allelic disorders reflecting mutation in the URO (uromodulin) gene encoding Tamm-Horsfall glycoprotein (54). Although the precise relationship between mutations (frequently affecting cysteine residues in this disulfide bond-rich protein) and progressive renal failure will await a clearer understanding of the function of Tamm-Horsfall glycoprotein, severe impairment of renal uric acid clearance is identifiable in affected individuals early in life, prior to other renal functional defects (51,52). Delineation of the mechanism involved in diminished urate clearance in patients with these disorders may shed light on molecular processes involved in regulating normal urate handling. Moreover, whether more subtle alterations in expression of the URO gene than have been identified to date could account for a more substantial proportion of patients with familial or even sporadic gout with impaired renal uric acid excretion is currently under investigation.

The second advance of potentially great impact in this area comes from the identification and characterization of URAT1, a highly specific urate-anion exchanger localized to the luminal membrane of proximal renal tubular epithelial cells. The physiological properties of this exchanger with respect to transport of endogenous ions and drug agents with known uricoretentive and uricosuric properties accord well with a role for URAT1 as a regulator of blood urate levels (55). Moreover, mutations in SLC22A12, the gene encoding URAT1, have been identified in affected members of families with inherited tubular defects resulting in hypouricemia, increased urate clearance, susceptibility to exercise-induced acute renal failure, and chronic renal dysfunction, strongly supporting a role for URAT1 in the normal process of net uric acid reabsorption (56).

INBORN ERRORS OF HUMAN PURINE METABOLISM

Delineation of the pathways of purine metabolism and the regulation of purine nucleotide and urate synthesis in humans has been facilitated considerably by the identification and analysis of genetic defects affecting enzymes catalyzing some of the component reactions. The clinical phenotypes associated with one or another of these hereditary enzyme defects are rather diverse and overlapping, but a convenient classification is possible based on the major clinical manifestations associated with each defect (Table 2).

Table 2 Phenotypic Classification of Inborn Errors of Human Purine Metabolism

1. Gout with uric acid overproduction; uric acid urolithiasis common
    - Neurobehavioral or neurodevelopmental impairment common
        - Severe HPRT deficiency (Lesch-Nyhan syndrome and variants)
        - PRPP synthetase superactivity (defective allosteric regulation)
    - Neurological impairment uncommon
        - Partial deficiency of HPRT (Kelley-Seegmiller syndrome)
        - PRPP synthetase overactivity (excessive synthesis of normal enzyme)
2. Urolithiasis
    - APRT deficiency (2,8-dihydroxyadenine stones)
    - Xanthine oxidase deficiency (hereditary xanthinuria)
3. Immunodeficiency disease
    - Adenosine deaminase (ADA) deficiency and variants
    - Purine nucleoside phosphorylase (PNP) deficiency
4. Myopathy
    - Myoadenylate deaminase deficiency
5. Psychomotor retardation, seizures, autistic behavior
    - Adenylosuccinate lyase deficiency

Abbreviations: APRT, adenine phosphoribosyltransferase; HPRT, hypoxanthine-guanine phosphoribosyltransferase; PRPP, 5-phosphoribosyl-1-pyrophosphate.

Most directly germane to the subject of gout are the two X chromosome-linked disorders HPRT deficiency (35,36) and PRPP synthetase overactivity (37,38). As discussed above, accelerated purine nucleotide and urate production, hyperuricemia, and hyperuricosuria occur in each of these disorders, in major part as a consequence of increased availability of PRPP (7,8,15,41,57). These derangements readily explain the metabolic features of these disorders but not the distinctive neurological syndromes encountered in infants or young boys with more severe or complete defects in these enzymes.

Fully expressed, the Lesch-Nyhan syndrome, including mental retardation, dystonia/hypotonia, and self-injurious behavior in addition to hyperuricemia, is a devastating disorder of male infancy or early childhood, but components of the syndrome may appear in varying combinations and with varying severities (42,43). Overall, the extent of neurobehavioral expression is better correlated with the severity of disruption of HPRT function than with location of mutation in the HPRT gene (43). Patients with HPRT deficiency presenting after puberty are usually free of neurological abnormalities and are most often detected among patients with early-onset gout in association with hyperuricosuria or uric acid urolithiasis (57). Among affected families, widely varying levels of residual HPRT activity are detectable in screening assays, but substantial intracellular deficiency of HPRT function is invariable.

As is the case in HPRT deficiency, all patients with overactivity of PRPP synthetase overproduce purine nucleotides and urate and are thus at risk for gouty arthritis and uric acid urolithiasis, features comprising the sole manifestations of the disorder in most patients presenting as adults (58). Affected male infants and children, however, show a more serious disorder combining the consequences of greatly accelerated purine nucleotide and urate production with neurodevelopmental impairment and, most commonly, sensorineural hearing loss (44). Among families with affected children, women heterozygous for X-linked PRPP synthetase overactivity may be affected with metabolic and/or neurologic features, although usually later in life than their hemizygous affected male family members and in a more attenuated form (44).

PRPP synthetase overactivity results from excessive activity of the PRS1 isoform (59,60). In each family with the infantile-onset phenotype, a point mutation in the PRS1 gene encoding an overactive mutant PRS1 isoform has been demonstrated. In contrast, most families with later-onset PRPP synthetase overactivity have an excess of structurally and functionally normal PRS1, which, in turn, results from accelerated rate of transcription of the PRPS1 gene (59–61). The genetic basis of this unusual inherited defect remains uncertain.

Urolithiasis is the major clinical manifestation of two autosomally transmitted inborn errors of purine metabolism, deficiencies of adenine APRT and of XO (Fig. 3). In APRT deficiency, salvage of adenine, largely derived from 5′-methylthioadenosine phosphorolysis, is impaired. Adenine thus undergoes conversion (catalyzed by the dehydrogenase form of XO) to 2, 8-dihydroxyadenine, a poorly soluble metabolic dead-end product that undergoes urinary excretion, predisposing affected individuals to recurrent urinary tract stone formation (62). Although up to 1% of the population in many parts of the world carries a mutant allele for APRT deficiency, disease expression appears to be less common than expected except in Japan, where both type I and type II deficiencies are expressed as stone disease, occasionally associated with chronic renal failure (63). Purine nucleotide and urate overproduction is not a feature of APRT deficiency, as is the case with deficiency of HPRT, the other major purine base salvage enzyme.

Deficiency of XO, known as hereditary xanthinuria, is a rare disorder, typically manifested by urinary tract xanthine stone disease (12). A xanthine crystal deposition myopathy has also been described in some xanthinuric patients (64). Urinary tract stones may, of course, comprise a major problem in the management of patients with gout unassociated with a hereditary enzyme defect or in patients with HPRT deficiency or PRPP synthetase overactivity, but, in most such individuals, arthritis or neurological features are usually more prominent than stone disease.

A third clinical phenotype associated with hereditary defects in purine metabolic enzymes is immunodeficiency disease. Deficiencies in the activity of adenosine deaminase (ADA), the enzyme catalyzing conversion of adenosine (and deoxyadenosine) to inosine (and deoxyinosine) (Fig. 3), are associated with lymphopenia and impaired immune function, ranging from severe combined immunodeficiency disease expressed in infants or young children with virtually complete lack of ADA activity to milder immune deficits presenting in adults with residual but reduced ADA activity (65). Recurrent infection dominates the clinical picture of ADA deficiency, but osteochondral defects and central nervous system and hepatic abnormalities have also been described in some affected families.

A second purine enzyme defect predisposing to immune dysfunction (mainly involving cell-mediated processes) and infection is deficiency of PNP (66). The lymphopenia encountered in each of these autosomal recessive disorders is related to the accumulation to lymphocytotoxic levels of derivatives of deoxynucleosides (deoxyATP in ADA deficiency and deoxyGTP in PNP deficiency) normally converted to deoxybases by the respective enzyme.

Inherited deficiency of myoadenylate deaminase (adenylate deaminase; MADD) (Fig. 3) is by far the most common purine enzyme deficiency state, with heterozygous carrier frequencies of over 10% in both Caucasians and African Americans (67). A metabolic myopathy, documented in some persons homozygous for MADD deficiency, comprises a fourth clinical phenotype associated with a purine enzyme defect. Clinical expression of this disorder, however, appears far more rarely than would be expected from a genotype with a 1% or more prevalence in the population. Of interest, it has been suggested that heterozygosity for MADD deficiency may be cardioprotective (68). Among individuals with congestive heart failure, survival appears prolonged among MADD deficiency heterozygotes compared with persons with normal enzyme activity. A possible basis for this finding is the greater availability of adenosine for its cardiotonic effects among persons whose adenylate deaminase deficiency favors conversion of AMP to adenosine rather than to IMP.

A final clinical phenotype associated with a defective purine metabolic enzyme is psychomotor retardation, epilepsy, and autistic behavior described among patients homozygous for deficiency of adenylosuccinate lyase. This enzyme catalyzes two reactions in purine nucleotide biosynthesis (Fig. 3).

REFERENCES

1. Hall AP, Barry PE, Dawber TR, et al. Epidemiology of gout and hyperuricemia: a long-term population study. Am J Med 1967; 42:27–37.
2. Campion EW, Glynn RJ, DeLabry LO. Asymptomatic hyperuricemia: risks and consequences in the normative aging study. Am J Med 1987; 82:421–426.
3. Mikkelsen WM, Dodge HJ, Valkenburg H. The distribution of serum uric acid values in a population unselected as to gout or hyperuricemia: Tecumseh, Michigan 1959–60. Am J Med 1965; 39:242–251.
4. Johnson RJ, Cameron JS. Uric acid in cardiovascular and renal disease. Semin Nephrol 2005; 25:1–66.
5. Ames BN, Cathcart R, Schwiers EE, et al. Uric acid provides an antioxidant defense in humans against oxidant- and radical-caused aging and cancer: a hypothesis. Proc Natl Acad Sci USA 1981; 78:6858–6862.
6. Hooper DC, Scott GS, Zborek A, et al. Uric acid, a peroxynitrite scavenger, inhibits CNS inflammation, blood-CNS barrier permeability changes and tissue damage in a mouse model of multiple sclerosis. FASEB J 2000; 14:691–698.
7. Wyngaarden JB, Kelley WN. Gout and Hyperuricemia. New York: Grune & Stratton, 1976 and references therein.
8. Becker MA. Phosphoribosylpyrophosphate synthetase and the regulation of phosphoribosylpyrophosphate production in human cells. Prog Nucl Acid Res Mol Biol 2001; 69:115–148.
9. Holmes EW, Jr. Regulation of purine synthesis de novo. In: Kelley WN, Weiner IM, eds. Uric Acid. New York: Springer-Verlag, 1978:21–41.
10. Smith JL, Zaluzec EJ, Wery J-P, et al. Structure of the allosteric regulatory enzyme of purine biosynthesis. Science 1994; 264:1427–1433.
11. Krahn JM, Kim JH, Burns MR, et al. Coupled formation of an amidotransferase interdomain ammonia channel and a phosphribosyltransferase active site. Biochemistry 1996; 36:11061–11068.
12. Raivio KO, Saksela M, Lapatto R. Xanthine oxidoreductase-role in human pathophysiology and in hereditary xanthinuria. In: Scriver CR, Beaudet AL, Sly WS, Valle D, eds. The Metabolic and Molecular Bases of Inherited Disease. 8th ed. New York: McGraw-Hill, 2001:2639–2652.
13. McCord JM. Oxygen derived free radicals in postischemic tissue injury. N Engl J Med 1985; 312:159–162.
14. Woolliscroft JO, Fox IH. Increased body fluid purine levels during hypotensive events: evidence for ATP degradation. Am J Med 1986; 81:472–478.
15. Becker MA, Kim M. Regulation of purine synthesis de novo in human fibroblasts by purine nucleotides and phosphoribosylpyrophosphate. J Biol Chem 1987; 262:14531–14537.

16. Itakura M, Sabina RL, Heald PW, et al. Basis for the control of purine biosynthesis by purine ribonucleotides. J Clin Invest 1981; 67:994–1002.
17. Holmes EW, Wyngaarden JB, Kelley WN. Human glutamine phosphoribosylpyrophosphate amidotransferase: two molecular forms interconvertible by purine nucleotide and phosphoribosylpyrophosphate. J Biol Chem 1973; 248:6035–6040.
18. Holmes EW, McDonald JA, McCord JM, et al. Human glutamine phosphoribosylpyrophosphate amidotransferase: kinetic and regulatory properties. J Biol Chem 1973; 248:144–150.
19. Iwahana H, Oka J, Mizusawa N, et al. Molecular cloning of human amidophosphoribosyltransferase. Biochem Biophys Res Commun 1993; 190:192–200.
20. Becker MA, Meyer LJ, Huisman WH, et al. Human erythrocyte phosphoribosylpyrophosphate synthetase. Subunit analysis and states of subunit association. J Biol Chem 1977; 252:3911–3918.
21. Meyer LJ, Becker MA. Human erythrocyte phosphoribosylpyrophosphate synthetase. Dependence of activity on state of subunit association. J Biol Chem 1977; 252:3919–3925.
22. Nosal JM, Switzer RL, Becker MA. Overexpression, purification, and characterization of recombinant human 5-phosphoribosyl-1-pyrophosphate synthetase isozymes I and II. J Biol Chem 1993; 268:10168–10173.
23. Yen RCK, Raivio KO, Becker MA. Inhibition of phosphoribosylpyrophosphate synthesis by 6-methylthioinosinate. J Biol Chem 1981; 256:1839–1845.
24. Fox IH, Kelley WN. Human phosphoribosylpyrophosphate synthetase: distribution, purification, and properties. J Biol Chem 1971; 246:5739–5748.
25. Hershfield MS, Seegmiller JE. Regulation of de novo purine biosynthesis in human lymphoblasts: coordinate control of proximal (rate-determining) steps and the inosinic acid branch point. J Biol Chem 1976; 251:7348–7354.
26. Fox IH. Degradation of purine nucleotides. In: Kelley WN, Weiner IM, eds. Uric Acid. New York: SpringerVerlag, 1978:93–124.
27. Wu X, Muzny DM, Lee CC, Caskey CT. Two independent mutational events in the loss of urate oxidase during hominid evolution. J Mol Evol 1992; 34:78–84.
28. Watanabe S, Kang DH, Feng L, et al. Uric acid, hominid evolution, and the pathogenesis of salt sensitivity. Hypertension 2002; 40:355–360.
29. Sorensen LB. Degradation of uric acid in man. Metabolism 1959; 68:687–703.
30. Seegmiller JE, Grayzel AI, Laster L, et al. Uric acid production in gout. J Clin Invest 1961; 40:1304–1314.
31. Perez-Ruiz F, Calabozo M, Garcia-Erauskin G, et al. Renal underexcretion of uric acid is present in patients with apparent high urinary uric acid output. Arthritis Rheum 2002; 47:610–613.
32. Becker MA. Clinical aspects of monosodium urate monohydrate crystal deposition disease (gout). Rheum Dis Clin North Am 1988; 14:377–394.
33. Simkin PA. Urate excretion in normal and gouty men. Adv Exp Med Biol 1977; 76B:41–45.
34. Scott JT. Drug-induced gout. Balliere's Clin Rheumatol 1991; 5:39–60.
35. Seegmiller JE, Rosenbloom FM, Kelley WN. Enzyme defect associated with sex linked human neurological disorder and excessive purine synthesis. Science 1967; 155:1682–1684.

36. Kelley WN, Rosenbloom FM, Henderson JF, et al. A specific enzyme defect in gout associated with overproduction of uric acid. Proc Natl Acad Sci USA 1967; 57:1735–1739.
37. Sperling O, Boer P, Persky-Brosh S, et al. Altered kinetic property of erythrocyte phosphoribosylpyrophosphate synthetase in excessive purine production. Rev Eur Etud Clin Biol 1972; 17:703–706.
38. Becker MA, Meyer LJ, Wood AW, et al. Purine overproduction in man associated with increased phosphoribosylpyrophosphate synthetase activity. Science 1973; 179:1123–1126.
39. Faller J, Fox IH. Ethanol-induced hyperuricemia: evidence for increased urate production by activation of adenine nucleotide turnover. N Engl J Med 1982; 307:1598–1602.
40. Choi HK, Atkinson K, Karlson EW, et al. Alcohol intake and risk of incident gout in men: a prospective study. Lancet 2004; 363:1277–1281.
41. Becker MA, Losman MJ, Kim M. Mechanisms of accelerated purine nucleotide synthesis in human fibroblasts with superactive phosphoribosylpyrophosphate synthetases. J Biol Chem 1987; 262:5596–5602.
42. Puig JG, Torres RJ, Mateos FA, et al. The spectrum of hypoxanthine-guanine (HPRT) deficiency: clinical experience based on 22 patients from 18 Spanish families. Medicine 2001; 80:102–112.
43. Jinnah HA, Gregorio LD, Harris JC, et al. The spectrum of inherited mutations causing HPRT deficiency:75 new cases and a review of 196 previously reported cases. Mutat Res 2000; 463:309–326.
44. Becker MA, Puig JG, Mateos FA, et al. Inherited superactivity of phosphoribosylpyrophosphate synthetase: association of uric acid overproduction and sensorineural deafness. Am J Med 1988; 85:383–390.
45. Hershfield MS, Seegmiller JE. Regulation of de novo purine synthesis in human lymphoblasts: similar rates during growth by normal cells and mutants deficient in hypoxanthine-guanine phosphoribosyltransferase. J Biol Chem 1977; 252:6002–6010.
46. Fox IH, Palella TD, Kelley WN. Hyperuricemia: a marker for cell energy crisis. N Engl J Med 1987; 317:111–112.
47. Fox IH. Adenosine triphosphate degradation in specific disease. J Lab Clin Med 1985; 106:101–110.
48. Roch-Ramel F, Diezi J. Renal transport of organic ions and uric acid. In: Schrier RW, Gottschalk CE, eds. Diseases of the Kidney. 6th ed. Boston: Little, Brown and Company, 1996:231–249.
49. Gibson T, Waterworth R, Hatfield P, et al. Hyperuricemia, gout and kidney function in New Zealand Maori men. Br J Rheumatol 1984; 23:276–282.
50. Rieselbach RE, Sorensen LB, Shelp WD, et al. Diminished renal urate secretion per nephron as a basis for primary gout. Ann Intern Med 1970; 73:359–366.
51. Calabrese G, Simmonds HA, Cameron JS, et al. Precocious familial gout with reduced fractional urate clearance and normal purine enzymes. Q J Med 1990; 78:441–445.
52. Moro E, Ogg CS, Simmonds HA, et al. Familial juvenile gouty nephropathy with renal urate hypoexcretion preceding renal disease. Clin Nephrol 1991; 35:263–269.
53. Dahan K, Fuchshuber A, Adamis S, et al. Familial juvenile hyperuricemic nephropathy and autosomal dominant medullary cystic kidney disease type 2: two facets of the same disease? J Am Soc Nephrol 2001; 12:2348–2357.

54. Hart TC, Gorry MC, Hart PS, et al. Mutations of the UMOD gene are responsible for medullary cystic kidney disease 2 and familial juvenile hyperuricaemic nephropathy. J Med Genet 2002; 39:882–892.
55. Enomoto A, Kimura H, Chairoungdua C, et al. Molecular identification of a renal urate-anion exchanger that regulates blood urate levels. Nature 2002; 417:447–452.
56. Ichida K, Hosoyamada M, Hisatome I, et al. Clinical and molecular analysis of patients with renal hypouricemia in Japan- Influence of URAT1 gene on urinary urate excretion. J Am Soc Nephrol 2004; 15:164–173.
57. Kelley WN, Greene ML, Rosenbloom FM, et al. Hypoxanthine-guanine phosphoribosyltransferase deficiency in gout. Ann Intern Med 1969; 70:155–206.
58. Becker MA. Clinical aspects of monosodium urate monohydrate crystal deposition disease (gout). Rheum Dis Clin North Am 1988; 14:377–394.
59. Becker MA, Smith PR, Taylor W, et al. The genetic and functional basis of purine nucleotide feedback-resistant phosphoribosylpyrophosphate synthetase superactivity. J Clin Invest 1995; 96:2133–2141.
60. Becker MA, Taylor W, Smith PR, et al. Overexpression of the normal PRS1 isoform underlies catalytic superactivity of human phosphoribosylpyrophosphate synthetase. J Biol Chem 1996; 271:19894–19899.
61. Ahmed M, Taylor W, Smith PR, et al. Accelerated transcription of PRPS1 in X- linked overactivity of normal human phosphoribosylpyrophosphate synthetase. J Biol Chem 1999; 274:7482–7488.
62. Sahota A, Tischfield JA, Kamatani N, et al. Adenine Phosphoribosyltransferase deficiency and 2,8-dihydroxyadenine lithiasis. In: Scriver CS, Beaudet AL, Sly WS, Valle D, eds. The Metabolic and Molecular Bases of Inherited Disease. 8th ed. New York: McGraw-Hill, 2001:2571–2584.
63. Kamatani N, Hakoda M, Otsuka S, et al. Only three mutations account for almost all alleles accounting for adenine phosphoribosyltransferase deficiency in Japanese patients. J Clin Invest 1992; 90:130–135.
64. Chalmers RA, Watts RWE, Bitensky L, et al. Microscopic studies of crystals in skeletal muscle from two cases of xanthinuria. J Pathol 1969; 99:45–56.
65. Hershfield MS, Mitchell BS. Immunodeficiency diseases caused by adenosine deaminase deficiency and purine nucleoside phosphorylase deficiency. In: Scriver CS, Beaudet AL, Sly WS, Valle D, eds. The Metabolic and Molecular Bases of Inherited Disease. 8th ed. New York: McGraw-Hill, 2001:2585–2625.
66. Stoop JW, Zegers BJM, Hendrickx GFM, et al. Purine nucleotide phosphorylase deficiency associated with selective cellular immunodeficiency. N Engl J Med 1977; 296:651–655.
67. Sabina RL, Holmes EW. Myoadenylate deaminase deficiency. In: Scriver CS, Beaudet AL, Sly WS, Valle D, eds. The Metabolic and Molecular Bases of Inherited Disease. 8th ed. New York: McGraw-Hill, 2001:2627–2638.
68. Loh E, Rebbeck TR, Mahoney PD, et al. A common variant in the AMPD1 gene predicts prolonged survival in patients with heart failure. Circulation 1999; 29:1422–1425.
69. Van den Berghe G, Jaeken J. Adenylosuccinate lyase deficiency. In: Scriver CS, Beaudet AL, Sly WS, Valle D, eds. The metabolic and Molecular Bases of Inherited Disease. 8th ed. New York: McGraw-Hill, 2001:2585–2625.

13

Biochemistry of Calcium Pyrophosphate Dihydrate Deposition

Lawrence M. Ryan and Jill C. Costello
Division of Rheumatology, Department of Medicine, Medical College of Wisconsin, Milwaukee, Wisconsin, U.S.A.

INTRODUCTION

Calcium pyrophosphate dihydrate (CPPD) crystals form extracellularly, most commonly in cartilage matrix. The essential anionic component of CPPD crystals is inorganic pyrophosphate (PPi). Each unit cell of crystalline CPPD contains one pyrophosphate (P_2O_7) for every 2 calciums and 2 waters of hydration, yielding a structural formula of $Ca_2P_2O_7 \cdot 2H_20$. Theoretically, perturbations of matrix or elevations of either calcium or PPi concentrations within cartilage could favor CPPD crystal formation and growth. Changes in organic matrix components and in PPi have been most prominently implicated in the pathogenesis of CPPD formation, while there is little support for elevations of ionized calcium as a predisposing factor. Subsequent discussion will focus on PPi metabolism and matrix factors that may influence crystal formation.

INTRACELLULAR INORGANIC PYROPHOSPHATE

Intracellular PPi is a byproduct of multiple synthetic reactions with enormous quantities generated by cellular metabolism. For instance, calculated PPi production by the liver in the process of synthesizing albumin alone generates 30 grams of intracellular PPi daily (1). It has been hypothesized that the hydrolysis of intracellular PPi serves to drive synthetic reactions by removal of a coproduct. In order to maintain synthetic rates (protein, nucleotide, lipids, etc.),

PPi must not accumulate within cellular synthetic compartments. Ubiquitous intracellular pyrophosphatases (PPi-ase) prevent accumulation by hydrolyzing PPi into 2 molecules of inorganic phosphate (Pi) in the general reaction: PPi$\rightarrow$2Pi. As the prefix "pyro" implies, PPi is a high-energy molecule. Hydrolysis of PPi is exothermic, yielding from 4 to 6 Cal/mole, similar to energy release during hydrolysis of the pyrophosphate bonds contained in ATP. Indeed, PPi may represent the primary energy source in primordial organisms, a contention that has not been universally accepted. However, the hydrolysis of PPi within cells does not go to completion. Measurable PPi is present in all cells thus far tested. An alternative mechanism for lowering PPi concentration aside from hydrolysis revolves around the protein ANK, which may play a role in further reducing intracellular PPi concentrations by transporting PPi that escapes hydrolysis to the extracellular space. Upregulation of ANK has been described in growth factor stimulated fibroblasts, cells that require enhanced synthetic capacity (2).

In some tissues and cell compartments, PPi serves specific functions unrelated to its passive role in promoting synthetic reactions. Within the hepatopancreas of mollusks, intracellular granules concentrate toxic metal cations as complexes with PPi (3). These granules seem to serve as a detoxification system, ridding the blood of environmental pollutants absorbed by these organisms. Mitochondrial PPi content is quite high in multiple species, particularly in liver where concentrations of several μmol PPi/g of protein have been measured. Within mitochondria, PPi aids ferric ion mobilization and nucleotide transport and possibly prevents calcium phosphate precipitates from forming or growing as reviewed elsewhere (4). In platelets, storage granules contain PPi as well as ADP and ATP. PPi released from these granules during clotting accounts for the higher levels of PPi in serum compared to those in uncoagulated plasma (5).

Elevated PPi levels have been reported in tissue from some patients with either sporadic or familial CPPD crystal deposition disease (6,7). This increase was noted in non-articular cells, implying a generalized metabolic aberration underlying CPPD deposition. Unexpectedly, intracellular PPi levels correlated with activity levels of ecto-nucleoside triphosphate pyrophosphohydrolase (NTPPPH), an extracellular PPi-generating ecto-enzyme that catalyzes breakdown of nucleoside triphosphate, such as ATP, into nucleoside monophosphate (AMP) and PPi. Transfection studies indicate that a specific NTPPPH ectoenzyme, PC-1 or ENNP1, generates both extracellular and intracellular PPi (8,9). Although primarily an ectoenzyme that would be expected to generate only extracellular PPi, presumably PC-1 produces intracellular PPi prior to reaching its cell membrane destination. A second NTPPPH, B10, is not an ectoenzyme, and also increases intracellular PPi levels by generating PPi from ATP. ANK, a putative PPi transporter, affects intracellular PPi concentrations. A loss of function mutation in *ank* leads to increased intracellular PPi levels and decreased extracellular PPi levels in cell cultures (10). Forced expression of wild type *ank* has opposite effects. Transforming growth factor β (TGFβ) stimulation of chondrocytes increases intracellular PPi levels, an increase antagonized by interleukin 1β (11). Chondrocyte PPi content is dependent upon mitochondrial ATP production, since it is diminished by treatment of cultured cells with antimycin, oligomycin, and nitric oxide in sufficient quantities to diminish chondrocyte oxidative phosphorylation (12). Thus, many factors interact to determine intracellular PPi concentrations including PPi transporters, cellular synthetic activity, PPi hydrolytic enzymes, cytokines, and growth factors.

EXTRACELLULAR INORGANIC PYROPHOSPHATE

Production

Extracellular PPi is necessary for the formation of CPPD crystals, which with rare exception are exclusively observed in extracellular spaces, primarily near chondrocytes or areas of chondroid metaplasia. Compelling evidence points to elevation of extracellular PPi concentration as the underlying metabolic abnormality in most cases of CPPD deposition disease. Unlike in gout where systemic elevation of the anion urate leads to crystal formation, plasma levels of PPi are normal in patients with CPPD deposition disease (13). However, synovial fluid PPi concentration is elevated in CPPD-containing joint fluids compared to concentrations in fluids from normal individuals and those in fluids from patients with a variety of other forms of inflammatory and non-inflammatory arthritis (14–16). The observed elevation is not due to dissolution of CPPD crystals within the specimens. There is a consistent gradient between synovial fluid and plasma PPi concentrations, levels in plasma averaging 2 μM, and those in joint fluid 20 μM (17). This gradient suggests a local origin of the PPi in synovial fluid. Homeostatic mechanisms control extracellular PPi levels within narrow boundaries unless pathologic processes supervene.

The source of the extracellular PPi that participates in crystal formation is the chondrocyte. Chondrocytes are unique in their ability to spontaneously generate substantial quantities of PPi, with lesser amounts being produced by synovial cells, osteoblasts, and cells of tendons and ligaments (18,19). Chondrocytes from aged animals produce much more PPi than do young animals. This age-related increase may account for the increased prevalence of CPPD deposits with aging (20,21). Factors that induce hypertrophic changes in cultured chondrocytes also enhance PPi production, a correlate of the histological hypertrophy seen in chondrocytes adjacent to CPPD deposits in pathologic specimens (22–24). As chondrocytes endure in culture and assume a fibroblastic phenotype, the capacity for PPi elaboration diminishes.

The mechanisms by which chondrocytes generate extracellular PPi have been extensively studied. A widely accepted model is depicted in Figure 1. Factors known to enhance or diminish extracellular PPi formation by cultured cells and tissues are summarized in Table 1.

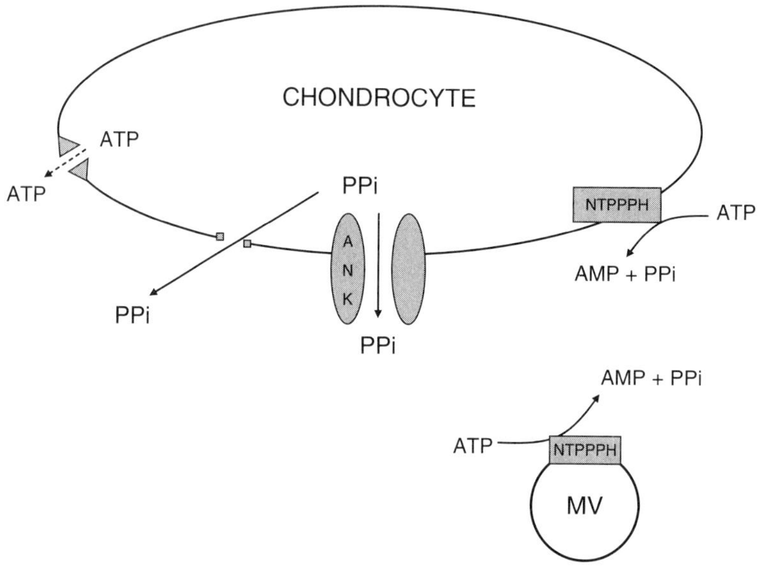

Figure 1 Extracellular inorganic pyrophosphate (PPi) may occur by transport of intracellular PPi across the chondrocyte plasma membrane by ANK, a putative anion transporter. Alternatively, extracellular PPi can be generated by ectoenzymes exhibiting nucleoside triphosphate pyrophosphohydrolase (NTPPPH) activity. NTPPPH generates PPi from nucleoside triphosphates including ATP. NTPPPH ectoenzyme is concentrated on chondrocyte membranes and on vesicles within cartilage matrix variously referred to as matrix vesicles (MV) or articular cartilage vesicles.

Table 1 Factors Affecting Chondrocyte Extracellular Pyrophosphate

Increase ePPi	Decrease ePPi
TGF-β	IGF-1
BMP-2	Basic fibroblast growth factor
BMP-4	Interleukin-1β
Retinoic acid	TNF-α
Ascorbic acid	Adenylyl cyclase activation
Thyroid hormone	Increased ANK protein
Osteopontin	Probenecid
PKC activation	PGE_1, PGE_2
	Decreased ANK protein

Abbreviations: BMP, bone morphogenetic protein; ePPi, extracellular pyrophosphate; IGF-1, insulin-like growth factor-1; PGE_1, prostaglandin E_1; PGE_2, prostaglandin E_2; PKC, protein kinase C; TGF-β, transforming growth factor-β; TNF-α, tumor necrosis factor-α.

One source of extracellular PPi is intracellular PPi. Enormous quantities of PPi are generated as byproducts of intracellular synthetic reactions. However, the bulk of intracellular PPi is hydrolyzed and PPi that escapes hydrolysis cannot diffuse across biomembranes (such as the chondrocyte plasma membrane). The multipass membrane protein ANK seems to serve as a conduit for PPi egress. In addition, a portion of extracellular PPi is generated by the action of chondrocyte ectoNTPPPH on extracellular nucleoside triphosphates such as ATP. Vesicular structures within matrix termed variously matrix vesicles or articular cartilage vesicles also are enriched in NTPPPH and able to generate extracellular PPi.

Many factors modify chondrocyte extracellular PPi elaboration. Perhaps the most potent stimulus is TGF-β, which increases PPi in media surrounding chondrocytes when supplied exogenously (25–28). Other TFG family members have also been studied. Bone morphogenetic proteins-2 and -4 enhance PPi elaboration from immortalized enchondral chondrocytes, in a process antagonized by basic fibroblast growth factor (29). Other stimuli of extracellular PPi production include retinoic acid, ascorbate, and thyroid hormone (22,23,30). Soluble factors impairing PPi generation include insulin-like growth factor-1 (IGF-1), some isoforms of parathyroid hormone-related peptide, interleukin-1β, and tumor necrosis factor-α (31). IGF-1 is a particularly important inhibitor of the TGFβ-induced stimulation of extracellular PPi production (32). The effect of IGF-1 on lowering ePPi levels is restrained by a matrix protein termed cartilage intermediate layer protein (CILP) that is restricted in tissue distribution to cartilage (33). The blocking activity resides in the N-terminus of CILP. CILP excess is seen in articular cartilage of patients with CPPD deposition disease, where it may permit tonic and unrestrained TGF-β stimulation of extracellular PPi formation by interfering with the inhibitory effect of IGF-1 (34). Similar failure to repress PPi formation may be associated with the parallel increase in CILP and in PPi production observed with aging (35,36). Chondrocyte insensitivity to IGF-1 may account for increased levels of PPi in synovial fluids of patients with osteoarthritis and be responsible for the frequent finding of CPPD crystals in osteoarthritic joints (15,17,37–40).

Transduction mechanisms involved in extracellular PPi production in cartilage include the adenylyl cyclase and protein kinase C (PKC) signaling pathways. Adenylyl cyclase activation diminishes and PKC activation enhances ePPi elaboration (41). Interestingly, IGF-1 treatment of cultured chondrocytes increases intracellular cAMP levels, providing a potential mechanistic explanation for its effect on PPi generation.

Physiologic Role

Extracellular PPi concentrations modulate BCP crystal formation. Mutant and knockout murine models demonstrate that excess BCP deposition occurs when extracellular PPi production is impaired. Progressive murine ankylosis (*ank/ank*) mice express a truncated form of ANK protein, the putative PPi transporter (10).

The *ank/ank* mice exhibit extensive articular calcification resulting in ankylosis and degeneration of axial and peripheral joints. Fibroblasts from mutant animals retain excess concentrations of intracellular PPi and are unable to generate normal quantities of extracellular PPi. The phenotype of the intact *ank/ank* animal can be rescued by transgenic expression of wild type *ank*. The production of normal ANK protein prevents the loss of joint mobility and BCP deposits seen in the homozygous mutant. ANK protein is located in the cell membrane and has the predicted structure of a multi-pass membrane protein. ANK effects of lowering intracellular PPi and raising extracellular PPi are reversed by probenecid, a weak organic anion that inhibits anion transport that is known to impair extracellular PPi production by chondrocytes (10,42). A similar and even more severe phenotype of articular BCP deposition is observed in the tiptoe walking (ttw) mouse. A nonsense mutation results in a truncated form of PC-1, the PPi-generating ectoenzyme with NTPPPH activity (43). Loss of PC-1 function is attended with decreased extracellular PPi and hypermineralization in the form of BCP. PC-1 null mice exhibit the same phenotype and display impaired production of extracellular PPi by cultured osteoblasts (44). This phenotype can be rescued by cross breeding PC-1 null mice with mice deficient in the tissue nonspecific form of alkaline phosphatase (45). Alkaline phosphatase has PPi-ase activity at physiologic pH. Presumably the deficiency in PPi generation caused by absence of PC-1 is rectified by diminished hydrolysis in the crossbred mice.

Patients with hypophosphatasia have elevated extracellular PPi levels and osteomalacic bone changes (46,47). A model of the human disease is created in alkaline phosphatase (tissue nonspecific isoenzyme) knock-out mice. Histologically the initial mineral formation within matrix vesicles of bone is normal. However, once the trilaminar vesicle membrane is breached by crystal growth or membranolytic effects of intravesicular BCP, then PPi adsorbs to crystal surface. This is followed by arrest of BCP crystal growth (48,49). Quite possibly the excess PPi surrounding the small BCP crystals at the point of matrix vesicle permeability adsorbs to the crystal surface preventing further BCP growth. It is well recognized that PPi adsorbs onto BCP crystals. In fact, this provides the basis for using radiolabeled PPi complexes as bone scanning agents. PPi analogues, the bisphosphonates, also adhere to BCP surface.

Therefore, it appears that excess extracellular PPi concentrations limit BCP formation whereas inadequate levels are associated with increased BCP deposition. Although this is true, the situation is more complicated. Complex interrelationships exist among PPi, osteopontin, ANK, PC-1, and alkaline phosphatase (50). It is likely that increased osteopontin, diminished alkaline phosphatase, and increased ePPi levels (the latter via increased PC-1 and/or increased ANK) act in concert to retard BCP mineralization (45,50,51). ANK plays a less important role in controlling matrix vesicle related mineralization than do the other factors. Linked regulatory mechanisms are shared by osteopontin and PPi (44).

Non-articular physiologic effects of extracellular PPi are also elucidated by observed pathologic changes in animal models. PC-1 deficient mice exhibit arterial calcification (52). More importantly a human disease, formerly termed "idiopathic" infantile arterial calcification, has been described and can be explained by extracellular PPi deficiency. Affected children suffer from premature arterial calcification and periarticular BCP deposits. Pathogenesis was unraveled in a rapid sequence of studies. Reduced levels of urinary PPi were first reported in these children (53). Deficiency of PC-1 was next detected in affected individuals (54). Finally, specific mutations within predicted functional domains of PC-1 were identified in 8 of 11 affected kindreds studied (55). It would appear the extracellular PPi functions to prevent BCP formation in media and internal elastic fibers of arteries. An in vitro study strengthens this contention. Cultured rat aortic rings are rendered resistant to calcification in the presence of hyperphosphatemia and hypercalcemia by a soluble, endogenous, PPi-ase sensitive factor, namely extracellular PPi (56). Aortic rings injured by abrasion were more prone to mineralization, and they too were protected from calcification when exogenous PPi was added to the culture media.

Role of Extracellular PPi in CPPD Crystal Formation

Clinical observations support a central role of elevated extracellular PPi levels in predisposing to CPPD crystal formation. Studies by numerous investigators have determined that synovial fluid PPi levels are consistently elevated in patients with CPPD crystal deposition disease and in asymptomatic patients with metabolic diseases associated with chondrocalcinosis (14–17,57,58). Synovial fluids containing CPPD crystals have higher levels of PPi-generating NTPPPH activity and of substrate for NTPPPH (ATP) than do fluids from normal or osteoarthritic patients (17,59,60). NTPPPH activity is increased in cartilage from affected patients compared to normal as is the content of mRNA encoding for the PPi transporter ANK (34,61). Putative gain of function mutations of *ank* have been described in several families affected with CPPD deposition disease and transcriptional upregulation is also described (62–65). Moreover, chondrocytes derived from CPPD-containing cartilage produce more PPi than normal (34). CPPD deposition is an age-related phenomenon, and in vitro cartilage PPi elaboration correlates positively with donor age (20). CPPD deposits occur with increased frequency in patients with hypophosphatasia in which circulating PPi levels are high (46). Taken together these correlative studies suggest an important link between excess extracellular PPi and CPPD crystal formation.

MATRIX CHANGES AND CPPD CRYSTAL DEPOSITION

With few exceptions, CPPD crystals are observed in matrix adjacent to hypertrophic-appearing chondrocytes (24,66). An abnormal cartilage matrix surrounds CPPD crystal deposits (24). The matrix exhibits loss of safranin-O staining, implying depletion of proteoglycans, which deter calcium crystal formation in vitro. Collagen content around crystal deposits is not altered, but fibers are fragmented and type I collagen is expressed. In addition, immunohistologic studies identified abundant quantities of the calcium-binding protein S-100 (67,68). Crystal deposits stain strongly with Sudan-III, a staining pattern that disappears following lipid extraction (69). It is uncertain whether matrix alteration results in or results from crystal deposition.

VESICLES WITHIN CARTILAGE MATRIX

Membrane-bound vesicles within cartilage matrix have been referred to as articular cartilage vesicles or matrix vesicles. They are structurally and biochemically similar to matrix vesicles within growth plate cartilage that are sites of BCP formation. Articular cartilage vesicles are enriched in enzymes that generate Pi and PPi from organic substrates (70). They also have specific calcium binding proteins and channels, such as annexin V. NTPPPH is prominently concentrated in articular cartilage vesicles. In the presence of exogenous ATP as a substrate for NTPPPH, CPPD crystals form within the vesicles (71–73). The PPi content of the articular cartilage vesicles-generated CPPD crystals is derived from ATP, demonstrating that ATP has been hydrolyzed to PPi by NTPPPH activity. CPPD crystal formation within these vesicles occurs at physiologic pH and ionic concentrations, in sharp contrast to the extremes of pH, ion concentration, and temperature required for CPPD crystal formation in inorganic solutions. Initial characterization of articular cartilage vesicles was done on vesicles released spontaneously into chondrocyte conditioned culture media or enzymatically released from cartilage. Morphologically and functionally identical vesicles form CPPD crystals in the perichondrocytic matrix of intact articular cartilage explants supplemented with ATP (73). Osteoarthritic cartilage contains more vesicles than does normal cartilage (74). No differences are seen in CPPD crystal formation between articular cartilage vesicles from osteoarthritic cartilage and from normal cartilage (75). Calcium-containing crystals in human osteoarthritic cartilage have been found to be associated with matrix vesicles (76). Articular cartilage vesicles may well play a role in formation of both CPPD and BCP crystals in articular cartilage.

Transglutaminase (TGase) enzymes are found within articular cartilage vesicles (77,78). One function of TGase is to form intra- or intermolecular isopeptide bonds within or between extracellular proteins. TGase substrates are plentiful in calcifying cartilage and include collagens, osteopontin, SPARC (osteonectin), bone sialoprotein, and α_2 HS-glycoprotein. Two forms of TGase observed in articular cartilage are tissue TGase (type 2 TGase) and factor XIIIa (78,79). Both are increased in cartilages from aged animals compared to juvenile animals. These enzymes may profoundly alter pericellular matrix by crosslinking protein components, thereby altering function. In addition to their role in modifying matrix, TGases activate TGF-β, thus enhancing extracellular PPi production by chondrocytes (79). Moreover, TGase type 2 is important for chondrocyte hypertrophy in response to retinoic acid. This hypertrophic phenotype is commonly observed in areas of pathologic cartilage calcification (80). By whatever mechanism, overexpression of these TGase enzymes induces abnormal mineralization in knee meniscal cells (81).

REFERENCES

1. Russell RGG. Metabolism of inorganic pyrophosphate (PPi). Arthritis Rheum 1976; 19:465–478.
2. Guo Y, Hsu KW, Feng SY, et al. Polypeptide growth factors and phorbol ester induce progressive ankylosis (Ank) gene expression in murine and human fibroblasts. J Cell Biochem 2001; 84:27–38.
3. Howard B, Mitchell PC, Ritchie A, et al. The composition of intracellular granules from the metal-accumulating cells of the common garden snail (Helix aspersa). Biochem J 1981; 194:507–511.
4. Mansurova SE. Inorganic pyrophosphate in mitochondrial metabolism. Biochimica et Biophysica Acta 1989; 977:237–247.
5. Ryan LM, Lynch MP, McCarty DJ. Inorganic pyrophosphate levels in blood platelets from normal donors and patients with calcium pyrophosphate dihydrate crystal deposition disease. Arthritis Rheum 1983; 26:564–566.
6. Ryan LM, Wortmann RL, Karas B, et al. Pyrophosphohydrolase activity and inorganic pyrophosphate content of cultured human skin fibroblasts. Elevated levels in some patients with calcium pyrophosphate dihydrate deposition disease. J Clin Invest 1986; 77:1689–1693.
7. Lust G, Faure G, Netter P, Seegmiller JE. Increased pyrophosphate in fibroblasts and lymphoblasts from patients with hereditary diffuse articular chondrocalcinosis. Science 1981; 214:809–810.
8. Terkeltaub R, Rosenbach M, Fong F, Goding J. Causal link between nucleotide pyrophosphohydrolase overactivity and increased intracellular inorganic pyrophosphate generation demonstrated by transfection of cultured fibroblasts and osteoblasts with plasma cell membrane glycoprotein-1: relevance to calcium pyrophosphate dihydrate crystal deposition disease. Arthritis Rheum 1994; 37:934–941.
9. Johnson K, Vaingankar S, Chen Y, et al. Differential mechanisms of inorganic pyrophosphate production by plasma cell membrane glycoprotien-1 and B10 in chondrocytes. Arthritis Rheum 1999; 42:1986–1997.
10. Ho AM, Johnson MD, Kingsley DM. Role of the mouse *ank* gene in control of tissue calcification and arthritis. Science 2000; 289:265–270.
11. Lotz M, Rosen F, McCabe G, et al. Interleukin 1 beta suppresses transforming growth factor-induced inorganic pyrophosphate (PPi) production and expression of the PPi-generating enzyme PC-1 in human chondrocytes. Proc Natl Acad Sci USA 1995; 92:10364–10368.
12. Johnson K, Jung A, Murphy A, et al. Mitochondrial oxidative phosphorylation is a downstream regulator of nitric oxide effects on chondrocyte matrix synthesis and mineralization. Arthritis Rheum 2000; 43:1560–1570.
13. Ryan LM, Kozin F, McCarty DJ. Quantification of human plasma inorganic pyrophosphate I. Normal values in osteoarthritis and calcium pyrophosphate dihydrate crystal deposition disease. Arthritis Rheum 1979; 22:886–891.

14. Silcox DC, McCarty DJ. Elevated inorganic pyrophosphate concentrations in synovial fluids in osteoarthritis and pseudogout. J Lab Clin Med 1974; 83:518–531.
15. Altman RD, Muniz OE, Pita JC, Howell DS. Articular chondrocalcinosis: microanalysis of pyrophosphate in synovial fluid and plasma. Arthritis Rheum 1973; 16:171–178.
16. Pattrick M, Hamilton E, Hornby J, Doherty M. Synovial fluid pyrophosphate and nucleoside triphosphate pyrophosphatase: comparison between normal and diseased and between inflamed and non-inflamed joints. Ann Rheum Dis 1991; 50:214–218.
17. Rachow JW, Ryan LM, McCarty DJ, Halverson PB. Synovial fluid inorganic pyrophosphate concentration and nucleotide pyrophosphohydrolase activity in basic calcium phosphate deposition arthropathy and Milwaukee shoulder syndrome. Arthritis Rheum 1988; 31:408–413.
18. Howell DS, Muniz O, Pita JC, Enis JE. Extrusion of pyrophosphate into extracellular media by osteoarthritic cartilage incubates. J Clin Invest 1975; 56:1473–1480.
19. Rosenthal AK, McCarty BA, Cheung HS, Ryan LM. A comparison of the effect of transforming growth factor B1 on pyrophosphate elaboration from various articular tissues. Arthritis Rheum 1993; 36:539–542.
20. Rosenthal AK, Ryan LM. Ageing increases growth factor-induced inorganic pyrophosphate elaboration by articular cartilage. Mech Ageing Dev 1994; 75:35–44.
21. Rosen F, McCabe G, Quach J, et al. Differential effects of aging on human chondrocyte responses to transforming growth factor: increased pyrophosphate production and decreased cell proliferation. Arthritis Rheum 1997; 40:1275–1281.
22. Rosenthal AK, Henry LA. Retinoic acid stimulates pyrophosphate elaboration by cartilage and chondrocytes. Calcif Tiss Int 1996; 59:128–133.
23. Rosenthal AK, Henry LA. Thyroid hormones induce features of the hypertrophic phenotype and stimulate correlates of CPPD crystal formation in articular chondrocytes. J Rheumatol 1999; 26:395–401.
24. Ishikawa K, Masuda I, Ohira T, Yokoyoma M. A histologic study of calcium pyrophosphate dihydrate crystal-deposition disease. J Bone Joint Surg 1989; 71-A:875–886.
25. Rosenthal AK, Cheung HS, Ryan LM. Transforming growth factor B1 stimulates inorganic pyrophosphate elaboration by porcine cartilage. Arthritis Rheum 1991; 34:904–911.
26. Rosenthal AK, Rosier TA, Ryan LM. TGF beta levels in synovial fluid. Arthritis Rheum 1993; 36:S161.
27. Fava R, Olsen N, Keski-Oja J, et al. Active and latent forms of transforming growth factor beta activity in synovial effusions. J Exp Med 1989; 169:291–296.
28. Punzi L, Oiviero F, Ramonda R. Transforming growth factorβ-1 levels in synovial fluid of osteoarthritis with or without calcium pyrophosphate dihydrate crystals [comment]. J Rhematol 2003; 30:420–421.
29. Terkeltaub RA, Johnson K, Rohnow D, et al. Bone morphogenetic proteins and bFGF exert opposing regulatory effects on PTHrP expression and inorganic pyrophosphate elaboration in immortalized murine endochondral hypertrophic chondrocytes (MCT cells). J Bone Miner Res 1998; 13:931–941.
30. Ryan LM, Kurup I, Cheung HS. Stimulation of cartilage inorganic pyrophosphate elaboration by ascorbate. Matrix: Collagen Related Res 1991; 11:276–281.

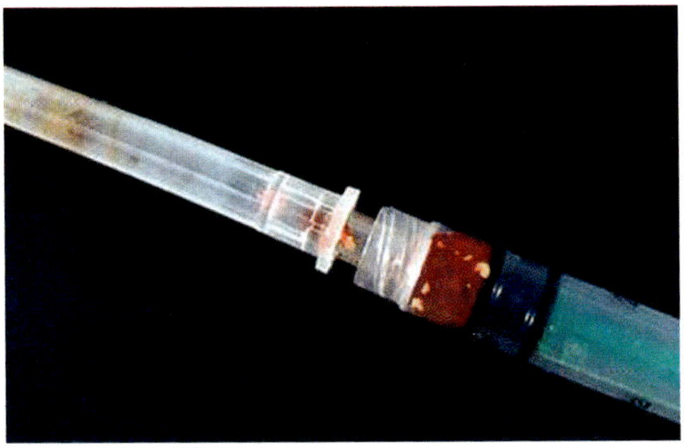

Figure 9.1 White aggregates of tophaceous material in bloody synovial fluid. (*See page 158.*)

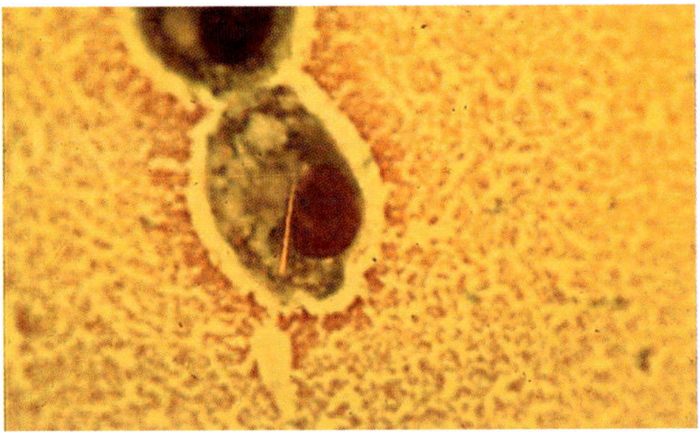

Figure 9.3 Monosodium urate crystal in Wright's stained synovial fluid macrophage. (*See page 160.*)

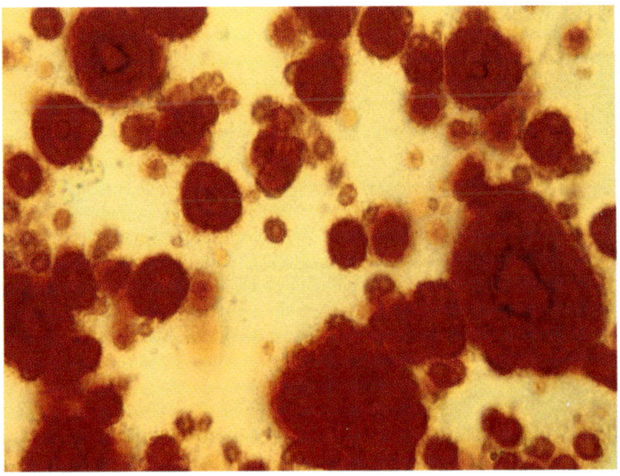

Figure 9.4 Alizarin red stained clumps of apatite. (*See page 161.*)

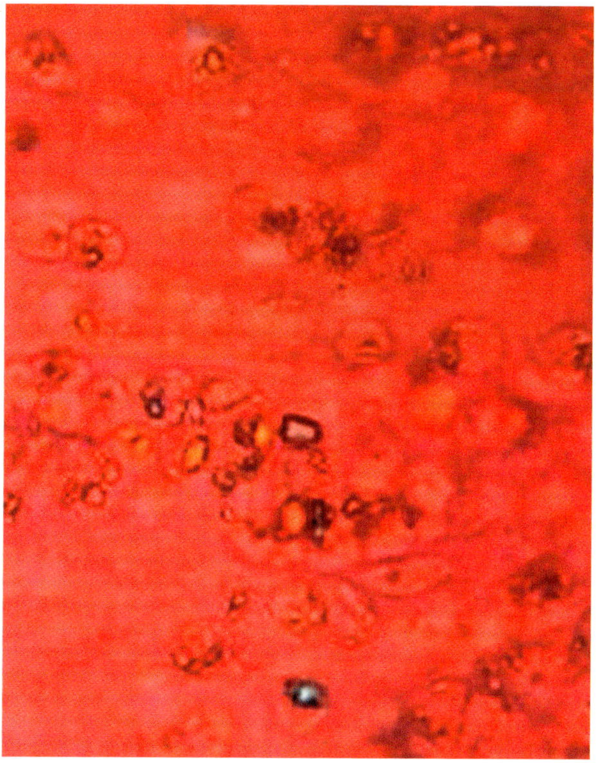

Figure 9.6 Calcium pyrophosphate dihydrate (CPPD) crystals with compensated polarized light. (*See page 162.*)

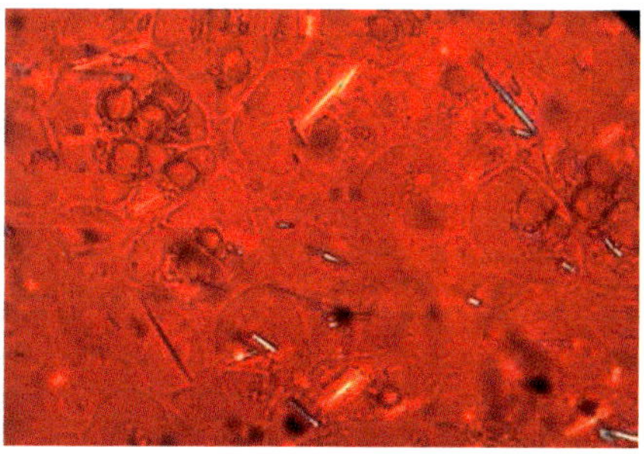

Figure 9.7 Monosodium urate crystals with compensated polarized light. (*See page 163.*)

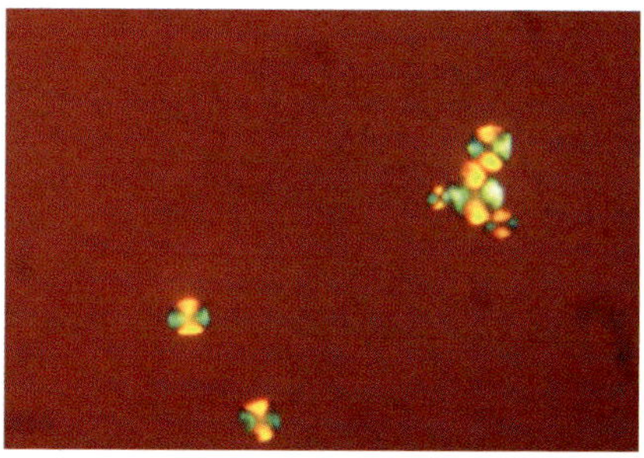

Figure 9.10 Maltese cross-like lipid liquid crystals seen with compensated polarized light. (*See page 165.*)

(A)

(B)

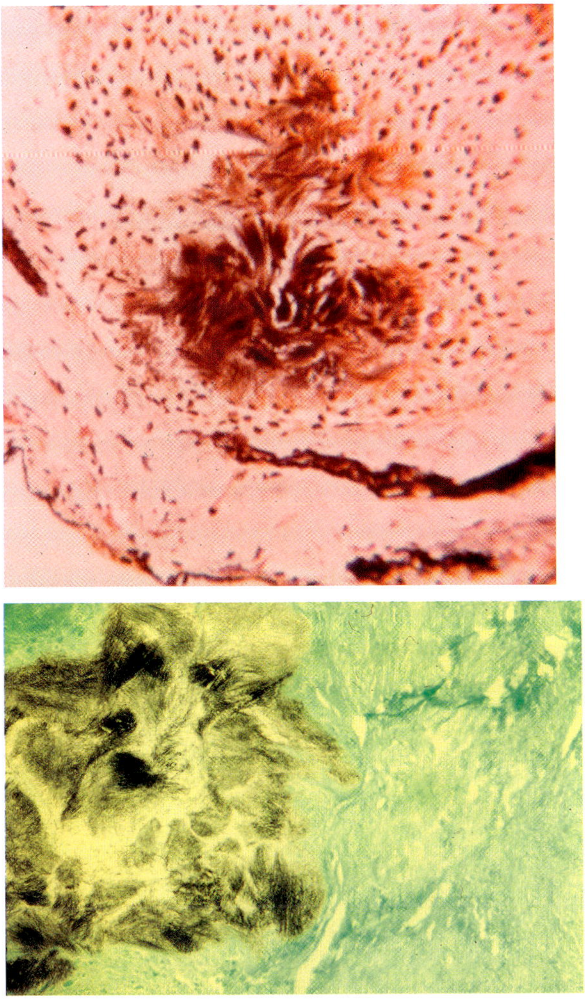

Figure 18.6 (**A**) A synovial tophus with crystals stained brown with De Golantha stain 400X. (**B**) Gomori methanamine silver staining monosodium urate crystals black. 100X. (*See page 295.*)

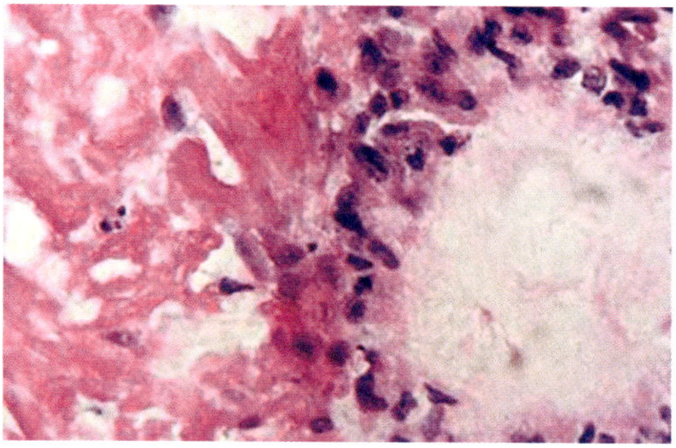

Figure 18.8 Fibrin overlying tophus site which may have recently released crystals into the joint space. 400X. (*See page 296.*)

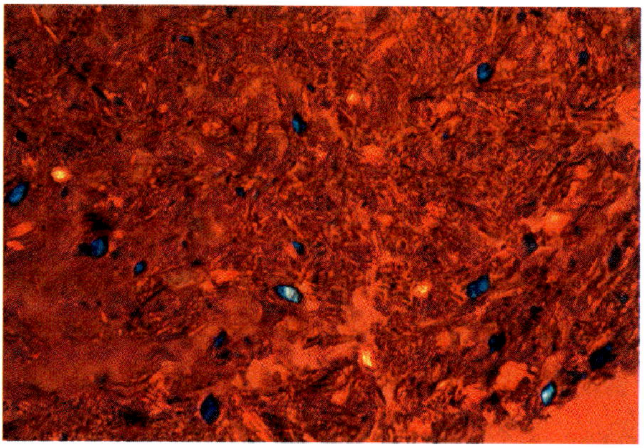

Figure 18.28 Calcium pyrophosphate dihydrate crystals in biopsy from parotid area mass. H&E, compensated polarized light, 400X. (*See page 312.*)

31. Terkeltaub RA. Inorganic pyrophosphate generation and disposition in pathophysiology. Am J Physiol Cell Physiol 2001; 281:C1–C11.
32. Olmez U, Ryan LM, Kurup IV, Rosenthal AK. Insulin-like growth factor-1 suppresses pyrophosphate elaboration by transforming growth factor beta1-stimulated chondrocytes and cartilage. Osteoarthritis Cartilage 1994; 2:149–154.
33. Johnson K, Farley D, Hu S-I, Terkeltaub R. One of two chondrocyte-expressed isoforms of cartilage intermediate-layer protein functions as an insulin-like growth factor 1 antagonist. Arthritis Rheum 2003; 48:1302–1314.
34. Hirose J, Ryan L, Masuda I. Up-regulated expression of cartilage intermediate-layer protein and ANK in articular cartilage from patients with calcium pyrophosphate dihydrate crystal deposition disease. Arthritis Rheum 2002; 46:3218–3229.
35. Lorenzo P, Bayliss MT, Heinegard D. A novel cartilage protein (CILP) present in the mid-zone of human articular cartilage increases with age. J Biol Chem 1998; 273:23463–23468.
36. Hirose J, Masuda I, Ryan LM. Expression of cartilage intermediate layer protein/nucleotide pyrophosphohydrolase parallels the production of extracellular inorganic pyrophosphate in response to growth factors and with aging. Arthritis Rheum 2000; 43:2703–2711.
37. Dore S, Pelletier JP, DiBattista JA, et al. Human osteoarthritic chondrocytes possess an increased number of insulin-like growth factor 1 binding sites but are unresponsive to its stimulation. Arthritis Rheum 1994; 37:253–263.
38. Tardif G, Reboul P, Pelletier JP, et al. Normal expression of type 1 insulin-like growth factor receptor by human osteoarthritic chondrocytes with increased expression and synthesis of insulin-like growth factor binding proteins. Arthritis Rheum 1996; 39:968–979.
39. Gibilisco PA, Schumacher HR, Hollander JL, Soper KA. Synovial fluid crystals in osteoarthritis. Arthritis Rheum 1985; 28:511–515.
40. Derfus BA, Kurian JB, Butler JJ, et al. The high prevalence of pathologic calcium crystals in pre-operative knees. J Rheumatol 2002; 29:570–574.
41. Ryan LM, Kurup IV, Cheung HS. Transduction mechanisms of porcine chondrocyte inorganic pyrophosphate elaboration. Arthritis Rheum 1999; 42:555–560.
42. Rosenthal AK, Ryan LM. Probenecid inhibits transforming growth factor beta1 induced pyrophosphate elaboration by chondrocytes. J Rheumatol 1994; 21:896–900.
43. Okawa A, Nakamura I, Goto S, et al. Mutation in Npps in a mouse model of ossification of the posterior longitudinal ligament of the spine. Nature Genetics 1998; 19:271–273.
44. Johnson K, Goding J, Van Etten D, et al. Linked deficiencies in extracellular PPi and osteopontin mediate pathologic calcification associated with defective PC-1 and ANK expression. J Bone Miner Res 2003; 18:994–1004.
45. Hessle L, Johnson KA, Anderson CA, et al. Tissue-nonspecific alkaline phosphatase and plasma cell membrane glycoprotein-1 are central antagonistic regulators of bone mineralization. Proc Natl Acad Sci USA 2002; 99:9445–9449.
46. Russell RGG, Bisaz S, Donath A, et al. Inorganic pyrophosphate in plasma in normal persons and in patients with hypophosphatasia, osteogenesis imperfecta, and other disorders of bone. J Clin Invest 1971; 50:961–969.
47. Whyte MP. Hypophosphatasia and the role of alkaline phosphatase in skeletal mineralization. Endocr Rev 1994; 15:439–461.

48. Anderson HC, Hsu HHT, Morris DC, et al. Matrix vesicles in osteomalacic hypophosphatasia bone contain apatite-like mineral crystals. Am J Pathol 1997; 151:1555–1561.
49. Fedde KN, Blair L, Silverstein J, et al. Alkaline phosphatase knock-out mice recapitulate the metabolic and skeletal defects of infantile hypophosphatasia. J Bone Mineral Res 1999; 14:2015–2026.
50. Harmey D, Hessle L, Narisawa D, et al. Concerted regulation of inorganic pyrophosphate and osteopontin by Akp2, Enpp1, and Ank. Am J Pathol 2004; 164:1199–1209.
51. Johnson KA, Hessle L, Vaingankar S, et al. Osteoblast tissue-nonspecific alkaline phosphatase antagonizes and regulates PC-1. Am J Physiol Regul Integr Comp Physiol 2000; 279:R1365–R1377.
52. Hosoda Y, Yoshimura Y, Higaki S. A new breed of mouse showing multiple osteochondral lesions—twy mouse. Ryumachi 1981; 21S:157–164.
53. Rutsch F, Schaurte P, Kalhoff H, et al. Low levels of urinary inorganic pyrophosphate indicating systemic pyrophosphate deficiency in a boy with idiopathic infantile arterial calcification. Acta Paediatr 2000; 89:1265–1269.
54. Rutsch F, Vaingankar S, Johnson K, et al. PC-1 nucleoside triphosphate pyrophosphohydrolase deficiency in idiopathic infantile arterial calcification. Am J Pathol 2001; 158:543–554.
55. Rutsch F, Ruf N, Vaingankar S, et al. Mutations in ENPP1 are associated with "idiopathic" infantile arterial calcification. Nat Genet 2003; 34:379–381.
56. Lomashvili KA, Cobbs S, Hennigar RA, et al. Phosphate-induced vascular calcification: Role of pyrophosphate and osteopontin. J Am Soc Nephrol 2004; 15:1392–1401.
57. Russell RGG, Fleisch H, Bisaz S. Inorganic pyrophosphate in plasma, urine, and synovial fluid of patients with pyrophosphate arthropathy (chondrocalcinosis or pseudogout). J Clin Invest 1970;899–902.
58. Doherty M, Chuck A, Hosking D, Hamilton E. Inorganic pyrophosphate in metabolic diseases predisposing to calcium pyrophosphate dihydrate crystal deposition. Arthritis Rheum 1991; 34:1297–1303.
59. Rachow JW, Ryan LM. Adenosine triphosphate pyrophosphohydrolase and neutral inorganic pyrophosphatase in pathologic joint fluids: Elevated pyrophosphohydrolase in calcium pyrophosphate dihydrate deposition disease. Arthritis Rheum 1985; 28:1283–1288.
60. Ryan LM, Rachow JW, McCarty DJ. Synovial fluid ATP: a potential substrate for the production of inorganic pyrophosphate. J Rheumatol 1991; 18:716–720.
61. Tenenbaum J, Muniz O, Schumacher HR, et al. Comparison of pyrophosphohydrolase activities from articular cartilage in calcium pyrophosphate deposition disease and primary osteoarthritis. Arthritis Rheum 1981; 24:492–500.
62. Pendleton A, Johnson M, Hughes A, et al. Mutations in ANKH cause chondrocalcinosis. Am J Hum Genet 2002; 71:933–940.
63. Williams C, Zhang Y, Timms A, et al. Autosomal dominant familial calcium pyrophosphate dihydrate deposition disease is caused by mutation in the transmembrane protein ANKH. Am J Hum Genet 2002; 71:985–991.
64. Williams CJ, Pendleton A, Bonavita G, et al. Mutations in the amino terminus of ANKH in two US families with calcium pyrophosphate dihydrate crystal deposition disease. Arthritis Rheum 2003; 48:2627–2631.

65. Zhang Y, Johnson K, Wordsworth P, et al. ANKH mutations cause both familial and sporadic calcium pyrophosphate dihydrate chondrocalcinosis and increase ANKH transcription/translation. Arthritis Rheum 2004; 50:S240.
66. Dijkgraaf LC, Liem RSB, de Bont LGM, Boering G. Calcium pyrophosphate dihydrate crystal deposition disease: A review of the literature and a light and electron microscopic study of a case of the temporomandibular joint with numerous intracellular crystals in the chondrocytes. Osteoarthritis Cartilage 1995; 3:35–45.
67. Boskey AL, Bullough PG. Cartilage calcification: normal and aberrant. Scan Electron Microsc 1984; 2:943–952.
68. Masuda I, Ishikawa K, Usuku G. A histologic and immunohistochemical study of calcium pyrophosphate dihydrate crystal deposition disease. Clin Orthop 1991; 263:272–287.
69. Ohira T, Ishikawa K, Masuda I, et al. Histologic localization of lipid in the articular tissues in calcium pyrophosphate dihydrate crystal deposition disease. Arthritis Rheum 1988; 31:1057–1062.
70. Masuda I, Hamada J, Haas AL, Ryan LM, McCarty DJ. A unique ectonucleotide pyrophosphohydrolase associated with porcine chondrocyte-derived vesicles. J Clin Invest 1995; 95:699–704.
71. Wortmann RL, Chowdhury M, Rachow JW. ATP-dependent mineralization of hyaline articular cartilage matrix vesicles. Adv Exp Med Biol 1989; 253A:81–85.
72. Derfus BA, Rachow JW, Mandel NS, et al. Articular cartilage vesicles generate calcium pyrophosphate dihydrate-like crystals in vitro. Arthritis Rheum 1992; 35:231–240.
73. Ryan LM, Kurup IV, Derfus BA, Kushnaryov VM. ATP-induced chondrocalcinosis. Arthritis Rheum 1992; 35:1520–1525.
74. Derfus BA, Kurtin SM, Camacho NP, et al. Comparison of matrix vesicles derived from normal and osteoarthritic human articular cartilage. Conn Tiss Res 1996; 35:337–342.
75. Derfus B, Kranendonk S, Camacho N, et al. Human osteoarthritic cartilage matrix vesicles generate both calcium pyrophosphate dihydrate and apatite In vitro. Calcif Tissue Int 1998; 63:258–262.
76. Kirsch T, Swoboda B, Nah H-D. Activation of annexin II and V expression, terminal differentiation, mineralization, and apoptosis in human osteoarthritic cartilage. Osteoarthritis Cartilage 2000; 8:294–302.
77. Rosenthal AK, Derfus BA, Henry LA. Transglutaminase activity in aging articular chondrocytes and articular cartilage vesicles. Arthritis Rheum 1997; 40:966–970.
78. Rosenthal AK, Masuda I, Gohr CM, et al. The transglutaminase Factor XIIIA, is present in articular chondrocytes. Osteoarthritis Cartilage 2001; 9:578–581.
79. Rosenthal AK, Gohr CM, Henry LA, Le M. Participation of transglutaminase in the activation of latent transforming growth factor beta 1 in aging articular cartilage. Arthritis Rheum 2000; 43:1729–1733.
80. Johnson KA, Van Etten D, Nanda N, et al. Distinct transglutaminase 2-independent and transglutaminase 2-dependent pathways mediate articular chondrocyte hypertrophy. J Biol Chem 2003; 278:18824–18832.
81. Johnson K, Hashimoto S, Lotz M, et al. Interleukin-1 induces pro-mineralizing activity of cartilage tissue transglutaminase and factor XIIIa. Am J Pathol 2001; 159:149–163.

14

Biochemistry of Basic Calcium Phosphate (Apatite)-Associated Syndromes

Eamonn S. Molloy
Department of Molecular and Cellular Therapeutics, Royal College of Surgeons of Ireland, Dublin, Ireland
Geraldine M. McCarthy
Department of Molecular and Cellular Therapeutics, Royal College of Surgeons of Ireland and Mater Misericordiae University Hospital, Dublin, Ireland

INTRODUCTION

Basic calcium phosphate (BCP) crystals include hydroxyapatite, octacalcium phosphate, tricalcium phosphate and magnesium whitlockite, although the most abundant of these crystal species in apatite-associated syndromes is hydroxyapatite. Hydroxyapatite is represented by the formula $Ca_{10}(PO_4)_6(OH)_2$ and generally occurs in the partially carbonate-substituted form. Octacalcium phosphate ($Ca_8H_2(PO_4)_6 \cdot 5H_2O$) and tricalcium phosphate ($Ca_3(PO_4)_2$) also occur. Although these crystals may form deposits that are asymptomatic, they are associated with a number of clinical syndromes (see Chapter 7). In vitro experiments have demonstrated a number of effects of BCP crystals that may contribute to the pathogenesis of these BCP crystal–associated syndromes (1). This chapter reviews the biochemical basis that underlies these clinical and laboratory observations.

COMPOSITION OF BCP DEPOSITS

Whereas urate and calcium pyrophosphate dihydrate (CPPD) crystals are readily identifiable by polarising light microscopy, detection of BCP crystals is more difficult. Individual hydroxyapatite crystals may be as small as 1.0 nm, but more usually clump together to form small aggregates of non-birefringent material. Initial reports of hydroxyapatite in synovial fluid identified small, spherical electron-dense particles, varying in diameter from 0.15 to 0.8 μm by high-resolution scanning electron microscopy (2). These particles had calcium/phosphate ratios very close to that of pure crystalline calcium hydroxyapatite. The majority of BCP crystal clusters are less than 100 nm in diameter, and concentrations of crystals range from 2 to 120 μg per mL of synovial fluid (3). BCP crystals appear as spheroid-shaped masses 1.9 to 15.6 μm in diameter in synovial fluid from patients with Milwaukee shoulder syndrome (4). Crystals were frequently associated with collagen types I, II, and III and collagenase and proteases. The crystals in all cases have been identified as hydroxyapatite by energy dispersive analysis and X-ray diffraction (4). Using Fourier transform infrared spectroscopy, particulates of apatite with octacalcium phosphate or tricalcium phosphate were identified in joint fluids from four patients with Milwaukee shoulder syndrome and a subcutaneous tissue aspirate from a child with dermatomyositis and calcinosis. Apatite was the predominant form of BCP found in all cases, with octacalcium phosphate also detected in all but one case in which tricalcium phosphate was found. Apatite was invariably characterised as hydroxyapatite with carbonate partially substituted for phosphate (5).

In one analysis of 36 cases of acute calcific periarthritis, hydroxyapatite, octacalcium phosphate, or tricalcium phosphate were not identified. Instead the deposits consisted of carbonate apatite (6). These results were attributed to the use of Raman spectroscopy and radiographic fluorescence spectrometry facilitating differentiation of carbonate apatite from hydroxyapatite. This differentiation was noted to be more difficult with previously used techniques such as radiographic diffraction and infrared absorption spectroscopy.

Magnesium whitlockite is another form of BCP, similar to tricalcium phosphate. Magnesium whitlockite crystals have a distinct cuboid morphology and are 50 to 500 nm in size, with Ca:P ratios of 1.30 to 1.47 on X-ray microanalysis and variable magnesium content (7). Magnesium whitlockite was found in normal and osteoarthritic hyaline cartilages but not osteophytic cartilage and was not correlated with the presence of fibrillation, suggesting that it is not likely to play a pathogenic role in osteoarthritis (7). Magnesium whitlockite crystals can stimulate cell proliferation as well as stimulate synthesis and secretion of matrix metalloproteinases in human fibroblasts in vitro (8). However, they are less stimulatory than BCP crystals in which magnesium is not substituted for calcium. It is uncertain whether magnesium whitlockite significantly contributes to the pathogenesis of apatite-associated rheumatic syndromes.

Given that octacalcium phosphate can be hydrolysed to form apatite, it may constitute an intermediate phase in BCP crystal formation, thus explaining its less frequent occurrence in biological samples, as compared to hydroxyapatite (9). Although it is possible to generate hydroxyapatite crystals without the formation of a precursor phase, that process is dependent on well-defined physicochemical conditions which may not occur in biological systems (10). In addition there is evidence to suggest that octacalcium phosphate is involved as a precursor to apatite formation in vivo, particularly in the early stages of mineralization. Formation of calcium-deficient apatites by the hydrolysis of octacalcium phosphate could explain the non-stoichiometric composition of human mineralised tissue, as this process has been shown to lead to formation of octacalcium phosphate-hydroxyapatite epitaxial layers and could give rise to heterogeneous composition of BCP crystal deposits (10).

However, octacalcium phosphate can occasionally be the predominant constituent of BCPs found in arthritic joint fluids (11). Four cases of BCP crystal-associated arthritis with multiple joint involvment have been described. Three of four patients had erosions and radiographically visible calcinosis. Transmission electron microscopy revealed long thin curved needles or feathery foamy chunks typical of octacalcium phosphate in contrast to the short needles of apatite. Why the generally less stable octacalcium phosphate persisted in these cases is not clear. The suggestion in this report of an association between octacalcium phosphate predominance and more extensive disease has not been confirmed elsewhere. However, it raises an interesting hypothesis, that differences in relative proportions of various BCP crystal species may influence the phlogistic and/or degenerative potential of BCP crystal deposits. Certain observations lend some support to this theory (12). The inflammatory potential of BCP crystals in the rat air pouch model differ among various crystal species and according to crystal features such as specific surface area and Ca:P ratio which correlates with crystal solubility.

EFFECT OF CRYSTAL CHARACTERISTICS

Significant morphological variation has been noted among BCP crystals identified in joint fluids (13). Crystals may be punctate, rod-shaped, thicker "boat-like" structures, or needle shaped. Larger crystals may have the suggestion of an internal structure at high magnification. Crystals may be rare or sufficiently profuse to make the joint aspirate cloudy. Elemental analysis also shows variation with some apatites having Ca:P ratios well below the expected 1.67:1, suggesting the presence of some amorphous or poorly crystalline salts. The degree of substitution of carbonate in apatite also varies (13). It is not known whether these variables correlate with pathogenic effects of crystals or associate with specific clinical syndromes. In one study the particles in a given synovial fluid are of a similar size, but the smallest BCP crystal particles were found in an acutely inflamed joint (4).

Recent evidence suggests that certain particle characteristics correlate to the pathogenic potential of BCP crystals. Nine different BCP crystal preparations were compared in the ability to stimulate tumor necrosis factor-α (TNF-α) release from macrophages and to induce human fibroblast mitogenesis (14). Crystal preparations were characterized in terms of particle morphology, size, surface pore diameter and surface area by X-ray diffraction, Raman spectroscopy, scanning electron microscopy and gas absorption analysis. There was a wide variation in response to different BCP preparations in terms of both TNF-α production and fibroblast mitogenesis, but both of these effects were tightly correlated. In addition, the crystals that appeared smaller and more needle-shaped had a greater effect than those that were larger and rounder. TNF-α production and fibroblast mitogenesis were also correlated with particle size and mean surface pore diameter (14). Thus such crystal characteristics may influence the pathogenic potential of these crystals in BCP crystal-associated diseases.

CRYSTAL FORMATION

It was previously assumed that intra-articular BCP crystal deposition was merely a consequence of damage to subchondral bone. However, the fact that BCP crystal deposition occurs in osteoarthritis, but only rarely in other arthropathies that involve damage to juxta-articular bone (i.e., rheumatoid arthritis), suggests that a more specific mechanism exists for the generation of BCP crystals in osteoarthritis. It appears that BCP (and CPPD) crystal formation occurs as a result of a complex interplay of factors that disturb tightly regulated homeostatic balances within the joint.

Regulation of Extracellular Inorganic Pyrophosphate

Matrix vesicles are extracellular cell-derived membrane-enclosed structures approximately 100 nm in diameter, initially described in epiphyseal growth plates. They are involved in hydroxyapatite deposition as part of the process of endochondral ossification which results in the formation of mature bone from cartilage (15). Matrix vesicles are generated by polarised budding and release from the membrane surface of chondrocytes into the extracellular matrix, but can also be derived from osteoblasts and odontoblasts. Matrix vesicles have been implicated in the formation of both BCP and calcium pyrophosphate dihydrate crystals.

The generation of calcium-containing crystals from matrix vesicles is critically dependent on the metabolism of extracellular inorganic pyrophosphate. Not only is this PPi the anionic component of CPPD, it also is a potent inhibitor of apatite crystal nucleation. Extracellular inorganic pyrophosphate (PPi) homeostasis is controlled by complex mechanisms, recently reviewed in detail (16). The most important of these are the nucleotide triphosphate pyrophosphohydrolase (NTPPPH) and alkaline phosphatase enzymes, found in matrix vesicles and a number of cell types including chondrocytes.

The NTPPPHases break down ATP to form adenosine monophosphate (AMP) and PPi. Plasma cell membrane glycoprotein 1 (PC-1), also known as nucleotide pyrophosphatase/phosphodiesterase 1 (NPP1), accounts for 50% of NTPPPH activity in human chondrocytes. Extracellular PPi is cleaved by the action of alkaline phosphatases, of which tissue non-specific alkaline phosphatase is the most important. In addition to PPi cleavage, alkaline phosphatases can split terminal phosphates from ATP, ADP, and AMP, which reduces the availability of ATP for the production of PPi by NTPPPH enzymes and increases the availability of inorganic phosphate (Pi) required for hydroxyapatite crystallisation. However, it is the hydrolysis of PPi to Pi that is critical to the ability of alkaline phosphatases to promote BCP crystal generation and CPPD crystal dissolution (16).

Examination of osteoarthitic cartilage reveals a 10- to 20-fold increase in the number of chondrocytes that stain positive for alkaline phosphatase activity when compared to normal articular cartilage. NTPPPH activity is also increased in osteoarthritic cartilage, but less so in the absence of CPPD crystals. PC-1 mRNA is not upregulated in osteoarthritic cartilage, but another NTPPPH, CILP/NTPPPH, is increased 6-fold and 3-fold with and without CPPD crystals, respectively (16).

Other enzymes that may influence matrix calcification include the transglutaminases (TGases), which cleave Pi from ATP and GTP (16). Type 2 (or tissue) TGase and the tissue form of factor XIII (FXIIIa) are expressed by chondrocytes and upregulated in osteoarthritis. TGases have also been implicated in apoptosis, can promote cell death of hypertrophic chondrocytes, and can lead to TGFβ activation (17,18). Given that TGase inhibitors significantly suppress chondrocyte ePPi elaboration, the net effect of TGase activity would be to increase extracellular PPi levels and thus inhibit BCP crystal formation but promote CPPD crystal formation. The presence of other enzymes, such as pyrophosphatase, which cleave PPi, could facilitate apatite deposition. Such activities have be found within matrix vesicles from osteoarthritic cartilage (16). The precise involvement of these enzymes in calcium crystal formation in osteoarthritis has yet to be elucidated.

The involvement of PC-1 and TNAP in matrix calcification is underlined by in vivo models of calcium-crystal deposition. PC-1 knockout mice exhibit the same phenotype as the naturally occurring tiptoe-walking mouse (ttw), with prominent calcification of the ligaments of the axial skeleton due to apatite crystal deposition, resulting in myelopathy and abnormal gait. A nonsense mutation in the gene encoding PC-1 is responsible for the ttw phenotype (19). In addition, susceptibility to and severity of ossification of the posterior longitudinal ligament of the spine in humans is associated with a PC-1 gene polymorphism, and mutations in PC-1 are also associated with idiopathic infantile arterial calcification which leads to arterial and, in some cases, periarticular calcification (20,21). Chondrocalcinosis, poorly mineralized bones, and spontaneous fractures develop in humans with hypophosphatasia, an inherited deficiency of alkaline phosphatase that causes PPi accumulation (22). TNAP knockout mice develop a syndrome that resembles hypophosphatasia (23). ANK is a multipass transmembrane protein thought to facilitate PPi efflux from the intracellular to the extracellular compartment. ANK knockout mice develop murine progressive ankylosis, characterised by spontaneous ankylosis of peripheral and axial joints with BCP containing tissue (24). This phenotype is similar to but less severe than the PC-1 knockout mice, emphasising the role of ANK in augmenting extracellular PPi levels. Mutations in the ANK gene have been associated with familial and sporadic chondrocalcinosis, but have not yet been sought in apatite-associated rheumatic syndromes (25,26). Interestingly, while bone mineralization in PC-1/TNAP double knockout mice is normal (27), ANK deletion does not fully rescue the phenotype of TNAP knockout mice (28). This was attributed to the fact that unlike PC-1 and TNAP, ANK did not localise to the matrix vesicles.

While lowering extracellular PPi concentrations may be an effective therapeutic strategy to inhibit BCP crystal formation, excess PPi is equally undesirable as it would result in CPPD crystal deposition. Prevention of the degenerative consequences of calcium-containing crystals likely requires maintenance of ePPi concentration within a narrow physiological range (29).

Matrix Vesicles in Osteoarthritis

Ultrastructural studies of cartilage obtained from patients with osteoarthritis have demonstrated apatite and apatite-like crystals in association with matrix vesicles (30). Matrix vesicles derived from human osteoarthritic cartilage can generate calcium-containing crystals in vitro (31). Progressive calcium precipitation over 96 hours via ATP-dependent and ATP-independent mechanisms was documented by a radiometric biomineralization assay. Crystals generated were examined by Fourier transform infrared spectroscopy. Crystals formed in the presence of ATP resembled CPPD, whereas the crystals produced by the ATP-independent mechanism resembled carbonate-substituted apatite. Evidence was also provided to explain the co-occurrence of CPPD and BCP crystals within the same osteoarthritic joint. They identified heavy and light matrix vesicle fractions. The heavy vesicle fractions had higher alkaline phosphatase and NTPPPH activities than the light vesicle fractions. When ATP was available to generate PPi, CPPD crystals were precipitated by both vesicle fractions. However, in the absence of ATP, only the high vesicle fractions generate BCP crystals. Compared with analogous fractions derived from mature porcine cartilage, the mean NTPPPH activity was 11-fold lower and the mean alkaline phosphatase activity 6-fold higher in human high vesicle fraction from osteoarthritic cartilage and the mean NTPPPH activity 7-fold lower in human low vesicle fraction (31). This suggests that the balance of NTPPPH/AP activity in osteoarthritis may be tilted toward alkaline phosphatase activity, thus favouring BCP crystal formation.

In calcific tendonitis, another clinical manifestation of BCP crystal deposition, tenocytes undergo chondrogenic differentiation and generate a cartilaginous matrix containing matrix vesicles (32). These matrix vesicles then initiate BCP crystal deposition like that which occurs at the growth plate (33).

Chondrocyte Apoptosis

Nitiric oxide has an apoptotic on human chondrocytes which is associated with degradation of the pericellular matrix (34). Because articular cartilage is not vascularized and does not contain phagocytes, the chondrocyte-derived apoptotic bodies accumulate within the chondrocyte lacunae and remain within the articular cartilage unless surrounding extracellular matrix is degraded and release into the synovial cavity occurs. Chondrocyte-derived apoptotic bodies resemble matrix vesicles and contain NTPPPH and alkaline phosphatase activities and are capable of ATP-dependent and independent mineralization and thus CPPD and BCP crystal deposition (34). BCP crystals upregulate inducible nitric oxide synthase and NO production from osteoarthritic synovial fibroblasts and therefore may potentially further aggravate deposition of calcium-containing crystals within the joint (35).

Role of Cytokines and Growth Factors

Evidence is accumulating regarding the role of cytokines such as transforming growth factor-β1 (TGF-β1), interleukin-1β (IL-1β) and TNF-α in the pathogenesis of osteoarthritis (36). IL-1β and TNF-α have been identified in synovial fluid and articular cartilage from patients with osteoarthritis. IL-1β is felt to be the key cytokine involved in progression of osteoarthritis, whereas TNF-α is involved at disease onset. TGF-β1 and IL-1β, in particular, have been implicated in the regulation of calcium crystal formation (16). TGF-β1 augments extracellular PPi production by increasing NTPPPH activity and decreasing alkaline phosphatase activity and up regulates ANKH mRNA expression in human chondrocytes (37–39). IL-1β diminishes basal NTPPPH activity by half, and completely inhibits the effects of TGF-β_1 on extracellular PPi production (40). IL-1β and TNF-α also reduce ANK mRNA expression in rat chondrocytes (41). In addition, insulin-like growth factor-1, an anabolic factor produced by articular chondrocytes, reduces TGF-β1-induced PPi production, potentially favouring BCP crystal formation (42).

Therefore, increased expression of these cytokines in osteoarthritis may influence the type of crystals deposited within the joint, with TGF-β1 favouring CPPD crystal formation and IL-1β favouring BCP crystal generation. In this context it is interesting to note that BCP crystals upregulate IL-1β expression by human fibroblasts, suggesting that BCP crystals may create an environment within the joint that predisposes to further BCP crystal deposition (43).

Other Factors that Influence BCP Crystal Formation

Hormonal influences are also involved in the regulation of this complex process. For example, thyroxine leads to increased NTPPPH activity and extracellular PPi accumulation by articular chondrocytes (44). Parathyroid hormone-related peptide (PTHrP) expression is increased in osteoarthritic cartilage. One PTHrP isoform, PTHrP 1-173, attenuates PPi without affecting NTPPPH activity (45). Interestingly, this PTHrP isoform is increased by TGF-β and down regulated by IL-1β. PThrP also promotes chondrocyte proliferation, thus inhibiting chondrocyte differentiation and matrix vesicle generation (46).

Osteopontin is an acidic phosphoglycoprotein that is thought to inhibit soft tissue calcification. Osteopontin, which is upregulated in osteoarthritis, can inhibit hydroxyapatite formation, but must be in its phosphorylated form to do so (47–49). Osteopontin is a substrate for the ecto-protein kinases, a group of enzymes that utilise extracellular nucleotides to phosphorylate cell surface receptors and matrix proteins, thus potentially reducing the pool of nucleotides available for extracellular PPi generation (16). Fibronectin is a glycoprotein found in cartilage and upregulated in osteoarthritis (50). Fibronectin is involved in chondrocyte adhesion through binding cell-surface integrins, but there is also evidence to suggest that it can promote BCP crystal precipitation (51,52).

Proteoglycans, key constituents of the extracellular matrix, potently inhibit BCP crystal formation (53–55). This may occur by linking of functional groups on aggrecan to growth sites on crystal surfaces via calcium ion bridges. Hyaluronan, a normal constituent of proteoglycan aggregates, can also inhibit BCP crystal growth (55). Aggrecan, chondroitin sulphate, and core protein moieties of proteoglycan exert a similar degree of inhibition of BCP crystal growth (53). This inhibition is markedly diminished following enzymatic breakdown of these components (56). The degradation of proteoglycans by the action of mineral metalol-proteinases (MMPs) produced by matrix vesicles, chondrocytes, and synoviocytes within the joint could release this restraint on cartilage mineralization. BCP crystals have not only been demonstrated to induce expression and release of MMPs from chondrocytes and synoviocytes, but also to downregulate the tissue inhibitors of MMPs (TIMPs), which further shifts the MMP/TIMP balance in favour of protease activity.

A more speculative theory of BCP crystal formation involves nanobacteria, tiny cell-walled bacteria recently isolated from human blood, which have the ability to produce carbonate apatite (57). They stimulate intra- and extracellular calcification when cultured with fibroblasts and form carbonate apatite in serum-free media. Apatite is formed at physiologic concentrations of calcium and phosphate; this crystal formation is inhibited by irradiation. Although there is some debate as to the existence of nanobacteria (58), they have subsequently been identified in calcified arteries and cardiac valves and renal stones (59–62). As carbonate apatite has been identified as the principal mineral in acute calcific periarthritis (9), it is possible that nanobacteria may contribute to the formation of apatite deposits in this condition.

REFERENCES

1. Molloy ES, McCarthy GM. Basic calcium phosphate crystals and pathways to joint degeneration. Curr Opin Rheumatol 2006; 18:187–192.
2. Dieppe PA, Crocker P, Huskisson EC, Willoughby DA. Apatite deposition disease. A new arthropathy. Lancet 1976; 1:266–269.
3. Swan A, Chapman B, Heap P, et al. Submicroscopic crystals in osteoarthritic synovial fluids. Ann Rheum Dis 1994; 53:467–470.
4. Halverson PB, Cheung HS, McCarty DJ, et al. "Milwaukee shoulder"—association of microspheroids containing hydroxyapatite crystals, active collagenase, and neutral protease with rotator cuff defects. II. Synovial fluid studies. Arthritis Rheum 1981; 24:474–483.
5. McCarty DJ, Lehr JR, Halverson PB. Crystal populations in human synovial fluid. Identification of apatite, octacalcium phosphate, and tricalcium phosphate. Arthritis Rheum 1983; 26:1220–1224.
6. Hamada J, Ono W, Tamai K, et al. Analysis of calcium deposits in calcific periarthritis. J Rheumatol 2001; 28:809–813.
7. Scotchford CA, Ali SY. Magnesium whitlockite deposition in articular cartilage: a study of 80 specimens from 70 patients. Ann Rheum Dis 1995; 54:339–344.
8. Ryan LM, Cheung HS, LeGeros RZ, et al. Cellular responses to whitlockite. Calcif Tissue Int 1999; 65:374–377.
9. Johnsson MS, Nancollas GH. The role of brushite and octacalcium phosphate in apatite formation. Crit Rev Oral Biol Med 1992; 3:61–82.
10. Nelson DG, McLean JD. High-resolution electron microscopy of octacalcium phosphate and its hydrolysis products. Calcif Tissue Int 1984; 36:219–232.
11. Schumacher HJ, Rothfuss S, Lehr JR, et al. Octacalcium phosphate as a sole or predominant calcium phosphate crystal in joint fluid. Arthritis Rheum 1988; 31:S19.
12. Prudhommeaux F, Schiltz C, Liote F, et al. Variation in the inflammatory properties of basic calcium phosphate crystals according to crystal type. Arthritis Rheum 1996; 39:1319–1326.
13. Schumacher HR, Cherian PV, Reginato AJ, et al. Intra-articular apatite crystal deposition. Ann Rheum Dis 1983; 42:54–59.
14. Nadra I, Boccaccini AR, Whelan L, et al. Basic calcium phosphate crystal induced human fibroblast mitogenesis is tightly correlated to macrophage pro-inflammatory activation which is determined by the same particle characteristics. Arthritis Rheum 2004; 50:S333.

15. Anderson HC. Matrix vesicles and calcification. Curr Rheumatol Rep 2003; 5:222–226.
16. Picher M, Graff RD, Lee GM. Extracellular nucleotide metabolism and signaling in the pathophysiology of articular cartilage. Arthritis Rheum 2003; 48:2722–2736.
17. Nurminskaya M, Magee C, Nurminsky D, Linsenmayer TF. Plasma transglutaminase in hypertrophic chondrocytes: expression and cell-specific intracellular activation produce cell death and externalization. J Cell Biol 1998; 142:1135–1144.
18. Melino G, Piacentini M. 'Tissue' transglutaminase in cell death: a downstream or a multifunctional upstream effector? FEBS Lett 1998; 430:59–63.
19. Okawa A, Nakamura I, Goto S, et al. Mutation in Npps in a mouse model of ossification of the posterior longitudinal ligament of the spine. Nat Genet 1998; 19:271–273.
20. Koshizuka Y, Kawaguchi H, Ogata N, et al. Nucleotide pyrophosphatase gene polymorphism associated with ossification of the posterior longitudinal ligament of the spine. J Bone Miner Res 2002; 17:138–144.
21. Rutsch F, Ruf N, Vaingankar S, et al. Mutations in ENPP1 are associated with 'idiopathic' infantile arterial calcification. Nat Genet 2003; 34:379–381.
22. Jones AC, Chuck AJ, Arie EA, et al. Diseases associated with calcium pyrophosphate deposition disease. Semin Arthritis Rheum 1992; 22:188–202.
23. Fedde KN, Blair L, Silverstein J, et al. Alkaline phosphatase knock-out mice recapitulate the metabolic and skeletal defects of infantile hypophosphatasia. J Bone Miner Res 1999; 14:2015–2026.
24. Ho AM, Johnson MD, Kingsley DM. Role of the mouse ank gene in control of tissue calcification and arthritis. Science 2000; 265:289–270.
25. Pendleton A, Johnson MD, Hughes A, et al. Mutations in ANKH cause chondrocalcinosis. Am J Hum Genet 2002; 71:933–940.
26. Zhang Y, Johnson K, Wordsworth P, et al. ANKH mutations cause both familial and sporadic calcium pyrophosphate dihydrate chondrocalcinosis and increase ANKH transcription/translation. Arthritis Rheum 2004; 50:S240.
27. Hessle L, Johnson KA, Anderson HC, et al. Tissue-nonspecific alkaline phosphatase and plasma cell membrane glycoprotein-1 are central antagonistic regulators of bone mineralization. Proc Natl Acad Sci USA 2002; 99:9445–9449.
28. Harmey D, Hessle L, Narisawa S, et al. Concerted regulation of inorganic pyrophosphate and osteopontin by akp2, enpp1, and ank: an integrated model of the pathogenesis of mineralization disorders. Am J Pathol 2004; 164:1199–1209.
29. Ryan LM. The ank gene story. Arthritis Res 2001; 3:77–379.
30. Ali SY, Griffiths S. Formation of calcium phosphate crystals in normal and osteoarthritic cartilage. Ann Rheum Dis 1983; 42:45–48.
31. Derfus B, Kranendonk S, Camacho N, et al. Human osteoarthritic cartilage matrix vesicles generate both calcium pyrophosphate dihydrate and apatite in vitro. Calcif Tissue Int 1998; 63:258–262.
32. Sarkar K, Uhthoff HK. Ultrastructural localization of calcium in calcifying tendinitis. Arch Pathol Lab Med 1978; 102:266–269.
33. Anderson HC. Vesicles associated with calcification in the matrix of epiphyseal cartilage. J Cell Biol 1969; 41:59–72.
34. Hashimoto S, Ochs RL, Rosen F, et al. Chondrocyte-derived apoptotic bodies and calcification of articular cartilage. Proc Natl Acad Sci USA 1998; 95:3094–3099.

35. Whelan L, O'Byrne JM, Sallis JD, McCarthy GM. Basic calcium phosphate crystals stimulate nitric oxide synthase and modulate bcl-2/bax expression in human synovial fibroblasts. Arthritis Rheum 2002; 46:S140.
36. Goldring MB. The role of cytokines as inflammatory mediators in osteoarthritis: lessons from animal models. Connect Tissue Res 1999; 40:1–11.
37. Lotz M, Rosen F, McCabe G, et al. Interleukin 1 beta suppresses transforming growth factor-induced inorganic pyrophosphate (PPi) production and expression of the PPi-generating enzyme PC-1 in human chondrocytes. Proc Natl Acad Sci USA 1995; 92:10364–10368.
38. Rosen F, McCabe G, Quach J, et al. Differential effects of aging on human chondrocyte responses to transforming growth factor beta: increased pyrophosphate production and decreased cell proliferation. Arthritis Rheum 1997; 40:1275–1281.
39. Hirose J, Ryan LM, Masuda I. Up-regulated expression of cartilage intermediate-layer protein and ANK in articular hyaline cartilage from patients with calcium pyrophosphate dihydrate crystal deposition disease. Arthritis Rheum 2002; 46:3218–3229.
40. Lotz M, Blanco FJ, von Kempis J, et al. Cytokine regulation of chondrocyte functions. J Rheumatol Suppl 1995; 43:104–108.
41. Bianchi A, Perrey J, Morin S, et al. Growth factors and cytokines modulate progressive ankylosis gene expression in rat chondrocytes—ank induction by TGFb depends on PKC pathway and ePPi level. Arthritis Rheum 2004; 50:S248.
42. Olmez U, Ryan LM, Kurup IV, Rosenthal AK. Insulin-like growth factor-1 suppresses pyrophosphate elaboration by transforming growth factor beta1-stimulated chondrocytes and cartilage. Osteoarthritis Cartilage 1994; 2:149–154.
43. Morgan MP, Whelan LC, Sallis JD, et al. Basic calcium phosphate crystal-induced prostaglandin E2 production in human fibroblasts: role of cyclooxygenase 1, cyclooxygenase 2, and interleukin-1beta. Arthritis Rheum 2004; 50:1642–1649.
44. Rosenthal AK, Henry LA. Thyroid hormones induce features of the hypertrophic phenotype and stimulate correlates of CPPD crystal formation in articular chondrocytes. J Rheumatol 1999; 26:395–401.
45. Terkeltaub R, Lotz M, Johnson K, et al. Parathyroid hormone-related proteins is abundant in osteoarthritic cartilage, and the parathyroid hormone-related protein 1-173 isoform is selectively induced by transforming growth factor beta in articular chondrocytes and suppresses generation of extracellular inorganic pyrophosphate. Arthritis Rheum 1998; 41:2152–2164.
46. Kronenberg HM, Lee K, Lanske B, Segre GV. Parathyroid hormone-related protein and Indian hedgehog control the pace of cartilage differentiation. J Endocrinol 1997; 154:S39–S45.
47. Attur MG, Dave MN, Clancy RM, et al. Functional genomic analysis in arthritis-affected cartilage: yin-yang regulation of inflammatory mediators by alpha 5 beta 1 and alpha V beta 3 integrins. J Immunol 2000; 164:2684–2691.
48. Hunter GK, Hauschka PV, Poole AR, et al. Nucleation and inhibition of hydroxyapatite formation by mineralized tissue proteins. Biochem J 1996; 317:59–64.
49. Jono S, Peinado C, Giachelli CM. Phosphorylation of osteopontin is required for inhibition of vascular smooth muscle cell calcification. J Biol Chem 2000; 275:20197–20203.
50. Burton-Wurster N, Lust G. Deposition of fibronectin in articular cartilage of canine osteoarthritic joints. Am J Vet Res 1985; 46:2542–2545.

51. Loeser RF. Integrin-mediated attachment of articular chondrocytes to extracellular matrix proteins. Arthritis Rheum 1993; 36:1103–1110.
52. Daculsi G, Pilet P, Cottrel M, Guicheux G. Role of fibronectin during biological apatite crystal nucleation: ultrastructural characterization. J Biomed Mater Res 1999; 47:228–233.
53. Eanes ED, Hailer AW, Midura RJ, Hascall VC. Proteoglycan inhibition of calcium phosphate precipitation in liposomal suspensions. Glycobiology 1992; 2:571–578.
54. Dziewiatkowski DD, Majzncrski LL. Role of proteoglycans in endochondral ossification: inhibition of calcification. Calcif Tissue Int 1985; 37:560–564.
55. Paschalakis P, Vynios DH, Tsiganos CP, et al. Effect of proteoglycans on hydroxyapatite growth in vitro: the role of hyaluronan. Biochim Biophys Acta 1993; 1158:129–136.
56. Eanes ED, Hailer AW. Effect of ultrafilterable fragments from chondroitinase and protease-treated aggrecan on calcium phosphate precipitation in liposomal suspensions. Calcif Tissue Int 1994; 55:176–179.
57. Kajander EO, Ciftcioglu N. Nanobacteria: an alternative mechanism for pathogenic intra- and extracellular calcification and stone formation. Proc Natl Acad Sci USA 1998; 95:8274–8827.
58. Cisar JO, Xu DQ, Thompson J, et al. An alternative interpretation of nanobacteria-induced biomineralization. Proc Natl Acad Sci USA 2000; 97:11511–11515.
59. Miller VM, Rodgers G, Charlesworth, et al. Evidence of nanobacterial-like structures in calcified human arteries and cardiac valves. Am J Physiol Heart Circ Physiol 2004; 287:H1115–H1124.
60. Jelic TM, Malas AM, Groves SS, et al. Nanobacteria-caused mitral valve calciphylaxis in a man with diabetic renal failure. South Med J 2004; 97:194–198.
61. Kajander EO, Ciftcioglu N, Aho K, Garcia-Cuerpo E. Characteristics of nanobacteria and their possible role in stone formation. Urol Res 2003; 31:47–54.
62. Khullar M, Sharma SK, Singh SK, et al. Morphological and immunological characteristics of nanobacteria from human renal stones of a north Indian population. Urol Res 2004; 32:190–195.

15

Pathophysiology of Crystal-Induced Arthritis

Nicola Dalbeth and Dorian O. Haskard
Faculty of Medicine, Eric Bywaters Centre, Imperial College London, London, U.K.

INTRODUCTION

This chapter outlines current understanding of the pathophysiology of crystal arthritis. We focus first on the cellular response to monosodium urate (MSU) crystals, and propose a unifying model of gout involving the differential role of mononuclear phagocytes in regulation of the inflammatory response. In this context we then discuss the inflammatory responses to calcium pyrophosphate and basic calcium phosphate (BCP) crystals.

GOUT AND THE INFLAMMATORY RESPONSE TO MONOSODIUM URATE CRYSTALS

Initiation of the Acute Gout Attack

The acute attack of gout has all the hallmarks of an acute inflammatory response. Histological examination of the synovium in acute gout shows lining layer hyperplasia and intense infiltration of the membrane by neutrophils, monocyte-macrophages, and lymphocytes (1,2). Acute attacks of gout are often triggered by intercurrent events, such as trauma, surgery, excess alcohol intake, or drugs which alter (especially lower) serum urate levels. These triggers may stimulate de novo formation of MSU crystals or may promote release of microcrystals from preformed deposits within the joint. Although supersaturation of interstitial fluid with MSU is required for the development of crystals, other factors such as local temperature and pH within the joint also influence whether crystal formation occurs (3). Debris or other factors within the synovial cavity may provide an initial nucleus for early crystal development (4). In addition, MSU crystal nucleation may be stabilised by albumin and by antibodies (5,6). Depletion of endogenous mast cells has been found to significantly inhibit neutrophil influx in the murine MSU crystal induced peritonitis model, suggesting a role for crystal-induced mast cell degranulation in initiating inflammation (7). Mast cells contain preformed proinflammatory substances including histamine, cytokines, and enzymes, all of which may contribute to the promotion of down-steam inflammatory cascades.

Leukocyte Recruitment

A central component of acute inflammation involves the activation of vascular endothelial cells, leading to vasodilatation with increased blood flow, increased permeability to plasma proteins, and the recruitment of leukocytes into the tissues. Initial endothelial activation with expression of adhesion molecules such as E-selectin, intercellular adhesion molecule-1 (ICAM-1) and vascular cell adhesion molecule-1 (VCAM-1) may be caused by factors such as tumour necrosis factor-α (TNF-α) released by mast cells (7) (see above), and it is likely that endothelial activation is then amplified by factors released by leukocytes entering the tissues and encountering crystals. Experiments using human umbilical vein endothelial cells have shown that MSU-stimulated monocyte supernatants induce expression of E-selectin, ICAM-1, and VCAM-1, and that this effect is entirely attributable to release of TNF-α and interleukin-1β (IL-1β) (8). Moreover, in a pig model of MSU, induced arthritis, blockade of TNF-α significantly inhibited E-selectin expression and neutrophil recruitment (Fig. 1) (8). Leukocyte recruitment is also likely to be enhanced by the local generation of chemotactic factors, such as C5a, and chemokines (e.g., IL-8). In urate crystal-induced arthritis in rabbits, inflammation was inhibited using an anti-IL-8 antibody (9). Furthermore, neutrophil influx following injection of MSU crystals into a murine subcutaneous air pouch was found to be attenuated in mice deficient in the murine homologue of IL-8 receptor (10).

Amplification

Native uncoated MSU crystals can activate neutrophils, but may also be directly membranolytic (11). However, a number of interstitial fluid proteins bind MSU crystals, including immunoglobulins (IgG and IgM), adhesion proteins (i.e., fibronectin), and complement proteins, resulting in protection from lysis, activation of inflammatory cascades such as complement and kininogen, and direct interactions with specific cell surface receptors (6,11–19). This in turn results in the release of soluble cellular products which further amplify the

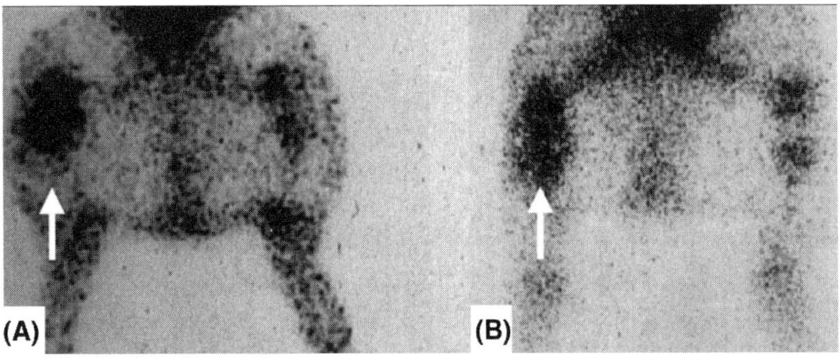

Figure 1 Imaging E-selectin expression in monosodium urate (MSU) crystal–induced arthritis in the pig. Scintigraphic images of anti-E-selectin monoclonal antibody (mAb) uptake in untreated and anti-TNF-α-treated pigs. Scintigraphic images of the hind limbs and abdomen of (**A**). an untreated and (**B**). an anti-TNF-α-treated animal were taken 24 hours after the intra-articular injection of MSU crystals into the right knee and saline solution into the left knee. There is marked uptake of anti-E-selectin mAb into the inflamed joint of the untreated animal, particularly in the region of the joint space (**A**, *arrow*). In contrast, anti-E-selectin mAb uptake in the injected knee of an anti-TNF-α treated animal demonstrates a pattern of uptake that is both less intense and less focal. *Source*: Adapted from Ref. 8.

inflammatory response, leading to both local arthritis and the systemic acute phase response.

Intense infiltration of neutrophils into both synovial membrane and fluid is the hallmark of acute gout, and these cells provide the main cellular mechanism of inflammatory amplification. In the dog, MSU crystal-induced synovitis can be inhibited by depletion of neutrophils, and this can be reversed by neutrophil reconstitution (20). A number of neutrophil surface receptors are probably involved in mediating responses to MSU crystals, and these include CR3 (CD11b/CD18) and FcγRIII (CD16), which bind crystal-bound iC3b and IgG, respectively (21–23). The consequences of neutrophil interaction with MSU crystals include the synthesis and release of a large variety of mediators that promote vasodilatation, erythema, and pain associated with the acute gout attack. These include reactive oxygen species such as superoxide, hydrogen peroxide, and singlet oxygen, nitric oxide, leukotriene B4, prostaglandin (PG) E2, anti-microbial peptides, enzymes, IL-1, and chemoattractants, including S100A8, S100A9, and IL-8 (24–31).

Infiltrating monocytes also amplify the inflammatory response in acute gout. Following exposure to MSU crystals, monocytes become activated, resulting in expression of a number of proinflammatory genes, including those of IL-1, TNF-α, IL-6, IL-8, and cyclooxygenase-2 (32–36).

Although the generation of acute inflammatory mediators is usually associated with infiltrating leukocytes, resident stromal cells may contribute mediators to the response. For example, synovial fibroblasts can phagocytose MSU crystals and respond by releasing arachadonic acid metabolites such as PGE2 (37).

Termination of the Acute Gout Attack

Even in the absence of treatment, the acute inflammatory response in gout is typically self-limiting over 7 to 14 days. Furthermore, it is well recognized that MSU crystals can be found in the asymptomatic joints of patients with hyperuricaemia (38–40). These observations imply a balance between the factors within the joint that maintain the non-inflamed state in the presence of MSU crystals and the pro-inflammatory response that accompanies an acute gout attack.

Changes in Proteins that Coat MSU Crystals

Changes in the interstitial fluid proteins that coat MSU crystals may significantly modify leukocyte responses during the course of the inflammatory reaction. For example, coating with either Apolipoprotein-B-100 or Apolipoprotein-E can reduce the responsiveness of neutrophils to MSU crystals (41–43). Apolipoprotien-E has been detected on the surface of MSU crystals recovered from patients with gout, and is probably synthesised locally in synovium (43). Similar coating has been demonstrated on MSU crystals in resolving air-pouch inflammation (44).

Role of the Hypothalamic-Pituitary Axis

The anti-inflammatory properties of the melanocortins, such as adrenal corticotropic hormone (ACTH)1–39 and α-melanocyte stimulating hormone (MSH), may contribute to the resolution phase of acute gout. Melanocortin type 3 receptor (MC3-R) expression has been demonstrated in a murine model of MSU crystal-induced peritonitis, and on macrophages isolated from rat knee joints. In a dose that does not increase circulating corticosteroids, ACTH has an anti-inflammatory effect on MSU-induced arthritis in the rat knee joint. ACTH1-39 is also effective in adrenalectomized rats, confirming that this effect is not due to stimulation of adrenal corticosteroids. This effect is dependent on signalling through the MC3-R, as the ACTH1-39 effect can be blocked by a selective MC3-R antagonist and can be reproduced by a MC3-R agonist (45).

Role of Peroxisome Proliferator-Activated Receptor-γ

Spontaneous resolution of the acute attack may also involve induction of specific intracellular anti-inflammatory pathways. One such example is the induction of the transcription factor peroxisome proliferator-activated receptor-γ (PPAR-γ), which functions as an important negative regulator of the inflammatory response. PPAR-γ expression can be detected in monocytes by immunohistochemistry twelve hours after exposure to MSU crystals. A natural ligand of PPAR-γ,

15-deoxy-PGJ2, is capable of inhibiting the production of TNF-α and IL-1β by MSU-stimulated monocytes, and also inhibits early cellular infiltration in the air pouch model (46).

Role of Monocyte-Macrophage Differentiation

Several observations imply that differentiated macrophages may play an important role in the resolution of the acute gout attack. MSU crystals can be found in asymptomatic joints of patients with hyperuricaemia and interval gout, and are usually present within macrophages and almost never within neutrophils (47,48). This suggests that macrophages can interact with MSU crystals within the joint without triggering an inflammatory response. Within air pouches injected with MSU crystals, macrophage accumulation continues even after hours when neutrophil infiltration has resolved (48,49).

The effect of differentiation upon the response of monocyte-macrophages to MSU crystals has been studied using a panel of mouse cell lines fixed at different stages of maturation (defined by expression of the markers F4/80 and BM 8) (50). There was close correlation between level of expression of the surface markers and capacity to phagocytose latex beads or MSU crystals. However, TNF-α production was not linked to phagocytic activity, since those cell lines at an intermediate level of maturation expressed the highest concentrations of TNF-α. In contrast, the most mature macrophage lines (MH-S and IC-21) failed to produce TNF-α despite efficient phagocytosis of MSU crystals (Fig. 2). Following exposure to MSU crystals, culture supernatants from partially differentiated macrophages, but not from the fully differentiated cell lines, stimulate endothelial activation. Zymosan, an alternative phagocytic stimulus, leads to TNF-α production by IC-21 cells, indicating particle specificity of the response. Furthermore, in co-culture experiments release of TNF-α by the IC-21 cells in response to zymosan is inhibited by a soluble factor released in response to MSU crystals, suggesting that the response to MSU crystals is actively anti-inflammatory rather than neutral.

These experiments using mouse cell lines have now been extended to a model in which human monocytes are differentiated in vitro to macrophages in the presence of autologous serum (51). Following exposure to MSU crystals, undifferentiated peripheral blood monocytes secrete the cytokines TNF-α, IL-1β, and IL-6, induce endothelial activation, and promote neutrophil adhesion to endothelial cells under shear flow in vitro. However, differentiation of monocytes into mature macrophages over five days leads to the loss of the capacity to release proinflammatory cytokines capable of activating endothelial cell adhesion molecule expression.

High levels of transforming growth factor-β1 (TGF-β1) in the synovial fluid of patients with acute gout and administration of TGF-β1 significantly inhibit leukocyte infiltration into air pouches injected with MSU crystals (52,53). TGF-β1 has been identified as a key soluble factor in the suppression of MSU-induced inflammation by differentiated macrophages (54). As

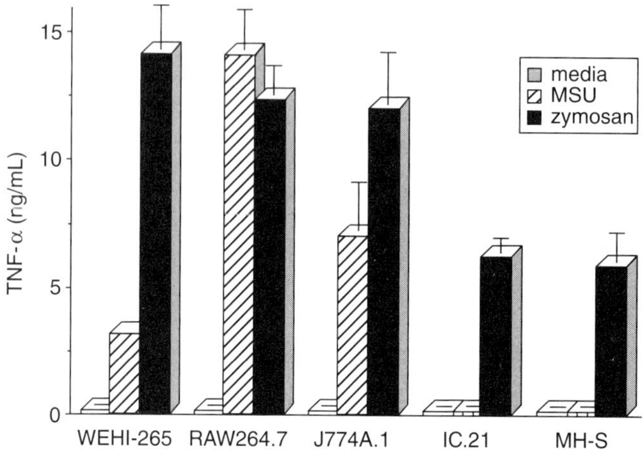

Figure 2 Secretion of TNF-α by macrophage cell lines in response to monosodium urate (MSU) crystals or zymosan. TNF-α as measured by ELISA in culture supernatants was collected from five phagocytically competent macrophage cell lines cultured for 16 hours in the presence of media alone, MSU crystals (0.5 mg/mL), or unopsonized zymosan particles (0.4 mg/mL). The mature macrophage cell lines IC-21 and MH-S secreted TNF-α in response to zymosan but not to MSU crystals. All these cell lines efficiently phagocytosed MSU crystals. Values are means ± SD of triplicates. *Source*: Adapted from Ref. 50.

monocytes differentiate in vitro towards a macrophage end-point, the loss of the capacity to secrete proinflammatory cytokines in response to MSU crystals is paralleled by a gain in the capacity to release TGF-β1 (Fig. 3). Functional effects of TGF-β1 in this model system include the suppression of monocyte proinflammatory cytokine release in response to MSU crystals, endothelial cell activation in response to monocyte-derived cytokines, and macrophage release of TNF-α in response to zymosan. However, not all effects of TGF-β1 are suppressive, and this growth factor may contribute to fibroblast proliferation and the physical encasing of crystals away from contact with leukocytes. Certainly synovial tissue taken from patients with acute gout demonstrates marked fibroblast proliferation within the lining layer (2).

Taken together, these data support a role for monocyte differentiation in the resolution of acute inflammation in gout. A hypothetical model of the role of monocyte-macrophage differentiation in gout is shown in Fig. 4. As with any in vitro model, the interpretation of the data needs to be qualified by the possibility that macrophage differentiation in vitro may not faithfully reproduce the in vivo situation. In this respect it is reassuring that monocytes and macrophages derived from a skin blister model shows the same disparity in cytokine secretion in response to MSU crystals as in vitro differentiated

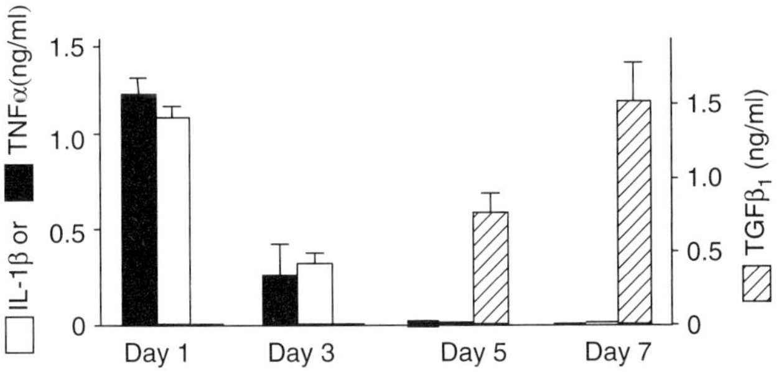

Figure 3 Differential cytokine production depending on stage of macrophage maturation. Human blood monocytes were cultured in vitro for various durations, during which they differentiated to macrophages. At various time points of in vitro differentiation (days 1, 3, 5, and 7), cells were stimulated a further 24 hours with monosodium urate (MSU) crystals (0.5 mg/mL), after which the presence of cytokines in culture supernatants was measured by ELISA. Day 1 monocytes produced TNF-α and IL-1β in response to MSU crystals. However, differentiated macrophages released TGF-β1 but not TNF-α or IL-1β in response to MSU crystals. Values are the mean ± SEM of triplicates. *Source*: Adapted from Ref. 54.

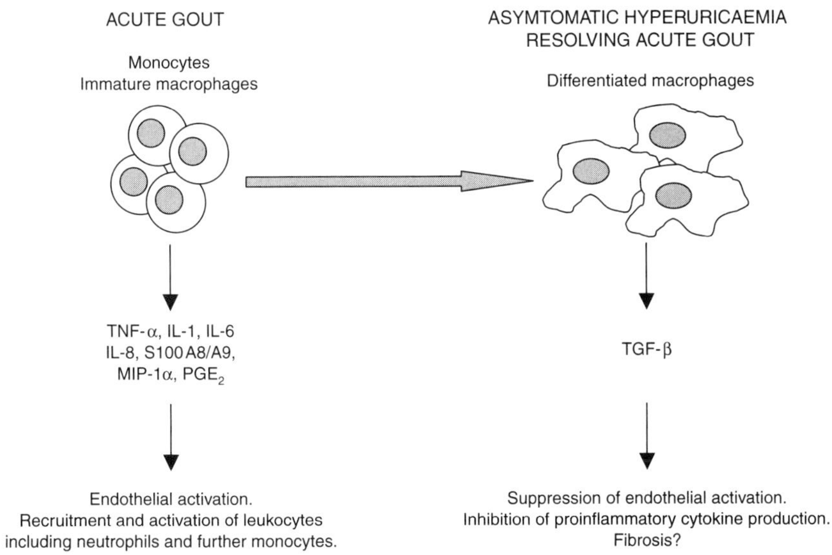

Figure 4 Model of the differential roles of monocytes and macrophages in the inflammatory response to monosodium urate crystals. The model proposes that monocytes play a central role in stimulating and amplifying an acute attack of gout, whereas differentiated macrophages may play an anti-inflammatory role in terminating an acute attack and in preserving the asymptomatic state through production of TGF-β.

cells, with the macrophage end-point appearing rather earlier in vivo (40 hours as opposed to five days), consistent with the kinetics of a typical gout attack (54).

Tophaceous Gout

In some individuals, persistent hyperuricaemia leads to the formation of tophaceous deposits of MSU crystals, typically in subcutaneous and periarticular areas. Tophus development may occur due to the formation of crystals at a rate that exceeds the handling capacity of tissue macrophages or possibly the failure of macrophages to differentiate to an anti-inflammatory end-point.

Microscopically, tophi are granulomas of mono- and multi-nucleated macrophages surrounding a core of debris and MSU crystals, encased by dense connective tissue (55). The gradation of size and urate content of gouty tophi suggests a progressive enlargement and maturation. Within the tophus, macrophages express mature, late differentiation markers and show high levels of apoptosis. However, in associated perivascular regions, there is a predominance of mono-nucleated monocyte-macrophages expressing surface markers of recent migration (56). These data suggest that development of the gouty tophus is a dynamic process with a low level continuous recruitment, pro-inflammatory activation, maturation, and turnover of monocyte-macrophages. This view is supported by the detection of TNF-α in tophaceous tissue (33,56).

Tophi are frequently associated with erosion of cartilage and bone. A number of factors have been identified within tophaceous material that may contribute to such erosive disease. Monocyte-macrophages within the gouty tophus produce matrix metalloproteinase (MMP)-2 (gelatinase-A) and MMP-9 (gelatinase-B) (56). These enzymes are capable of degrading type IV and type V collagen, elastin, and gelatin. MMP-9 expression is induced in macrophages by MSU crystals in vitro in a dose-dependent manner (57). Resident stromal cells also produce MMPs on exposure to MSU crystals, with synovial fibroblasts producing MMP-1 (collagenase) and chondrocytes producing MMP-3 (stromelysin 1) (58–60). Release of such enzymes may play a role in degradation of matrix in articular structures adjacent to the tophus.

CALCIUM PYROPHOSPHATE DIHYDRATE CRYSTAL-RELATED INFLAMMATION

Many of the cellular responses discussed above in relation to MSU crystals also apply to calcium pyrophosphate dihydrate (CPPD) crystals. The development of acute flares of pseudogout may be related to development of new CPPD crystals within the joint or, more likely, shedding of preformed crystals from cartilage (61). CPPD crystals activate the classical and alternative complement pathways in vitro, and evidence of complement activation is present in the synovial fluid of patients with pseudogout, but not chronic pyrophosphate arthropathy (13,15,62). Alterations in coating proteins may also modify the inflammatory response; in particular, coating with IgG strongly potentiates the neutrophil response to CPPD crystals (63,64).

CPPD crystals induce acute inflammation in the rat air pouch model, with associated elevations in pouch fluid TNF-α, PGE2, and leukocyte infiltration (65). These crystals stimulate mononuclear phagocytes to produce proinflammatory soluble mediators such as TNF-α, IL-6, and IL-8 (34,66,67). CPPD crystals also interact with fibroblasts to promote the production of mediators such as PGE2 and MMPs and induce neutrophil activation, with release of lysosomal products and proinflammatory cytokines and chemokines (26,28,30,68–70). TNF-α may, in turn, accentuate the activation of neutrophils in response to CPPD crystals, leading to further amplification of the inflammatory response (71).

The mechanisms of resolution of the acute attack in pseudogout, and maintenance of CPPD crystals within the asymptomatic joint, are currently unknown. Interestingly, TGF-β may promote the formation of CPPD crystals through elaboration of inorganic pyrophosphate from hyaline cartilage and fibrocartilage (72).

CPPD crystals may also induce matrix degradation through stimulation of MMPs and PGs from stromal cells such as osteoblasts, fibroblasts, and chondrocytes (68–70,73). Stimulation of IL-1 production from mononuclear cells by CPPD crystals acts synergistically with the crystals themselves to promote collagenase and PGE2 production from chondrocytes (74).

BASIC CALCIUM PHOSPHATE-RELATED ARTHROPATHIES

As with other crystals, triggering of acute inflammation by BCP crystals may be due to de novo formation of crystals, crystal shedding from preformed deposits, or alterations in the resident cellular or soluble components of the synovial environment. BCP crystals can be coated with immunoglobulins and complement components within the joint and induce complement activation in vitro (13,75).

BCP crystals are also phagocytosed by resident synoviocytes and influxing leukocytes. However, following phagocytosis, BCP crystals may be solubilized by dissolution within the acidic phagolysosome. This dissolution of BCP crystals leads to increased intracellular calcium concentrations, and activation of calcium dependent signalling pathways within the cell (76).

The physicochemical properties of BCP crystals significantly influence the ability of crystals to induce an inflammatory response. In the rat air pouch model, the degree of inflammation induced by injection of BCP crystals correlates with the specific surface area of the crystals and also the Ca:P ratio (which corresponds to crystal solubility) (77). Overall, the degree of inflammation induced by injection of BCP crystals into the air pouch is lower than that induced by injection of MSU or CPPD crystals (65,78). There have been varying reports regarding the ability of BCP crystals to induce monocyte/macrophage production of proinflammatory cytokines such as TNF-α and IL-6 in vitro (33,34,66,79). Overall, BCP crystals do induce proinflammatory cytokine production from these cells, but to a lesser extent than MSU crystals. Again, the ability of these crystals to activate monocyte-macrophages in vitro is dependent on the biochemical and crystalline structural properties of the particles (80). For example, in vitro studies of macrophages indicate that small needle-shaped particles of hydroxyapatite induce much higher levels of TNF-α than large spherical particles (79). This is in contrast to MSU crystals, where crystal size does not appear to significantly influence the production of TNF-α from mononuclear phagocytes (51).

Phagocytosis of BCP crystals by neutrophils leads to neutrophil activation with release of inflammatory oxygen metabolites and enzymes. The neutrophil response is again influenced by the crystalline structural properties of BCP crystals (81). In addition, low concentrations of hydroxyapatite crystals can prime neutrophils to respond to other stimuli, suggesting that these crystals may act to amplify inflammatory responses within the joint (82).

Synovial lining layer hyperplasia is a characteristic feature of BCP crystal-associated arthropathies. Calcium-containing crystals, particularly those of hydroxyapatite, have striking mitogenic effects on synovial fibroblasts and chondrocytes (83,84). This mitogenic response to BCP crystals is associated with intracellular crystal dissolution within the acidic phagolysosome and agents that raise lysosomal pH, such as ammonium chloride, chloroquine, and bafilomycon A1, suppress intracellular crystal dissolution, and also inhibit mitogenesis (85,86).

BCP crystal arthropathies are frequently associated with degradation of intra-articular matrix. Fibroblasts respond to BCP crystals by production of a number of MMPs, including collagenase 1 (MMP-1), stromeolysin 1 (MMP-3), gelatinase B (MMP-9), collagenase 3 (MMP-13), and matrix metalloprotease-8 (MMP-8) (69,70,87). As with other crystal related arthropathies, release of these enzymes may play a key role in cartilage and bone destruction in BCP crystal-induced disease. Unlike cell proliferation, the induction of MMP-1 production by fibroblasts does not depend on intracellular BCP crystal dissolution (86). Stimulation of IL-1 and COX-2 release from synovial fibroblasts by BCP crystals may also contribute to both the inflammatory response and also matrix degradation (88).

BCP crystals may be frequently identified within asymptomatic uninflamed joints, suggesting that controls exist within the joint to prevent triggering of the inflammatory response. As with MSU crystals, coating of BCP crystals by specific proteins may contribute to this protective effect. Addition of serum and plasma inhibits the ability of hydroxyapatite crystals to activate neutrophils. The coating of crystals by α2-HS glycoprotein is particularly effective in reducing BCP crystal induced neutrophil activation (89).

REFERENCES

1. Agudelo CA, Schumacher HR. The synovitis of acute gouty arthritis. A light and electron microscopic study. Hum Pathol 1973; 4:265–279.
2. Schumacher HR. Pathology of the synovial membrane in gout. Light and electron microscopic studies. Interpretation of crystals in electron micrographs. Arthritis Rheum 1975; 18:771–782.
3. Tak HK, Cooper SM, Wilcox WR. Studies on the nucleation of monosodium urate at 37 degreesc. Arthritis Rheum 1980; 23:574–580.
4. McGill NW, Dieppe PA. Evidence for a promoter of urate crystal formation in gouty synovial fluid. Ann Rheum Dis 1991; 50:558–561.
5. Perl-Treves D, Addadi L. A structural approach to pathological crystallizations. Gout: the possible role of albumin in sodium urate crystallization. Proc R Soc Lond B Biol Sci 1988; 235:145–159.
6. Kam M, Perl-Treves D, Caspi D, Addadi L. Antibodies against crystals. Faseb J 1992; 6:2608–2613.
7. Getting SJ, Flower RJ, Parente L, et al. Molecular determinants of monosodium urate crystal-induced murine peritonitis: a role for endogenous mast cells and a distinct requirement for endothelial-derived selectins. J Pharmacol Exp Ther 1997; 283:123–130.
8. Chapman PT, Yarwood H, Harrison AA, et al. Endothelial activation in monosodium urate monohydrate crystal-induced inflammation: in vitro and in vivo studies on the roles of tumor necrosis factor alpha and interleukin-1. Arthritis Rheum 1997; 40:955–965.
9. Nishimura A, Akahoshi T, Takahashi M, et al. Attenuation of monosodium urate crystal-induced arthritis in rabbits by a neutralizing antibody against interleukin-8. J Leukoc Biol 1997; 62:444–449.
10. Terkeltaub R, Baird S, Sears P, et al. The murine homolog of the interleukin-8 receptor CXCR-2 is essential for the occurrence of neutrophilic inflammation in the air pouch model of acute urate crystal-induced gouty synovitis. Arthritis Rheum 1998; 41:900–909.
11. Kozin F, Ginsberg MH, Skosey JL. Polymorphonuclear leukocyte responses to monosodium urate crystals: modification by adsorbed serum proteins. J Rheumatol 1979; 6:519–526.
12. Terkeltaub R, Tenner AJ, Kozin F, Ginsberg MH. Plasma protein binding by monosodium urate crystals. Analysis by two-dimensional gel electrophoresis. Arthritis Rheum 1983; 26:775–783.
13. Hasselbacher P. C3 activation by monosodium urate monohydrate and other crystalline material. Arthritis Rheum 1979; 22:571–578.
14. Giclas PC, Ginsberg MH, Cooper NR. Immunoglobulin G independent activation of the classical complement pathway by monosodium urate crystals. J Clin Invest 1979; 63:759–764.
15. Doherty M, Whicher JT, Dieppe PA. Activation of the alternative pathway of complement by monosodium urate monohydrate crystals and other inflammatory particles. Ann Rheum Dis 1983; 42:285–291.
16. Tramontini N, Huber C, Liu-Bryan R, et al. Central role of complement membrane attack complex in monosodium urate crystal-induced neutrophilic rabbit knee synovitis. Arthritis Rheum 2004; 50:2633–2639.

17. Damas J, Remacle-Volon G, Adam A. The role of the kinin system in various inflammatory models in the rat. Int J Tissue React 1984; 6:391–399.
18. Damas J, Remacle-Volon G. Influence of a long-acting bradykinin antagonist, Hoe 140, on some acute inflammatory reactions in the rat. Eur J Pharmacol 1992; 211:81–86.
19. Antommattei O, Heimer R, Baker DG, Schumacher HR, Jr. Binding of synovial fluid proteins to monosodium urate crystals in vitro. Clin Exp Rheumatol 1990; 8:29–34.
20. Phelps P, McCarty DJ, Jr. Crystal-induced inflammation in canine joints II. Importance of polymorphonuclear leukocytes. J Exp Med 1966; 124:115–126.
21. Terkeltaub RA, Sklar LA, Mueller H. Neutrophil activation by inflammatory microcrystals of monosodium urate monohydrate utilizes pertussis toxin-insensitive and -sensitive pathways. J Immunol 1990; 144:2714–2719.
22. Onello E, Traynor-Kaplan A, Sklar L, Terkeltaub R. Mechanism of neutrophil activation by an unopsonized inflammatory particulate Monosodium urate crystals induce pertussis toxin-insensitive hydrolysis of phosphatidylinositol 4,5-bisphosphate. J Immunol 1991; 146:4289–4294.
23. Barabe F, Gilbert C, Liao N, et al. Crystal-induced neutrophil activation VI. Involvment of FcgammaRIIIB (CD16) and CD11b in response to inflammatory microcrystals. FASEB J 1998; 12:209–220.
24. Abramson S, Hoffstein ST, Weissmann G. Superoxide anion generation by human neutrophils exposed to monosodium urate. Arthritis Rheum 1982; 25:174–180.
25. Simchowitz L, Atkinson JP, Spilberg I. Stimulation of the respiratory burst in human neutrophils by crystal phagocytosis. Arthritis Rheum 1982; 25:181–188.
26. Naccache PH, Grimard M, Roberge CJ, et al. Crystal-induced neutrophil activation I. Initiation and modulation of calcium mobilization and superoxide production by microcrystals. Arthritis Rheum 1991; 34:333–342.
27. Gilbert C, Poubelle PE, Borgeat P, et al. Crystal-induced neutrophil activation: VIII. Immediate production of prostaglandin E2 mediated by constitutive cyclooxygenase 2 in human neutrophils stimulated by urate crystals. Arthritis Rheum 2003; 48:1137–1148.
28. Roberge CJ, Grassi J, De Medicis R, et al. Crystal-neutrophil interactions lead to interleukin-1 synthesis. Agents Actions 1991; 34:38–41.
29. Roberge CJ, de Medicis R, Dayer JM, et al. Crystal-induced neutrophil activation V. Differential production of biologically active IL-1 and IL-1 receptor antagonist. J Immunol 1994; 152:5485–5494.
30. Hachicha M, Naccache PH, McColl SR. Inflammatory microcrystals differentially regulate the secretion of macrophage inflammatory protein 1 and interleukin 8 by human neutrophils: a possible mechanism of neutrophil recruitment to sites of inflammation in synovitis. J Exp Med 1995; 182:2019–2025.
31. Ryckman C, Gilbert C, De Medicis R, et al. Monosodium urate monohydrate crystals induce the release of the proinflammatory protein S100A8/A9 from neutrophils. J Leukoc Biol 2004; 76:433–440.
32. di Giovine FS, Malawista SE, Nuki G, Duff GW. Interleukin 1 (IL 1) as a mediator of crystal arthritis. Stimulation of T cell and synovial fibroblast mitogenesis by urate crystal-induced IL 1. J Immunol 1987; 138:3213–3218.

33. di Giovine Fs, Malawista SE, Thornton E, Duff GW. Urate crystals stimulate production of tumor necrosis factor alpha from human blood monocytes and synovial cells. Cytokine mRNA and protein kinctics, and cellular distribution. J Clin Invest 1991:87.
34. Guerne PA, Terkeltaub R, Zuraw B, Lotz M. Inflammatory microcrystals stimulate interleukin-6 production and secretion by human monocytes and synoviocytes. Arthritis Rheum 1989; 32:1443–1452.
35. Terkeltaub R, Zachariae C, Santoro D, et al. Monocyte-derived neutrophil chemotactic factor/interleukin-8 is a potential mediator of crystal-induced inflammation. Arthritis Rheum 1991; 34:894–903.
36. Pouliot M, James MJ, McColl SR, et al. Monosodium urate microcrystals induce cyclooxygenase-2 in human monocytes. Blood 1998; 91:1769–1776.
37. Wigley FM, Fine IT, Newcombe DS. The role of the human synovial fibroblast in monosodium urate crystal-induced synovitis. J Rheumatol 1983; 10:602–611.
38. Gordon TP, Bertouch JV, Walsh BR, Brooks PM. Monosodium urate crystals in asymptomatic knee joints. J Rheumatol 1982; 9:967–969.
39. Pascual E. Persistence of monosodium urate crystals and low-grade inflammation in the synovial fluid of patients with untreated gout. Arthritis Rheum 1991; 34:141–145.
40. Pascual E, Batlle-Gualda E, Martinez A, et al. Synovial fluid analysis for diagnosis of intercritical gout. Ann Intern Med 1999; 131:756–975.
41. Terkeltaub R, Curtiss LK, Tenner AJ, Ginsberg MH. Lipoproteins containing apoprotein B are a major regulator of neutrophil responses to monosodium urate crystals. J Clin Invest 1984; 73:1719–1730.
42. Terkeltaub R, Martin J, Curtiss LK, Ginsberg MH. Apolipoprotein B mediates the capacity of low density lipoprotein to suppress neutrophil stimulation by particulates. J Biol Chem 1986; 261:15662–15667.
43. Terkeltaub RA, Dyer CA, Martin J, Curtiss LK. Apolipoprotein (apo) E inhibits the capacity of monosodium urate crystals to stimulate neutrophils. Characterization of intraarticular apo E and demonstration of apo E binding to urate crystals in vivo. J Clin Invest 1991; 87:20–26.
44. Ortiz-Bravo E, Sieck MS, Schumacher HR, Jr. Changes in the proteins coating monosodium urate crystals during active and subsiding inflammation. Immunogold studies of synovial fluid from patients with gout and of fluid obtained using the rat subcutaneous air pouch model. Arthritis Rheum 1993; 36:1274–1285.
45. Getting SJ, Christian HC, Flower RJ, Perretti M. Activation of melanocortin type 3 receptor as a molecular mechanism for adrenocorticotropic hormone efficacy in gouty arthritis. Arthritis Rheum 2002; 46:2765–2775.
46. Akahoshi T, Namai R, Murakami Y, et al. Rapid induction of peroxisome proliferator-activated receptor gamma expression in human monocytes by monosodium urate monohydrate crystals. Arthritis Rheum 2003; 48:231–239.
47. Agudelo CA, Weinberger A, Schumacher HR, et al. Definitive diagnosis of gout by identification of urate crystals in asymptomatic metatarsophalangeal joints. Arthritis Rheum 1979; 22:559–560.
48. Pascual E, Jovani V. A quantitative study of the phagocytosis of urate crystals in the synovial fluid of asymptomatic joints of patients with gout. Br J Rheumatol 1995; 34:724–726.

49. Schiltz C, Liote F, Prudhommeaux F, et al. Monosodium urate monohydrate crystal-induced inflammation in vivo: quantitative histomorphometric analysis of cellular events. Arthritis Rheum 2002; 46:1643–1650.
50. Yagnik DR, Hillyer P, Marshall D, et al. Noninflammatory phagocytosis of monosodium urate monohydrate crystals by mouse macrophages. Implications for the control of joint inflammation in gout. Arthritis Rheum 2000; 43:1779–1789.
51. Landis RC, Yagnik DR, Florey O, et al. Safe disposal of inflammatory monosodium urate monohydrate crystals by differentiated macrophages. Arthritis Rheum 2002; 46:3026–3033.
52. Fava R, Olsen N, Keski-Oja J, et al. Active and latent forms of transforming growth factor beta activity in synovial effusions. J Exp Med 1989; 169:291–296.
53. Liote F, Prudhommeaux F, Schiltz C, et al. Inhibition and prevention of monosodium urate monohydrate crystal-induced acute inflammation in vivo by transforming growth factor beta1. Arthritis Rheum 1996; 39:1192–1198.
54. Yagnik DR, Evans BJ, Florey O, et al. Macrophage release of transforming growth factor beta1 during resolution of monosodium urate monohydrate crystal-induced inflammation. Arthritis Rheum 2004; 50:2273–2280.
55. Palmer DG, Highton J, Hessian PA. Development of the gout tophus. An hypothesis. Am J Clin Pathol 1989; 91:190–195.
56. Schweyer S, Hemmerlein B, Radzun HJ, Fayyazi A. Continuous recruitment, co-expression of tumour necrosis factor-alpha and matrix metalloproteinases, and apoptosis of macrophages in gout tophi. Virchows Arch 2000; 437:534–539.
57. Hsieh MS, Ho HC, Chou DT, et al. Expression of matrix metalloproteinase-9 (gelatinase B) in gouty arthritis and stimulation of MMP-9 by urate crystals in macrophages. J Cell Biochem 2003; 89:791–799.
58. Hasselbacher P. Stimulation of synovial fibroblasts by calcium oxalate and monosodium urate monohydrate. A mechanism of connective tissue degradation in oxalosis and gout. J Lab Clin Med 1982; 100:977–985.
59. McMillan RM, Vater CA, Hasselbacher P, et al. Induction of collagenase and prostaglandin synthesis in synovial fibroblasts treated with monosodium urate crystals. J Pharm Pharmacol 1981; 33:382–383.
60. Liu R, Liote F, Rose DM, et al. Proline-rich tyrosine kinase 2 and Src kinase signaling transduce monosodium urate crystal-induced nitric oxide production and matrix metalloproteinase 3 expression in chondrocytes. Arthritis Rheum 2004; 50:247–258.
61. Doherty M, Dieppe PA. Acute pseudogout: "crystal shedding" or acute crystallization? Arthritis Rheum 1981; 24:954–957.
62. Doherty M, Richards N, Hornby J, Powell R. Relation between synovial fluid C3 degradation products and local joint inflammation in rheumatoid arthritis, osteoarthritis, and crystal associated arthropathy. Ann Rheum Dis 1988; 47:190–197.
63. Nagase M, Baker DG, Schumacher HR, Jr. Immunoglobulin G coating on crystals and ceramics enhances polymorphonuclear cell superoxide production: correlation with immunoglobulin G adsorbed. J Rheumatol 1989; 16:971–976.
64. Burt HM, Jackson JK. Enhancement of crystal induced neutrophil responses by opsonisation of calcium pyrophosphate dihydrate crystals. Ann Rheum Dis 1993; 52:599–607.

65. Watanabe W, Baker DG, Schumacher HR, Jr. Comparison of the acute inflammation induced by calcium pyrophosphate dihydrate, apatite and mixed crystals in the rat air pouch model of a synovial space. J Rheumatol 1992; 19:1453–1457.
66. Meng ZH, Hudson AP, Schumacher HR, Jr., et al. Monosodium urate, hydroxyapatite, and calcium pyrophosphate crystals induce tumor necrosis factor-alpha expression in a mononuclear cell line. J Rheumatol 1997; 24:2385–2388.
67. Liu R, O'Connell M, Johnson K, et al. Extracellular signal-regulated kinase 1/extracellular signal-regulated kinase 2 mitogen-activated protein kinase signaling and activation of activator protein 1 and nuclear factor kappaB transcription factors play central roles in interleukin-8 expression stimulated by monosodium urate monohydrate and calcium pyrophosphate crystals in monocytic cells. Arthritis Rheum 2000; 43:1145–1155.
68. McCarty DJ, Cheung HS. (PG) E2 Prostaglandin generation by cultured canine synovial fibroblasts exposed to microcrystals containing calcium. Ann Rheum Dis 1985; 44:316–320.
69. Reuben PM, Wenger L, Cruz M, Cheung HS. Induction of matrix metalloproteinase-8 in human fibroblasts by basic calcium phosphate and calcium pyrophosphate dihydrate crystals: effect of phosphocitrate. Connect Tissue Res 2001; 42:1–12.
70. Cheung HS, Halverson PB, McCarty DJ. Release of collagenase, neutral protease, and prostaglandins from cultured mammalian synovial cells by hydroxyapatite and calcium pyrophosphate dihydrate crystals. Arthritis Rheum 1981; 24:1338–1344.
71. Burt HM, Jackson JK. The priming action of tumour necrosis factor-alpha (TNF-alpha) and granulocyte-macrophage colony-stimulating factor (GM-CSF) on neutrophils activated by inflammatory microcrystals. Clin Exp Immunol 1997; 108:432–437.
72. Rosenthal AK, Cheung HS, Ryan LM. Transforming growth factor beta 1 stimulates inorganic pyrophosphate elaboration by porcine cartilage. Arthritis Rheum 1991; 34:904–911.
73. Bouchard L, de Medicis R, Lussier A, et al. Inflammatory microcrystals alter the functional phenotype of human osteoblast-like cells in vitro: synergism with IL-1 to overexpress cyclooxygenase-2. J Immunol 2002; 168:5310–5317.
74. Dayer JM, Evequoz V, Zavadil-Grob C, et al. Effect of synthetic calcium pyrophosphate and hydroxyapatite crystals on the interaction of human blood mononuclear cells with chondrocytes, synovial cells, and fibroblasts. Arthritis Rheum 1987; 30:1372–1381.
75. Schumacher HR, Cherian PV. Transmission electron microscopic studies on articular calcium crystals and associated protein coatings. Scan Electron Microsc 1984; Pt 2:965–968.
76. Evans RW, Cheung HS, McCarty DJ. Cultured canine synovial cells solubilize 45Ca-labeled hydroxyapatite crystals. Arthritis Rheum 1984; 27:829–832.
77. Prudhommeaux F, Schiltz C, Liote F, et al. Variation in the inflammatory properties of basic calcium phosphate crystals according to crystal type. Arthritis Rheum 1996; 39:1319–1326.
78. Nagase M, Baker DG, Schumacher HR, Jr. Prolonged inflammatory reactions induced by artificial ceramics in the rat air pouch model. J Rheumatol 1988; 15:1334–1338.

79. Laquerriere P, Grandjean-Laquerriere A, Jallot E, et al. Importance of hydroxyapatite particles characteristics on cytokines production by human monocytes in vitro. Biomaterials 2003; 24:2739–2747.
80. Harada Y, Wang JT, Doppalapudi VA, et al. Differential effects of different forms of hydroxyapatite and hydroxyapatite/tricalcium phosphate particulates on human monocyte/macrophages in vitro. J Biomed Mater Res 1996; 31:19–26.
81. Nagase M, Nishiya H, Abe Y. The effect of crystallinity on hydroxyapatite-induced production of reactive oxygen metabolites by polymorphonuclear leukocytes. FEBS Lett 1993; 325:247–250.
82. Nagase M, Nishiya H, Noda M. Priming effect of hydroxyapatite on the chemiluminescence response in human polymorphonuclear leukocytes. FEBS Lett 1994; 349:13–16.
83. Cheung HS, Story MT, McCarty DJ. Mitogenic effects of hydroxyapatite and calcium pyrophosphate dihydrate crystals on cultured mammalian cells. Arthritis Rheum 1984; 27:668–674.
84. Mitchell PG, Struve JA, McCarthy GM, Cheung HS. Basic calcium phosphate crystals stimulate cell proliferation and collagenase message accumulation in cultured adult articular chondrocytes. Arthritis Rheum 1992; 35:343–350.
85. Cheung HS, McCarty DJ. Mitogenesis induced by calcium-containing crystals. Role of intracellular dissolution. Exp Cell Res 1985; 157:63–70.
86. McCarthy GM, Cheung HS, Abel SM, Ryan LM. Basic calcium phosphate crystal-induced collagenase production: role of intracellular crystal dissolution. Osteoarthritis Cartilage 1998; 6:205–213.
87. Bai G, Howell DS, Howard GA, et al. Basic calcium phosphate crystals up-regulate metalloproteinases but down-regulate tissue inhibitor of metalloproteinase-1 and -2 in human fibroblasts. Osteoarthritis Cartilage 2001; 9:416–422.
88. Morgan MP, Whelan LC, Sallis JD, McCarthy CJ, Fitzgerald DJ, McCarthy GM. Basic calcium phosphate crystal-induced prostaglandin E2 production in human fibroblasts: role of cyclooxygenase 1, cyclooxygenase 2, and interleukin-1beta. Arthritis Rheum 2004; 50:1642–1649.
89. Terkeltaub RA, Santoro DA, Mandel G, Mandel N. Serum and plasma inhibit neutrophil stimulation by hydroxyapatite crystals. Evidence that serum alpha 2-HS glycoprotein is a potent and specific crystal-bound inhibitor. Arthritis Rheum 1988; 31:1081–1089.

16

Physiologic Aspects of Urate Homeostasis

Peter A. Simkin

Division of Rheumatology, Department of Medicine, University of Washington School of Medicine, Seattle, Washington, U.S.A.

INTRODUCTION

In normal men, the urate concentration of plasma averages approximately 5.5 ± 0.5 mg/dL, whereas that of children and women is lower by about 1 mg/dL. These levels fluctuate considerably in any individual but always remain in a rough, overall balance in which the amount of dietary and metabolic urate entering the system is equaled by the sum of the urinary uric acid together with the urate of gastrointestinal secretions that is lysed by the uricase of local flora and excreted as allantoin:

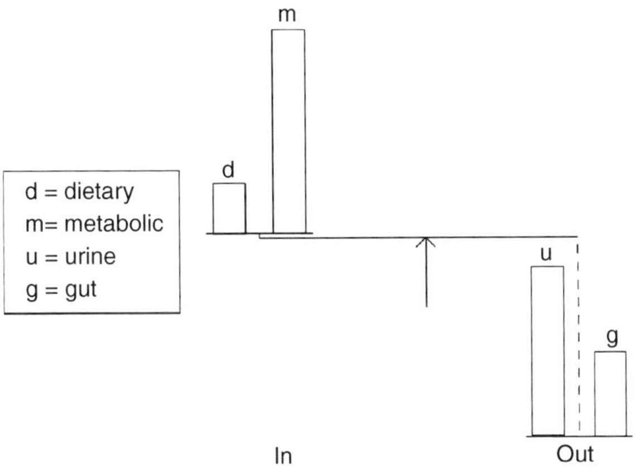

The load may be lowered a little (but not much) by decreasing the dietary intake or a lot by defective xanthine oxidase, the enzyme responsible for urate synthesis. This occurs rarely in nature in the form of xanthinuria but often in practice as a result of xanthine oxidase inhibition by allopurinol. Conversely, the load will increase with a purine-rich diet, with excessive breakdown of purine nucleotides (i.e., ATP, GTP, etc.), with accelerated catabolism of cells (as in the tumor lysis syndrome), or with the rare metabolic defects causing true overproduction of urate (see also Chapter 12). Each of the above factors affects the size of the urate burden that is ultimately processed by the kidney or the gut. Ultimately, however, the most significant determinants of hypo- and hyperuricemia are not in the load but in the way it is handled.

In normal people, approximately 70% of the daily purine load leaves the body through the kidneys as urinary uric acid (1,2). Not only are they the primary pathway of elimination, but the kidneys are also the site of the sometime complications of stones and renal insufficiency that figure prominently in the morbidity of hyperuricemia. It is therefore not surprising that most of the available physiologic information pertains to renal function. The gut contributes significantly to normal elimination, however, and it becomes the principal pathway of purine elimination when the kidneys start to fail (3). Together the kidneys and the gut employ specific transport systems to clear urate from the plasma and preserve physiologic balance in each person. "Compartmentalization and transport between compartments are the essence of physiology" (4). Current understanding of these systems (and their failings) will be reviewed briefly in this chapter.

THE TRANSPORTERS

The past decade has seen impressive progress in the recognition and characterization of urate transporters (5–7). These developments permit anatomic localization of tissue distribution. What organs contain which transporters? Where along the length of the nephron are the opposing carriers involved in tubular reabsorption and secretion? Will differences in the density and distribution of transporters provide logical explanations for the now-baffling degree of interspecies variation in urate disposal? These and other relevant questions can be addressed when the specific mediators of reabsorption and secretion are known. The current understanding of the transporters is illustrated nicely in the schematic Figure 1 (7).

The known structure of transporter proteins also permits the remarkable feat of inserting the cRNA encoding the relevant genes into eggs of the African frog, Xenopus, and observing the ultimate expression of those genes by transporters on the limiting membrane (8). There, each carrier may be studied in isolation, the affinity of competing substrates can be quantified, and the potential bidirectional effects of relevant agents can be examined.

URAT1

The most important tubular transporter was discovered in the sequence of the human genome (8). As previously postulated, it is an exchanger that swaps urate for other anions in both directions across the apical (luminal) membrane of

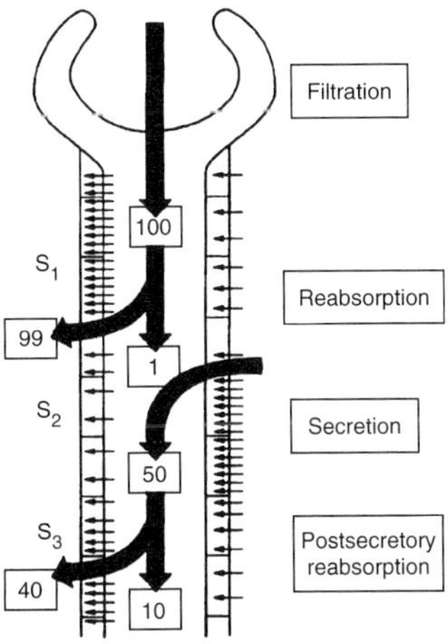

Figure 1 Model of urate transport in a schematic nephron. Free filtration is followed by nearly complete reabsorption, significant secretion, and further reabsorption. As the small arrows indicate, these processes are largely coextensive, although they are generally considered to be sequential. *Source*: From Ref. 7.

proximal tubular cells (9). The exchanges are apparently not mole for mole, and the avidity varies greatly among substrates, but the system can be "cis-inhibited" by known uricosuric agents (i.e., probenecid, sulfinpyrazone, benzbromarone, etc.) within the lumen. These drugs occupy the available transporters. As a result, less urate is absorbed, and the net result is an increased renal clearance and a fall in the serum concentration of urate ions. Conversely, the same system may be "trans-stimulated" by intracellular anions such as pyrazinamide, lactate, and nicotinamide which can drive more effective reabsorption. In either direction, urate is traded for another organic ion, and the same ion (i.e., lactate) may cause net influx or efflux from the cell depending on its concentration gradient across the limiting membrane. Drugs or agents with affinity for URAT1 are uricosuric when acting from the lumen and are antiuricosuric when acting from the intracellular space (8).

This concept provides an attractive explanation for the classic "paradox" of bidirectional pharmacodynamics of salicylate or probenecid (10). Like essentially all other uricosuric drugs, these agents are highly protein bound and therefore will largely bypass glomerular filtration (11). As organic acid transporters (OATs) carry them from the surrounding interstitium into the tubular cells, the intracellular concentration exceeds that within the lumen, thus trans-stimulating reabsorption and retaining urate. At higher concentrations, however, these agents ultimately reach the lumen, engage the transporters there and produce a net uricosuria.

OAT1

Organic acid transporters clear most of the drugs that leave the body through the kidney. Probenecid was developed originally to inhibit these carriers, to slow the renal clearance of penicillin, and to thereby extend the duration of action of this vital drug when it was a new agent in scant supply (12). It did that (as it also extends the half life of indomethacin and a host of other drugs), but it eventually found its principal role as a uricosuric inhibitor of what we now know to be URAT1.

The prototypic organic acid transporter substrate is para amino hippurate (PAH), an agent that is secreted so completely that its clearance has long been used as a determinant of the renal plasma flow. Its principal carrier, OAT1, has been cloned and the inhibition profiles of uricosuric and antiuricosuric agents as well as the potential capacity for urate secretion have been determined (13). OAT1 is found throughout the proximal tubular cell including the cytoplasm and the apical and basolateral "business sides" involved in reabsorption and secretion. OAT1 is able to carry urate to a degree that potentially can exceed the amount filtered at the glomerulus. Both benzbromarone and probenecid inhibit this carrier, and presumably are themselves carried by it. However, pyrazinamide and salicylate provide a higher degree of inhibition. The last point is perhaps the most interesting. It has long been recognized that salicylate (itself a uricosuric) interfered with the uricosuric properties of probenecid. Pyrazinamide too has been found to block the uricosuria not only of probenecid but also benzbromarone and sulfasalazine (14,15). These protein-bound drugs escape filtration at the glomerulous and must then be secreted into the tubular lumen before they can begin to inhibit reabsorption as uricosuric agents. Although it seems logical to suggest that salicylate and pyrazinamide (PZA) may block this necessary transport of uricosurics, and thus nullify their pharmacologic effects, such a competitive inhibition has not been found (16). Thus, the trans-stimulation of PZA appears able to trump the cis-inhibition of uricosurics. The manner of this strange competition has not yet been characterized, but it seems logical to suspect that it may largely be spatial. If sufficient URAT1 transporters can be stimulated by PZA within the juxta-glomerular proximal tubule, then urate reabsorption may be essentially complete before effective uricosuria can begin (i.e., the uricosuric belatedly arrives after the urate has left the tubule).

These concerns are also relevant to what happens when kidneys begin to fail. Although uricosuric agents offer highly effective control over the hyperuricemia of patients with normal renal function, they are generally ineffective in renal insufficiency (Fig. 2) (17). Although there has been little quantitative study of this phenomenon, the anecdotal evidence is so strong that it is recognized in the prescribing information for all of these drugs. The truism seems puzzling since gram amounts of urate are still filtered and reabsorbed daily by even the marginal kidney, uricosurics are known to inhibit URAT1-mediated reabsorption, and that process should remain susceptible to pharmacologic suppression. Why, then, don't uricosurics work?

A plausible explanation begins with the fact that uricosurics work from within the tubular lumen and require specific tubular secretion before they can begin to inhibit reabsorption (11). As weak organic acids, they are secreted by organic acid transporters (perhaps sharing the same pathway with urate ions). For

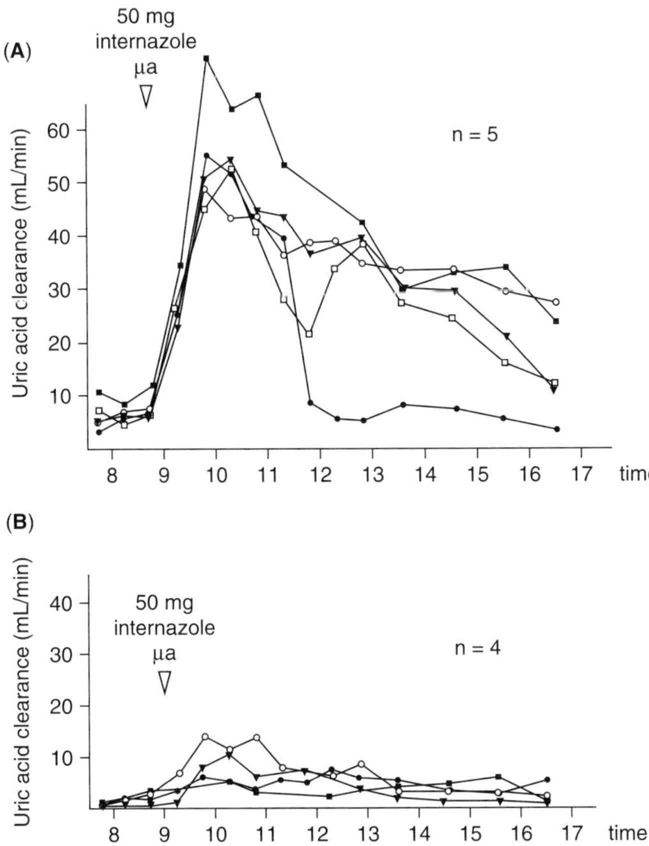

Figure 2 Uric acid clearance after a 50 mg oral dose of the uricosuric drug irtemazole. Panel (**A**) shows response in five hyperuricemic men with normal renal function. Panel (**B**) shows lack of response in four patients with renal insufficiency. *Source*: From Ref. 17.

reasons that remain unclear, organic acid transporter function may be affected disproportionately by renal impairment (18). Thus, for instance, removal of one and a half kidneys in sheep (a 75% reduction in mass) leads to only a 43% decrease in glomerular filtration because of "compensatory hypertrophy" in the remaining kidney. At the same time, however, tubular secretion of probenecid decreases by 90% (19). This peculiar phenomenon appears to pertain in people as well with the end result being renal "resistance" to uricosuric agents despite seemingly modest overall renal compromise. For no reason that is yet apparent, OAT1 function may be more affected by renal disease than are OAT2, OAT3, and OAT4 (20). If probenecid is predominantly secreted by OAT1 while benzbromarone is secreted by, for instance, OAT3, this would explain why the latter is more effective in patients with renal impairment.

The shared liability among present uricosurics of high protein binding and necessary secretion appears to present an opportunity for pharmacologic exploitation. Any inhibitor of URAT1 that is filtered freely at the glomerulus should be an effective uricosuric, almost irrespective of renal function. Such an advance would bypass the need for active secretion and might add greatly to the therapeutic options for hyperuricemia.

hUAT

The transporter termed hUAT is widely distributed among human tissues and is thought to be the principal carrier responsible for the "housekeeping" function of exporting intracellular urate (21). The previously discussed transporters, URAT1 and OAT1, carry urate into tubular cells from their luminal (apical) and interstitial (basolateral) sides respectively. Once within the cell, however, these polar ions ultimately confront another sparsely permeable lipid bilayer on the opposite side which they must also pass to complete the trans-cellular passage required by either reabsorption or secretion. hUAT is a voltage-dependant carrier that belongs to a hexose-binding class of proteins called galectins, a surprising finding since the other members of this group are cytosolic rather than membrane constituents and they are not known to be transporters. Like the other urate carriers, hUAT is blocked by pyrazinoate but apparently not by probenecid. It is also blocked by oxonic acid, an agent used widely to inhibit uricase but not known to interfere significantly with transcellular transport of urate.

The wide tissue distribution of this carrier, its high specificity for urate, and the obvious need for cellular export in both reabsorption and secretion all make this an interesting molecule. However, it has not been clearly linked to pathophysiologic or pharmacologic events in human subjects.

Carrier Confusion

The bidirectionality of tubular urate transport, the wide species variation among potential animal models, and the general inaccessibility of proximal tubules have always led to confusion, and sometimes dissention, among students of urate transport. To date, three transporters (URAT1, hOAT1, and hUAT) have been characterized in elegant detail and the amount of relevant data has been greatly amplified. But questions still remain. We still do not know if all of the relevant transporters have been identified. Will OAT3 or some other presently unidentified carrier turn out to be a major player in the human scene (22). We know little about what happens beneath the cell membrane. How will PDZ or other proteins link the transcellular passage of urate to the intracellular signaling cascades involved in the transport of other solutes (23,24)? Several metabolites identified as inhibitors or activators of specific transporters (i.e., lactate, acetoacetate, betahydroxybutyrate, nicotinamide, etc.) are linked intimately to NAD/NADH ratios in their own metabolism. As long ago as 1923, it was found that lactate infusions caused urate retention while pyrurate led to uricsuria (25).

$$\frac{\text{NADH}}{\text{NAD}^+} \approx \frac{\text{lactate}}{\text{pyruvate}} \approx \frac{\beta\text{OH butyrate}}{\text{actetaccate}} \approx \frac{\text{ethanol}}{\text{acetaldehyde}}$$

Just where does the intracellular redox potential fit in the overall picture of urate transport and how can we assess it in vivo? Does it drive the voltage sensitive transporter UAT? Intriguing hypotheses have been proposed to link the transport of urate with that of sodium and glucose (26,27). Are these concepts clear enough to logically explain the known associations with hypertension, insulin resistance, and the other manifestations of the metabolic syndrome?

THE TRANSPORT

Filtration

Were urate to be highly protein-bound, it would bypass filtration at the glomerulus, as uricosurics do, and it would then have to be secreted into the renal tubules before it could be excreted in the urine. Thus there has been considerable investigation and some controversy over the question of protein binding (28). For the most part, however, the issue is whether the amount bound is small or none. Micropuncture studies of glomerular filtrates have offered little support for the concept, many of the positive studies were carried out under unphysiologic conditions, and most studies of uric acid excretion now operate under the assumption that any binding present is small enough to be neglected.

Reabsorption

As the glomerular filtrate enters the tubule, it starts down a passage lined on all sides by URAT1 transporters. The great majority of filtered urate ions will not get through this gantlet. Instead they will intersect with a transporter and be extracted to enter the lining cells and begin their return trip to the plasma. As they pass down the tubule, the escapees will be joined by secreted urate ions, but the total reaching the end of the nephron will be 5% to 10% of the number originally filtered. To distinguish between these two sources of urinary uric acid, pyrazinamide was given with the thought that it blocked tubular secretion, thereby dropping the surviving percentage to approximately 1% (29). We now know that this drug not only blocks secretion, but it also stimulates URAT1 mediated reabsorption. Thus, it has again become unclear just how many filtered ions might pass all the way through in the absence of pharmacologic interference. By any measure, though, the number must be small. A number of factors affect the odds of completing this passage successfully. These include the number of competing ions, the number of receptors, transit times, and the "receptivity" of the receptors.

If there is a large but fixed number of carriers and a variable number of ions, the chance of any individual ion's escape increases exponentially as the capture of other ions occupies the available receptors and thus saturates the uptake capacity (30). Recapture will be avid when low concentrations exist, whereas most will pass through when there are high concentrations. Just such an exponential pattern occurs in the excretion of uric acid (31). The most extreme example occurs in the tumor lysis syndrome where a cataclysmic release of nuclear purines creates massive loads of filtered urate that overwhelm the tubular reabsorptive capacity of entirely normal kidneys (32). Precipitation of this burden can then create a crystalline sludge that obstructs the collecting system and leads to renal failure.

A similar problem occurs in patients with congenital hypouricemia due to structurally defective URAT1 reabsorbers. When these individuals exercise strenuously, they release a flood of adenine nucleotides that on hepatic conversion to urate then overwhelms the meager reabsorptive capacity with subsequent obstructive renal injury (33).

The number of receptors may prove to be the most critical factor in the regulation of the serum urate concentration. Women have lower serum urate concentrations because they have a lower reabsorptive capability than men, and this may simply represent a lower number of URAT1 transporters as appears to be the case in normal, female mice (34,35). Conversely, genetic predispositions toward hyperuricemia such as that which is prevalent among Filipino and Polynesian men could simply reflect an increase in the number of otherwise normal transporters (36).

Intuitively, it seems appropriate that slowly moving ions might be picked off more readily while those moving faster could be flushed on past the waiting transporters. Consistent with this concept is the finding that renal clearance of urate is higher at more rapid rates of glomerular filtration and urine flow (Fig. 3) (16,37–40). Osmotic diuresis increases clearance as do pathologic states of volume expansion such as in the syndrome of inappropriate anti-diuretic hormone (SIADH) (41,42). Conversely, dehydration may slow the flow and lead to

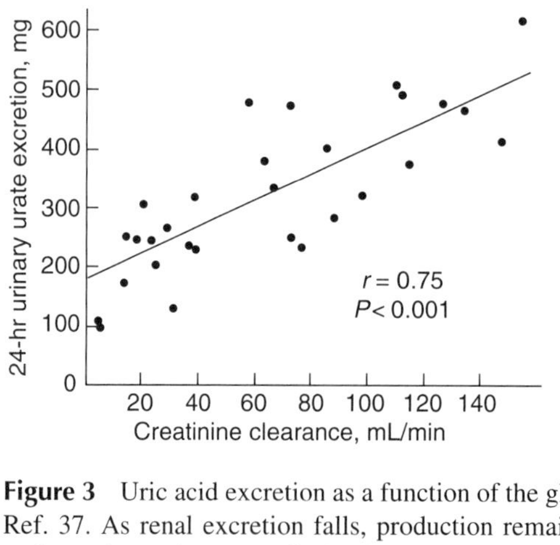

Figure 3 Uric acid excretion as a function of the glomerular filtration rate. *Source*: From Ref. 37. As renal excretion falls, production remains constant and the gut becomes the major pathway for urate elimination (3).

hyperuricemia through excessive reabsorption of both filtered and secreted urate within the tubules (43).

The simple presence of a URAT1 receptor in the luminal membrane does not mean that it will avidly react with urate. These carriers are anion exchangers and they will not take on an urate ion unless they have an appropriate intracellular anion such as lactate, pyrazinamide, or (less likely) chloride to swap for it. In the present era, URAT1 transporters can be, and have been, expressed on the limiting membranes of Xenopus eggs (8). In that setting it is reasonably straightforward to establish a hierarchy of ionic interactions with the carrier from both the inside and the outside of the cell. It is not as easy to apply those findings to intact humans.

Clearance

The renal clearance of any solute is the theoretical volume of plasma that is cleared of that solute per unit of time (i.e., mL/min). It is determined by dividing the excretion rate (mg/min) by the plasma concentration (mg/mL). Since tubular reabsorption is by far the most important determinant of that fraction of filtered urate that will be cleared by the kidney, this seems an appropriate place to consider clearance.

Like the excretion rates they are in part derived from, clearance rates may vary widely in any individual as well as in normal and gouty populations (44,45). Largely for this reason, and perhaps because some data were collected during the transient uricosuria that may accompany acute gouty arthritis, some who conducted early studies found no significant difference in clearance between normal and gouty subjects and therefore believed the kidney had no responsibility for hyperuricemia. To resolve the issue of how this solute was "handled," six different groups independently employed the same protocol to examine uric acid excretion both in normal and in gouty men with at least two different serum urate concentrations in each individual. The level was raised by milkshakes laden with yeast RNA and lowered by allopurinol, an agent known to be without effect on renal function. At each data point, every subject had his glomerular filtration rate (GFR) measured by inulin clearance, and it was therefore possible to exclude subjects with significant impairment in renal function and to express the remaining excretion rates per 100 mL/min GFR (since GFR parallels body size, and body size correlates positively with the excretion rate of any physiologic solute, this is an important correction). In sum, it was possible to compare 80 data points from 36 normal men to 120 observations in 73 gouty men (46).

Several aspects of the central figure (excretion rate versus plasma urate) merit consideration (Fig. 4). First, the differences between normal and gouty men were striking. The average gouty individual excreted only 71% as much uric acid as normal at any serum concentration and required a serum concentration 1.7 mg/dL higher to attain the normal rate of uric acid excretion. Second, in each group the slope of the relationship was exponential. This means that the clearance went up with urate loads, went down with allopurinol, and was not a constant characteristic of each person. Such a slope is, of course, predictable for the

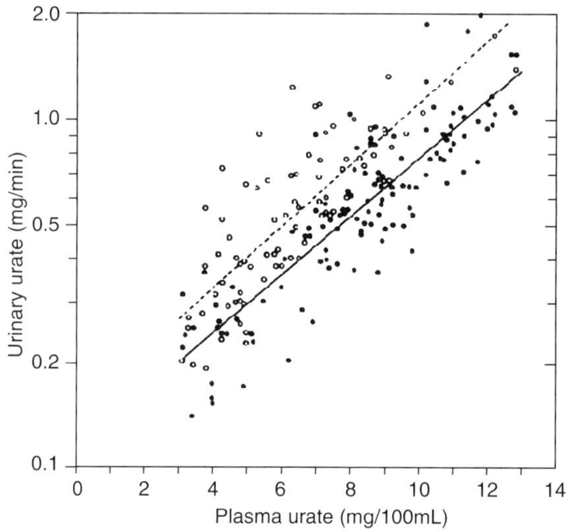

Figure 4 Meta-analysis of uric acid excretion (mg/min/dLGFR) at varying concentrations of serum urate in normal (*open symbols*) and gouty men (*closed symbols*). The regression lines through each data set are exponential and they are parallel to each other. *Source*: From Ref. 46.

relation between a rising filtered load and a fixed number of transporters. As the burden rises toward saturation, the chances become better that individual ions will escape reabsorption. Third, the slopes of the two groups were parallel. This means that kidneys of the gouty subjects responded to additional increments or decrements in filtered load in the same manner as did normal men. This suggests that the transporters themselves are normal and the groups differ only in numbers of URAT1 carriers (more in hyperuricemic men). The point is important because it suggests that mutations in URAT1 may not be necessary to explain more avid tubular reabsorption of filtered urate.

Parenthetically, this analysis pertains only to men since no women or children were studied by the same protocol. Had that been done, it seems highly probable that their data also would have been parallel but above and to the left of the normal men. This is the expected position if they do, indeed, have the same transporters as men but in lesser numbers.

One final point deserves mention with respect to clearance. Data has been reported from 25 gouty subjects before and after their hyperuricemia was effectively controlled by allopurinol over several months (47). In contrast to the findings discussed above, serum urate fell but the uric acid clearance at follow-up was unchanged from that at the start of therapy. This then suggests that over time there was a proportional decrease in the number of transporters. This finding complements less systematic evidence in the opposite direction that people with sustained hyperuricemia "handle" their problem more efficiently than those with acute hyperuricemia. If subsequent studies substantiate these impressions, the necessary conclusion will be that the number of transporters is regulated and is inducible by changes in either direction (48). This may substantiate the prediction that "the serum urate is controlled by URAT1 and vice versa" (49).

Secretion

Although tubular secretion of urate unquestionably occurs, this process has been difficult to quantify because of concurrent reabsorption by coextensive tubular transporters (Fig. 1). The seeming folly of this arrangement continues to mystify all students of the issue. As discussed already with pyrazinamide, pharmacologic attempts to dissect these processes have been complicated because essentially all agents found to inhibit secretion will also affect reabsorption and vice versa. Clearly, much secreted urate is reabsorbed and this process blunts the secretory contribution to urinary uric acid. In fact, post secretory reabsorption is often defined as the fourth component of renal urate transport (the first component being filtration, the second reabsorption, and the third secretion). Although this has been conceptually useful, it implies a sequence of processes that probably does not correspond to the anatomic distribution of transporters. The distinction will be most useful if the "fourth component" can ultimately be ascribed to a transporter other than URAT1.

Perhaps the best quantitative evidence of tubular secretion comes from those rare people with genetic hypouricemia who seem to have a true "Dalmatian defect." In other words, their tubules reabsorb almost no urate. They regularly have a clearance ratio (C urate/GFR) that is greater than 1.0, and probenecid is

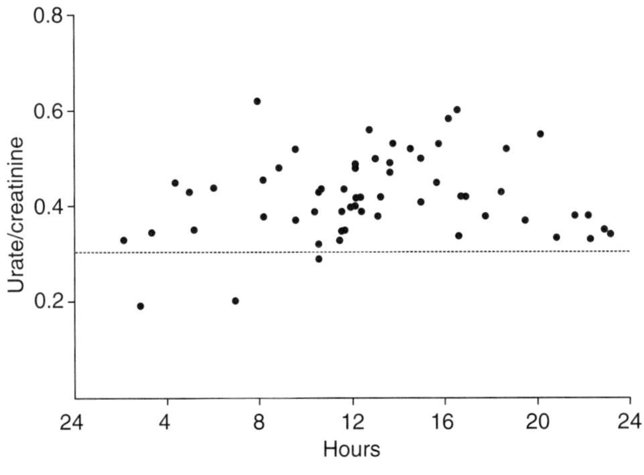

Figure 5 Urate/creatinine ratios in random urine samples from a patient with renal hypouricemia. The dashed line is at 0.31—the same ratio in serum. All points above this line evince clear tubular secretion, although the extent of secretion varies widely. *Source*: From Ref. 52.

antiuricosuric rather than uricosuric (50–52). Sixty random urine specimens were collected from such a person over the course of four weekends. The urinary uric acid/creatinine ratio was plotted against the time of day and against the same ratio in her serum, which was relatively stable at 0.31. Urine ratios greater than 0.31 (57 of 60) indicate net secretion during the time of that collection (Fig. 5). The sample ratios varied widely with an overall pattern of diurnal variation that peaked in the mid-afternoon and reached nadir values in the small hours of the morning (53). No patterns of diet or activity were found to explain the marked variability. Comparable variation occurs in the constant kenneled environment of Dalmatian dogs and in the 24-hour excretion of uric acid in normal and in hyperuricemic people. No one presently understands these fluctuations or the normal variation in serum urate values, but the data imply a parallel and determining variability in the tubular secretion of urate.

HYPOURICEMIA

Hypouricemia is usually defined as a serum urate concentration less than 2.0 mg/dL. It can result from inherited defects or be acquired. Although it is relatively uncommon, a substantial literature has accumulated (54,55).

Inborn Hypouricemia

Most reports are anecdotal observations of patients found incidentally in evaluations for other problems. All such individuals have normal uric acid excretion rates, thus excluding the xanthine oxidase deficiency state of xanthinuria, with high rates of renal clearance and without evidence of other transport problems (although hypouricemia may also occur as part of a juvenile Fanconi syndrome). Acute, exercise-induced renal failure is the only unequivocal clinical association in these otherwise healthy people (33).

Although almost all of these patients are well, their defects are of interest because of the insights they afford into mechanisms of tubular transport. Traditional pharmacologic modifiers, largely pyrazinamide and probenecid, have been used to recognize several mechanistic subsets among patients who share the same clinical presentation.

Of these, the most common is defective tubular reabsorption. Such individuals commonly have fractional excretion of 30% to 50% of the GFR (as opposed to the normal 5% to 10%), thus implying that at least 50% to 70% of the filtered urate is still reabsorbed. Probenecid remains modestly uricosuric, and pyrazinamide produces little or no antiuricosuric response. Limited family studies suggest that this defect is transmitted as an autosomal recessive trait. Thus, the evidence points toward a defect in the gene responsible for production of the URAT1 transporter. This is just what has been found in Japanese studies with the majority of cases derived from a single mutation (56,57). Almost all of the variants cause changes in a "PDZ binding region" at the carboxyl terminal of the transporter. PDZ proteins are abundant in the proximal tubule of the kidney where they are thought to form a scaffold beneath the membrane that optimally supports, positions, and activates membrane carriers (i.e., URAT1) for optimal function (49). Addition of a PDZ protein has now been shown to upregulate URAT1 activity in vitro. This work implies that additional hypouricemic individuals may ultimately be identified who have entirely normal URAT1 but a defective PDZ protein. To date, this is the only form of hypouricemia that has been clearly associated with a molecular defect in a specific transporter.

Other, as yet unexplained patterns have also been described. These include cases in which significant reabsorption occurs but both probenecid and pyrazinamide are without effect (a finding supporting the existence of an additional postsecretory reabsorptive pathway), cases where pyrazinamide normally inhibits net secretion but uricosurics are without effect, instances of apparent hypersecretion where pyrazinamide essentially eliminates all urinary uric acid while uricosurics are exceptionally effective, and individuals whose baseline clearance of urate exceeds the GFR and both pyrazinamide and uricosurics cause a fall in uric acid clearance (Fig. 6) (52). This last form is of special interest because it parallels the much studied pattern of the Dalmatian dog.

Dalmatian Dogs

Although the present review focuses on human physiology, the intriguing defects of Dalmatian dogs deserve mention here (58). Like the human hypouricemia

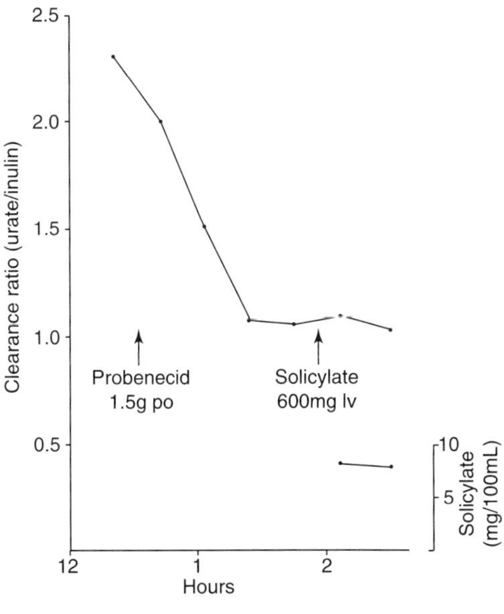

Figure 6 Effects of probenecid and subsequent salicylate infusion on the fractional excretion (urate clearance/inulin clearance) in a patient with renal hypouricemia. Probenecid inhibits secretion and salicylate confers no further effect. *Source*: From Ref. 52.

illustrated in Figure 6, these animals have almost total lack of urate reabsorption, but tubular secretion continues (regularly demonstrated by urate clearance findings in excess of the GFR), and probenecid causes a fall rather than a rise in uric acid excretion. Concurrently, these animals have impaired hepatic uricolysis in vivo despite abundant uricase activity in homogenized liver, in vitro. Thus, there is clear evidence of impaired membrane transport of urate in both the kidney and the liver. In classic (but widely overlooked) cross transplantation experiments between Dalmatians and mongrels, implanted kidneys assumed the urate transport behavior of the host animal (59). Thus Dalamatian kidneys began to reabsorb filtered urate in mongrel hosts, and mongrel kidneys stopped doing so after they were implanted in Dalmatians. Further organ exchanges then found the liver to be the determining organ. Dalmatian livers led mongrels to stop reabsorbing uric acid while mongrel livers enabled Dalmatians to start doing so (Fig. 7) (60). These experiments show that expression of this autosomal recessive trait is somehow determined by the liver and is not inherent in the kidney cells alone. This implies that a hepatic hormone (as yet undiscovered, but tentatively called uratin) regulates URAT1-mediated tubular reabsorption (58).

Years ago, it was suggested that urate reabsorption might be "controlled by chemicals" and that "blood-borne uricosuric" or "antiuricosuric factors" possibly existed (61,62). More recently, the theory "that URAT1 regulates urate levels and vice versa" has been proposed. It seems likely that this additional level of control is exercised by the liver through the hormone uratin. Such a system in people could have profound implications for our understanding of hyperuricemia as well as hypouricemia and could prove to be an important target for pharmacologic intervention.

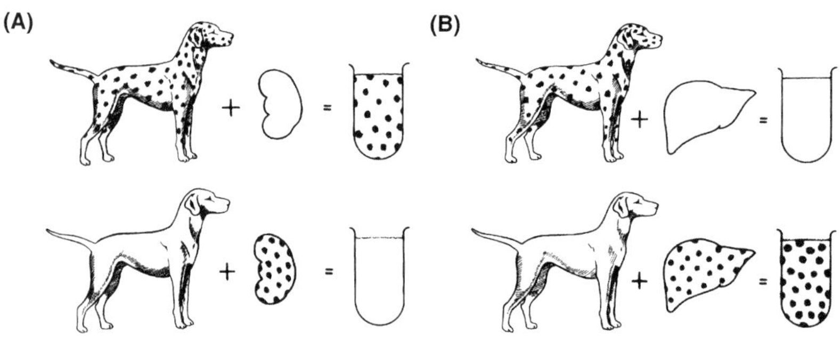

Figure 7 Cartoons depicting effects on uric acid excretion of cross-transplantation experiments between mongrel and Dalmatian dogs. With renal transplants (**A**), the transplanted kidney assumes the properties of the host and exhibits hyperuricosuria (*spotted sample*) in the Dalmatian and relative hypouricosuria (*clear sample*) in the mongrel. With hepatic transplants (**B**), the recipient assumes the excretion properties of the donor.

Acquired Hypouricemia

Additional opportunities for study of excretory mechanisms arise when hypouricemia develops in the course of other diseases (63–65). Some of these such as SIADH and diabetes seem consistent with increased tubular flow or osmotic diuresis. Others occurring with malignancy are intriguing in that their hypouricemia has been noted to go away in disease remission and recur when the tumor recurs. This pattern has suggested the presence of a humoral or perhaps a nutritional factor. Similar concerns arise with the association with several forms of liver disease.

In addition, acquired hypouricemia may appear in concert with other defects in tubular reabsorption as the Fanconi syndrome which also may occur in malignancies, with drug toxicity, and in other forms of tubular injury (66). The shared vulnerability of multiple reabsorptive systems suggests that they may also share intracellular signaling pathways which, when subjected to specific insult, might then affect the handling of multiple solutes.

EXTRARENAL DISTRIBUTION OF URATE

For the most part, human interstitial fluids, including synovial fluid, are fully equilibrated with plasma. A conspicuous exception occurs when the small urate ions (158 Kd) are largely excluded from the cerebrospinal fluid together with the panoply of other solutes that are denied access by the "blood brain barrier" (67). There the physiologic concentration of urate is approximately 20% of concurrent plasma levels. It is unlikely that this exclusion reflects carrier-mediated outward transport. The cerebral spinal fluid is largely formed in the choroid plexus through water specific channels (primarily aquaporin 4) and cleared by nonselective outflow through lymphatic and other channels (68,69). Thus the urate clearance from plasma into the CSF is greatly exceeded by the outward clearance from cerebral spinal fluid back to plasma, and the balance of these two clearance rates determines the 20% concentration ratio of cerebral spinal fluid to serum.

Perspiration is the one other extracellular fluid from which urate is largely excluded. In contrast, urea is abundant in sweat. The classic "uremic frost" of terminal renal disease is crystalline urea alone. The mechanism of urate exclusion has yet to be established but it is presumed to be passive.

The concentration of urate in intracellular water has not been studied systematically in all tissues of the body. The normal, 70-kg adult carries approximately 25 L of intracellular and 17 L of extracellular fluid. If one takes a serum concentration of 6 mg/dL as the level throughout the latter compartment, this space then contains 1 g of the normal body pool of 1.8 g. The approximately 800 mg remaining must be intracellular, but in which cells? Clearly, the liver (where it is made) and the kidney (where it is extensively transported) must contain substantial intracellular urate. Red blood cells have been studied and clearly contain urate, but the possible modes of ingress and egress have been controversial (especially in Dalmatian dogs). Skeletal muscle may be responsible for large surges of urate production secondary to surges of adenine nucleotide released during exhaustive exercise. The specific conversion from nucleotide to uric acid, however, probably occurs in the liver rather than the muscle cells.

Gastrointestinal Elimination

Turnover studies have found that the average person produces approximately 1200 mg of urate a day and eliminates the same amount to remain in metabolic balance (3). Of this, approximately 800 mg is excreted through the kidney by complex systems as discussed above. The remaining 400 mg are eliminated through the gastrointestinal tract. Four hundred milligrams per day represents the content of more than 7 L of plasma. Uricase in commensal, intestinal bacteria converts the urate to allantoin which is largely reabsorbed and excreted by the kidneys. Thus a substantial degree of uricolysis occurs even though we lack the capacity to do this for ourselves. The fraction of urate removed by intestinal lysis falls with hypouricemia and rises to become the major elimination route in the hyperuricemia of chronic, renal insufficiency. This pattern suggests that intestinal catabolism is a passive reflection of the serum urate concentration rather than specific transport.

Saliva is by far the most accessible and perhaps the most relevant secretion of the gastrointestinal tract. There, the concentration of urate is usually equivalent to that of plasma, and the daily flow of 600 to 1000 mL is insufficient to account for more than a fraction of the urate that is broken down in the gut (70). Saliva is of interest, however, because it is the one site where urate confers measurable benefits (71). Together with ascorbic acid, urate is one of the two scavengers that are thought to mop up the free radicals produced by normal oral flora. As such, it is considered an important factor in the control of tooth decay.

Urate is present in bile but does not seem to be concentrated there (72). The succus entericus and pancreatic fluid are more difficult to sample and do not seem to have been studied. One experiment found significant clearance into a lavaged 50-cm segment of canine gut similar to that in a study with "enterolavage" in humans (73,74). The intestine stands second only to the liver in its content of the urate-generating enzyme xanthine oxidase (75). It remains possible that some urate may escape the local flora, be reabsorbed in the intestine, and return to the circulating pool. In either secretion or reabsorption of urate, it should be clear that this hydrophilic ion is unlikely to diffuse alone through the lipid barriers of cellular membranes. Either active (energy requiring) or passive (facilitated diffusion) mechanisms must be involved, but to date, these systems have not been defined.

Synovial Fluid

Gouty arthritis results when urate crystals precipitate from supersaturated synovial fluid. Thus the intrasynovial kinetics and concentration of urate have been of obvious interest to rheumatologists, although relatively little experimental work has been done. In a study of saline "effusions" in normal knees, the transynovial exchange rate of endogenous urate entering the joint was determined concurrently with the rate at which ^{14}C labeled urate left. The clearance of tritiated water was also studied (and taken as a measure of effective synovial plasma flow) along with exchange rates for a number of other small solutes (76). Taken together, the data indicated that transvascular exchange is driven primarily by bidirectional diffusion between plasma and synovial fluid. The urate data suggested, however, that the process may not be entirely symmetrical. Urate clearance out exceeded that into the joint in 5 of 6 experiments. The mean difference was not significant, but the trend is consistent with modest diffusive ingress limited by protein binding of plasma urate and/or egress augmented by non-diffusive lymphatic efflux from the joint.

These speculations become more interesting when seen in the light of the best available data from 66 synovial effusions, 63 from knees sampled in clinical practice from ambulatory patients (77). The findings from that study were summarized in the following simple tabulation of mean urate concentrations in serum and synovial fluid:

	N	Serum	sf	*p*
"Inflammatory"	29	5.59	5.04	<0.0001
Gout	18	9.57	10.17	0.479
"Noninflammatory"	19	5.81	5.51	0.388

Most of the "inflammatory" fluids were from patients with rheumatoid disease while most of the "noninflammatory" samples were from osteoarthritic individuals. In the inflamed knees, as in the small kinetic trial, the synovial fluid urate may be lower because urate diffuses into the joint more slowly than water while both water and urate are cleared in part by equal, convective, lymphatic efflux. An alternative possibility is that urate is cleaved to allantoin as it scavenges free radicals in these inflamed joints. The anomalous findings of higher synovial fluid urate levels in gouty subjects are plausibly explained by dissolution of synovial tophi in three of their 18 patients, whereas the relative equilibration in the "noninflammatory" fluids is consistent with less lysis of urate and/or reduced lymphatic egress in these more quiet joints.

Two other series of synovial samples are particularly noteworthy. In the knees of 21 resting, hospitalized patients with no articular disease, evidence of full equilibration between plasma and synovial fluid was found (78). Comparable equilibration was also observed in the knees of 52 non-gouty persons which were aspirated post-mortem (79). These investigators found similar parity between plasma and synovial fluid samples taken from the ankles and first metatarsophalangeal joints of the same bodies. Thus, these findings stand against the possibility of sustained, relative hyperuricemia in these more gout-prone joints. Intriguingly, however, 12 individuals had higher urate levels in the first metatarsophalangeal joint than in concurrent plasma or in the synovial fluid of any other joint that was sampled.

Each of the series reviewed above was conducted in individuals whose joints were most probably at equilibrium at the time of aspiration. It remains possible, however, that transient, activity-related fluctuations in intra-articular urate may play a significant role in the pathophysiology of gouty synovitis (80,81). This hypothesis begins with the observation that the first metatarsophalangeal joint, the "target joint" of so much gouty arthritis, is also the bunion joint. As such, it has more radiographic evidence of osteoarthritis than does any other weight-bearing joint. Here then, as in the interphalangeal osteoarthritis of postmenopausal women, gout appears to have a clear predilection for peripheral (colder), osteoarthritic joints. Secondly, gouty arthritis is often brought on by excessive or unusual use of these joints. When this occurs the disease flares not during the period of overuse but during the early hours of the following morning. This classical constellation of events may be related to the fact that urate moves more slowly between synovial fluid and plasma than does water (the relative rate was $49 \pm 1\%$ in 51 normal human knees) (80). When the osteoarthritic joint is used (or abused), an effusion

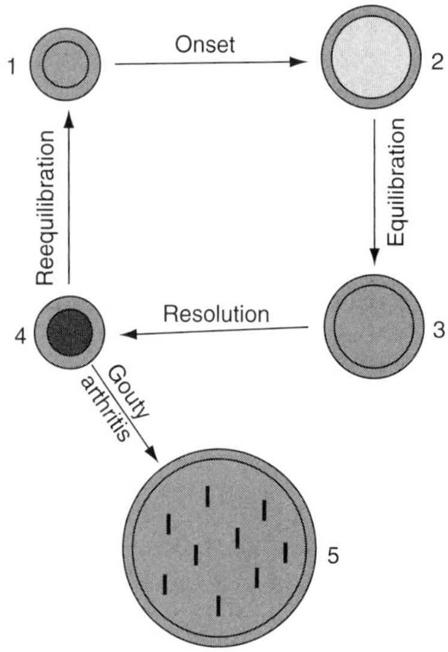

Figure 8 Effect of synovial permeability on intrasynovial urate. Urate concentration in the plasma (*outer ring*) and in the joint (*inner circle*) is represented by intensity of shading. At rest (1), the concentrations are the same. During the onset of an effusion (2), water enters the joint space more rapidly than urate, thus transiently lowering the intrasynovial urate concentration. As the effusion persists (3), reequilibration of the two spaces will occur. During resolution of effusion (4), water will leave more rapidly than urate and the intrasynovial concentration of urate will therefore exceed that of the plasma. At this point, crystals may precipitate and induce gouty arthritis (5) or reequilibration may occur with a return to the original conditions (1). *Source*: From Ref. 81.

may develop. During this period of enlargement the synovial fluid urate level will be less than that in perfusing plasma, because water enters faster. As joint use continues, the fluids will equilibrate and the total urate within the joint will parallel the effusion volume. When the joint is put to rest at night, water will leave more rapidly, the effusion will resolve, and the synovial fluid urate level will exceed that in any other interstitial compartment. If this passive process leads to supersaturation, crystals may precipitate with ensuing gouty arthritis (Fig. 8).

REFERENCES

1. Sorensen LB. The elimination of uric acid in man. Scand J Clin Lab Invest 1960; 12:1–214.
2. Scott JT, Holloway VP, Glass HI, Arnot RN. Studies of uric acid pool size and turnover rate. Ann Rheum Dis 1969; 28:366–373.
3. Sorensen LB. Role of the intestinal tract in the elimination of uric acid. Arthritis Rheum 1965; 8:694–706.
4. Benos DJ. Introduction to medical physiology: cellular membranes and transmembrane transport of solutes and water. Am J Physiol 1996; 271:S2–S9.
5. Rafey MA, Lipkowitz MS, Leal-Pinto E, Abramson RG. Uric acid transport. Curr Opin Nephrol Hypertens 2003; 12:511–516.
6. Bieber JD, Terkeltaub RA. Gout: on the brink of novel therapeutic options for an ancient disease. Arthritis Rheum 2004; 50:2400–2414.
7. Sica DA, Schoolwerth AC. Renal handling of organic anions and cations: excretion of uric acid. In: Brenner BM, Rector FC, eds. Brenner and Rector's the Kidney. Philadelphia: Saunders, 2004:644–662.
8. Enomoto A, Kimura H, Chairoungdua A, et al. Molecular identification of a renal urate anion exchanger that regulates blood urate levels. Nature 2002; 417:447–452.
9. Guggino SE, Martin GJ, Aronson PS. Specificity and modes of the anion exchanger in dog renal microvillus membranes. Am J Physiol 1983; 244:F612–F621.
10. Yu TF, Gutman AB. Paradoxical retention of uric acid by uricosuric drugs in low dosage. Proc Soc Exp Biol Med 1955; 90:542–547.
11. Fanelli GM, Jr. Uricosuric agents. Arthritis Rheum 1975; 18:853–858.
12. Cunningham RF, Israili ZH, Dayton PG. Clinical pharmacokinetics of probenecid. Clin Pharmacokinet 1981; 6:135–151.
13. Ichida K, Hosoyamada M, Kimura H, et al. Urate transport via human PAH transporter hOAT1 and its gene structure. Kidney Int 2003; 63:143–155.
14. Yu TF, Perel J, Berger L, et al. The effect of the interaction of pyrazinamide and probenecid on urinary uric acid excretion in man. Am J Med 1977; 63:723–728.
15. Roch-Ramel F, Guisan B. Renal transport of urate in humans. News Physiol Sci 1999; 14:80–84.
16. Meisel AD, Diamond HS. Inhibition of probenecid uricosuria by pyrazinamide and para-aminohippurate. Am J Physiol 1977; 232:F222–F226.
17. Kamilli I, Gresser U, Pellkofer T, et al. Uricosuric effect of irtemazole in hyperuricemic patients without and with renal insufficiency. J Rheumatol 1989; 48:307–312.
18. Hasannejad H, Takeda M, Taki K, et al. Interactions of human organic anion transporters with diuretics. J Pharmacol Exp Ther 2004; 308:1021–1029.

19. Guerrini VH, Filippich LJ, English PB, et al. Pharmacokinetics of cefotaxime and probenecid in sheep with normal and reduced renal function. J Vet Pharmacol Ther 1984; 7:283–291.
20. Sakurai Y, Motohashi H, Ueo H, et al. Expression levels of renal organic anion transporters (OATs) and their correlation with anionic drug excretion in patients with renal diseases. Pharm Res 2004; 21:61–67.
21. Leal-Pinto E, Cohen BE, Lipkowitz MS, Abramson RG. Functional analysis and molecular model of the human urate transporter/channel, hUAT. Am J Physiol Renal Physiol 2002; 283:F150–F163.
22. Koepsell H, Endou H. The SLC22 drug transporter family. Pflugers Arch 2004; 447:666–676.
23. Kay BK, Kehoe JW. PDZ domains and their ligands. Chem Biol 2004; 11:423–425.
24. Brone B, Eggermont J. PDZ proteins retain and regulate membrane transporters in polarized epithelial cell membranes. Am J Physiol Cell Physiol 2005; 288:C20–C29.
25. Gibson HV, Doisy EA. A note on the effect of some organic acids upon the uric acid excretion of man. J Biol Chem 1923; 55:605–610.
26. Quinones Galvan A, Natali A, Baldi S, et al. Effect of insulin on uric acid excretion in humans. Am J Physiol 1995; 268:E1–E5.
27. Johnson RJ, Kivlighn SD, Kim YG, et al. Reappraisal of the pathogenesis and consequences of hyperuricemia in hypertension, cardiovascular disease, and renal disease. Am J Kidney Dis 1999; 33:225–234.
28. Steele TH. Pyrazinamide suppressibility of urate excretion in health and disease: Relationship to urate filtration. In: Silbernagl S, Lang F, Greger R, Stuttgart GT, eds. Amino Acid Transport and Uric Acid Transport, 1976:248.
29. Steele TH. Urate secretion in man: the pyrazinamide suppression test. Ann Intern Med 1973; 79:734–737.
30. Berliner RW, Hilton JG, Yu TF, Kennedy TJ. The renal mechanism for urate excretion in man. J Clin Invest 1950; 29:396–401.
31. Fontenaille C, Guiheneuc P, Heron B, et al. Renal excretion of urate in normal and gouty subjects at high, normal and low plasma urate levels. Biomedicine 1974; 21:382–385.
32. Cheson BD, Dutcher BS. Managing malignancy-associated hyperuricemia with rasburicase. J Support Oncol 2005; 3:117–124.
33. Yeun JY, Hasbargen JA. Renal hypouricemia: prevention of exercise-induced acute renal failure and a review of the literature. Am J Kidney Dis 1995; 25:937–946.
34. Anton FM, Garcia Puig J, Ramos T, et al. Sex differences in uric acid metabolism in adults: evidence for a lack of influence of estradiol-17 beta (E2) on the renal handling of urate. Metabolism 1986; 35:343–348.
35. Hosoyamada M, Ichida K, Enomoto A, et al. Function and localization of urate transporter 1 in mouse kidney. J Am Soc Nephrol 2004; 15:261–268.
36. Simmonds HA, McBride MB, Hatfield PJ, et al. Polynesian women are also at risk for hyperuricaemia and gout because of a genetic defect in renal urate handling. Br J Rheumatol 1994; 33:932–937.
37. Emmerson BT. Hyperuricemia, Gout, and the kidney. In: Schrier RW, ed. Disease of the Kidney and the Urinary Tract. Philadelphia: Lippincott, Williams and Wilkins, 2001:2255–2279.
38. Perez-Ruiz F, Nolla JM. Usefulness of Simkin's Index and the Cockroft-Gault equation to classify patients with gout using spot blood and urine samples. Arthritis Rheum 2003; 48:S533.

39. Engle JE, Steele TH. Variation of urate excretion with urine flow in normal man. Nephron 1976; 16:50–56.
40. Diamond HS, Lazarus R, Kaplan D, Halberstam D. Effect of urine flow rate on uric acid excretion in man. Arthritis Rheum 1972; 15:338–346.
41. Skeith MD, Healey LA, Cutler RE. Urate excretion during mannitol and glucose diuresis. J Lab Clin Med 1967; 70:213–220.
42. Rizos E, Liamis G, Elisaf M. Multiple metabolic abnormalities in a patient with the syndrome of inappropriate antidiuresis. Nephron 2002; 91:339–340.
43. Marangella M. Uric acid elimination in the urine. Pathophysiological implications. Contrib Nephrol 2005; 147:132–148.
44. Pak CY, Peterson R, Poindexter JR. Adequacy of a single stone risk analysis in the medical evaluation of urolithiasis. J Urol 2001; 165:378–381.
45. Ricos C, Jimenez CV, Hernandez A, et al. Biological variation in urine samples used for analyte measurements. Clin Chem 1994; 40:472–477.
46. Simkin PA. Uric acid excretion in patients with gout. Arthritis Rheum 1979; 22:98–99.
47. Perez-Ruiz F, Calabozo M, Erauskin GG, et al. Renal underexcretion of uric acid is present in patients with apparent high urinary uric acid output. Arthritis Rheum 2002; 47:610–613.
48. Simkin PA. New standards for uric acid excretion and evidence for an inducible transporter. Arthritis Rheum 2003; 49:375–376.
49. Anzai N, Miyazaki H, Noshiro R, et al. The multivalent PDZ domain-containing protein PDZK1 regulates transport activity of renal urate-anion exchanger URAT1 via its C terminus. J Biol Chem 2004; 279:45942–45950.
50. Praetorius E, Kirk JE. Hypouricemia: with evidence for tubular elimination of uric acid. J Lab Clin Med 1950; 35:865–868.
51. Khachadurian AK, Arslanian MJ. Hypouricemia due to renal uricosuria. A case study. Ann Intern Med 1973; 78:547–550.
52. Simkin PA, Skeith MD, Healey LA. Suppression of uric acid secretion in a patient with renal hypouricemia. Adv Exp Med Biol 1974; 41:723–728.
53. Tiselius HG, Larsson L. Urinary excretion of urate in patients with calcium oxalate stone disease. Urol Res 1983; 11:279–283.
54. Sperling O. Renal hypouricemia: classification, tubular defect and clinical consequences. Contrib Nephrol 1992; 100:1–14.
55. Gaspar GA, Puig JG, Mateos FA, et al. Hypouricemia due to renal urate wasting: different types of tubular transport defects. Adv Exp Med Biol 1986; 195:357–363.
56. Ichida K, Hosoyamada M, Hisatome I, et al. Clinical and molecular analysis of patients with renal hypouricemia in Japan-influence of URAT1 gene on urinary urate excretion. J Am Soc Nephrol 2004; 15:164–173.
57. Komoda F, Sekine T, Inatomi J, et al. The W258X mutation in SLC22A12 is the predominant cause of Japanese renal hypouricemia. Pediatr Nephrol 2004; 19:728–733.
58. Simkin PA. The Dalmatians defect: a hepatic endocrinopathy of urate transport. Arthritis Rheum 2005; 52: 2257–2262.
59. Appleman RM, Hallenbeck GA, Shorter RG. Effect of reciprocal allogeneic renal transplantation between Dalmatian and non-dalmatian dogs on urinary excretion of uric acid. Proc Soc Exp Biol Med 1966; 121:1094–1097.

60. Kuster G, Shorter RG, Dawson B, Hallenbeck GA. Uric acid metabolism in dalmatians and other dogs. Role of the liver. Arch Intern Med 1972; 129:492–496.
61. Weiner IM. Urate transport in the nephron. Am J Physiol 1979; 237:F85–F92.
62. Roch-Ramel F, Peters G. Urinary excretion of uric acid in nonhuman mammalian species. In: Kelley WNW IW, ed. In: Uric Acid. Springer-Verlag: New York, 1978:211–255.
63. Bairaktari ET, Kakafika AI, Pritsivelis N, et al. Hypouricemia in individuals admitted to an inpatient hospital-based facility. Am J Kidney Dis 2003; 41:1225–1232.
64. Ramsdell CM, Kelley WN. The clinical significance of hypouricemia. Ann Intern Med 1973; 78:239–242.
65. Michelis MF, Warms PC, Fusco RD, Davis BB. Hypouricemia and hyperuricosuria in Laennec cirrhosis. Arch Intern Med 1974; 134:681–683.
66. Izzedine H, Launay-Vacher V, Isnard-Bagnis C, Deray G. Drug-induced Fanconi's syndrome. Am J Kidney Dis 2003; 41:292–309.
67. Alho H, Leinonen JS, Erhola M, et al. Asay of antioxidant capacity of human plasma and CSF in aging and disease. Restor Neurol Neurosci 1998; 12:159–165.
68. Speake T, Freeman LJ, Brown PD. Expression of aquaporin 1 and aquaporin 4 water channels in rat choroid plexus. Biochim Biophys Acta 2003; 1609:80–86.
69. Edsbagge M, Tisell M, Jacobsson L, Wikkelso C. Spinal CSF absorption in healthy individuals. Am J Physiol Regul Integr Comp Physiol 2004; 287:R1450–R1455.
70. Sculley DV, Langley-Evans SC. Periodontal disease is associated with lower antioxidant capacity in whole saliva and evidence of increased protein oxidation. Clin Sci (Lond) 2003; 105:167–172.
71. Diab-Ladki R, Pellat B, Chahine R. Decrease in the total antioxidant activity of saliva in patients with periodontal diseases. Clin Oral Investig 2003; 7:103–107.
72. Kountouras J, Magoula I, Tsapas G, Liatsis I. The effect of mannitol and secretin on the biliary transport of urate in humans. Hepatology 1996; 23:229–233.
73. Knapowski J, Adam W, Arasimowicz C, Weiss K. Intestinal excretion of uric acid in dogs. Acta Med Pol 1963; 29:201–207.
74. Kelley RA, Hill LD. Acute renal insufficiency and the role of potassium with treatment by intestinal lavage. J Urol 1951; 66:645–660.
75. Qu XW, Rozenfeld RA, Huang W, et al. The role of xanthine oxidase in platelet activating factor induced intestinal injury in the rat. Gut 1999; 44:203–211.
76. Simkin PA, Pizzorno JE. Transynovial exchange of small molecules in normal human subjects. J Appl Physiol 1974; 36:581–587.
77. Beutler AM, Keenan GF, Soloway S, et al. Soluble urate in sera and synovial fluids from patients with different joint disorders. Clin Exp Rheumatol 1996; 14:249–254.
78. Weinberger A, Wysenbeck A, Agam G, et al. Synovial fluid urate concentration in normouricemic and hyperuricemic subjects without joint diseases. Clin Chim Acta 1981; 111:279–280.
79. Culora G, Gallagher PJ. Gouty arthropathy and synovial uric acid. Br J Rheumatol 1992; 31:791–792.
80. Simkin PA. The pathogenesis of podagra. Ann Intern Med 1977; 86:230–233.
81. Simkin PA. Role of local factors in the precipitation of urate crystals. In: Kelley WN, Weiner IM, eds. Uric Acid. Springer-Verlag: New York, 1978:379–395.

17

Biological Effects of Calcium-Containing Crystals

Herman S. Cheung
Department of Biomedical Engineering, University of Miami and Miami VA Medical Center, Miami, Florida, U.S.A.

INTRODUCTION

Crystalline calcium pyrophosphate dihydrate (CPPD) and basic calcium phosphate (BCP) are the two most common forms of pathologic articular mineral found in articular tissues. Each occurs frequently in patients with osteoarthritis, and each may be phlogistic, causing acute attacks of pseudogout in the case of CPPD crystals and acute calcific periarthritis in the case of BCP crystals (1–3).

Evidence for a causal role of crystals in cartilage degeneration is primarily inferential, based on correlative data. However, clinical observations and experimental evidence of their in vitro effects support the thesis that articular crystals promote cartilage degeneration. More definitive investigations of causality are impeded by the lack of a suitable animal model for studying non-inflammatory aspects of crystal deposition, and the slow pace of degeneration (1,4).

At concentrations found in pathologic human joint fluids, CPPD and BCP crystals exert biological effects on cultured cells in a manner similar to growth factors like platelet-derived growth factor (PDGF), epidermal growth factor (EGF), and serum. It has been demonstrated that both crystals stimulate fibroblast, synoviocyte, and chondrocyte mitogenesis in vitro, stimulate the production of prostaglandin (PGE_2) via the phospholipase A_2/cyclo-oxygenase (COX) pathway, activate phospholipase C and inositol phospholipid hydrolysis, induce the expression of the proto-oncogenes c-fos and c-myc, induce the synthesis and secretion of matrix metalloproteinases (MMPs) 1, 3, 8, 9, and 13, and down-regulate tissue inhibitors of metalloproteinase (TIMP) (1,4–12). In contrast to other mitogenic and growth factors, BCP crystal-elicited signal transduction pathways have not been completely studied. However, some of the component molecules involved in calcium-containing crystal signal transduction mechanisms have now been identified.

CLINICAL ASSOCIATION OF CALCIUM-CONTAINING CRYSTALS AND OSTEOARTHRITIS

Correlative data indicate that CPPD and BCP crystals are more common in degenerative joints than in normal joints or joints affected with inflammatory forms of arthritis. In addition, osteoarthritis is both more common and more severe in patients with calcium-containing crystals. One or both crystals are present in up to 60% of fluid from knees of patients with advanced osteoarthritis (13–16). The presence of CPPD crystals predicts a poor clinical and radiographic outcome (17). Similarly a prospective study of radiographic chondrocalcinosis in Slovakian kindred with autosomal dominant CPPD deposition demonstrated that radiographic evidence of crystal deposition antedated radiographic evidence of degeneration (16). Although there is no satisfactory animal model of crystal deposition disease, there are useful models of osteoarthritis. In the two studies of the anterior cruciate injury model, BCP crystals have been detected early, at a time when they might contribute to ongoing cartilage damage (15,18).

Studies of synovial fluid containing CPPD crystals suggest associated chondrolytic activity in the involved joints, usually of a greater magnitude than seen in fluids from patients with osteoarthritis but no crystals. Patients with acute "pyrophosphate arthropathy" (CPPD in joint fluids and osteoarthritis) had the highest synovial fluid proteoglycan fragment concentrations of six disease categories evaluated (15,19–21). Moreover, these CPPD-containing fluids also had the highest levels of MMP-1, MMP-3, and the highest ratio of MMP-3 to TIMP, all factors, which would support increased matrix catabolism (21). Although these studies do not prove a causative role of the crystals in osteoarthritis, they strongly support an association of accelerated matrix degradation with the presence of calcium-containing crystals.

BIOLOGIC EFFECTS OF CALCIUM-CONTAINING CRYSTALS

Perhaps the most compelling argument favoring a causative role for crystals in osteoarthritis stems from their in vitro effects on articular tissues. Crystals can cause the degeneration of articular tissues in three separate pathways. First, in the "direct" pathway, crystals induce fibroblast-like synoviocytes to proliferate and produce metalloproteinases and prostaglandins (PGE2). Second, the "paracrine pathway" centers on the interaction between crystals and macrophages/monocytes which leads to synthesis and release of cytokines which can reinforce the action of crystals on synoviocytes and/or induce chondrocytes to secrete enzymes and which eventually cause the degeneration of articular tissues (1). Finally, the "biomechanical" pathway involves structural changes in joints resulting from articular calcification. These can lead to altered loading of the joint causing injury to the cartilage matrix. The injured cartilage matrix then may fail under normal loading. Chondrocytes respond to this by elaborating MMPs and altered attempts at repair (22).

Direct Pathway

Much of the research was stimulated by recognition of the Milwaukee shoulder syndrome as a paradigm for non-inflammatory yet destructive arthritis associated with synovial fluid BCP crystals and active proteases (23,24). Subsequent studies revealed that both BCP and CPPD crystals could elicit mitogenesis, synthesis, and secretion of proteases, and synthesis and secretion of PGE2 by articular tissues (1).

Crystal-Induced Mitogenesis

Synovial lining proliferation is observed in crystal-associated arthritis, and the crystals themselves induce mitogenesis in this tissue (23,25,26). The increased cellularity of the synovium in turn enhances the capacity for cytokine and protease secretion, both of which can promote chondrolysis.

A variety of calcium-containing crystals stimulate (^{3}H)-thymidine incorporation into phagocytic cells, whereas other crystals have weak or no mitogenic properties (25,27). Particularly well studied has been the mitogenic response to BCP crystals. At concentrations routinely observed in pathologic joint fluids, these crystals are endocytosed and then are solubilized in the acidic environment of the phagolysosome. Mitogenesis induced by these crystals can be inhibited by preventing endocytosis or by raising lysosomal pH. The latter effect can be produced by lysosomotropic agents NH_4Cl or chloroquine or by the specific vacuolar ATPase inhibitor, bafilomycin (28,29). Cells that are exposed to such inhibitors remain responsive to other mitogenic stimuli (i.e., serum).

Calcium-containing crystals also induce mitogenesis through diacylglycerol, a hydrolysis product of phospholipase C action on phosphatidylinositol 4,5-bisphosphate. Elevated phospholipase C activity and diacylglycerol accumulation are observed in cells exposed to BCP crystals, a response similar to that observed when cells are stimulated with PDGF (9,30). A downstream effector of diacylglycerol-induced mitogenesis may be protein kinase C (PKC), since down-regulation of that activity inhibits the mitogenic response to crystals (9,31–33).

Proto-oncogenes are important in the control of cell proliferation. BCP crystals induce c-fos and c-myc expression in fibroblasts (9,31). Transcription of c-fos begins within minutes and peaks at 30 minutes after stimulation with BCP.

Messenger RNA for c-myc accumulates within 1 hour with maximal levels at 3 hours. In PKC down-regulated cells, there is an attenuated proto-oncogene response to BCP, reinforcing the importance of PKC in regulating BCP-induced biologic responses.

Members of the extra cellular signal-regulate kinase (ERK) family of Ser/Thr kinases are key regulators of a variety of signal transduction cascades and play a central role in cellular responses to many environmental agents. One of the ERK family is termed p42/p44 MAPK. To explore the link of activation of PKC and p42/44 MAPK in crystal induction of MMP, fibroblasts have been treated with the C inhibitors staurosporine or Bis-I. These inhibitors suppress BCP crystal-induced MMP-1 and -3 transcripts and protein expression in a dose-dependent fashion (34). Crystal-induced PKC activation requires an influx of extracellular calcium (Ca^{2+}), as crystal stimulation in a Ca^{2+}-free environment inhibits PKC translocation. PKC-α is the only Ca^{2+}-dependent isozyme activated. A preferential inhibitor of Ca^{2+}-dependent PKC isozymes, Gö 6976, is most effective at blocking crystal-induced PKC translocation and MMP-1 expression. Crystal-induced activation of p44/42 MAPK is independent of PKC-α because the PKC inhibitors, Bis I and Gö6976, exert no effect on p44/42 MAPK, and conversely, the p44/42 MAPK inhibitors, PD098058 and U0126, have no effect on PKC. Therefore, crystal stimulation of MMP-1 and MMP-3 mRNA and protein expressions are dependent upon the Ca^{2+}-dependent PKC signal transduction pathway, and the PKC-α isozyme is specifically involved in the pathway (33).

However, the possibility that another PKC isozyme that is not sensitive to the Ca^{2+}-dependent PKC inhibitors might be required for the crystal-induced activation of the p44/42 signal transduction pathway can not be ruled out (32). Evaluation of the PKC isozymes from all the PKC sub-families shows that only PKC-α and PKC-μ are expressed in human fibroblasts. The fact that PKC-α is Ca^{2+}-dependent and PKC-μ is Ca^{2+}-independent, and that they belong to two different PKC sub-families, suggests differential roles for these isozymes in crystal-induced cell activation (35). Inhibition of PKC-μ synthesis and activity by antisense oligodeoxynucleotides and H-89, respectively, results in the inhibition of p44/42 MAPK activation, thus demonstrating that p44/42 MAPK activity is dependent upon PKC-μ. Inhibition of PKC-μ also results in the inhibition of MMP-1 and MMP-3 mRNA and protein expression as a result of p44/42 MAPK inhibition (32).

These data lead to the hypothesis that BCP crystals activate cells via two independent pathways. One pathway is the Ca^{2+}-dependent PKC pathway characterized by PKC-α and modulated by mobilized intracellular Ca^{2+} generated by the sequential hydrolysis of PLC-PIP_2-IP_3 (36–39), by transient opening of the Ca^{2+} channel, and by crystal endocytosis and dissolution (2,28,40,41). The mobilized Ca^{2+} in the cytosol then modifies the activation of PKC-α by diacylglycerol and induces its translocation to the plasma membrane where it becomes physiologically active (42). Some of the mobilized Ca^{2+}

diffuses through the nuclear pores into the nucleus where it enhances the crystal induction of c-fos mRNA (43–45). It has been shown that PKC isozymes can either act in the cytoplasm and cause nuclear effects indirectly by triggering signaling pathways directed towards the cell nucleus or PKC itself can act in the cell nucleus (46).

The other pathway is the Ca^{2+}-independent p44/42 MAPK pathway, which is mediated by the Ca^{2+}-independent PKC-μ. Crystals activate the sequential hydrolysis of PLC-PIP_2 producing diacylglycerol which activates PKC-μ which, in turn, activates p44/42 MAPK generated from the Ras-Raf-MEK-P44/42 MAPK signaling cascade (33,34,47). The activated and phosphorylated p44/42 MAPK then migrates to the nucleus to mediate crystal-induced cellular responses. It appears that these two pathways, although independent, complement each other for the efficient regulation of cellular responses to crystal stimulation (Fig. 1).

Crystal-Induced MMP Synthesis

The original and subsequent reports of Milwaukee shoulder syndrome indicated the presence of active neutral protease and collagenase in synovial fluids from affected individuals (23,24). Such proteases were felt to explain the profound rotator cuff and cartilage destruction observed. Due to the consistent finding of BCP crystals in all and the coexistence of CPPD crystals in half of these joint fluids, it was postulated that these particulates might induce protease secretion by

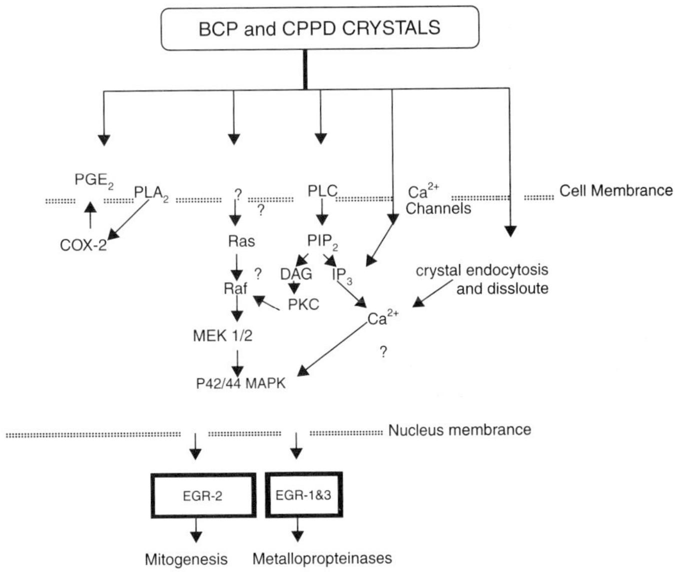

Figure 1 In vitro biologic effect of basic calcium phosphate (BCP) and calcium pyrophosphate dihydrate (CPPD) crystals.

synovial lining cells. When natural and synthetic BCP and CPPD crystals are incubated with human and canine synovial cells in culture, neutral protease and collagenase activities can be identified in the media after 8 hours and peak levels measured at 24 hours (48).

Other studies have confirmed that both BCP and CPPD crystal induce the synthesis of MMP-1, -3, -8, -9 and -13 in cultured cells (10–12,49). Furthermore, it has been observed that although BCP crystal upregulate expression and synthesis of MMP, the crystals also downregulate TIMP significantly (10). Since the in vivo degradative effect of MMPs is dependent on the presence of TIMP, this would explain the earlier observation that the CPPD-containing fluids have the highest levels of MMP-1, MMP-3, and the highest ratio of MMP-3 to TIMP, and support the thesis that crystals increase matrix catabolism (21).

Transcriptional regulation of MMPs is dependent upon multiple DNA binding elements located in their promoters. The promoters of the MMP-1 and MMP-3 genes contain a previously mentioned binding site for AP-1 known as the TRE, named for its ability to mediate induction of transcription in response to TPA and other PKC activating agents (50,51). Transcriptional activation of MMP genes by growth factors and cytokines is preceded by a rapid transient increase in AP-1 protein expression (40,41). It has been determined that an AP-1 site is located in the promoters of all the MMPs except for MMP-2, whereas MMP-1 and MMP-3 each have a second AP-1 site.

Transfections with hMMP1 luciferase reporter plasmids in synoviocytes reveals that the induction of hMMP1 promoter by BCP crystals is mainly mediated through the -72AP-1 element. Elimination of the -72AP-1 element either by mutation or deletion almost completely abolishes the induction of hMMP1 promoter activity by BCP crystals. Interestingly, a mutation at the -88PEA-3 site also abolishes the induction of hMMP1 promoter. Further mutation at the -181AP-1 site resumes the induction indicating that the -181AP-1 element has an effect opposite to the -72AP-1 element. The effect of -181AP-1 can be inactivated either by a mutation at this -181AP-1 site or by the -88PEA-3 element. In addition, dominant-negative Ras, Raf, and MEK1/2 can block the induction of hMMP1, and a MEK1/2 specific inhibitor (UO126) can block the induction of hMMP1 and c-fos by BCP crystals (52). Treatment of fibroblasts with crystals results in the activation of both AP-1 and NFκB (8). These data indicate that multiple elements, including at least AP-1 and PEA-3, are involved in the induction of the hMMP1 gene expression by BCP crystals and that the induction follows the Ras/MAPK/c-fos/AP-1/MMP1 signaling pathway (51).

Crystal Activation of Early Growth Response Genes

Early Growth Response (EGR) genes were identified originally based on their rapid induction of gene expression in quiescent fibroblasts stimulated by serum (52). While the amino acid sequences of four family members are distinct, they all interact with the Sp1-type of DNA target element. EGR protein alters gene transcription through mechanisms dependent on both co-activators and co-repressors. Transcriptional co-activators such as CREB-binding protein (CBP) and p300 can interact directly with the activation domain of EGR1 and increase its trans-activating activity (53). EGR proteins serve as sensors of extracellular signaling pathways that play key roles in regulating cell proliferation, differentiation, and function. BCP crystals can induce the message levels of EGR-1 and -3 that peak at about one hour. In contrast, the message levels of EGR-2 increase steadily and peak at 24 hours after BCP crystals stimulation. This induction is dependent on the crystal concentration and can be abolished by either phosphocitrate, p44/42 MAPK inhibitor U0126, or calcium chelators EGTA and TMB-8, but not by SAPK2/p38 and the PKC inhibitor Bis-I. The induction of Egr2 expression significantly enhances the binding of transcription factors such as c-fos, SRF, and c-myc to enhancer elements and activates the p44/42 MAPK signaling pathway. Thus, crystals induce Egr-2 transcription through a PKC-α-independent p44/42 MAPK pathway, and that induction of Egr2 may subsequently activate genes regulated by SRF, c-myc, and c-fos, which may play key roles in regulating fibroblast proliferation (54). Preliminary data exist that suggest that the activation EGR-1 and EGR-3 leads to the induction of MMPs, while activation of EGR-2 results in cell proliferation. This suggests there is differential regulation of crystal induction of MMP synthesis and mitogenesis by these early responding genes (Fig. 2).

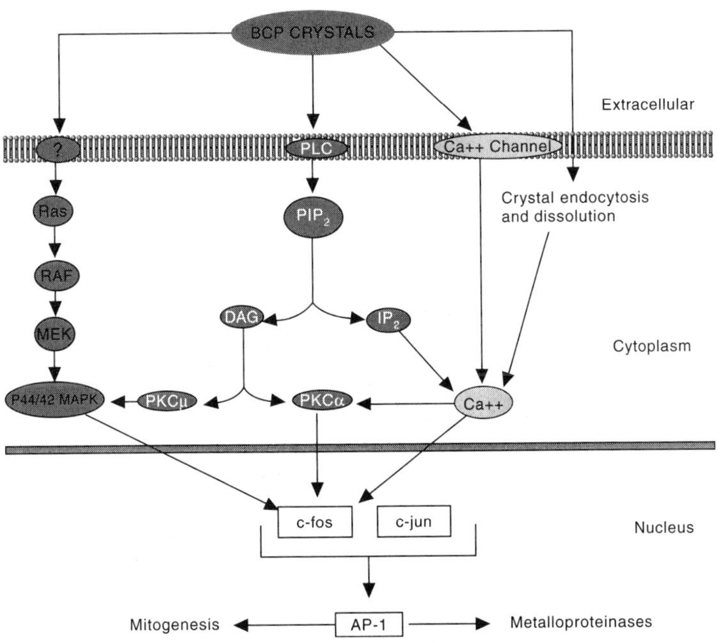

Figure 2 Mechanism of crystal-induced cell activation.

Indirect Pathway

Both BCP and CPPD crystals exert a number of biologic responses that may injure articular structures. Crystals provoke prostaglandin generation, especially PGE2 (5,6,55). Phosphatidylcholine and phosphatidylethanolamine are the major sources of arachidonic acid for PGE2 synthesis, confirming that the phospholipase A2/cyclooxygenase pathway is the predominant route for PGE2 production (56). BCP crystals upregulate COX enzymes (in particular COX-2), which in turn induce production of PGE2 and expression of IL-β in fibroblasts. This suggests that BCP crystals might amplify of the PGE2 production through the induction of the COX enzymes and the pro-inflammatory cytokine IL-1β (6).

TGF-β is present in synovial fluids from patient with various arthritic conditions (10). Recently, synovial fluids from patients with CPPD deposits have significantly higher levels of TGF-β than those in fluids from patients with osteoarthritis or rheumatoid arthritis (57). TGF-β is a stimulator of inorganic pyrophosphate extrusion from chondrocytes (58). Therefore TGF-β can potentially promote new CPPD crystal formation.

Neutrophils play an important role during acute episodes of pseudogout and likely BCP-induced periarthritis as well. Indeed, neutrophils were found attached to superficial deposits of CPPD crystals in three cartilage specimens from patients with pseudogout (59). The adjacent matrix was eroded. Mechanisms of matrix damage during acute episodes of crystal-induced arthritis include release of leukotrienes, lysosomal proteases, chemotactic factors, fibronectin fragments, and active oxygen species. These mechanisms are probably not prominent in non-inflammatory arthritis associated calcium-containing crystals. CPPD and BCP crystals are known to induce the release of IL-6 and, to a lesser extent, IL-1β by synovial cells (60).

Both CPPD and BCP crystals can be phlogistic and membranolytic. To date, however, the molecular mechanism of crystal-induced membranolysis is unclear. The molecular dynamics of the interactions between crystal and the phospholipid bilayer have been studied (61). These interactions between the surface of CPPD and the extracellular layer of the hydrated dimyristoyl phosphatidylcholine phospholipid bilayer may lead to decoupling of the external layer from the intracellular side of the membrane. In turn, a local thinning of the layer on the intracellular side of the membrane occurs, which leads to membranolysis. This favors water penetration that leads to membranolysis. The (010) crystal surface of CPPD is responsible for the interaction with the phospholipid bilayer that leads to crystal-induced membranolysis This process is very similar to the lysis induced by melittin in bee and snake venom (61). Curiously, when the [010] CPPD crystal surface binds to an anti-calcification agent such as phosphocitrate, crystal growth is retarded or ceases (62).

BCP crystals also stimulate the endocytotic activity of cells. Since calcium-containing crystals are associated with many different macromolecules including DNA fragments andcytokines, these particulate may be endocytosed together with crystals disturbing the homeostasis of normal molecular signaling. This finding could be important for our understanding of the potential pathological role of crystals in crystal arthropathy (63).

MECHANISMS OF CRYSTAL-INDUCED CELL ACTIVATION

Role of Calcium (Ca^{2+}) Influx

Treatment of human fibroblasts with BCP crystals induces a rapid transient rise of intracellular Ca^{2+} levels within seconds followed by a slow, sustained increase within 60 minutes after stimulation. Experiments involving crystal stimulation of cells in Ca^{2+}-free media and pretreatment of cells to prevent intracellular crystal dissolution suggest that the initial transient rise in intracellular Ca^{2+} is due to Ca^{2+} influx from outside the cell, whereas the second sustained rise is due to crystal dissolution (45).

One possible result of the influx of Ca^{2+} from outside to inside the cell is the activation of the protein kinase Pyk2, followed by signaling through the Ras cascade to induce p42/44 MAPK pathway (38,39,64,65). Another possibility is that the rise in intracellular Ca^{2+} that occurs upon crystal treatment of cells is responsible for the activation of cAMP response element binding protein (CREB), a key transcriptional regulator of the c-fos gene that is important for mediating c-fos activation in response to elevated levels of intracellular calcium (66,67). CREB binds to the CRE element in the c-fos promoter, a DNA binding site with similarity to the TPA response element (TRE) AP-1 binding site (68).

Role of p42 and p44 Mitogen-Activated Protein (MAP) Kinase Pathway

Three distinct ERK-dependent signaling cascades have been identified in mammalian cells, all playing an important role in signal transduction cascades. They can be distinguished based on the particular ERK members activated: p42/p44 MAPKs (ERK2/ERK1), p38 MAPK, or p46/p54 SAPK/JNKs. p38 MAPK and the SAPK/JNKs mediate signals in response to cytokines and environmental stress. The p42/p44 MAPK pathway was the first identified and is the best understood ERK-based signaling pathway (64,65). This pathway is required for extracellular stimulation of growth and Ras transformation of cells. The p42/p44 MAPKs are believed to regulate proliferation by a mechanism that involves activation of genes associated with cell proliferation, including primary response genes such as c-fos and c-jun.

BCP and CPPD crystals, activate MAPK p42–p44 but not p38 protein kinase cascade pathway (48). Both crystals also cause phosphorylation of the nuclear transcription factor CREB. This occurs on serine 133, a residue essential for CREB's ability to transactivate. Treatment of cells with PD98059, an inhibitor of MEK1, an upstream activator of MAPKs, U0126 (a novel inhibitor of

MEK1 and MEK2), or phosphocitrate significantly inhibited the crystal-activation of p42/p44 MAP kinases, CREB serine 133-phosphorylation, c-fos, and cell proliferation in a dose-dependent fashion. This indicates that the MAPK pathway is the mediator of crystal-induced signals to the nucleus (47).

To determine the role of the p42/44 MAPK signal transduction pathway in crystal-induced expression of matrix MMPs, fibroblasts have been treated with PD98059, an agent that blocks the induction of crystal-stimulated MMP-1 and -3 expression. Both PD98059 and phosphocitrate reduce the level of crystal-induced MMP-1 and -3 mRNA expression to that observed in non-stimulated cells. Similarly, PD98059 treatment of cells blocks the EGF- and crystal-induced increase in MMP-1 and -3 protein expression. These results suggest that the p42/44 MAPK pathway is the important signal transduction pathway of crystal- and EGF-induced MMP-1 and MMP-3 expression.

REFERENCES

1. Cheung HS. Calcium crystal effects on the cells of the joint: implications for pathogenesis of the disease. Curr Opin Biol 2000; 12:223–227.
2. Halverson PB. BCP crystal deposition disease and calcinosis. In: Koopman WJ, ed. Arthritis and Allied Conditions. Philadelphia, PA: Lippincott Williams and Wilkins, 2001:2372.
3. Ryan LM, Kurup IV, Cheung HS. Transduction mechanisms of chondrocyte inorganic pyrophosphate elaboration. Arthritis Rheum 1999; 42:555–560.
4. Ryan LM, Cheung HS. Role of crystals in osteoarthritis. In: Brandt KD, ed. Rheumatic Disease of America. Philadelphia: W.B. Saunders Co., 1999:257–267.
5. McCarty DJ, Cheung HS. Prostaglandin (PG)E_2 generation by cultured canine synovial fibroblasts exposed to microcrystals containing calcium. Ann Rheum Dis 1985; 44:316–320.
6. Morgan MP, Whelan LC, Sallis JD, et al. Basic calcium phosphate crystal-induced prostaglandin E2 production in human fibroblasts: role of cyclooxygenase 1, cyclooxygenase 2, and interleukin-1beta. Arthritis Rheum 2004; 50:1642–1649.
7. Cheung HS, Mitchell P, Pledger WJ. Induction of expressions of c-fos and c-myc proto-oncogenes by BCP crystals: effect of beta-interferon. Cancer Res 1989; 49:134–138.
8. McCarthy GM, Mitchell PG, Struve JA, Cheung HS. Basic calcium phosphate crystal cause coordinate induction and secretion of collagenase and stromelysin. J Cell Physiol 1992; 153:140–146.
9. Mitchell PG, Pledger WJ, Cheung HS. Molecular mechanisms of basic calcium phosphate crystal-induced mitogenesis, role of protein kinase C. J Biol Chem 1989; 264:14071–14077.
10. Bai G, Howell DS, Roos BA, et al. Crystals upregulate metalloproteinases and downregulate tissue inhibitor of metalloproteinase in human fibroblasts. OA & Cartilage 2001; 9:416–422.
11. McCarthy GM, Macius AM, Christopherson PA, et al. BCP crystals induced synthesis and secretion of 92 kDa gelatinase (gelatinaseB/matrix metalloprotease 9) in human fibroblasts. Ann Rheum Dis 1998; 57:56–60.

12. Reuben PM, Wenger L, Cruz M, Cheung HS. Induction of metalloproteinase-8 in human fibroblasts by basic calcium phosphate crystals: effect of phosphocitrate. Connect Tissue Res 2001; 42:1 12.
13. Gibilisco PA, Schumacher HR, Hollander JL, Soper KA. Synovial fluid crystals in osteoarthritis. Arthritis Rheum 1985; 28:511–515.
14. Klashman DJ, Moreland LW, Ike RW, Kalunian KC. Occult presence of CPPD crystals in patients undergoing arthroscopic knee irrigation for refractory pain related to osteoarthritis. Arthritis Rheum 1994; 37:S240.
15. Schumacher HR, Rubinow A, Rothfuss S, et al. Apatite crystal clumps in synovial fluid are an early finding in canine osteoarthritis. Arthritis Rheum 1994; 37:S346.
16. Zitnan D, Sitaz S. Natural course of articular chondrocalcinosis. Arthritis Rheum 1976; 19:363–390.
17. Ledingham J, Regan M, Jones A, Doherty M. Factors affecting radiographic progression of knee osteoarthritis. Ann Rheum Dis 1995; 54:53–58.
18. Altman RD, Cheung H. Synovial fluid basic calcium phosphate (BCP) crystals in an osteoarthritic (OA) canine model. OA & Cartilage 1997; 5:48.
19. Carroll G, McCappin S, Bell M, et al. Comparison of keratan sulphate concentrations and the size distribution of proteoglycans in the synovial fluid of patients with osteoarthritis and pyrophosphate arthropathy. Rheumatol Int 1991; 11:63–68.
20. Carroll G, Stuart RA, Armstrong JA, et al. Hydroxyapatite crystals are a frequent finding in osteoarthritic synovial fluid. J Rheumatol 1991; 18:861–866.
21. Lohmander LS, Hoerrner LA, Lark MW. Metalloproteinases, tissue inhibitor, and proteoglycan fragments in knee synovial fluid in human osteoarthritis. Arthritis Rheum 1993; 36:181–189.
22. Kapadia RD, Badger AM, Levin JM, et al. Meniscal ossification in spontaneous OA in guinea pig. OA & Cartilage 2000; 8:374–377.
23. Garancis JC, Cheung HS, Halverson PB, McCarty DJ. "Milwaukee shoulder": association of microspheroids containing hydroxyapatite crystals, active collagenase and neutral proteases with rotator cuff defects. III. Morphologic and biochemical studies of an excised synovium showing chondromatosis. Arthritis Rheum 1981; 24:484–491.
24. Halverson PB, Cheung HS, McCarty DJ, et al. The "Milwaukee shoulder": association of microspheroids containing hydroxyapatite crystals, active collagenase and neutral protease with rotator cuff defects. II. Synovial fluid studies. Arthritis Rheum 1981; 24:474–483.
25. Cheung HS, Story MT, McCarty DJ. Mitogenic effects of hydroxyapatite and calcium pyrophosphate dihydrate crystals on cultured mammalian cells. Arthritis Rheum 1984; 27:668–674.
26. McCarthy GM, Mitchell PG, Cheung HS. The mitogenic response to BCP crystals is accompanied by collagenase induction and secretion in human fibroblasts. Arthritis Rheum 1991; 34:1021–1030.
27. Ryan LM, Cheung HS, LeGeros RZ, et al. Cellular responses to whitlockite. Calcif Tissue Int 1999; 65:374–377.
28. Cheung HS, McCarty DJ. Mitogenesis induced by calcium-containing crystals: role of intracellular dissolution. Exp Cell Res 1985; 157:63–70.
29. McCarthy GM, Cheung HS, Abel SM, Ryan LM. BCP crystal-induced collagenase production: role of intracellular crystal dissolution. OA & Cartilage 1998; 6:205–213.

30. Rothenberg RJ, Cheung H. Rabbit synoviocyte inositol phospholipid metabolism is stimulated by hydroxyapatite crystals. Am J Physiol 1988; 254:C554–C559.
31. McCarthy GM, Augustine JA, Balwin AS, et al. Molecular mechanism of BCP crystal-induced activation of human fibroblasts. Role of nuclear factor κB activator protein 1 and protein kinase C. J Biol Chem 1998; 273:35161–35169.
32. Reuben PM, Sun Y, Cheung HS. Basic calcium phosphate crystals activate p44/42 MAPK signal transduction pathway via protein kinase Cmu in human fibroblasts. J Biol Chem 2004; (279):35719–35725.
33. Reuben P, Brogley M, Sun Y, Cheung HS. Molecular mechanism of the induction of metalloproteinases 1 and 3 in human fibroblasts by basic calcium phosphate crystals. Role of calcium-dependent protein kinase C-α. J Biol Chem 2002; 277:15190–15198.
34. Brogley M, Cruz M, Cheung HS. Basic calcium phosphate crystal induction of MMP-1 and MMP-3 expression is dependent upon a p42/44 mitogen-activated protein kinase signal transcution pathway. J Cell Physiol 1999; 180:215–234.
35. Johannes F-J, Prestle J, Eis S, et al. PKCμ is a novel, atypical member of the Protein Kinase C family. J Biol Chem 1994; 269:6140–6148.
36. Berridge MJ. Inositol triphosphate and diacylglycerol: two interacting second messengers. Annu Rev Biochem 1987; 56:59–93.
37. Griendling KK, Rittenhouse SE, Brock TA, et al. Sustained diacylglycerol formation from inositol phospholipids in angiotensin II-stimulated vascular smooth muscle cells. J Biol Chem 1986; 261:5901–5906.
38. Rasmussen H. The calcium messenger system. Part 1. N Engl J Med 1986; 314:1094–1101.
39. Rasmussen H. The calcium messenger system. Part 2. N Engl J Med 1986; 314:1164–1170.
40. Berbow U, Brinckerhoff CE. The AP-1 site and MMP gen regulation: what is all the fuss about? Matrix Biol 1997; 15:519–526.
41. Brinckerhoff CE. Regulation of metalloproteinase gene expression: implication for osteoarthritis. Crit Rev Eukaryot Gene Expr 1992; 2:145–164.
42. Echevarria W, Leite MF, Guerra MT, et al. Regulation of calcium signals in the nucleus by a nucleoplasmic reticulum. Nat Cell Biol 2003; 5:440–446.
43. Allbritton NL, Oancea E, Kuhn MA, Meyer T. Source of nuclear calcium signals. Proc Natl Acad Sci USA 1994; 91:12458–12462.
44. Lipp P, Thomas D, Berridge MJ, Bootman MD. Nuclear calcium signaling by individual cytoplasmic calcium puffs. EMBO J 1997; 16:7166–7173.
45. Halverson PB, Greene A, Cheung HS. Intracellular calcium responses to BCP crystals in fibroblasts. OA Cartilage 1998; 6:324–329.
46. Buchner K. The role of Protein Kinase C in the regulation of cell growth and in signalling to the cell nucleus. J Cancer Res Clin Oncol 2000; 126:1–11.
47. Nair D, Misra RP, Sallis JD, Cheung HS. Phosphocitrate inhibits a basic calcium phosphate and calcium pyrophosphate dihydrate crystal-induced mitogen-activated protein kinase cascade signal transduction pathway. J Biol Chem 1997; 272:18920–18925.
48. Cheung HS, Halverson PB, McCarty DJ. Release of collagenase, neutral protease and prostaglandins from cultured mammalian cells by HA and CPPD crystals. Arthritis Rheum 1981; 24:1338–1344.

49. McCarthy GM, Westfall PR, Masuda I, et al. Basic calcium phosphate crystals activate human osteoarthritis synovial fibroblasts and induce matrix metalloproteinse-13 (collagenase-3) in adult porcine articular chondrocytes. Ann Rheum Dis 2001; 60:399–406.
50. Aho S, Rouda S, Kennedy SH, et al. Regulation of human interstitial collagenase (matrix metalloproteinase-1) promoter activity by fibroblast growth factors. Eur J Biochem 1997; 247:503–510.
51. Sun Y, Wenger L, Brinckerhoff CE, et al. BCP crystals induced matrix metalloprteinase-1 through RAS/MEK1/SRF/c-fos/AP-1/MMP-1. Pathway: involvement of transcription factor binding sites: PEA-3 and AP-1. J Biol Chem 2002; 277:1544–1552.
52. Lemaire P, Revelant O, Bravo R, Charnay P. Two mouse genes encoding potential transcription factors with identical DNA binding domains are activated by growth factors in cultured cells. Proc Natl Acad Sci USA 1988; 85:4691–4695.
53. Silverman E, Du J, Williams A, Wadgaonkar E. cAMP-response-element-binding-protein and p300 are transcriptional co-activators of EGR-1. Biochem J 1998; 336:183–189.
54. Zeng XR, Sun Y, Wenger L, Cheung HS. Induction of early growth response gene EGR2 by BCP crystals through calcium-dependent PKC-independent p42/4 MAPK pathway. Cell Tissue Organ 2003; 174:63–72.
55. Dyer JM, Vaquez V, Zavadi-Grob C, et al. Effect of synthetic CPPD and HA crystals on the interaction of human blood mononuclear cells with chondrocytes, synovial cells, and fibroblasts. Arthritis Rheum 1987; 30:1372–1381.
56. Rothenberg RJ. Modulation of prostaglandin E2 synthesis in rabbit synoviocytes. Arthritis Rheum 1987; 30:266–274.
57. Rosenthal AK, Rosier TA, Ryan LM. TGF-beta levels in synovial fluid. Arthritis Rheum 1993; 36:S162.
58. Rosenthal AK, McCarty BA, Cheung HS. Effect of transforming growth factor β1 on pyrophosphate metabolism in porcine articular tissue. Arthritis Rheum 1993; 36:539–542.
59. Ishikawa H, Ueba Y, Isobe T, Hirohata K. Interaction of polymorphonuclear leukocytes with CPPD crystals deposited in chondrocalcinosis cartilage. Rheumatol Int 1987; 7:217–221.
60. Guerne P, Terkeltaub R, Zuraw B, Lotz M. Inflammatory microcrystals stimulate interleukin-6-production and secretion by human monocytes and synoviocytes. Arthritis Rheum 1989; 32:1443–1452.
61. Wierzbicki A, Dalal P, Madura JD, Cheung HS. Molecular dynamics simulation of crystal induced membranolysis. J Phys Chem B 2003; 107:12346–12351.
62. Wierzbicki A, Cheung HS. Molecular modeling of inhibition of crystals of CPPD by phosphocitrate. J Mol Struct 1998; 454:287–291.
63. Sun Y, Zeng XR, Wenger L, Cheung HS. Basic calcium phosphate crystals stimulate the endocytotic activities of cells—inhibition by anti-calcification agents. Biochem Biophys Res Commun 2003; 312:1053–1059.
64. Marshall CJ. Specificity of receptor tyrosine kiae signaling: transient versus sustained extracellular signal-regulated kinase activation. Cell 1995; 80:179–185.
65. Neary JT. MAPK cascades in cell growth and death. News Physiol Sci 1997; 12:286–293.

66. Karin M. The regulation of AP-1 activity by mitogen-activated protein kinases. J Biol Chem 1995; 270:16483–16486.
67. Karin M, Liu Z, Zandi E. AP-1 function and regulation. Curr Opin Biol 1997; 9:240–246.
68. Angel P, Karin M. The role of jun, fos and the AP-1 complex in cell-proliferation and transformation. Biochem Biophys Acta 1991; 1072:129–157.

18

The Pathology of Crystal-Induced Arthropathies

H. Ralph Schumacher, Jr.

Division of Rheumatology, Department of Medicine, University of Pennsylvania and VA Medical Center, Philadelphia, Pennysylvania, U.S.A.

Robert L. Wortmann

Division of Rheumatology, Department of Medicine, University of Oklahoma College of Medicine, Tulsa, Oklahoma, U.S.A.

INTRODUCTION

Morphologic studies have contributed considerably to our understanding of crystal-induced arthritis. This chapter focuses on (i) findings in the joint while also addressing pathologic features of gout at other sites, (ii) changes induced by calcium pyrophosphate dihydrate (CPPD) crystal deposition, and (iii) the pathologic changes associated with basic calcium phosphate (BCP) crystals.

GOUT

Gout is the end result of the overproduction of urate and/or the under excretion of uric acid that produces hyperuricemia and permits the deposition of monosodium urate (MSU) crystals in various tissues, including the cartilage, bone, tendons, and synovium of joints. Chronic tophaceous gout can produce very destructive arthritis with bone cysts caused by tophi and chronic joint inflammation.

Synovium

Gross Pathology

Tophi appear as refractile white clumps embedded in the synovium and can fairly often be seen on synovial surfaces at either surgery or autopsy (Fig. 1) (1–3).

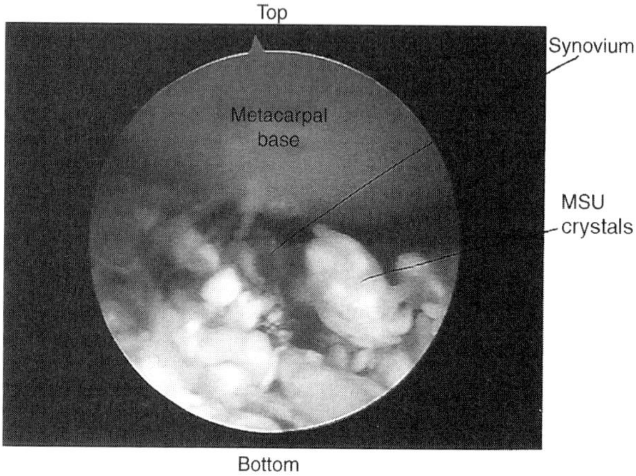

Figure 1 Creamy white masses of monosodium urate crystals are seen by arthroscopy at this metacarpal-phalangeal joint.

MSU crystal-containing tophi may be seen in the tips or stems of villi. Most are in the tissue and are not removed by irrigation (4–7). A diffuse crust of MSU crystals can also occasionally be seen over virtually the entire synovial and/or cartilage joint surface. There is still some uncertainty as to whether this surface deposition is an early event or whether tissue deposits always occur first.

Light Microscopy

During acute gouty arthritis an exudate containing polymorphonuclear leukocytes (PMNs) and fibrin adheres to the synovial surface. This is associated

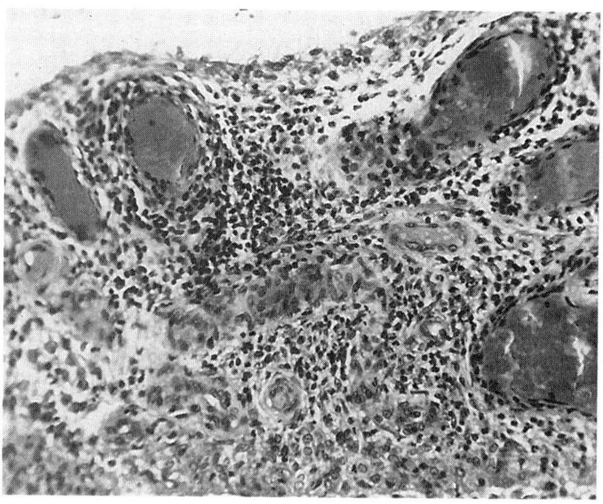

Figure 2 Acute and chronic inflammatory cells as well as congested vessels are seen in this synovial biopsy during acute gouty arthritis. H&E, 400X.

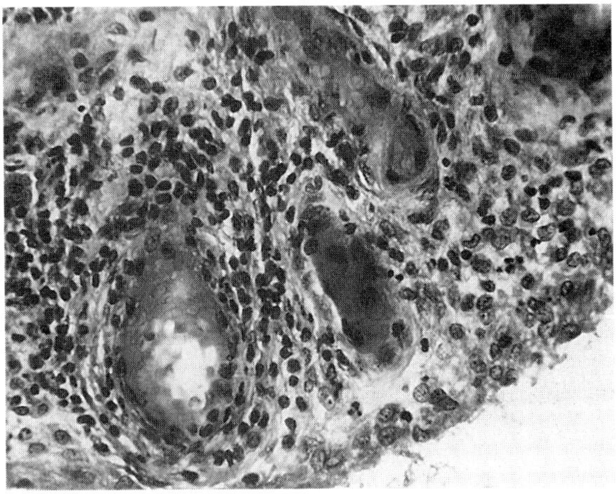

Figure 3 Chronic inflammation in synovium during low-grade, persistent symptoms. H&E, 400X.

with synovial lining cells proliferation in some areas (8). Diffuse and perivascular infiltration by PMNs is seen (Fig. 2). This is almost always associated with lymphocytes, macrophages, and plasma cells (Fig. 3). Vessels are congested and PMNs may be marginated in the lumens of venules. With synovial biopsy, PMN infiltration may be striking in area with an adjacent specimen showing mainly chronic inflammatory cells. Foreign body type giant cells have also been seen near the surface.

Tophi are commonly seen in synovium, for example, being found in 3 of 10 needle synovial biopsies in acute gouty arthritis and in 4 of 6 biopsies in another series (8,9). Tophi are also clearly present in asymptomatic joints between attacks (5).

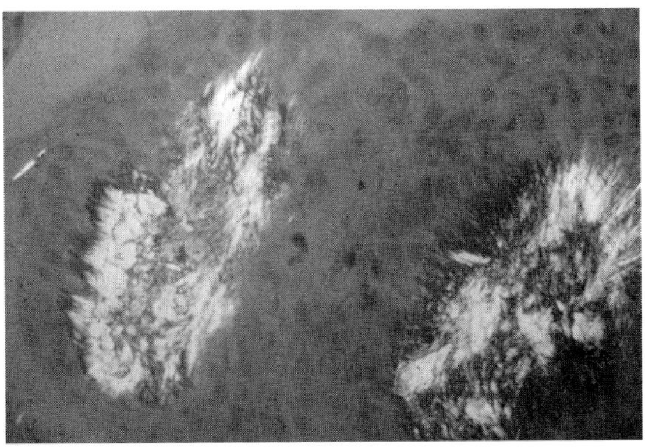

Figure 4 Synovial tophi as viewed with compensated polarized light after alcohol fixation. H&E, 400X.

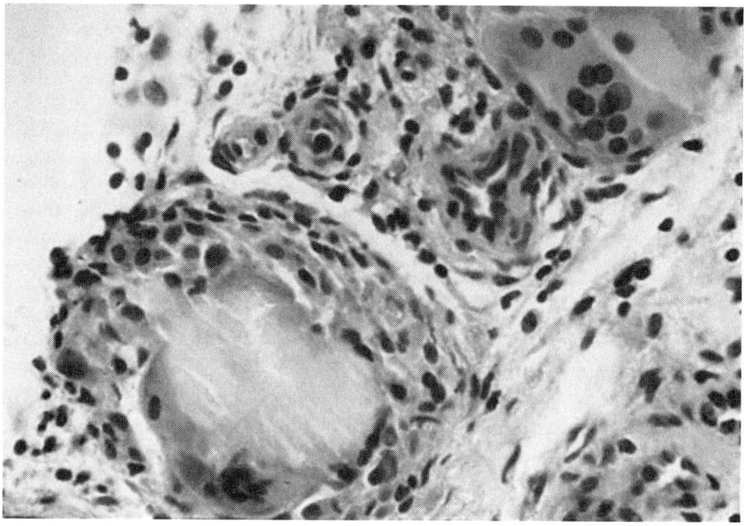

Figure 5 Site of synovial tophus from which crystals have been dissolved by formalin fixation. H&E, 400X.

Tophi consist of needle-shaped MSU crystals arranged radially (Fig. 4). Formalin-based fixatives can dissolve MSU crystals, but alcohol fixation preserves them intact (Fig. 5) (10). MSU crystals can also be easily identified in frozen sections or acetone-fixed tissue of stained sections examined with compensated polarized light. The DeGalantha stain or Gomori Methenamine silver stain also can be used to stain the crystals (Fig. 6) (11). When tophi dissolve in the fixation process, only the amorphous purple stained matrix remains. These areas could be confused with rheumatoid nodules, although clefts from which crystals have been dissolved can often be seen (5). The matrix material around the crystals has been shown to contain cholesterol and mucopolysaccharides (5). There is faint PAS staining and some metachromasia. Lipid stains show most lipid at the margins (5). Immunoglobulins have also been localized to tophi (Fig. 7) (12). Tophi may also occasionally calcify with deposition of hydroxyapatite.

The cells surrounding the tophus crystals are fibrocytes, macrophages, other mononuclear cells, and some foreign body giant cells. Acute inflammatory cells are strikingly absent around tophi. Many synovial tophi are very superficial and often rather thinly encapsulated with fibrous tissue. Fibrin-like material has been seen between some tophi and the joint space (Fig. 8) (8).

Electron Microscopy

During attacks of acute gouty arthritis, there is surface fibrin-like material and proliferation of lining cells with predominance of Type B and intermediate cells.

(A)

(B)

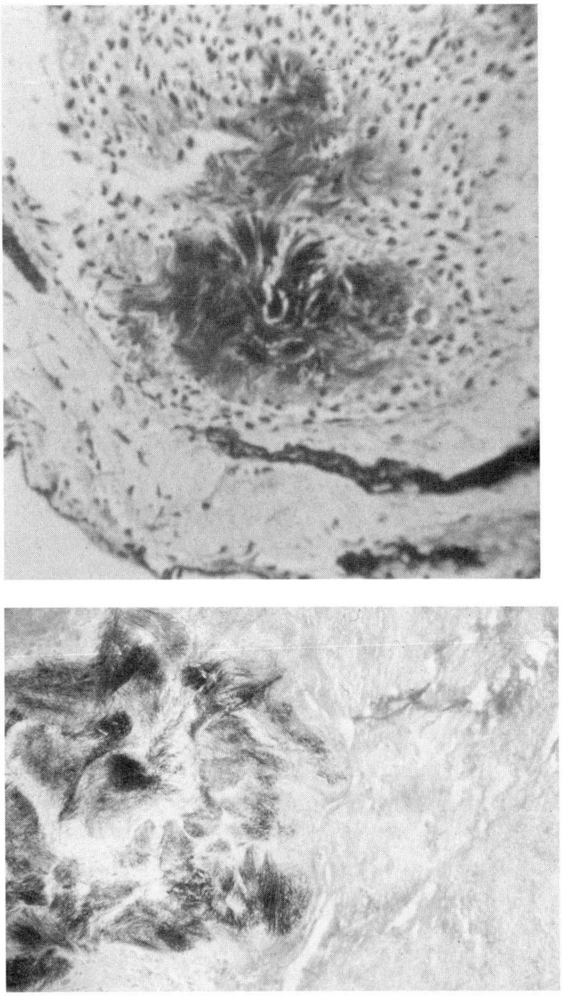

Figure 6 (*See color insert.*) (**A**) A synovial tophus with crystals stained brown with De Golantha stain. 400X. (**B**) Gomori methanamine silver staining monosodium urate crystals black. 100X.

Type B cells often have lipid deposits. The type A macrophage related cells have large vacuoles with granular material and cell debris and occasional definite crystal outlines in phagolysosomes (8). In experimental MSU crystal-induced synovitis, crystal phagocytosis by lining cells has also been seen (Fig. 9) (13). Inflammatory cells appear as described under light microscopy. Crystals are strikingly absent within PMNs infiltrating the synovium or in synovial vessels. Phagosomes within macrophages, however, contain cell fragments and intact PMNs. Extravasated erythrocytes and cell debris are found scattered through the interstitium.

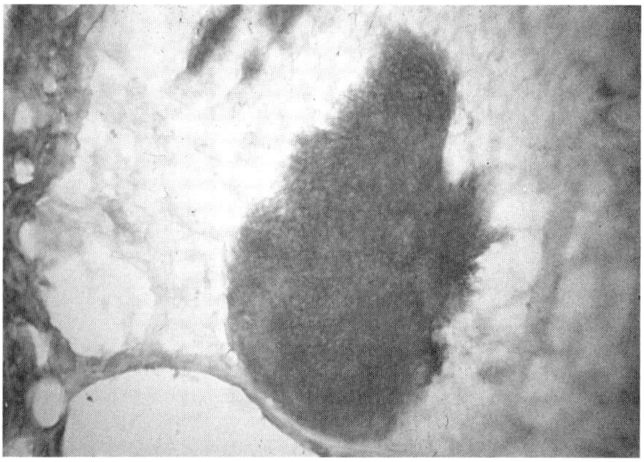

Figure 7 Immunoperoxidase stain for IgG in synovial tophus. 400X.

Some small vessels are congested while the lumens of others are packed with platelets, erythrocytes, and white blood cells. Gaps are observed between venular endothelial cells with emigrating erythrocytes and PMN, but very little endothelial cell necrosis is seen. Two patients have been described with dramatic but not further characterized electron dense deposits lying between endothelium and pericytes (Fig. 10) (8). Vascular basement membranes are often multilaminated.

PMNs in vessel lumens often contain foamy clear patches in the cytoplasm and fewer granules suggesting intraluminal degranulation (14). Some free dense bodies and fragmenting intraluminal PMNs can also be observed. Microtubules are easily seen in venular endothelium, pericytes, and lining cells regardless of whether the patient had taken clinically effective doses of colchicine.

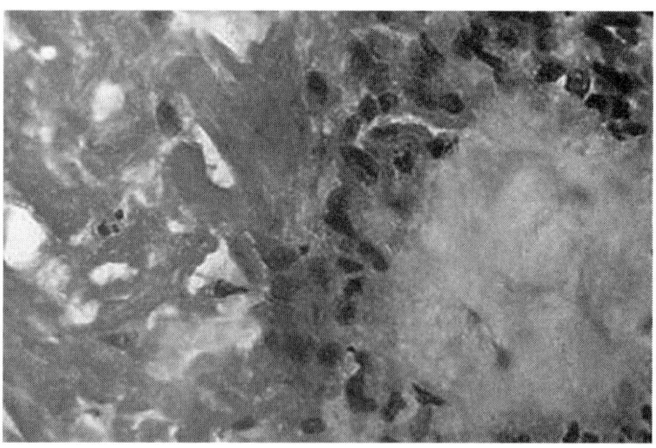

Figure 8 (*See color insert.*) Fibrin overlying tophus site which may have recently released crystals into the joint space. 400X.

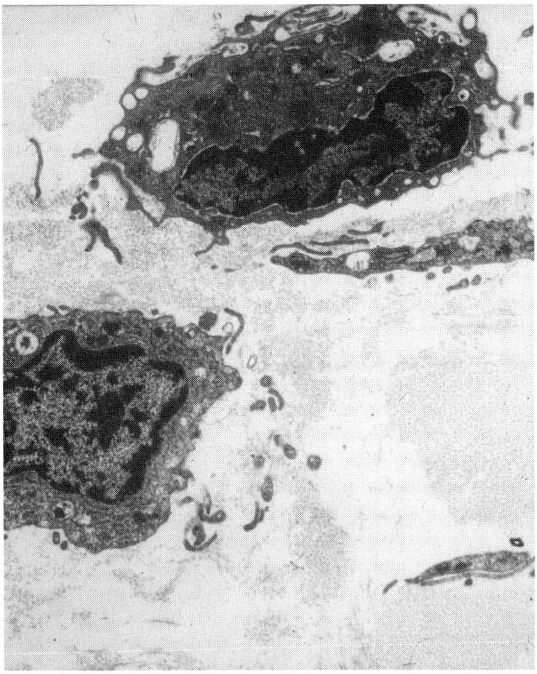

Figure 9 Monosodium urate crystals in superficial synovial lining cell. Electron micrograph, 15,000X.

With electron microscopy, a tophus shows parallel arrays of electron lucent crystal outlines lying in a finely granular material (Fig. 11). Cells adjacent to the crystals are fibrocyte-like and contain large lipid deposits. Occasional crystals seem to be in phagosomes within these cells. No intracytoplasmic crystals have been reported (8).

Scanning Electron Microscopy

These images show crystals on the synovial surface and occasionally within phagosomes in synovial lining cells (Fig. 12) (3).

Synovial Fluid

Findings in joint fluid can vary widely during apparent acute attacks of gouty arthritis. One study described leukocyte counts ranging from 1000 to 70,000 WBC/mm^3 with a mean of 13,317 WBC/mm^3 (15). The differential cell count showed 80% to 95% (mean of 71%) of the cells were PMNs.

MSU crystals are seen intra- and extracellularly during attacks of acute gouty arthritis. They may vary in size from large crystals that extend through a PMN membrane like a stick through an olive to tiny birefringent dots. Some PMNs are dead with pyknotic nuclei (16,17). Fragments of synovial tissue or

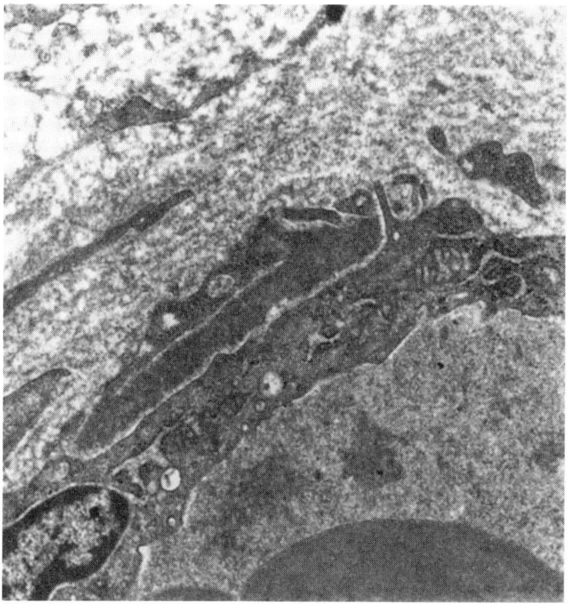

Figure 10 Synovial vessel in acute gout with subendothelial electron dense deposits. Electron micrograph, 20,000X.

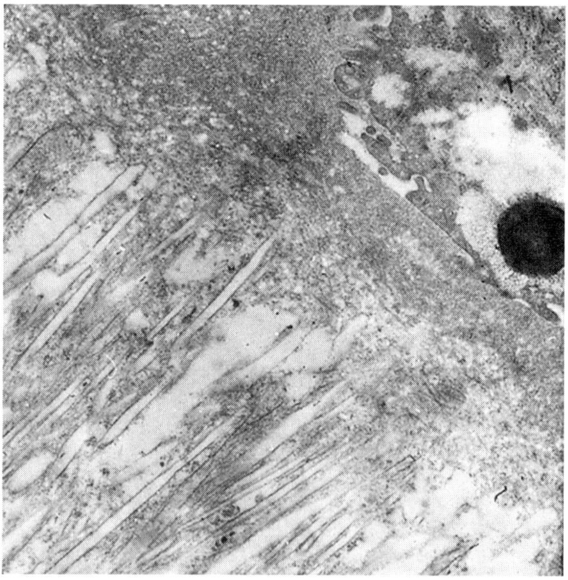

Figure 11 Electron micrograph of synovial tophus. Crystals are dissolved out but identified by the surface protein coats. 22,000X.

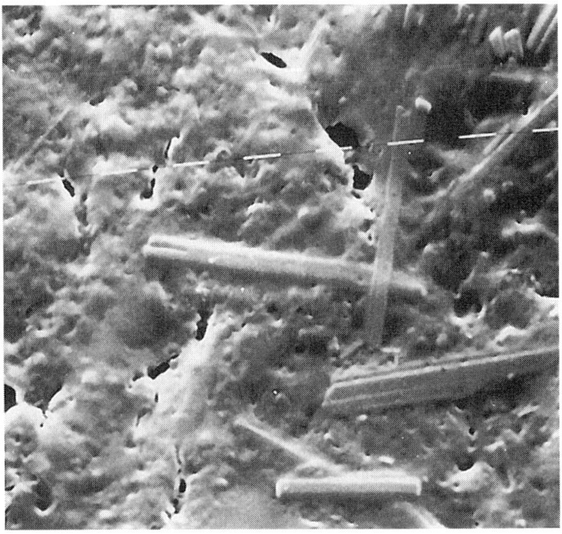

Figure 12 Scanning electron micrograph of monosodium urate crystals on the synovial surface.

cartilage can be found floating in gouty joint fluid. Either of these may contain masses of crystals. Fragments of synovium in the fluid may have attached dense microtophi-containing radially oriented arrays of crystals (Fig. 13).

Rarely MSU crystals are not identified in what otherwise seems to be typical acute gouty arthritis (18). Urate concentrations in synovial fluid are almost always identical to serum levels, although dissolution of crystals can reflect an increased total urate load (19). Crystals are also very commonly found in gouty synovial fluids in the interval between attacks (20,21). Untreated patients virtually always will have crystals in previously involved asymptomatic joints (20,22). Such crystals may be extracellular or phagocytized by mononuclear cells.

In specimens fixed with standard techniques, PMNs related to MSU crystals almost invariably show a striking patchy loss of cytoplasmic density (Fig. 14) (23). This is in contrast to PMNs from synovial fluid in patients with pseudogout or rheumatoid arthritis. The outlines of MSU crystals are formed by dense proteinaceous material lying on the crystal surface with the actual crystal dissolved by the fixative (8,23,24). Many crystals are located in phagosomes adjacent to dense bodies and finely granular material (Fig. 15). Other crystals seem to be totally free in the cytoplasm, but there is a strong possibility that some of these are artifacts (24). Large defects are often seen in phagosome membranes. Crystals in macrophages and synovial lining cells are not associated with membrane defects or loss in cytoplasmic density, but tiny crystal outlines can be seen (Fig. 16). Synovial macrophages have been seen to phagocytize crystal-laden PMN. Microtubules are easily seen in these large mononuclear cells.

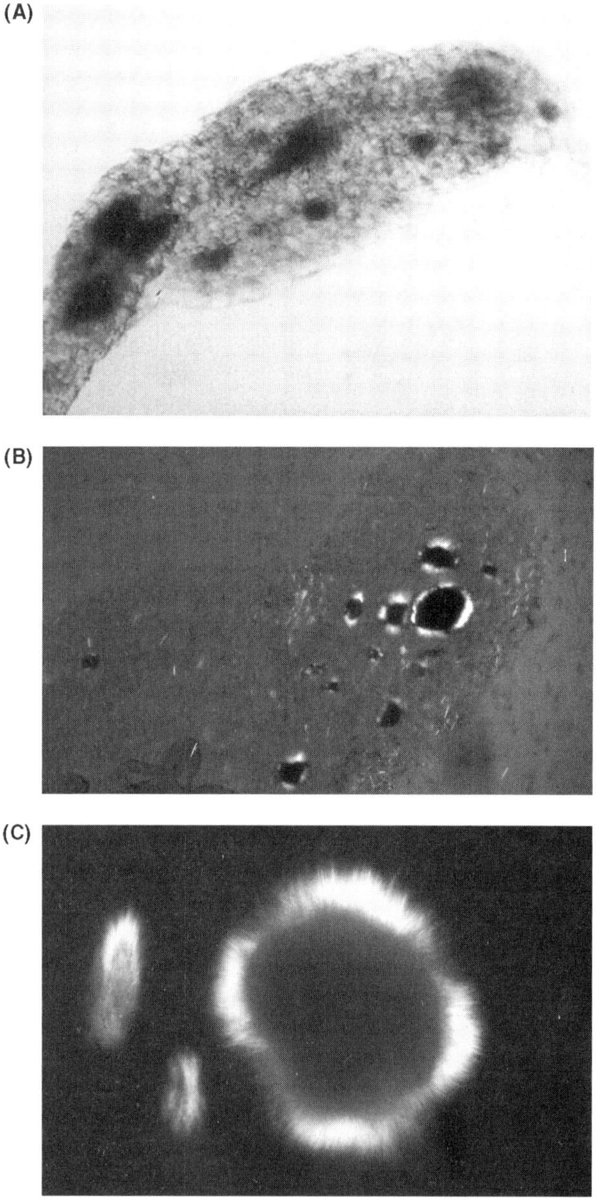

Figure 13 Synovial fragment found floating in synovial fluid. (**A**) Microtophi appear dense with regular light microscope. 100X. (**B**) Polarized light shows the crystals in the microtophi. 100X. (**C**) Oil immersion shows the radially arrayed crystals. 1000X.

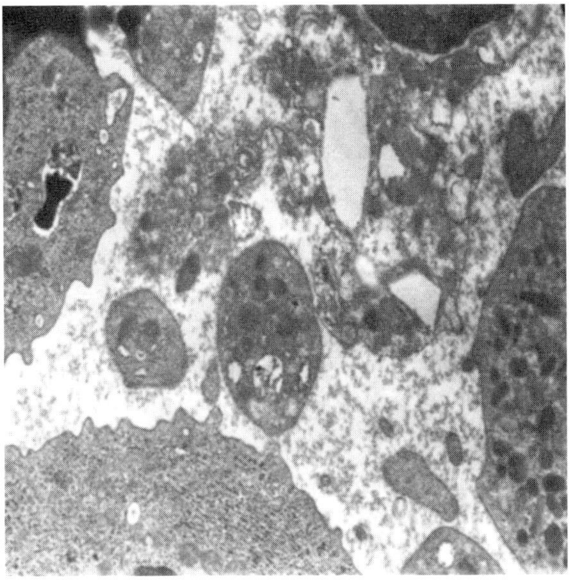

Figure 14 Degenerating neutrophil with monosodium urate crystal, loss of cytoplasmic detail, and apparent lysis of phagolysosome membrane. Electron micrograph, 11,000X.

Implications of Pathology of Synovium and Synovial Fluid

Morphologic studies have so far shown no differences between the arthritis in primary or secondary gout. Although not absolutely proved, most evidence suggests that tophi in the synovium antedate most attacks of gouty arthritis. These

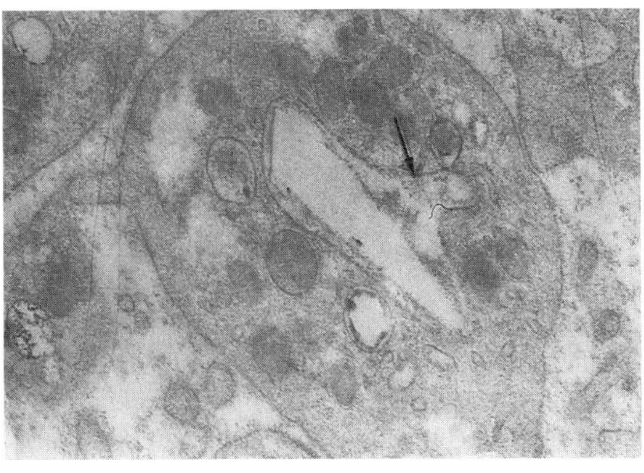

Figure 15 Monosodium urate crystal lying in phagolysome with site of emptying of lysosome into vacuole (*arrow*). 25,000X.

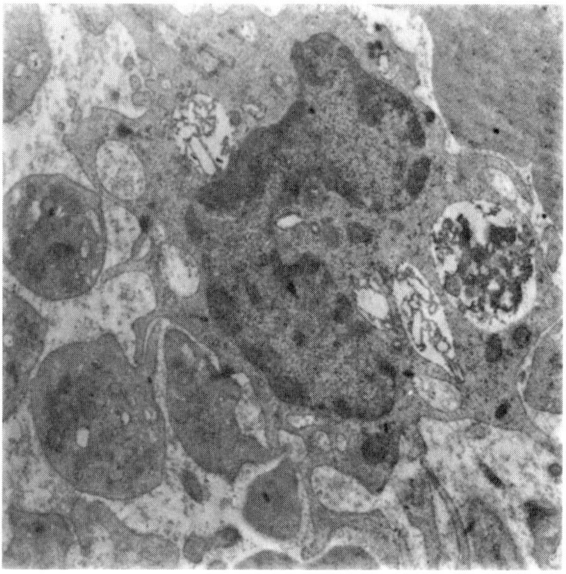

Figure 16 Very small monosodium urate crystal outlines in intact-looking macrophage. 19,000X.

tophi are often thinly encapsulated and may well be the site from which crystals break free into the joint, thereby initiating the acute arthritis. Support for this hypothesis is derived from experiments where an acute arthritis like that seen in human gout was induced following the injection of synthetic MSU crystals into human or animal (13,25).

The matrix in which the urate crystals reside may also play a role in precipitating crystals or maintaining the crystals (5,12). Changes in mucopolysaccharides, other connective tissue materials, serum urate levels, and serum binding factors may affect the local deposition of crystals. MSU crystal deposits have occurred at sites of local trauma such as a burn on the finger (Fig. 17) (26).

PMNs are essential for the production of the full syndrome of acute gouty arthritis (27). Phagocytosis of MSU crystals by PMNs produces rapid cell death with release of cell debris, enzymes, and crystals. These substances tend to perpetuate the inflammation (23). Crystal-laden phagolysosomes lyse in some synovial fluid cells. This is, at least in part, due to the effect of the negatively charged crystal on the membrane (28,29). PMNs in the synovial microvasculature and interstitium also seem to degranulate without direct contact with crystals. Crystals do not cause the same cell death in mononuclear cells.

Although PMNs contain myeloperoxidase that can digest crystals, the exact method for crystal clearing as well as the factors that lead to the spontaneous resolution of acute attacks are not yet clear. Alterations of proteins bound to the

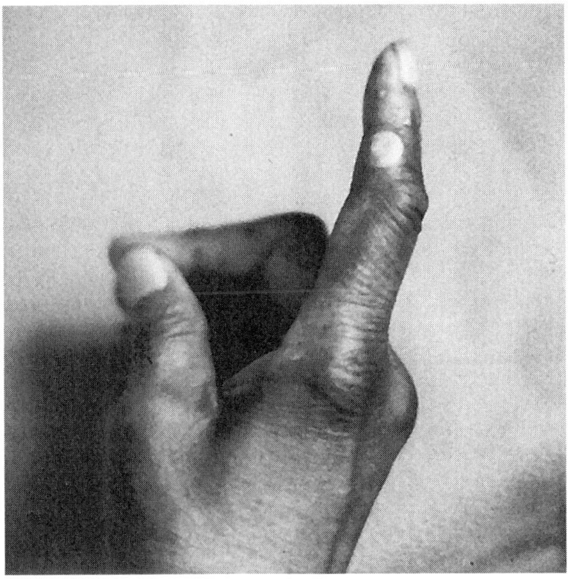

Figure 17 Synovial tophus rapidly developing on a finger at the exact site of a burn injury.

crystal surface can be a factor as could changes in cytokines produced as a result of mononuclear cell maturation (30–32).

The presence of chronic inflammatory cells in synovium even early in an acute attack is followed by persistent mild chronic inflammation even in asymptomatic intervals between attacks. This may play a part in the eventual joint destruction. Chronic inflammation has also been produced by injections of synthetic crystals into dog joints (13).

Immunologic mechanisms may contribute to gouty arthritis. There are dense deposits suggestive of immune complexes in vessel walls noted by EM (8). Gouty synovial fluids may contain complement-derived chemotactic factors (29). Immunoglobulins and complement have been identified in PMN phagosomes in synovial fluid in gout (33).

Bone and Cartilage

Tophi in subchondral bone are associated with collapse and resorption of trabeculae producing a punched out–like space as seen in X-rays (Fig. 18) and tissue specimens. Subperiosteal marginal MSU deposits have been illustrated (4,5,34,35). Crystals are phagocytized by adjacent mononuclear and giant cells. Bone sclerosis and osteophyte formation are typical adjacent to the tophi.

Cartilage surfaces in chronic gout may appear as diffusely dusted with white crystal deposits or speckled with nodular deposits (34). Such crystal deposits have been felt to begin in superficial cartilage and are accompanied by

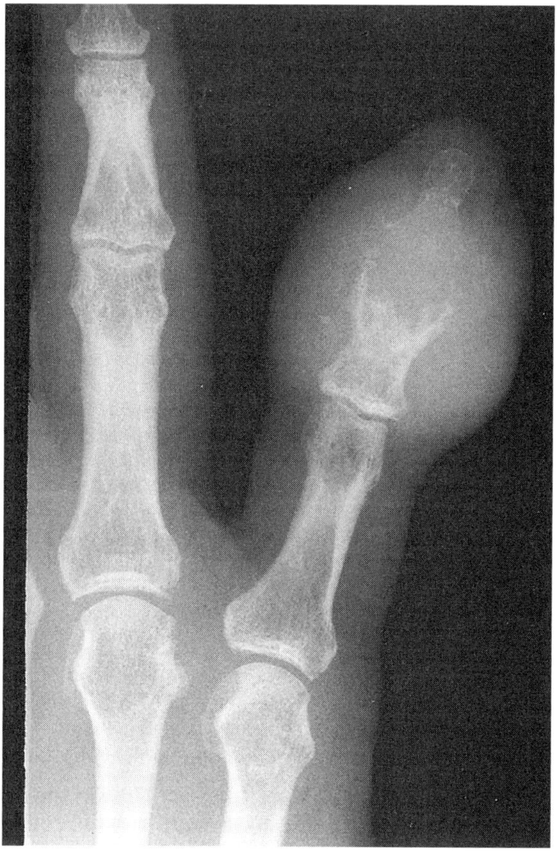

Figure 18 Bone loss is easily shown radiographically at this distal interphalangeal joint.

chondrocyte loss and fibrillation. In these cartilage sites and in the helix cartilage of the ear, cellular reaction is absent or minimal (34). Later cartilage can be focally eroded first with adjacent grossly normal areas. Pannus is not seen.

Synovial fluid cartilage fragments containing MSU crystals have been studied by polarized light (36). Sheets of crystals were arrayed along apparent collagen fibers, suggesting a role of the collagen matrix in the crystal localization.

Kidney

Kidney involvement in gout has been documented for years (37). Nephrosclerosis and renal vascular disease are common. Deposits of MSU can form microtophi in the interstitium with variable inflammatory reaction including giant cells. Concentrations of urate are highest in the papillae so MSU tophi are more

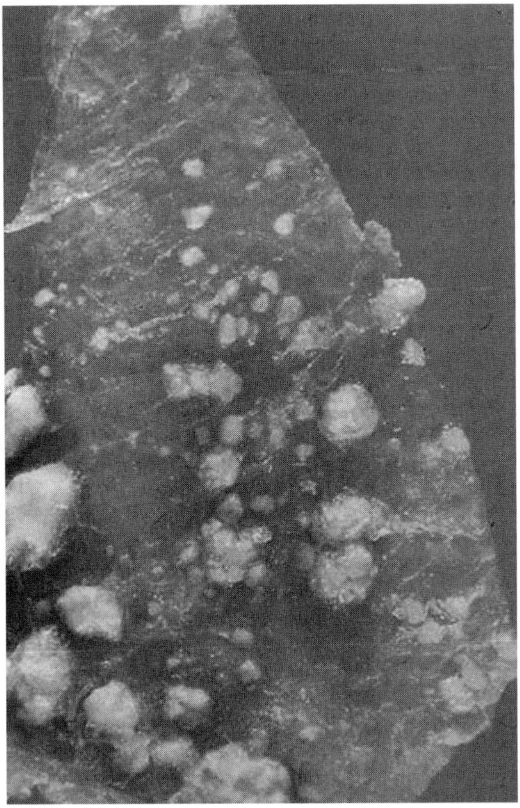

Figure 19 Undersurface of a non-inflamed blister-like tophus.

frequent there (38,39). Uric acid stones can form in the collecting system in acid urine in patients with increased uric acid excretion. Intraluminal casts of amorphous or crystalline uric acid have been demonstrated (38,40). There is some suggestion that renal tubular cells can phagocytize uric acid (41). Gouty patients also have an increased incidence of calcium oxalate stones. Lead nephropathy can show interstitial urates but is not specific histologically (39). There are other potentially important histologic changes including neutrophilic infiltrates from secondary infection, tubular atrophy, atrophy of loops of Henle, glomerulosclerosis, and hyalinization of arterioles (40,42).

Other Sites of Gouty Tophi

Gouty tophi have been demonstrated in connective tissues in many parts of the body. These include subcutaneous tissue, tendons, heart valves, larynx, sclera and cornea, middle ear, nasal septum, tongue, bronchi, buttocks, carpal tunnel, and even the penis (40).

Histopathologic findings at these sites have been limited but generally show findings similar to those in the synovium and without acute inflammation (40). Gross appearance in skin often shows tophaceous masses with no overt inflammatory reaction (Fig. 19).

CALCIUM PYROPHOSPHATE DIHYDRATE DEPOSITION

CPPD crystal deposition is believed to occur when excessive calcium or pyrophosphate ions accumulate. Factors that influence deposition of these include cartilage matrix vesicles, various ecto-enzyme activities, and the anion transporter ANK. The host response to these crystals leads to a variety of clinical and pathologic presentations generally restricted to the joints.

Gross Appearance

Joints with CPPD crystals can show white frosty appearing deposits coating cartilage and encrusting synovial villi when seen at arthroscopy or at surgery in advanced cases (Fig. 20)

Cartilage

CPPD crystals are most commonly found in articular cartilage (43–45). The distribution of these crystals generally is consistent with that seen radiographically (44). The heaviest deposits are distributed diffusely in fibrocartilaginous structures such as menisci (Fig. 21), but the midzonal and superficial areas

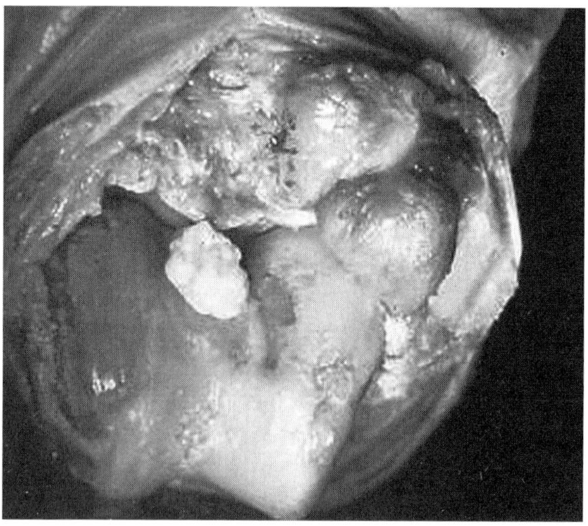

Figure 20 Gross appearance of massive white calcium pyrophosphate dihydrate crystals in knee synovium obtained at surgery.

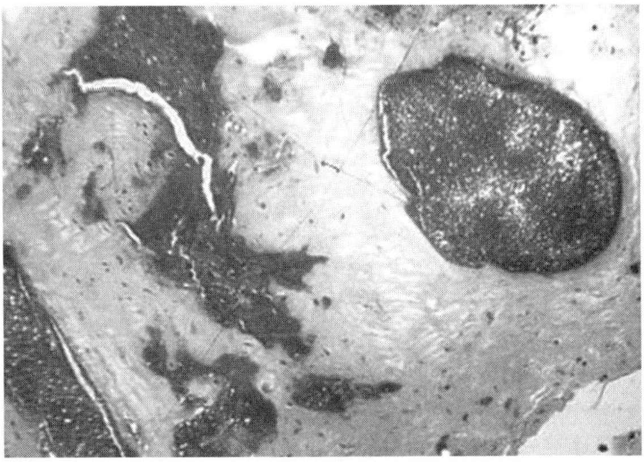

Figure 21 Calcium pyrophosphate dihydrate crystal clumps in hematoxyphilic matrix in midzone of meniscus. Hematoxylin and eosin stain, 400X.

of hyaline articular cartilages are also often affected as seen well with polarized light (Fig. 22). Isolated descriptions of CPPD crystals within chondrocytes have been reported, suggesting that chondrocytes may phagocytose crystals with resultant biologic consequences (46).

Light Microscopy

CPPD deposits typically are composed of various-sized microcrystalline aggregates with diameters varying from 15 mm to 0.6 cm. Small CPPD crystals (presumably the earliest to form) are found at the lacunar margin of chondrocytes. The surrounding matrix may appear normal or granular. Collagen fibril fragmentation may be seen in noncalcified areas of CPPD cartilage (47). Virtually all cartilages studied have also shown fibrillation as a degenerative

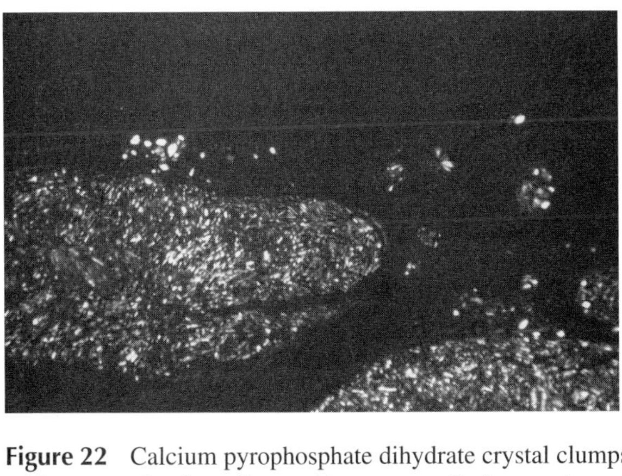

Figure 22 Calcium pyrophosphate dihydrate crystal clumps with plain polarized light in midzone meniscal cartilage with some small clumps closer to the surface at the top.

change. Larger superficial CPPD deposits are observed in more degenerative cartilages, presumably related to greater deposition. These are usually found at sites of surface ulcerations and fissuring and may be associated with chondrocyte "cloning."

Abnormal proteoglycan deposition is observed within chondrocytes in the immediate vicinity of early CPPD crystal deposits in familial and sporadic disease. The term "red cells" has been applied to these chondrocytes because of their appearance after staining with safranin-0, an appearance not seen if the tissue was pretreated with either papain or chondroitinase. "Red cells" remain a constant feature associated with evolving CPPD crystal deposits in fibrocartilage, hyaline cartilage, and in areas of synovium showing chondroid metaplasia. Red cells are not necessarily seen when the condition has matured (48).

Additional histologic findings include the absence of normal safranin-0 staining in the matrix in areas of early deposition, "packing" of the proteoglycan-denuded collagen fibers in these same areas, hypertrophy and mitotic activity of the "red cells," empty chondrocyte lacunae containing CPPD crystals, and mature CPPD deposits ringed with dense (proteoglycan-free) collagen, but with the crystals coated with a thin film of proteoglycan. No collagen or cells have been identified within these crystal masses by light microscopy. It is speculated that the cell-associated proteoglycan may indicate faulty release from the chondrocytes after synthesis or that it may enter these cells by endocytosis.

Fibrocartilage and hyaline articular cartilage (as well as synovium) from patients with CPPD deposits have been observed to contain excess lipid using Sudan III staining (49). Adjacent metaplastic chondrocytes also contain large Sudan III-positive granules. The relationship between lipid and mineralization is not clear, but lipid may bind calcium needed for CPPD formation.

In one study, the calcium-binding protein S-l00 was localized to CPPD-containing articular tissues, but not CPPD-free tissues from patients with osteoarthritis (50). Others, however, noted increased S-l00 protein in osteoarthritic joints in the absence of crystals (51).

Histologic abnormalities in joint tissues during attacks of acute pseudogout include neutrophil migration into the cartilage matrix (52). Intracellular CPPD crystals are observed within vacuoles of the invading neutrophils. The superficial cartilage is eroded, and collagen fibers are degraded. It is likely that the neutrophils generate enzymes and free oxygen radical species that damage the adjacent tissue.

Electron Microscopy

Cartilage in areas with CPPD crystals has been characterized by chondrocytes with large cytoplasmic processes, adjacent matrix vesicles, increased glycogen, often darkened cytoplasm with loss of organelles but others with profuse, rough endoplasmic reticulum, and lipid droplets (43,45,53,54). CPPD crystals appear uniformly dark or foamy with many adjacent to chondrocytes or debris from degenerated chondrocytes. Crystals are often dislodged during sectioning, but the

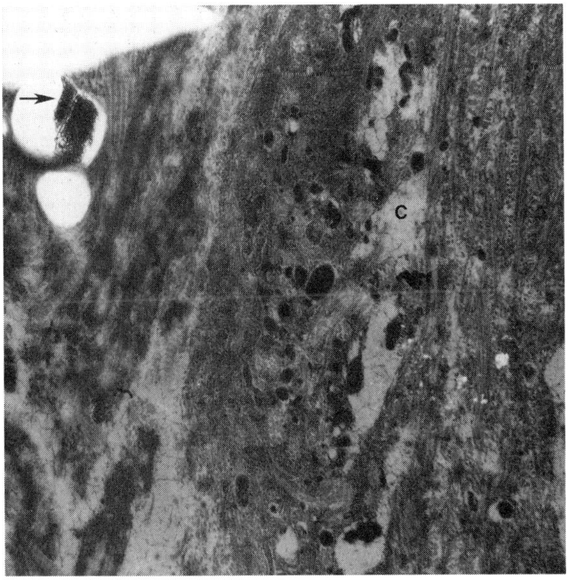

Figure 23 Tiny foamy calcium pyrohosphate dihydrate crystal (*arrow*) adjacent to necrotic chondrocyte (*C*). Electron micrograph, 6000X.

smallest similarly foamy crystals remain and lie in a finely grainy matrix often containing collagen fibers (Fig. 23). Matrix vesicles are prominent but CPPD have not been documented in matrix vesicles. Apatite crystals have been seen at that site in cartilage in patients with otherwise profuse CPPD (43).

Synovium and Periarticular Tissues

CPPD crystal deposition has also been localized to joint capsules, tendons, and in intraarticular ligaments (45,55). Of these, more common sites include the joint capsules of the shoulder and knee and the cruciate ligaments in the knee.

Light Microscopy

In synovium, CPPD crystals are often seen as birefringent tophus-like aggregates under the lining (Fig. 24). Crystals are not dissolved out by formalin but can be lost in decalcified specimens. Crystal sites are hematoxyphilic. Sites of chrondrometaplasia are often seen adjacent to deposits (Fig. 25), suggesting that some deposits are formed by these transformed cells. Other CPPD may be sequestered from joint fluid. Osteochondromatosis has been associated with CPPD deposition (56).

Early in an acute attack of pseudogout, the edematous synovium is infiltrated with PMNs. This is followed by mononuclear infiltration and fibroblastic proliferation. Synovial proliferation and infiltration with chronic

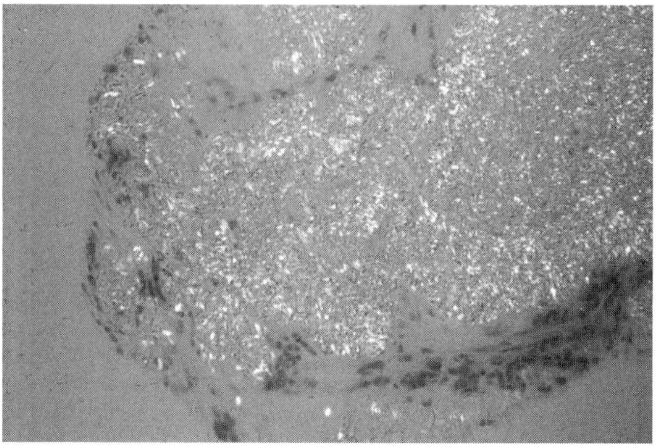

Figure 24 Calcium pyrophosphate dihydrate tophus filling synovial villus Safranin stain. Plain polarized light, 100X.

inflammatory cells in chronically symptomatic joints may resemble rheumatoid synovitis (55). In patients with pseudo-osteoarthritis undergoing knee replacement, synovial deposits tend to be focal and localized to avascular areas. Surgical samples excised from involved ligaments have shown chondrometaplasia and CPPD crystals.

Electron Microscopy

Dense, foamy CPPD crystals or the holes from which they have been dislodged can be seen in vacuoles of synovial macrophages, PMNs, synovial fibroblasts, or lying in the matrix (Fig. 26) (45,55,57,58). A dramatic finding in synovium is that

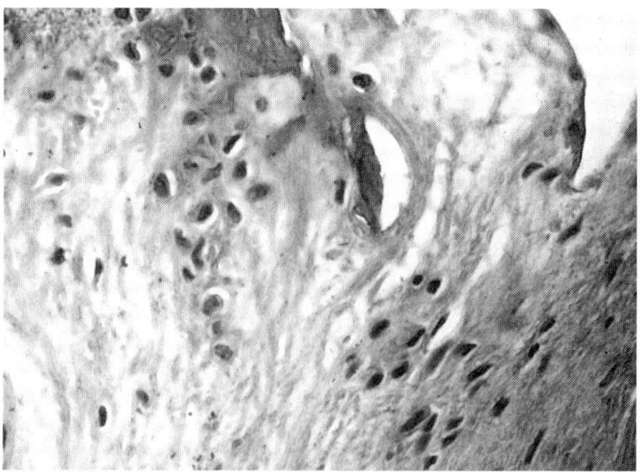

Figure 25 Synovium with chrondrometaplasia adjacent to calcium pyrophosphate dihydrate deposit (*arrow*). H&E, regular light, 400X.

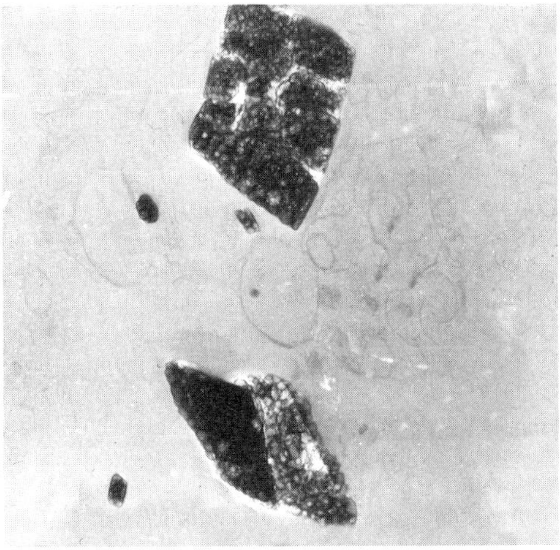

Figure 26 Calcium pyrophosphate dihydrate crystals in electron micrograph, 38,000X.

what appear to be tiny CPPD crystals can be seen lined up on or along collagen fibers (16), suggesting their role in crystal deposition or growth (Fig. 27).

Synovial Fluid

The positively birefringent CPPD crystals may be associated with fairly normal synovial fluid with a normal white blood cell count in the lanthanic (asymptomatic) or pseudo-osteoarthritic presentations. In other cases, they may be found phagocytosed and/or outside of PMNs with synovial fluid leukocyte counts ranging up to over 100,000 WBC/mm^3 in patients with pseudogout, pseudorheumatoid, or pseudoseptic presentations of CPPD crystal deposition.

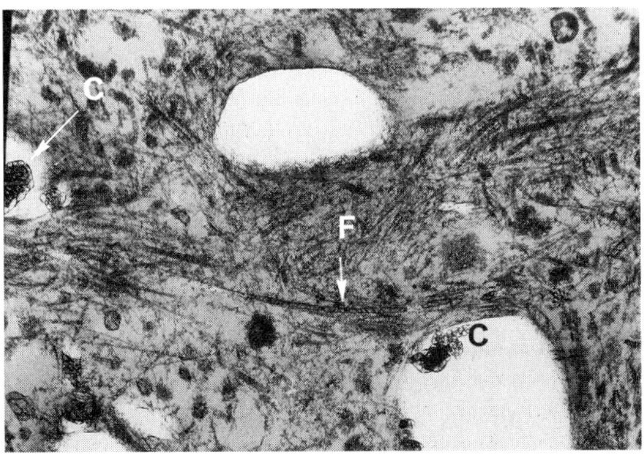

Figure 27 Calcium pyrophosphate dihydrate crystals (*C*) in synovium with some suggestion of early crystallization appearing to line up along collagen fibrils (*F*). Electron micrograph, 20,000X.

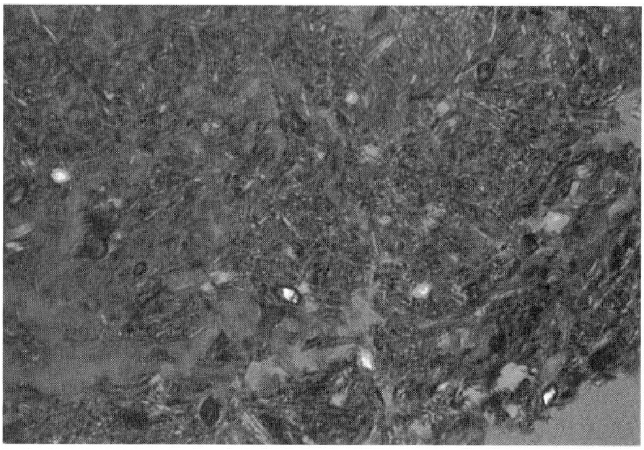

Figure 28 (*See color insert.*) Calcium pyrophosphate dihydrate crystals in biopsy from parotid area mass. H&E, compensated polarized light, 400X.

Unusual and Non-Articular Sites

Deposits of CPPD have been reported in dura mater, ligamenta flava, and the olecranon bursa, as well as in isolated tophi (44). On gross examination, larger CPPD accumulations appear as white chalky deposits and are difficult to distinguish from the tophaceous lesions of gout. A tophaceous CPPD deposit has been seen adjacent to a distal interphalangeal joint where it was mistaken for a tumor (59).

Superficial amyloid deposits have been observed adjacent to CPPD crystals (60). Cases of temporomandibular joint CPPD deposition were found to contain numerous crystals within chondrocytes and as tophus-like masses (Fig. 28) (61,62).

APATITE (BASIC CALCIUM PHOSPHATE)-ASSOCIATED ARTHROPATHIES

The most common crystal-associated arthropathies are those related to apatite (BCP) deposition. These crystals are those identified in calcific tendinitis and periarthritis, tumoral calcinosis, idiopathic calcification of spinal ligaments and disks, diffuse idiopathic skeletal hyperostosis, and Milwaukee shoulder syndrome.

In addition, BCP crystals are present in synovial fluids, cartilage (Fig. 29), and synovium (Fig. 30) in a large subset of patients with osteoarthritis. Apatite deposits are found around chondrocytes (63). Other apatite can be from bone fragments embedded in synovium in advanced osteoarthritis. Half of articular cartilages with advanced osteoarthritis contained hydroxyapatite-type crystals (64). Studies of synovial fluids from osteoarthritic knee joints reveal apatite crystals in approximately 30% to 60%, and such fluids more often contain both BCP and CPPD crystals than either species alone (65–67). The presence of

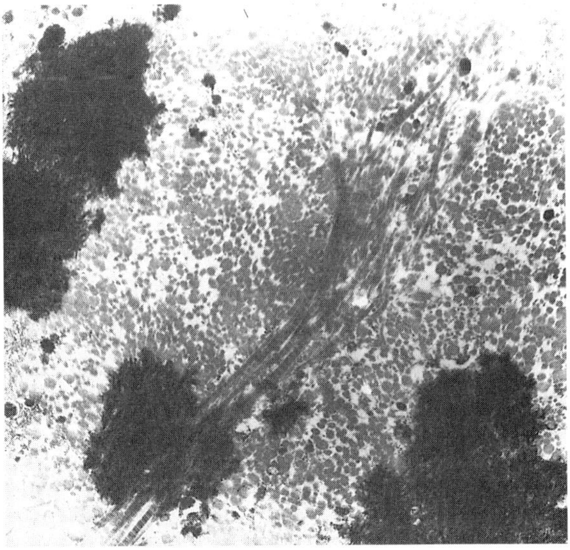

Figure 29 Masses of apatite in osteoarthritis articular cartilage. Electron micrograph, 22,000X.

BCP correlates with more severe radiographic joint degeneration and at times is associated with neuropathic-like arthropathy on X-ray (68). Synovial apatite deposits are also seen in some renal dialysis patients and in scleroderma or other connective tissue diseases embedded in the matrix or in phagocytic vacuoles (69–71). Apatite crystals are often present in synovial fluid rice bodies in rheumatoid arthritis (72). Materials associated with apatite deposits have received little study. Granular protein-like material is often present and can include immunoglobulins and complement (Fig. 31) (45,73).

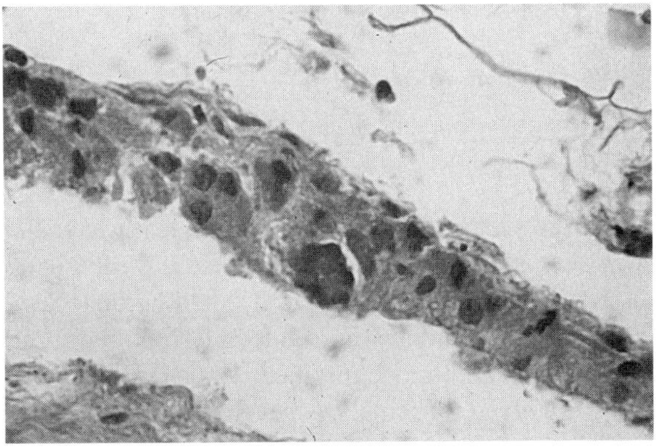

Figure 30 Hematoxyphilic chunk of apatite in synovial tissue among synovial lining cells (SLC) of a dialysis patient. H&E, 400X.

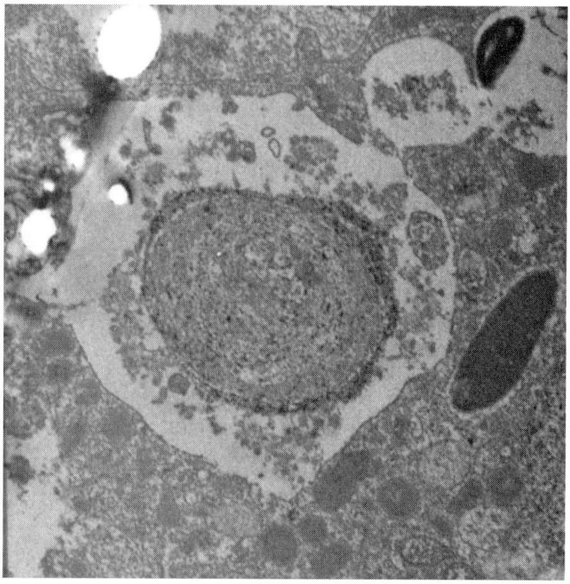

Figure 31 Apatite in proteinaceous matrix in synovial fluid vacuole during acute arthritis. Electron micrograph, 7500X.

A survey of a large number of pathologic nonarticular calcifications using crystallographic techniques showed no CPPD crystals (69). Identification of crystals in aortic plaques, costal cartilages, pancreas, and pineal glands obtained from pseudogout patients at necropsy showed only apatitedeposits. Therefore, BCP crystals are the crystals responsible for most non-articular calcifications.

Tendons with deposits of apatite often have hypovascular areas that are hematoxyphilic (74). As in synovium there may also be adjacent chondrometaplasia.

MILWAUKEE SHOULDER SYNDROME OR CUFF TEAR ARTHROPATHY

Gross Pathology

In one of the first reports of this arthropathy, a large, complete cuff tear was found in each patient at the time of surgery (75). In half the patients, the humeral head was fixed in a dislocated position and in the others it could be dislocated passively. In addition, the supraspinatus tendon was completely ruptured in all patients and the infraspinatus tendon in all but one instance. The teres minor and subscapularis tendons were also involved, but to a less severe degree. Seventy-five percent of the patients had pathology of the tendon of the long head of the biceps which was ruptured, dislocated, or frayed. The subdeltoid bursa was thickened, forming a large loose pouch around the head of the biceps, and contained variable amounts of clear to sanguineous synovial fluid. The articular cartilage was pebble-like. The collapsed articular surface, the major point of contact with the acromion, was eburnated and denuded of cartilage with small marginal osteophytes. The remainder of the humeral head was covered with degenerated cartilage and fibrous tissue, and the subchondral bone could be indented easily with a finger. The anterior acromial epiphysis had failed to fuse in three patients, which may have contributed to subacromial impingement.

Microscopy

Synovial biopsies obtained at the time of shoulder surgery have demonstrated increased numbers of villi, focal synovial lining cell hyperplasia, a few giant cells, fibrin, and BCP crystal deposits (76). Crystals being engulfed by synovial lining cells and histiocytes were observed with electron microscopy. Calcific deposits in synovial microvilli appeared to have access to the joint space through areas denuded of synovial lining cells.

The atrophic articular cartilage of the humeral head may be covered to a variable degree with a fibrous membrane. In these areas, the adjacent bone is osteoporotic and hypervascularized with evidence of attempts at repair in the areas of bony collapse. The cartilage may be completely denuded, and the bone is sclerotic at points of contact between the humeral head and scapula. Fragments of articular cartilage are found in the subsynovium, similar to those found in neuropathic joints.

REFERENCES

1. Van den Bosch F, Baeten D, Kruithof E, et al. Characteristic macro- and microscopic aspect of the synovial membrane in crystal induced arthritis. J Rheum 2001; 28:392–393.
2. Talbott JH, Gout. Grune & Stratton, NY 1957.
3. Hirohata K, Morimoto K. Ultrastructure of Bone and Joint Diseases. Tokyo: Igaku Shoin Ltd, 1971 p.107.
4. Sherman MS. Pathologic changes in gouty arthritis. Arch Pathol 1947; 42:557–559.
5. Sokoloff L. The pathology of gout. Metabolism 1957; 6:230–241.
6. Jayson MIV, Henderson DRF. Arthroscopy in the diagnosis of inflammatory joint disease. Rheumatol & Rehab 1973; 12:195–197.
7. Matsui N. Color atlas of arthroscopy. Med Postgraduates 1978; 16:465–466.
8. Agudelo CA, Schumacher HR. The synovitis of acute gouty arthritis A light and electron microscopic study. Hum Pathol 1973; 4:265–279.
9. Zevely HA, French AJ, Mikkelsen WM, Duff IF. Synovial specimens obtained by knee joint punch biopsy histologic study in joint diseases. Am J Med 1956; 20:510–519.
10. Simkin P, Bassett JE, Lee QP. Not water, but formalin, dissolves urate crystals in tophaceous tissue samples. J Rheumatol 1994; 21:2320–2321.

11. DeGalantha E. Technic for preservation and microscopic demonstration of nodules in gout. Am J Clin Path 1935; 5:165–166.
12. Hasselbacher P, Schumacher HR. Immunoglobulin in tophi and on the surface of monosodium urate monohydrate crystals. Arthritis Rheum 1978; 21:353–361.
13. Schumacher HR, Phelps P, Aqudelo CA. Urate crystal induced inflammation in dog joints: sequence of synovial changes. J Rheumatol 1974; 1:102–113.
14. Schumacher HR, Agudelo CA. Intravascular degranulation of neutrophils: an important factor in inflammation. Science 1972; 175:1139–1140.
15. Ropes MW, Bauer W. Synovial Fluid Changes in Joint Disease. Cambridge, MA: Harvard University Press, 1953 p.92.
16. Riddle JM, Bluhm GB, Barnhart MI. Ultrastructural study of leucocytes and urates in gouty arthritis. Ann Rheum Dis 1967; 26:389–401.
17. Schumacher HR, Reginato AJ. In: Atlas of Synovial Fluid Analysis and Crystal Identification. Philadelphia: Lea & Febiger, 1991:257.
18. Schumacher HR, Jimenez SA, Gibson T, et al. Acute gouty arthritis without urate crystals identified on initial examination of synovial fluid. Report of nine patients. Arthritis Rheum 1975; 18:603–612.
19. Tiliakos AN, Tiliakos NA. Total joint fluid urate in gout. J Clin Rheumatol 2004; 10:250–251.
20. Agudelo CA, Weinberger A, Schumacher HR, et al. Definitive diagnosis of gout by identification of urate crystals in asymptomatic metatarso phalangeal joints. Arthritis Rheum 1979; 22:559–560.
21. Weinberger A, Schumacher HR, Agudelo C. Urate crystals in asymptomatic metatarsophalangeal joints. Ann Int Med 1979; 91:56–57.
22. Li-Yu J, Clayburne G, Sieek M, Beuther A, Rull M, Eisner B, Schumacher HR. Can we determine when urate stores are depleted enough to prevent attacks of gout? J Rheumatol 2001; 28:577–580.
23. Schumacher HR, Phelps P:. Sequential changes in polymorphonuclear leucocytes after urate crystal phagocytosis: an electron microscopic study. Arthritis Rheum 1971; 14:513–526.
24. Bluhm GB, Riddle JM, Barnhart MI, et al. Crystal dynamics in gout and pseudogout. Med Times 1969; 97:135–144.
25. McCarty DJ. The inflammatory reaction to microcrystalline sodium urate. Arth Rheum 1965; 8:726–735.
26. Schumacher HR. Bullous tophi in gout. Ann Rheum Dis 1977; 36:91–93.
27. Phelps P. Polymorphonuclear leukocyte motility in vitro IV. Colchicines inhibition of chemotactic activity formation after phagocytosis of urate crystals. Arthritis Rheum 1970; 12:1–9.
28. Seegmiller JE. Toward a unitary concept of gout. Hosp Prac 1966; 1:33–39.
29. Naff GB, Byers PH. Complement as a mediator of inflammation in acute gouty arthritis I. Studies on the reaction between human serum complement and sodium urate crystals. J Lab Clin Med 1973; 81:747–760.
30. Cherian PV, Schumacher HR. Immunochemical and ultrastructural characterization of serum proteins associated with monosodium urate crystals in synovial fluid cells from patients with gout. Ultrastruct Pathol 1986; 10:209–219.
31. Kozin F, McCarty DJ. Protein absorption to monosodium urate, calcium pyrophosphate dihydrate and silica crystals. Arthritis Rheum 1976; 9:433–438.

32. Yagnik DR, Evans BJ, Florey O, et al. Macrophage release of transforming growth factor beta during resolution of monosodium urate monohydrate crystal-induced inflammation. Arthritis Rheum 2004; 50:2273–2280.
33. Barnett EV, Bienenstock J, Bluch KJ. Antinuclear factors in synovia. Possible participants in the rheumatoid inclusion body. JAMA 1966; 198:143–148.
34. Catto M. Pathology of gout. Scot Med J 1973; 18:232–238.
35. Lichtenstein L, Scott HW, Levin MH. Pathologic changes in gout. Survey of eleven necropsied cases. Am J Pathol 1956; 32:871–895.
36. Pascual E, Ordonez S. Orderly arrayed deposit of urate crystals in gout suggest epitaxial formation. Ann Rheum Dis 1998; 57:255–264.
37. Charcot JM. Clinical lectures on the diseases of old age. Translated by Leigh H, Hunt with additional lectures by Alfred L, Loomis. William Wood & Co., NY, 1881 from Wood's Library of Standard Medical Authors; the above quoted material is from pp. 56–57, Lecture, VI. Semeiology of Gout.—Uric Acid Diathesis.—Acute Gout.—Chronic Gout.
38. Emerson BT, Row PG. An evaluation of the pathogenesis of the gouty kidney. Kidney Int 1975; 8:65–71.
39. Emerson BT. Gout and renal disease. In: Smyth CJ, Helers VM, eds. Gout, Hyperuricemia & Other Crystal-Associated Arthropathies. New York: Marcel Dekker Inc, 1999:241–260.
40. Talbott JH, Yu T-F. Gout and Uric Acid Metabolism. New York: Stratton, 1976 p. 303.
41. Ball GV, Sorensen LB. Pathogenesis of hyperuricemia in saturnine gout. NEJM 1969; 280:1199–1202.
42. Gonick H, Rubini ME, Gleason IO, Sommers SC. The renal lesion in gout. Ann Int Med 1965; 62:667–674.
43. Reginato AJ, Schumacher HR, Martinez VA. The articular cartilage in familial chondrocalcinosis light and electron microscopic study. Arthritis Rheum 1974; 17:977–992.
44. Ryan L, McCarty DJ. Calcium pyrophosphate crystal deposition disease; pseudogout; articular chondrocalcinosis. In: McCarty DJ, ed. Arthritis and Allied Conditions. 11th ed. Philadelphia: Lea & Febiger, 1989:1711–1736.
45. Schumacher HR. Pathology of crystal deposition diseases. Rheum Dis Clin North Am 1988; 14:269–288.
46. Mitrovic D. Pathology of articular deposition of calcium salts and their relation to osteoarthritis. Ann Rheum Dis 1983; 42:19–26.
47. Bjelle A. Cartilage matrix in hereditary pyrophosphate arthropathy. J Rheumatol 1981; 8:959–964.
48. Ishikawa K, Masuda I, Ohira T, et al. A histopathological study of calcium pyrophosphate dihydrate crystal-deposition disease. J Bone Joint Surg 1989; 71A:866–875.
49. Ohira T, Ishikawa K, Masuda I, et al. Histologic localization of lipid in the articular tissues in calcium pyrophosphate dihydrate crystal deposition disease. Arthritis Rheum 1988; 31:1057–1062.
50. Masuda I, Ishikawa K, Usuku G, et al. A histologic and immunohistochemical study of calcium pyrophosphate dihydrate crystal deposition disease. Clin Orthop 1991; 263:272–287.
51. Chen F, Kerner MB, Dorfman HD, et al. The distribution of S-100 protein in articular cartilage from osteoarthritic joints. J Rheumatol 1990; 17:1676–1681.

52. Ishikawa K, Ueba Y, Isobe T, et al. Interaction of polymorphonuclear leukocytes with calcium pyrophosphate dihydrate crystals deposited in chondrocalcinosis cartilage. Rheumatol Int 1987; 7:217–221.
53. Ali SY, Griffiths S, Bayliss MT, et al. Ultrastructural studies of pyrophosphate crystal deposition in articular cartilage. Ann Rheum Dis 1983; 42:97–98.
54. Boivin G, Lagier R. An ultrastructural study of articular chondrocalcinosis in cases of knee osteoarthritis. Virchows Arch 1983; 400:13–29.
55. Schumacher HR. The synovitis of pseudogout: electron microscopic observations. Arthritis Rheum 1968; 11:4226–4435.
56. Wise CM, Wheeler GE, Irby MR, Schumacher HR. Synovial osteochondromatosis and pseudogout. J Rheumatol 1984; 11:229–232.
57. Schumacher HR. Ultrastructural findings in chondrocalcinosis and pseudogout. Arthritis Rheum 1976; 19:413–415.
58. Beutler A, Rothfuss S, Clayburne G, et al. Calcium pyrophosphate dihydrate crystal deposition in synovium. Arthritis Rheum 1993; 36:704–715.
59. Schumacher HR, Bonner H, Thompson JJ, et al. Tumor-like soft tissue swelling of the distal phalanx due to calcium pyrophosphate dihydrate crystal deposition. Arthritis Rheum 1984; 27:1428–1432.
60. Egan MS, Goldenberg DL, Cohen AS, et al. The association of amyloid deposits and osteoarthritis. Arthritis Rheum 1982; 25:204–208.
61. Dijkgraaf LC, Liem RS, de Bont GM, et al. Calcium pyrophosphate dihydrate crystal deposition disease: a review of the literature and a light and electron microscopic study of a case of the temporomandibular joint with numerous intracellular crystals in chondrocytes. Osteoarthritis Cartilage 1995; 3:35–45.
62. Li-Yu J, Schumacher HR, Gratwick G. Invasive tophaceous pseudogout in the temporomandibular joint: misdiagnosis as a tumor. J Clin Rheumatol 2000; 6:272–277.
63. Gordon GV, Villanueva T, Schumacher HR, Gohel V. Autopsy study correlating degree of osteoarthritis, synovitis and evidence of articular calcification. J Rheumatol 1984; 11:681–686.
64. Doyle DV. Tissue calcification and inflammation in osteoarthritis. J Pathol 1982; 136:199–216.
65. Derfus BA, Kurian JB, Butler JJ. The high prevalence of pathologic calcium crystals in preoperative knees. J Rheumatol 2002; 29:570–574.
66. Gibilisco PA, Schumacher HR, Jr., Hollander JL, Soper KA. Synovial fluid crystals in osteoarthritis. Arthritis Rheum 1985;511–515.
67. Swan A, Chapman B, Heap P, Seward H, Dieppe P. Submicroscopic crystals in osteoarthritic synovial fluids. Ann Rheum Dis 1994; 53:467–470.
68. Halverson PB, McCarty DJ. Patterns of radiographic abnormalities associated with basic calcium phosphate and calcium pyrophosphate dihydrate crystal deposition in the knee. Ann Rheum Dis 1986; 45:603–605.
69. Resnick D. Calcium hydroxyapatite crystal deposition disease. In: Resnick D, ed. Diagnosis of Bone and Joint Disorders. 4th ed. Philadelphia: WB Saunders, 2002:1619–1657.
70. Gatter RA, McCarty DJ. Pathological tissue calcification in man. Arch Pathol 1967; 84:346–353.
71. Reginato AJ, Schumacher HR. Synovial calcification in a patient with collagen-vascular disease: light and electron microscopic studies. J Rheumatol 1877; 4:261–271.

72. Li-Yu J, Clayburne GM, Sieck MS, et al. Calcium apatite crystals in synovial fluid rice bodies. Ann Rheum Dis 2002; 61:387–390.
73. Schumacher HR, Cherian PV. Transmission electron microscopic studies on articular calcium crystals and associated protein coatings. Scanning Electron Microsc 1984; 11:965–968.
74. Uhthoff HK, Sarkar K, Maynard JA. Calcifying tendonitis: A new concept of its pathogenesis. Clin Orthop 1976; 118:164–168.
75. Halverson PB. Basic calcium phosphate (apatite, octacalcium phosphate) crystal deposition diseases and calcinosis. In: Koopman WJ, Moorland LW, eds. Arthritis and Allied Conditions. 15th ed. Philadelphia: Lea & Febiger, 2005:2397–2416.
76. Halverson PB, Grancis JC, McCarty DJ. Histopathologic and ultrastructural studies of Milwaukee shoulder syndrome-a basic calcium phosphate crystal arthropathy. Ann Rheum Dis 1984; 43:734–741.

19

Management of Crystal-Induced Arthropathies

Robert L. Wortmann
Division of Rheumatology, Department of Medicine, University of Oklahoma College of Medicine, Tulsa, Oklahoma, U.S.A.

Lawrence M. Ryan
Division of Rheumatology, Department of Medicine, Medical College of Wisconsin, Milwaukee, Wisconsin, U.S.A.

INTRODUCTION

The goals in managing patients with gout and hyperuricemia are to terminate the acute attack as promptly as possible; to prevent recurrences of acute gouty arthritis; to prevent or reverse complications of the disease resulting from deposition of sodium urate or uric acid crystals in joints, kidneys, or other sites; and to prevent or reverse associated conditions, such as hypertension, obesity, hypertriglyceridemia, and alcoholism. Given that the cause of gout is known, it can be diagnosed with absolute certainty, and excellent therapies exist, then these goals should be achievable. Although more common, arthropathies caused by calcium pyrophosphate dihydrate (CPPD) crystal deposition are more difficult to treat because therapies that eliminate the cause (i.e., eliminate the crystals) are not available. Therefore the management of these diseases is more supportive and palliative in nature. Below the strategies available to help patients with various forms of crystal-induced arthropathy are reviewed.

MONOSODIUM URATE CRYSTAL DEPOSITION DISEASE: GOUT

Acute Gouty Arthritis

The acute gouty attack may be successfully treated with any of several drugs. These include colchicine, a nonsteroidal anti-inflammatory drug (NSAID), corticotropin (ACTH), or a corticosteroid preparation. Whereas these drugs relieve symptoms and help terminate the attack, their mechanisms of action do not correct the underlying hyperuricemia nor do they alter the progression of urate crystal deposition. The time of initiation of therapy is more important than the choice of drug. With any of these agents, the sooner the drug is started, the more rapidly a complete response will be attained. Thus, patients at risk should be advised to keep an oral agent close at hand at all times, and to use it at the first inkling of an attack. Generally, colchicine is preferred for patients in whom the diagnosis of gout is not crystal-proven, whereas NSAIDs are preferred when the diagnosis is known. If a patient cannot take medications by mouth or has active peptic ulcer disease, the choice is among intra-articular glucocorticoid, parenteral glucocorticoids, intramuscular ACTH, or intravenous colchicine. Local application of ice packs may help control the pain of an acute attack (1). In some cases, analgesics, including narcotics, may be added as well. Drugs that affect serum urate concentrations, including urate-lowering agents, should not be changed (either initiated or discontinued) during an acute attack. Just as sudden fluctuations in serum urate levels may precipitate an acute attack, an inflammatory reaction already in progress may be made substantially worse by a major fluctuation in the serum urate concentration.

Colchicine

Colchicine has been used to treat gout for more than 3000 years (2) and, as such, is recognized as the classic drug to use to treat acute gout attacks. It is the most specific agent available for the treatment of gout because its activities are effective predominantly in crystal-induced inflammation. This drug can be administered orally or by intravenous infusion. Orally, a dose of 0.5 or 0.6 mg is taken every one or two hours until one of three things occurs: (1) joint symptoms resolve; (2) gastrointestinal side effects develop; or (3) the patient has taken ten doses without relief. If ten doses are taken without benefit, one should discontinue the colchicine and question the accuracy of the diagnosis. Alternative regimens include a loading dose of 1.0 mg followed by 0.5 mg every two to six hours or 1.0 mg three times a day (3,4). Colchicine is most effective if initiated within the first 12 hours of an attack. Its efficacy is substantially reduced when administered 48 or more hours after the onset of an attack (5,6).

Colchicine has a low therapeutic index with steady-state plasma concentrations after acute treatment ranging between 0.5 and 3.0 ng/mL and with toxic effects occurring at approximately 3 ng/mL (7). Therefore, in most patients, the side effects precede or coincide with improvement in joint symptoms. Gastrointestinal side effects develop in 50% to 80% of patients and include cramping abdominal pain, increased peristalsis, diarrhea, nausea, or vomiting. The drug must be stopped promptly at the first sign of side effects (8).

Oral colchicine may be poorly tolerated by the elderly and those with renal insufficiency or liver disease, and therefore is best avoided in these patients (6–9). If employed in a setting of renal insufficiency, the dosage should be reduced. Colchicine therapy should be avoided in transplant patients with gout who are taking cyclosporine due to its potential to cause neuromyopathy (10,11).

Colchicine can also be administered intravenously. When used properly, the drug abolishes the acute attack with a low incidence of gastrointestinal side effects (provided that the patient is not also taking colchicine by mouth). An initial dose of 1 or 2 mg can be followed by one or two additional 1 mg doses administered at six hour intervals thereafter if needed. The total dose of intravenous colchicine should not exceed 4 mg (8). In those treated with intravenous colchicine, the use of oral colchicine must be avoided for 7 days because colchicine is retained in the white cells.

The colchicine for intravenous use should be diluted with 20 ml of normal saline before administration and given slowly into an established venous access to minimize sclerosis of the vein. Extravasation will cause extreme pain and severe tissue damage. In addition, oral colchicine should be discontinued and no additional colchicine should be given for at least 7 days because of slow excretion of this drug (3,12). The use of intravenous colchicine is discouraged by many and considered contraindicated by others. The reason for these cautions is due to its potential for serious adverse events including bone marrow suppression, oliguric renal failure, hepatic necrosis, severe diarrhea, seizures, and death (5,13,14). These have invariably occurred in patients who received inappropriate dosing.

Nonsteroidal Anti-inflammatory Drugs

For the majority of patients with gout, and especially for those in whom the diagnosis is confirmed by crystal identification, NSAIDs are preferred over colchicine due to their more favorable side effect profile and increased duration of efficacy (5,6). Currently there are numerous NSAIDs to select among. Traditional NSAIDs, such as indomethacin, naproxen, ibuprofen, and diclofenac, that inhibit both isoforms of cyclooxygenase (COX-1 and COX-2) and the relatively newer agents, such as celecoxib and etoricoxib, that are selective inhibitors of COX-2, are effective. In fact, with respect to the relief of pain and inflammation, there is no good evidence to indicate that one NSAID is more efficacious than another. This was demonstrated in a study that found comparable relief in patients treated with indomethacin or a selective COX-2 inhibitor, etoricoxib (15). Therefore, the choice of NSAID is made with consideration of the patient's history, associated diseases, risk of side effects, dosage frequency, and cost.

Traditional NSAIDs such as indomethacin 100 mg initially followed by 50 mg every 6 hours, naproxen 500 mg every 8 or 12 hours, and diclofenac sodium 50 mg every 8 hours are the more commonly used agents in the treatment of patients with gout. These doses should be administered until symptoms resolve and then gradually tapered over 5 to 7 days. As with other agents used to treat acute gouty arthritis, the sooner treatment is initiated after the signs of inflammation are recognized, the faster the attack will be eliminated. For this reason, patients are advised to have a supply of the NSAID with them at all times so they can begin treatment at the very first sign of a flare.

NSAIDs are relatively well tolerated by patients with gout. This may be in part because the symptoms of the attack are so severe that they overshadow milder side effects. More likely the tolerance is related to the short duration of use. Potential adverse events include nausea, dyspepsia, diarrhea, headache, and confusion. The use of these agents may induce fluid retention, hypertension, and elevation of serum creatinine. NSAIDs are relatively contraindicated in patients with renal insufficiency, should be used carefully in patients with comorbid medical conditions such as hypertension or heart failure, and are best avoided in individuals with previous or current peptic ulcer disease or gastric bleeding (6,9).

The risk for gastrointestinal events with NSAID treatment increases for those who are taking concurrent aspirin therapy, even at low cardioprotective doses. These patients warrant co-therapy with a proton pump inhibitor to reduce their risk for gastric symptoms and/or injury (16). The use of parenteral NSAID therapy, such as intramuscular ketorolac, carries the same risks as oral NSAIDs (5,6).

Corticosteroids and Corticotrophin

The use of corticosteroids administered systemically is usually reserved for patients who have refractory gout, who are intolerant of colchicine or NSAIDs, or who have medical conditions contraindicating the use of those agents (17,18). The occurrence of acute gouty attacks in patients receiving cyclosporine and maintenance prednisone at doses ranging from 7.5 to 15 mg a day indicates the need for the use of relatively large dose of corticosteroids in the treatment of acute gout (19). Prednisone is administered orally at a dose of 20 to 60 mg daily. Doses of methylprednisolone between 100 and 150 mg per day have also been recommended (20). The dose of either is then gradually tapered over the next 7 to 10 days, depending on rapidity of response.

Given parenterally, these agents are effective alternatives for patients who develop gout postoperatively or cannot use oral agents for any reason. Intramuscular administration of triamcinolone diacetate 60 mg or methylprednisolone acetate 40 mg daily, repeated every 1 to 4 days as needed, can be used to provide prompt control of gout symptoms (21). Intravenous methylprednisolone sodium succinate 40 to 60 mg also may be employed (22,23). Although not recommended as routine therapy, an intramuscular dose of corticotrophin (ACTH) gel (25 to 80 IU) is effective. In theory, corticotropin may be more effective than corticosteroids because, in addition to inducing endogenous corticosteroid production by the adrenal glands, it interferes with the acute inflammatory response through local activation of melanocortin receptor-3 (24). Although a single dose of parenteral corticosteroids or corticotropin gel may be all that is required, repeat administration as needed every 24 to 72 hours may be necessary to eliminate all signs of the flare (25).

Corticosteroids can also be administered intra-articularly (26,27). The route of administration is also useful in patients who cannot take oral agents, in older patients with multiple organ dysfunction, or in patients with organ transplants. Triamcinolone hexacetonide at doses of 10 to 40 mg or methylprednisolone acetate, 5 to 60 mg, have been effective. Higher doses are used according to the size of the joint and, perhaps, the degree of inflammation. Corticosteroid injections should be avoided if there is a possibility of a septic joint and given with care in those patients who are receiving concurrent anticoagulant therapy. In the latter situation, it is prudent to administer the injection using the smallest gauge needle possible (preferably smaller than 22 gauge), to manipulate the needle as little as possible, and to hold the pressure over the injection site for several minutes after instillation of the medication.

Patients treated with corticosteroids or corticotropin should be closely monitored for gout symptom flare during and following the dose tapering period. Side effects include fluid retention, glucose intolerance, electrolyte shifts, blood pressure elevation, and increased susceptibility to infection.

Preventing Further Attacks

Once an individual has suffered one attack of acute gouty arthritis, the likelihood of another attack is very high. In one study analyzing patients not treated with urate-lowering agents, 62% of the individuals experienced a recurrence within the first year of the initial attack, 78% by 2 years, and 89% by 5 years (28). In addition to relapse of acute attacks, without urate-lowering therapy tophi develop. Although tophi may not become apparent or appear for 3 to 10 yr (29,30), it is clear that they are growing undetected, yet eliciting the destructive chronic inflammatory response, long before becoming visible or palpable (31).

To eliminate acute attacks and tophi, it is necessary to return the total body pool of urate to normal (32–34). This is accomplished by maintaining serum urate levels consistently below 6.8 mg/dL, preferably at levels of 4 to 5 mg/dL (35,36). But precisely when urate-lowering therapy should be initiated is debated. Some believe that urate-lowering therapy be initiated after the first attack of gout, arguing that the disease has declared itself and will only progress (37,38). Because many patients do not experience a second attack for years, many authors maintain that long-term therapy is only required for those experiencing more than 2 to 4 episodes per year (39,40). The decision to initiate urate-lowering therapy should be made on a case by case basis. Some individuals find the first attack to be so debilitating and incapacitating that they want to do anything to avoid another. Others would rather see how long it takes before the second attack occurs. From an economic perspective, the cost of urate-lowering maintenance therapy in those with more than two attacks per year is considered to be less than that of acute attack management and treatment of NSAID-induced gastrointestinal adverse events (41).

Therapy with specific urate-lowering agents should be given until 2 to 3 weeks after all symptoms of a gout flare have resolved. In addition, when initiating urate-lowering maintenance therapy, patients should be made aware that this treatment may precipitate an acute gout attack. This fact is well recognized and probably occurs in at least 25% of patients (42,43). Lowering the serum urate level, by any means, can provoke a flare, and the more rapidly the urate is lowered, the more likely one will occur.

Prophylaxis

Several urate-lowering initiation strategies have been suggested to avoid acute flares. One is to initiate the urate-lowering agent at a low dose and then increase the dose by small increments every 7 to 14 days until the target serum urate level is attained. The other strategy involves the practice of giving low daily doses of colchicine or NSAID as prophylaxis. This approach is effective in preventing acute attacks in up to 85% (44). Prophylactic therapy is best initiated two weeks prior to starting the urate-lowering agent and then continued. How long to continue the prophylactic agent is difficult to tell, because patients with gout are at risk for an attack as long as there is excess urate in their bodies (32,45,46). Opinions vary from 3 to 12 months (47,48). One approach is to maintain the prophylactic therapy for 4 to 6 months after the patient's serum urate level reached and is sustained at the target value of 4.0 to 5.0 mg/dL and he or she has been free of attacks. Regardless of when the prophylactic agent is discontinued, the patient must be warned that a subsequent attack may occur and be instructed to take colchicine or an NSAID at the first hint of flare. Finally, prophylactic treatment is not recommended unless one also uses urate-lowering agents, because such treatment may block the acute inflammatory response but does not alter the deposition of crystals in tissues. With continued deposition, but without the warning signs of recurrent bouts of acute arthritis, tophi and destruction to cartilage and bone can occur insidiously and undetected.

The use of colchicine at 0.6 mg once to three times a day is generally well tolerated, although patients are at risk to develop an axonal neuromyopathy (49,50). This complication, which is reversible by discontinuing the drug, causes proximal muscle weakness with or without painful paresthesia and elevated serum levels of creatine phosphokinase. It most often develops in patients also using diuretics and with concurrent hypertension, renal dysfunction, or liver disease. Rhabdomyolysis may also occur, especially in patients concomitantly taking an HMG CoA reductase inhibitor (statin) or cyclosporin (50).

In patients who are unable to tolerate even one colchicine tablet per day, indomethacin, naproxen, or another NSAID has been used prophylactically at low doses with some success (i.e., indomethacin 25 mg two times a day or naproxen 250 mg twice a day) (36,47,51). A program of maintenance colchicine or an NSAID may make the difference between frequent incapacitation and uninterrupted daily activities.

CONTROL OF HYPERURICEMIA

Individuals taking urate-lowering agents should also understand that treatment must be continuous (i.e., lifelong) and not intermittent (5). The patient should also understand the purpose and importance of maintaining a serum urate level below 6.8 mg/dL. Lowering the serum urate level from 10.0 or 12.0 mg/dL to 7.5 or 8.0 mg/dL may look encouraging. However, such a change only retards the rate at which crystal deposition continues; it does not reverse the process. Accordingly, serum urate levels should be assessed on a regular basis to assure that appropriate levels (4.0 to 5.0 mg/dL) are being maintained.

In general, the lower the serum urate level achieved during antihyperuricemic therapy, the faster the reduction in tophaceous deposits. (52). Reduction to target levels may be achieved pharmacologically by the use of xanthine oxidase inhibitors or uricosuric agents. Xanthine oxidase, the enzyme that catalyzes the oxidation of hypoxanthine to xanthine and xanthine to uric acid, is inhibited by allopurinol oxypurinol and febuxostat. Probenecid, sulfinpyrazone, and benzbromarone are uricosuric agents that reduce serum urate concentrations by enhancing the renal excretion of uric acid. These antihyperuricemic drugs do not have anti-inflammatory properties. Each of these agents will be effective if used in sufficient dose to attain a sustained serum urate level of less that 6.8 mg/dL.

For those patients with gout who excrete less than 800 mg of uric acid per day and have normal renal function, reduction of serum urate concentration can be achieved equally well with a xanthine oxidase inhibitor or a uricosuric drug. These agents are equally effective in preventing deterioration of renal function in patients with primary gout (53).

Xanthine Oxidase Inhibitors

In most cases, a xanthine oxidase inhibitor is probably the drug of choice because it can be used with fewer restrictions compared with uricosuric agents. However, in certain situations, a xanthine oxidase inhibitor is clearly the drug of choice. Patients with gout who excrete larger quantities of urinary uric acid or who have a history of renal calculi of any type should be treated with a xanthine oxidase inhibitor. The incidence of renal calculi is about 35% in patients with primary gout who excrete more than 700 mg/day of uric acid (54). There is also greater risk for uric acid stones upon initiation of uricosuric therapy.

A final absolute indication for a xanthine oxidase inhibitor is the failure of uricosuric agents to produce a serum urate concentration lower than 6 mg/dL or patient intolerance to the uricosuric agent. Xanthine oxidase inhibitors and uricosuric agents may be used in combination for the patient with tophaceous gout in whom it is not possible to reduce the serum urate below 6 mg/dL with a single agent. In most settings, if a xanthine oxidase inhibitor does not cause the serum urate to fall below 6 mg/dL, it is the result of insufficient dosing or poor patient compliance.

Xanthine oxidase inhibitors are involved in relatively few drug-drug interactions. The most important of these are azathioprine and 6-mercaptopurine. In addition, allopurinol can reduce the activity of hepatic microsomal drug-metabolizing enzymes and prolong the half-lives of warfarin and theophylline.

The xanthine oxidase inhibitors include allopurinol, oxypurinol, and febuxostat (see Chapter 24). Each should be used at the lowest dose that lowers the serum urate level to the range of 4.0 to 5.0 mg/dL. Allopurinol can be started at doses of 100 mg a day and increased until the desired serum urate level is attained. The most frequently prescribed dose of allopurinol is 300 mg per day, but a maximum of 800 mg can be used. Recent evidence indicates that only 21 to 55% of gout patients reach an appropriate target serum urate level on 300 mg a day.

About 20% of patients who take allopurinol report side effects with 5% of patients discontinuing the medication. More common side effects include gastrointestinal intolerance and skin rashes. The occurrence of a rash does not necessarily mean that the drug be discontinued. If the rash is not severe, the allopurinol can be held temporarily and resumed after the rash has cleared. Oral and intravenous protocols for desensitization to allopurinol have been proven successful for some patients following cutaneous reactions (see Chapter 24) (55,56).

Other adverse reactions include fever, toxic epidermal necrolysis, alopecia, bone marrow suppression with leukopenia or thrombocytopenia, agranulocytosis, aplastic anemia, granulomatous hepatitis, jaundice, sarcoid-like reaction, and vasculitis. The most serve reaction is the allopurinol hypersensitivity syndrome that consists of a constellation of findings and may include fever, skin rash, eosinophilia, hepatitis, progressive renal insufficiency, and death (57,58). This is most likely to develop in individuals with pre-existing renal dysfunction and those taking diuretics.

Febuxostat is xanthine oxidase inhibitor with a chemical structure entirely different than allopurinol. It appears that febuxostat is an excellent alternative for patients who cannot tolerate allopurinol (59). In phase II clinical trials, febuxostat doses of 40, 80, and 120 mg successfully lowered serum urate levels below 6.0 mg/dL in 56%, 76%, and 94% of subjects, respectively (43). In a phase III trial, target serum urates were reached in 53% and 62% of subjects taking febuxostat 80 and 120 mg, respectively compared to 21% of patients taking 300 mg of allopurinol (60). In a phase III trial, the side effect profile for febuxostat and allopurinol were similar. No cases of hypersensitivity have been reported with the use of febuxostat.

Uricosuric Agents

In general, the candidate for uricosuric agents is the gouty patient who is younger than 60 years of age and has normal renal function (creatinine clearance greater than 80 ml/min), a 24-hour urinary uric acid excretion of less than 800 mg on a general diet, and no history of nephrolithiasis. Patients prescribed uricosuric agents should avoid salicylate use at doses greater than 81 mg per day (61).

Probenecid and sulfinpyrazone are the most widely used uricosuric agents available in the United States and Canada. Benzbromarone is used for this purpose in other countries as well (see Chapter 23). The maintenance dosage of probenecid ranges from 500 mg to 3 g per day and is administered on a twice or three times a day schedule. Acute gouty attacks may accompany the initiation of this medication, as with all other anti-hyperuricemic agents, and, as with any uricosuric agent, patients using probenecid are at increased risk for developing renal calculi. Gastrointestinal complaints, hypersensitivity, and rash limit its use in over 5% of patients. Although serious toxicity is rare, approximately one-third of individuals eventually become intolerant of probenecid and discontinue its use. Sulfinpyrazone is usually maintained at a daily dosage of 300 to 400 mg per day given in three to four divided doses. The rates of tolerability and types of adverse reactions are similar to those with probenecid. Benzbromarone is a more potent uricosuric (52). It is well tolerated and effective in cyclosporine-treated renal transplant patients.

Lowering Serum Urate Levels in Patients with Renal Insufficiency

Patients with gout and mild renal insufficiency may be given either type of agent, but probenecid and sulfinpyrazone would not be expected to work when the glomerular filtration rate is less than 30 mL/min. In contrast, the uricosuric agent benzbroarone can be used with moderate renal dysfunction (creatine clearance less than 25mi/min) (52). Allopurinol is effective in the presence of renal insufficiency, but doses may have to be decreased in that situation. It appears that febuxostat can be given to patients with mild to moderate renal insufficiency with-out dose adjustment. In general, the agent selected should be initiated at a low dose and gradually titrated until the desired target serum urate level is reached.

Management of Gout After Organ Transplantation

Gout after organ transplantation is a complex disease to manage. The use of glucocorticoids, azathioprine, or cyclosporine and the precarious status of renal function in many patients pose complex problems. For example, gout flare can occur even though patients are taking maintenance doses of prednisone (i.e., 7.5 to 15 mg per day) (19). In addition, use of NSAIDs or colchicine may be inappropriate in this setting because of their potential toxicities. However, colchicine can be used in prophylactic doses if renal function is normal and the patient is monitored closely. The combination of colchicine and cyclosporin can cause rhabdomyolysis (49). Intra-articular glucocorticoid injections may be most helpful, and one may be forced to rely more heavily on the use of pain medications in this setting.

When considering chronic therapy, it should be helpful to lower the doses of cyclosporine and eliminate the use of diuretics if possible. Uricosuric agents can be used safely if renal function is good. Of this class, only benzbromarone can be employed if renal insufficiency is present (52). Allopurinol can be used in patients with abnormal renal function, but the dose may need to be reduced depending on renal function. Febuxostat may be used with less dose modification. Both xanthine oxidase inhibitors, however, have potential severe interaction with azathioprine. Azathioprine is metabolized by xanthine oxidase. Because allopurinol, oxypurinol, and febuxostat inhibit that enzyme, the breakdown of azathioprine is slowed, increasing the effective dose. If care is not taken, significant bone marrow toxicity can result. If azathioprine and allopurinol are used together, they can be started at 25 and 50 mg/day, respectively (62). Complete blood counts and serum urate level concentrations should be monitored weekly, and the xanthine inhibitor dose should be adjusted to bring the serum urate concentration to less than 6 mg/dL. Mycophenolate mofetil, as an alternative to azathioprine, has been used effectively with allopurinol in some transplant patients (63).

ANCILLARY FACTORS

In addition to anti-inflammatory agents, colchicine prophylaxis, and urate-lowering therapy, other factors may be decisive in determining whether recurrent attacks, chronic gouty arthritis, or nephrolithiasis develop. Today, dietary purine restriction solely to control serum urate levels is rarely necessary. Although a diet totally restricted in purines can reduce the urinary excretion of uric acid by only 200 to 400 mg per day and lower the mean serum urate value by about 1 mg/dL (64), it is not a diet one can tolerate for long. In addition, the urate-lowering agents available are so effective that one rarely needs to consider this kind of dietary manipulation. Nevertheless, beneficial results have been reported with a diet of moderate calorie and carbohydrate restriction and increased proportional intake of protein and unsaturated fat (65).

Some subjects with gout are susceptible to acute attacks after the use of alcoholic beverages or consumption of rich foods. Others describe idiosyncratic responses, such as acute gout after ingesting a particular food, but such relationships are rare and questionable.

Diet is important with regards to other medical problems (66). Many gouty patients are obese, and restoration of ideal body weight through regulated caloric restriction is recommended. In addition, at least 75% of patients with primary gout have hypertriglyceridemia. The initial step in management of hypertriglyceridemia is reduction to ideal body weight and elimination of alcohol ingestion. Fenofibrate is an excellent agent for individuals with gout who require medication to treat their lipid abnormalities, because it has modest uricosuric properties (67).

About one-third of gouty subjects are hypertensive. Many hypertensive gouty patients require a thiazide diuretic. If this medication is needed to control hypertension, it should be used with the recognition that the dosage of the urate-lowering agent may need to be adjusted to maintain appropriate control of serum urate levels. The angiotensin receptor blocking agent losartan has modest uricosuric properties and should be considered for use in the patient with gout and hypertension (68,69).

Many patients with gout consume liberal amounts of alcohol. Acute excess alcohol intake is often followed by an acute attack. The added purine load resulting from regular ingestion of beer and, to a degree, liquor (but not wine taken in moderation) may also be a contributing factor (70). Compliance with medication may also be worse among patients who consume alcohol in excess.

Compliance and the Treatment of Gout

Because the processes involved in developing gout are so well understood, the diagnosis can be definitively established, and therapies available are so effective, gout should be a readily treated disease. However, too many patients, including those who are accurately diagnosed, do not do well. Failure of anti-hyperuricemic therapy to attain the target urate level is due to improper prescribing or poor compliance (71). It appears that too often patients are prescribed a urate-lowering agent at a certain strength and that dose is never changed. Noncompliance is well recognized as a problem when treating chronic asymptomatic conditions. Alcoholism can also be a factor. Perhaps most importantly, patients may be required to take up to three different medications on three different schedules to both control their symptoms and treat the disease.

It is believed that if patients understand why they are taking medications they are more likely to be compliant. To this end, an analogy has been developed that has helped some patients become more compliant (72). In this analogy urate crystals are compared to matches. The patient is told that "when the match strikes," it causes a gout attack. "To put out the fire" the patient takes an NSAID or colchicine, and this should be done at the first sign of an attack, because if treatment is delayed "more matches will catch fire." Although taking the anti-inflammatory medication resolves the attack, "the matches are still there." To eliminate future attacks the patient is given prophylactic colchicine, "which makes the matches damp and harder to strike," and a xanthine oxidase inhibitor or uricosuric agent "which actually removes the matches from the body."

Asymptomatic Hyperuricemia

The presence of hyperuricemia is rarely an indication for specific urate-lowering drug therapy, but it is not something that should be ignored. When encountered, it is appropriate that its cause is determined and that the patient is evaluated for associated conditions. Hyperuricemia may be the initial clue to the presence of a previously unsuspected disorder. In 70% of hyperuricemic patients, an underlying cause of the hyperuricemia can be readily defined by history and physical examination. The nature of the underlying cause may be useful in predicting the potential consequence, if any, of the elevated serum urate level.

The decision whether to treat hyperuricemia uncomplicated by articular gout, urolithiasis, or nephropathy is an exercise in clinical judgment about which there is less than universal agreement. When considering whether to treat asymptomatic hyperuricemia with urate-lowering agents, the following considerations are relevant: renal function is not adversely affected by elevated serum urate concentrations alone, and the renal disease that accompanies hyperuricemia most often is related to inadequately controlled hypertension or an inherited disorder. The critical question is whether correction of hyperuricemia has any effect on renal function or the development of hypertension or heart disease (see Chapter 5).

At this time, it seems prudent to not treat asymptomatic hyperuricemia with specific urate-lowering agents until symptoms attributable to the hyperuricemia develop. Rare exceptions include individuals with a known hereditary cause of uric acid overproduction of familial juvenile hyperuricemic nephropathy or patients at risk for tumor lysis syndrome. It is, however, strongly recommended that the cause of hyperuricemia be determined and any associated factors related to the process, such as obesity, hyperlipidemia, alcoholism, and especially hypertension, be addressed.

CALCIUM PYROPHOSPHATE DIHYDRATE CRYSTAL DEPOSITION DISEASE

Acute Pseudogout

There are no specific therapies for CPPD deposition disease. Pseudogout is currently managed with therapies similar to those used for acute gout. Oral colchicine is often used for acute pseudogout, but has not been rigorously studied in clinical trials. Intravenous colchicine has been proven effective in acute pseudogout attacks (73,74). It should be used judiciously because of its potentially life-threatening toxicities (75). NSAIDs remain a mainstay of therapy, but have not been studied in clinical trials. Intra-articular steroid injections remain the most logical and, perhaps, the most effective of the treatment choices for pseudogout patients. This treatment reduces the duration of the acute attack by one-half to one-third. Intra-articular therapy also eliminates concerns about side effects of NSAIDs and colchicine in this high-risk, primarily elderly population. Joint aspiration even without steroid injection may also be an effective therapy in acute pseudogout. Systemic steroids should not routinely be used in pseudogout attacks, but may be reserved for patients intolerant to other therapies. One small study suggested parenteral corticotropin was modestly effective in selected patients (76). Another report demonstrated a modest response to intramuscular triamcinolone (77). Although there is little concrete evidence that we can affect the frequency of acute attacks in pseudogout, some small studies suggest that oral colchicine may reduce the number of attacks in some patients (78).

Other Forms of CPPD Deposition Disease

Even less is known about therapy in chronic forms of CPPD deposition disease. NSAIDs remain the standard of care in most cases. Oral magnesium supplementation was used in a single small placebo-controlled clinical trial of crystal-proven patients (79). It did appear to improve pain and stiffness in some patients. However, the differences between magnesium-treated patients and those treated with placebo were not statistically significant. There is no evidence to support the use of systemic steroids for chronic symptoms in CPPD arthritis. Hydroxychloroquine was used in one small trial (80). Parenteral gold salts and other drugs used for rheumatoid arthritis have been tried for rheumatoid-like presentations of CPPD deposition, but have not been studied in clinical trials. Many patients with severe large joint disease ultimately require joint replacement.

BASIC CALCIUM PHOSPHATE ARTHROPATHY

Non-inflammatory Arthropathy

Treatment is generally unsatisfactory as many patients are unaware of the abnormalities until late in the disease. NSAIDs containing magnesium were anecdotally helpful for pain and proposed to reduce volume of joint effusion (81). Repeated aspiration with or without corticosteroid injection or tidal irrigation is frequently needed (82). Physical therapy including thermotherapy with heat, mobilizing exercise, isometric or strengthening exercise, and conditioning exercise can help to preserve the remaining function and maintain muscle strength. Shoulder arthroplasty has not been well studied in Milwaukee shoulder syndrome. In a case of rupture of the shoulder joint capsule, arthroplasty was required, and arthrodesis was performed in one case with a draining sinus (83).

Acute Inflammatory Arthritis and Periarthritis

For acute calcific periarthritis, use of ice and anti-inflammatory drugs such as NSAIDs or colchicine are helpful. With anti-inflammatory treatment, periarthritis resolves within a few weeks with an average duration of 4.9 days (84). During the acute period, mobilization to pain tolerance and isometric exercise is allowed (85). Calcific deposits that do not decrease in size with time, that are larger than 5 mm, and that continue to cause nocturnal pain may be removed by needle aspiration under fluoroscopic or ultrasonographic guidance followed by steroid injection (86). Mechanical disruption and dispersion of deposits with the needle facilitates dissolution. In some patients whose deposits remain symptomatic after acute attack, open or arthroscopic surgical removal becomes necessary. Ultrasound treatment over the calcified area for 6 weeks helps decrease the pain and resolve the calcification (87). Multiple studies have shown effectiveness of extracorporeal shock wave treatment (88–90). One controlled study has shown significant improvement in function without pain reduction in the treated group (91). Acupuncture anecdotally relieves pain in a large number of patients with chronic shoulder pain from periarthritis (92).

Diffuse Idiopathic Skeletal Hyoerostosis

Treatment of diffuse idiopathic skeletal hyoerostosis (DISH) is conservative. Osteophytectomy may be required in some cases. It should be noted that difficult intubation may be encountered, and hyperextended posture during surgery rarely results in spinal fracture-dislocation (93).

Tumoral Calcinosis

Surgical removal of the calcification may not be curative as the mass can recur.

Fibrodysplasia Ossificans Progressiva

Definitive treatment is lacking. Many case reports have shown improvement with different medications. Corticosteroids can be used to control inflammation in the early phase. Disodium etidronate (EHDP) is the most frequently employed with varying dosages and results (94–97). Whether it can prevent new lesion and resolve preexisting ossification is to be proved. As a result of long duration of treatment with etidronate, osteomalacia may develop. Isotretinoin was helpful in one observational study (98). Perivascular lymphocytic infiltration is the earliest pathologic finding in this condition, and these lymphocytes overexpressed bone morphogenetic protein-4 (BMP-4), a potent osteogenic morphogen (99). Interestingly, the progression in one patient was halted by bone marrow transplantation aimed at treating aplastic anemia (100). Based on the pathogenesis, rituximab is proposed to be helpful by inhibition of B lymphocytes (101). In an animal study, a BMP-4 antagonist, noggin mutein, abrogated cartilage formation and heterotopic ossification in BMP-4-induced heterotopic ossification in mice (102). Surgery is often followed by recurrence (95,96). Prevention of injuries should be underscored.

Calcinosis and Connective Tissue Diseases

There is no proven effective treatment of calcification in these conditions, but treatment of dermatomyositis may improve calcification. Reports of small numbers of patients have shown benefits from warfarin for calcification in scleroderma and dermatomyositis, probenecid and aluminum hydroxide in dermatomyositis, and diltiazem in limited scleroderma or other connective tissue diseases (103,104). Colchicine or NSAIDs have been helpful for the occasional acute inflammation event in dermatomyositis or scleroderma (105,106). Large deposits may require surgical excision. Since staphylococcal skin infections have been associated with accelerated calcification, prompt treatment of cutaneous infection seems warranted.

Myositis Ossificans

Multiple pharmacologic interventions have been used without clear benefits. Numerous types of NSAIDs, in particular indomethacin, and post-operative low-dose irradiation have been shown to be superior to placebo in terms of controlling inflammation and lowering the incidence of bone formation (107–109). Disodium etidronate has been used for acute lesion, but rebound ossification related to its use necessitates a prolonged duration of treatment (107). Two randomized controlled trials revealed contradictory outcome after spinal cord injuries (110,111). No study has established its long-term outcome. Currently, etidronate is not yet recommended as a standard treatment for acute heterotopic ossification after spinal cord injury (111). Surgical removal is often followed by recurrence.

REFERENCES

1. Schlesinger N, Detry MA, Holland BK, et al. Local ice therapy during bouts of acute gouty arthritis. J Rheumatol 2002; 29:331–336.
2. Molad Y. Update on colchicine and its mechanism of action. Curr Rheumatol Rep 2002; 4:252–256.
3. Kim KY, Schumacher H, Hunsche E, et al. A literature review of the epidemiology and treatment of acute gout. Clin Ther 2003; 25:1593–1617.
4. Ahern MJ, Reid C, Gordon TP, et al. Does colchicine work? The results of the first controlled study in acute gout Aust N Z J Med 1987; 17:301–304.
5. Emmerson BT. The management of gout. N Engl J Med 1996; 334:445–451.
6. Fam AG. "Problem" gout: clinical challenges, effective solutions. J Musculoskelet Med 1997; 14:63–77.
7. Iacobuzio-Donahue CA, Lee EL, Abraham SC, et al. Colchicine toxicity. Distinct morphologic findings in gastrointestinal biopsies. Am J Surg Path 2001; 25:1067–1970.
8. Wallace SL, Singer JZ. Review: systemic toxicity associated with the intravenous administration of colchicines—guidelines for use. J Rheumatol 1988; 15:495–500.
9. Dieppe PA. Investigation and management of gout in the young and the elderly. Ann Rheum Dis 1991; 50:263–266.
10. Beathge BA, Work J, Landreneau MD, et al. Tophaceous gout in patients with renal transplants treated with cyclosporine, A. J Rheumatol 1993; 20:718–720.
11. Gerster JC, Landry M, Dufresne L, et al. Imaging of tophaceous gout: computed tomography provider specific images compared to magnetic resonance imaging and ultrasonography. Ann Rheum Dis 2002; 61:2002–2007.
12. Evans TI, Wheeler MT, Small RE, et al. A comprehensive investigation of inpatient intravenous colchicine use shows more education is needed. J Rheumatol 1996; 23:143–148.
13. Rosenthal AK, Ryan LM. Treatment of refractory crystal-associated arthritis. Rheum Dis Clin North Am 1995; 21:151–161.
14. Wallace SL, Singer JZ. Review: systemic toxicity associated with the intravenous administration of colchicines—guidelines for use. J Rheumatol 1988; 15:495–499.

15. Schumacher HR, Jr., Boice JA, Daikh DI, et al. Randomized double blind trial of etoricoxib and indomethacin in treatment of acute gouty arthritis. BMJ 2002; 324:1488–1492.
16. Fendrick AM, Garabedian-Ruffalo SM. A clinician's guide to the selection of NSAID therapy. Pharm Ther 2002; 27:579–582.
17. Alloway JA, Moriarty MJ, Hoogland YT, Nashold DJ. Comparison of triamcinolone acetonide with indomethacin in the treatment of acute gouty arthritis. J Rheumatol 1993; 20:111–113.
18. Axelrod D, Preston S. Comparison of parenteral adrenocorticotropic hormone with oral indomethacin in the treatment of acute gout. Arthritis Rheum 1988; 33:803–805.
19. Clive DM. Renal transplant-associated hyperuricemia and gout. J Am Soc Nephrol 2000; 11:974–979.
20. Terkeltaub RA. Gout. N Engl J Med 2003; 349:1647–1655.
21. Siegel LB, Alloway JA, Nashel DJ. Comparison of adrenocorticotropic hormone and triamcinolone acetonide in the treatment of acute gouty arthritis. J Rheumatol 1994; 21:1325–1327.
22. Groff GD, Franck WA, Raddatz DA. Systemic steroid therapy for acute gout: a clinical trial and review of the literature. Semin Arthritis Rheum 1990; 19:329–336.
23. Fam AG. Current therapy of acute microcrystalline arthritis and the role of corticosteroids. J Clin Rheumatol 1997; 3:35–40.
24. Getting SJ, Christian HC, Flower RJ, Perretti M. Activation of melanocortin type 3 receptor as a molecular mechanism for adrenocorticotropic hormone efficacy in gouty arthritis. Arthritis Rheum 2002; 46:2765–2775.
25. Ritter J, Kerr LD, Valeriano-Marcet J, Spirea H. ACTH revisited: effective treatment for acute crystal induced synovitis in patients with multiple medical problems. J Rheumatol 1994; 21:696–699.
26. Schlesinger N, Schumacher HR, Jr. Gout: can management be improved? Curr Opin Rheumatol 2001; 13:240–244.
27. Schlesinger N, Baker DG, Schumacher HR, Jr. How well have diagnostic tests and therapies for gout been evaluated? Curr Opin Rheumatol 1999; 11:441–445.
28. McGill NW. Gout and other crystal-associated arthropathies. Baillieres Best Pract Res Clin Rheumatol 2000; 14:445–460.
29. Bull PW, Scott JT. Intermittent control of hyperuricemia in the treatment of gout. J Rheumatol 1989; 16:1246–1248.
30. Van Lieshout-Zuidema MF, Breedveld FC. Withdrawal of long term antihyperuricemic therapy in tophaceous gout. J Rheumatol 1993; 20:1383–1385.
31. Nakayama DA, Barthelemy C, Carrera G, et al. Tophaceous gout: a clinical and radiographic assessment. Arthritis Rheum 1984; 27:468–473.
32. Li-Yu J, Clayburne G, Sieck M, et al. Treatment of chronic gout. Can we determine when urate stores are depleted enough to prevent attacks of gout? J Rheumatol 2001; 28:577–580.
33. Chen LX, Schumacher HR. Diagnosis and management of gout. J Sci Commun 2003; 10:337–342.
34. Shoji A, Yamanaka H, Kamatani N. A retrospective study of the relationship between serum urate level and recurrent attacks of gouty arthritis: evidence for reduction of recurrent gouty arthritis with antihyperuricemic therapy. Arthritis Rheum 2004; 51:321–325.

35. McCarty DJ. Gout without hyperuricemia. JAMA 1994; 271:302–303.
36. Fam AG. Difficult gout and new approaches for control of hyperuricemia in the allopurinol-allergic patient. Curr Rheumatol Rep 2001; 3:29–35.
37. Wortmann RL. Gout and hyperuricemia. Curr Opin Rheumatol 2002; 14:281–286.
38. Palella TD, Kelley WN. An approach to hyperuricemia and gout. Geriatrics 1984; 39:89–102.
39. Baer AN. Treatment of Gout and Hyperuricemia. In: Bittar EE, Bittar N, eds. Molecular and Cellular Pharmacology. In: Principles of Medical Biology, Vol. 8C. Greenwich: JAI Press Inc, 1997:723–735.
40. Simkin PA. Management of gout. Ann Intern Med 1979; 90:812–816.
41. Ferraz MB, O'Brien B. A cost effectiveness analysis of urate lowering drugs in nontophaceous recurrent gouty arthritis. J Rheumatol 1995; 22:908–914.
42. Fam AG. Should patients with interval gout be treated with urate lowering drugs? J Rheumatol 1995; 22:1621–1623.
43. Becker MA, Schumacher HR, Jr., Wortmann RL, et al. Febuxostat, a novel nonpurine selective inhibitor of xanthine oxidase. Arthritis Rheum 2005; 52:916–923.
44. Kunck RW, Duncan G, Watson D, et al. Colchicine myopathy and neuropathy. N Engl J Med 1987; 316:1562–1565.
45. Schumacher HR, Smolyo AP, Tse RL, Maurer K. Arthritis associated with apatite crystals. Ann Intern Med 1977; 87:411–416.
46. Schumacher HR. Crystal-induced arthritis: an overview. Am J Med 1996; 100:46S–52S.
47. Fam AG. Gout in the elderly: clinical presentation and treatment. Drugs Aging 1998; 13:229–243.
48. Kot TV, Day RD, Brooks PM. Preventing acute gout when starting allopurinol therapy. Colchicine or NSAIDs? Med J Aust 1993; 159:182–184.
49. Chattopadhyay I, Shetty HMG, Routledge PA, et al. Colchicine induced rhabdomyolysis. Postgrad Med J 2001; 77:191–194.
50. Ferraz MB, O'Brien B. A cost effectiveness analysis of urate lowering drugs in nontophaceous recurrent gouty arthritis. J Rheumatol 1995; 22:908–913.
51. Wallace SL, Singer JZ. Therapy in gout. Rheum Dis Clin North Am 1988; 14:441–457.
52. Perez-Ruiz F, Calabozo C, Herrero-Betes A, et al. Improvement in renal function in patients with chronic gout after proper control of hyperuricemia and gouty bouts. Nephron 2000; 86:287–292.
53. Stamp L, Sharples K, Gow P, et al. The optional use of allopurinol: an audit of allopurinol use in South Auckland. Aust NZ J Med 2000; 30:567–572.
54. Simmonds HA, Sahota AS, Van Acker KJ. In: Scriver CR, Beaudet AC, Sly WS, Valle D, eds. The Metabolic and Molecular Bases of Inherited Disease. 7th ed. New York: McGraw-Hill, 1995:1655–1670.
55. Fam AG. Difficulty gout and new approaches for control of hyperuricemia to allopurinol-allergic patients. Curr Rheum Rep 2001; 3:29–37.
56. Hande KR, Noone RM, Stone WI. Severe allopurinol toxicity: description and guidelines for presentation in patients with renal insufficiency. Am J Med 1984; 76:47–53.
57. Singer JZ, Wallace SL. The allopurinol hypersensitivity syndrome: unnecessary morbidity and mortality. Arthritis Rheum 1986; 29:82–87.

58. Weiner JM, Mudge GH. In: Gillman AG, Rall TW, Nies AW, Taylor P, eds. The Pharmacologic Basis of Therapeutics. 8th ed. New York: Pergamon Press, 1990:920.
59. Becker MA, Schumacher HR, Jr., Wortmann RL, et al. Febuxostat, a novel nonpurine selective inhibitor of xanthine oxidase, therapy in allopurinol intolerant patients. Arthritis Rheum 2004; 50:S336.
60. Becker MA, Schumacher HR, Jr, Wortmann, et al. Febuxostat versus allopurinol in patients with hyperuricemia and gout. N Engl J Med 2005; 353:2450–2461.
61. Harris M, Bryant LR, Danaher P, Alloway JA. Effect of low dose daily aspirin on serum urate levels and urinary excretion in patients receiving probenecid for gouty arthritis. J Rheumatol 2000; 27:2873–2876.
62. Perez-Ruiz F, Alonso-Ruiz A, Calabozo M, Duruelo J. Treatment of gout after transplantation. Br J Rheumatol 1998; 37:580–586.
63. Jacobs F, Mamzer-Bruneel MF, Skhir H, et al. Safety of the mycophenolate mofetil-allopurinol combination in kidney transplant recipients with gout. Transplantation 1997; 64:1087–1091.
64. Maesaka JK, Fishbane S. Regulation of renal urate excretion: a critical review. Am J Kidney Dis 1998; 32:917–925.
65. Dessein PH, Shipton EA, Stanwix AE, et al. Beneficial effects of weight loss associated with moderate calorie/carbohydrate restriction, and increased proportional intake of protein and unsaturated fat on serum urate and lipoprotein levels in gout: a pilot study. Ann Rheum Dis 2000; 59:539–548.
66. Fam AG. Gout, diet and the insulin resistance syndrome. J Rheumatol 2002; 29:1350–1356.
67. Yamamoto T, Moriwaki Y, Takahashi S, et al. Effect of fenofibrate on plasma concentration and urinary excretion of purine bases and oxypurinol. J Rheumatol 2001; 28:2294–2297.
68. Minghelli G, Seydoux C, Goy JJ, Burnier M. Uricosuric effect of the angiotensin II receptor antagonist losartan in heart transplant recipients. Transplantation 1998; 66:268–271.
69. Wurzner G, Gerster JC, Chiolero A, et al. Comparative effects of losartan and irbesartan on serum uric acid in hypertensive patients with hyperuricaemia and gout. J Hypertens 2001; 19:1855–1860.
70. Choi H, Atkinson KK, Karlson E, et al. Alcohol intake and risk of incident gout in men. A prospective study. Lancet 2004; 363:1277–1281.
71. Stamp L, Sharples K, Gow P, Raill B. The optimal use of allopurinol: an audit of allopurinol use in South Auckland. Aust NZ J Med 2000; 30:567–572.
72. Wortmann RL. The treatment of gout: the use of an analogy. Am J Med 1998; 105:513–516.
73. Spilberg I, McLain D, Simchowitz L, et al. Colchicine and pseudo gout. Arthritis Rheum 1980; 23:1062–1063.
74. Tabatabia M, Cummings N. Intravenous colchicine in the treatment of acute pseudogout. Arthritis Rheum 1980; 23:370–374.
75. Roberts W, Liang M, Stem S. Colchicine in acute gout. JAMA 1987; 257:1920–1922.
76. Ritter J, Kerr L, Valeriano-Marcet J, et al. ACTH revisited: effective treatment for acute crystal induced synovitis in patients with multiple medical problems. J Rheumatol 1993; 21:696–699.

77. Roane D, Harris M, Cap enter M, et al. Prospective use of intramuscular triamcinolone in pseudogout. J Rheumatol 1997; 24:1168–1170.
78. Averellos A, Spliberg I. Colchicine prophylaxis in pseudogout. J Rheumatol 1986; 13:804–808.
79. Doherty M, Dieppe P. Double blind, placebo controlled trial of magnesium carbonate in chronic pyrophosphate arthropathy. Ann Rheum Dis 1983; 42:106–107.
80. Rothschild B, Yakubov L. Prospective 6-month, double-blind trial of hydroxychloroquine treatment fCJD. Compr Ther 1997; 23:327–331.
81. Patel KJ, Weidensaul D, Palma C, et al. Milwaukee shoulder with massive bilateral cysts: effective therapy for hydrops of the shoulder. J Rheumatol 1997; 24.2453–2479.
82. Weiss JJ, Good A, Schumacher HR. Four cases of "Milwaukee shoulder syndrome" with a description of clinical presentation and long term treatment. J Am Geriatrics Soc 1985; 33:202–205.
83. McCarty DJ, Swanson AB, Ehrhart RH. Hemorrhagic rupture of the shoulder. J Rheumatol 1994; 21:1134–1137.
84. Claudepierre P, Rahmouni A, Bergamasco P, et al. Misleading clinical aspects of hydroxyapatite deposits: a series of 15 cases. J Rheumatol 1997; 24:531–535.
85. Buschbacher RM. Shoulder girdle and arm. In: Buschbacher RM, ed. Diagnosis and Rehabilitation. 2nd ed. In: Practical guide to musculoskeletal disorders, 2nd ed. Boston: Butterworth-Heinemann, 2002:113–140.
86. Parlier-Cuau C, Champsaur P, Nizard R, et al. Percutaneous treatments of painful shoulder. Radiol Clin N Am 1998; 36:589–596.
87. Ebenbichler GR, Erdogmus CB, Resch KL, et al. Ultrasound therapy for calcific tendinitis of the shoulder. N Engl J Med 1999; 340:1533–1538.
88. Jakobeit C, Winiarski B, Jakobeit S, et al. Ultrasound-guided, high-energy extracorporeal—shock-wave treatment of symptomatic calcareous tendinopathy of the shoulder. ANZ J Surg 2002; 72:496–500.
89. Haupt G. Use of extracorporeal shock waves in the treatment of pseudoarthritis, tendinopathy and other orthopedic diseases. J Urol 1997; 158:4–11.
90. Rompe JD, Rumler F, Hopf C, et al. Extracorporeal shock wave therapy for calcifying tendinitis of the shoulder. Clin Orthop 1995; 321:196–201.
91. Pleiner J, Crevenna R, Langenberger H, et al. Extracorporeal shockwave treatment is effective in calcific tendonitis of the shoulder. A randomized controlled trial. Wein Klin Wochenschr 2004; 116:536–541.
92. Feng Z. Two-hundred and ten cases of shoulder periarthritis treated by needling lengxia and sanjian. J Trad Chin Med 2003; 23:201–202.
93. Israel Z, Mosheiff R, Gross E, et al. Hyperextension fracture-dislocation of the thoracic spine with paraplegia in a patient with diffuse idiopathic skeletal hyperostosis. J Spinal Disord 1994; 7:455–457.
94. Brantus JF, Meunier PJ. Effects of intravenous etidronate and oral corticosteroids in fibrodysplasia ossificans progressiva. Clin Orthop 1998; 346:117–120.
95. Smith R, Russell RG, Woods CG. Myositis ossificans progressiva. Clinical features of eight patients and their response to treatment. J Bone Joint Surg Br 1976; 58:48–57.
96. Bruni L, Giammaria P, Tozzi MC, et al. Fibrodysplasia ossificans progressiva. An 11-year-old boy treated with a diphosphonate. Acta Paediatr Scand 1990; 79:994–998.

97. Bar Oz B, Boneh A. Myositis ossificans progressiva: a 10-year follow-up on a patient treated with etidronate disodium. Acta Paediatr 1994; 83:1332–1334.
98. Jones G, Rocke DM. Multivariate survival analysis with doubly-censored data: application to the assessment of Accutane treatment for fibrodysplasia ossificans progressiva. Stat Med 2002; 21:2547–2562.
99. Shafritz AB, Shore EM, Gannon FH, et al. Overexpression of an osteogenic morphogen in fibrodysplasia ossificans progressiva. N Engl J Med 1996; 335:555–561.
100. Spruce WE, Forman SJ, Blume KG, et al. Successful second bone marrow transplantation in a patient with myositis ossificans progressiva and aplastic anemia. Am J Pediatr Hematol Oncol 1983; 5:337–340.
101. Altschuler EL. Consideration of Rituximab for fibrodysplasia ossificans progressiva. Med Hypoth 2004; 63:407–408.
102. Glaser DL, Economides AN, Wang L, et al. In vivo somatic cell gene transfer of an engineered Noggin mutein prevents BMP4-induced heterotopic ossification. J Bone Joint Surg Am 2003; 85:2332–2342.
103. Dolan AL, Kassimos D, Gibson T, Kingsley GH. Diltiazem induces remission of calcinosis in scleroderma. Br J Rheumatol 1995; 34:576–578.
104. Torralla TP, Li-Yu J, Navarra STGV. Successful use of diltiazem in calcinosis caused by connective tissue disease. J Clin Rheumatol 1999; 5:74–78.
105. Fuchs D, Fruchter L, Fishel B, et al. Colchicine suppression of local inflammation due to calcinosis in dermatomyositis and progressive systemic sclerosis. Clin Rheumatol 1986;527–530.
106. Rashad SM, Abdelaty BM, Rooney J, Schumacher HR. Acute inflammation at the site of calcification in limited cutaneous scleroderma. J Rheumatol 2002; 29:74–78.
107. van Kuijk AA, Geurts AC, van Kuppevelt HJ. Neurogenic heterotopic ossification in spinal cord injury. Spinal Cord 2002; 40:313–326.
108. Sell S, Willms R, Jany R, et al. The suppression of heterotopic ossifications: radiation versus NSAID therapy — a prospective study. J Arthroplasty 1998; 13:854–859.
109. Pakos EE, Ioannidis JP. Radiotherapy vs. nonsteroid anti-inflammatory drugs for the prevention of heterotopic ossification after major hip procedures: a meta-analysis of randomized trials. Int J Radiat Oncol Biol Phys 2004; 60:888–895.
110. Stover SL, Niemann KM, Miller JM. Disodium etidronate in the prevention of postoperative recurrence of heterotopic ossification in spinal-cord injury patients. J Bone Joint Surg Am 1976; 58:683–688.
111. Haran M, Bhuta T, Lee B. Pharmacological interventions for treating acute heterotopic ossification. Cochrane Database Syst Rev 2004; 18.

20

Colchicine

Brian F. Mandell

Department of Medicine and Rheumatic and Immunologic Diseases, Cleveland Clinic Lerner College of Medicine of Case Western Reserve University, Cleveland, Ohio, U.S.A.

INTRODUCTION

It is generally perceived that colchicine is an effective anti-inflammatory agent only in select conditions such as crystal-induced inflammatory disease, chronic pericarditis, and familial Mediterranean fever. Although there are case reports and small series suggesting therapeutic benefit in other disorders, compelling data to support these claims are lacking. If this selectivity is real, one explanation is that the drug may affect a unique pathophysiologic mechanism shared by crystal-induced arthritis and a few other disorders, but not function as a general anti-microtubule agent acting to depress oriented cellular motility (chemotaxis). Alternatively, the colchicine sensitive pathway may be utilized in other inflammatory conditions, but in these other disorders there are redundant colchicine insensitive pathways that mediate the inflammatory response.

Lore has arisen regarding the "appropriate" use and dosing of colchicine. Despite many textbook reiterations of the drug's selectivity and guidelines for its "appropriate" use, a dearth of adequate trial-based data exist to support these contentions. There has been only one randomized, placebo-controlled prospective study (43 patients) demonstrating a beneficial effect of oral colchicine in treating acute gout (1) and one randomized placebo-controlled trial to support its use as a prophylactic agent (2). Several other studies suggest that the chronic use of colchicine can decrease the frequency of acute gout attacks, but most of these reports lack appropriate randomization or placebo group controls. In addition, several trials were of limited duration and others included a large number of patients who were lost to follow-up. Nonetheless, colchicine is frequently employed orally and occasionally intravenously to treat acute gout attacks and in a low daily dosage as prophylaxis against attacks. Accumulated clinical experience supports these uses, but it is appropriate to reevaluate the frequently recommended details and complications of colchicine administration.

Side effects of chronic oral colchicine use are increasingly being reported, but the incidence of these toxicities is not well defined. Despite the limited amount of data, and perhaps over reliance on published adverse case reports, legitimate concerns have been raised regarding the poor risk-benefit ratio of intravenous administration as well as the use of chronic oral therapy in certain patient populations. A number of deaths have been reported following intravenous administration of colchicine, most due to inappropriate dosing. There have also been three retrospective case series published (3), or presented at national meetings, that have included approximately 300 unselected patients who received intravenous colchicine without suffering a significant frequency of severe drug-related adverse effects. Nonetheless, since colchicine is used to treat non-life threatening conditions, conservatism with regard to route of administration, dose, and monitoring for development of potential complications should be exercised.

PHARMACOLOGY

Colchicine is an alkaloid derived from several related plants including the meadow saffron *colchicum autumnale*. Recognized for its medicinal effect since at least the sixth century A.D., colchicine became a popular treatment for the gout in the 18th century. It may have been introduced into the United States by Benjamin Franklin. Historically colchicine has been empirically dosed orally and intravenously, without benefit of drug level monitoring or a surrogate marker of drug effect. It is 30% to 50% protein-bound in plasma (4), and is concentrated within cells due in part to intracellular binding to tubulin, and probably intercalation within membranes. Among circulating cells, high concentrations are found within erythrocytes and neutrophils (5). The membrane P-glycoprotein multiple resistance efflux transporter (MDR1 gene product) can actively pump colchicine out of cells (6). It has been proposed that the higher concentrations of drug that accumulate in neutrophils compared to those in lymphocytes is due to the absence of this transporter in neutrophils (6). The P-glycoprotein is present on many cell surfaces, including bile canalicular cells. A population heterogeneity in expression of this transporter may explain some of the inter-patient variability in efficacy, biliary excretion, and adverse event frequency.

The drug has a large volume of distribution and a slow terminal clearance $T_{1/2}$ of approximately 60 hours under steady state conditions. This is due in part to large intracellular stores. Following a single intravenous administration, colchicine can be found in leukocytes and urine for greater than 9 days. The clinical implication of prolonged intracellular colchicine deposition is that patients on long-term therapy are potentially predisposed to toxicity, particularly bone marrow suppression, from additional dosing boluses given for acute flares of gout.

Colchicine is absorbed predominantly from the jejunum and ileum. Bioavailability on initial oral dosing is approximately 50% (7,8). There may be significant but variable enterohepatic recirculation (8). The drug is metabolized in the liver, and excreted into bile. The fate of drug in the gastrointestinal tract is incompletely defined. Because colchicine is lipid soluble, it may enter intestinal lining cells and provoke the diarrhea and other gastrointestinal toxicity prominently observed following oral administration. There is significant fecal excretion of both the unmodified and metabolized drug. Renal excretion is considerably less, but that route is still an important pathway of excretion. Less than 25% of unmetabolized drug is excreted in the urine (9). The relative roles of renal versus gastrointestinal excretion following intravenous dosing have not been extensively studied.

Colchicine undergoes demethylation in the liver at several carbon atom rings and the demethylated forms are excreted in feces and urine. Human liver microsomal fractions can demethylate colchicine in vitro, and the P450 isoform CYP3A4 plays a prominent role in the metabolism of the drug (10). Thus, drugs that affect CYP3A4 such as the macrolide antibiotics (11), cyclosporine, and most of the statins (except fluvastatin) inhibit the metabolism of colchicine (11,12). In patients with familial Mediterranean fever, renal or liver dysfunction has been shown to impair colchicine clearance. This observation is not likely limited to patients with that disease. Colchicine crosses the placenta, and a high concentration has been reported to be present in breast milk from a patient taking 1 mg daily (13).

COMPLICATIONS OF THERAPY

The adverse effects of colchicine therapy, other than in cases of extreme toxicity, differ somewhat depending upon the route of administration. Gastrointestinal toxicity, predominantly diarrhea with cramping, is extremely common with oral dosing, but uncommon with IV administration (unless the drug is concomitantly taken orally). During chronic therapy with low doses (0.6 mg twice daily), continued use is frequently limited because of loose stools or diarrhea. In a clinical trial involving 22 patients with acute gout, a frequently utilized regimen (1 mg followed by 0.5 mg every two hours until relief or toxicity) universally caused diarrhea or vomiting at a median time of 24 hours. Relief of pain by 50% was attained in all patients, but in 13 of the 22, the positive effects occurred concurrently or after the onset of gastrointestinal toxicity (1).

Reversible bone marrow suppression, usually leukopenia, can occur with chronic or high dose acute therapy. Rash is uncommon. Alopecia and decreased sperm counts have been reported with chronic dosing.

Neuromuscular toxicity is infrequent, but is increasingly recognized as a complication of chronic or sometimes even short-term administration. Neuromyopathy can occur even when patients are taking low doses of colchicine. This reversible complication is characterized by a vacuolar myopathy, often with an axon loss neuropathy. Both may be a result of the anti-microtubule effects of high intracellular levels of colchicine that inhibit effective vacuolar fusion and neuronal transport. Reports have emphasized proximal skeletal muscle weakness and/or pain, usually with an elevated serum creatine phosphokinase level. Colchicine-associated neuromyopathy can occur in the setting of apparently normal renal function, but it is far more likely to occur in patients with renal insufficiency (14,15). This association could be due to decreased initial clearance of the drug, or conceivably some effect of renal insufficiency on P-glycoprotein mediated efflux of the drug from certain cells. Rhabdomyolysis has been described (16), although in several patients polypharmacy makes it difficult to discern if colchicine alone was the actual offending agent. Prominent injury to the respiratory muscles has been described (17). Drug interactions frequently play a role in the development of neuromuscular toxicity (18). Fortunately, most patients with neuromyopathy improve dramatically over several weeks following discontinuation of colchicine.

The early diagnosis of colchicine neuromyopathy rests on recognition of the syndrome by the clinician. Serum creatine phosphokinase elevations have ranged from minimal to greater than 50-fold times the upper limit of normal. Electromyography and nerve conduction studies may reveal a myopathy, with irritative features. There are frequently both proximal and distal abnormalities. These changes can also be seen with statin-induced myopathy. The coexistence of an axonal neuropathy, however, favors colchicine and not a statin as the etiology for the muscle symptoms in a patient using both agents. Myocardial involvement can occur. Biopsy may strongly suggest colchicine as the etiologic agent, unless other autophagic vacuolar myopathy-inducing drugs (i.e., hydroxychloroquine, amiodarone, vincristine) have also been consumed. Electron microscopy can reveal abnormal deposits termed colchicine bodies (Fig. 1), although this technique is not usually necessary for making the diagnosis. Withdrawal of the colchicine and monitoring the resolution of the creatine phosphokinase elevation and improved clinical course is sufficient to comfortably confirm the diagnosis. Some patients may tolerate reinstitution of the drug at a lower dose, or restarting the drug without the concomitant use of medications that influence colchicine clearance or distribution. However, avoiding the use of colchicine, if possible, is the optimal approach since the neuromyopathy may recur.

Acute colchicine overdose is a toxicological emergency, with a high mortality rate due to multiorgan failure. The drug quickly binds to plasma proteins and

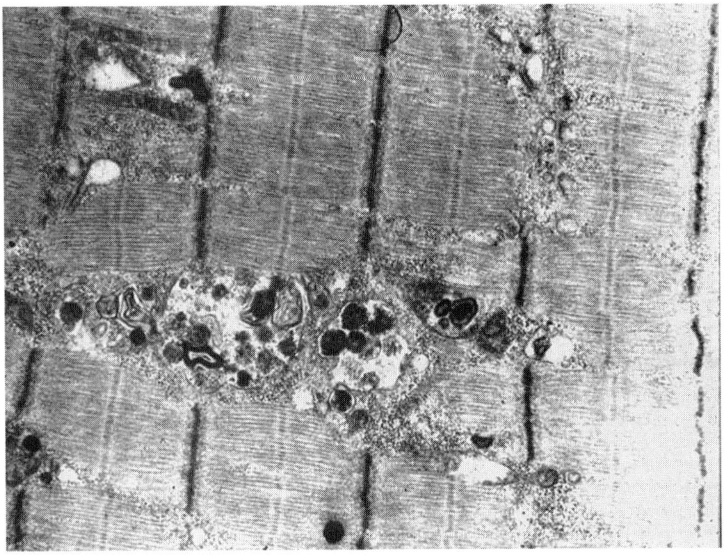

Figure 1 Electron micrograph of skeletal muscle reveals colchicine bodies in a patient with an axonal neuromyopathic complication from taking colchicine.

distributes within cells. It is not removed by filtration or dialysis. In the setting of acute ingestion, induced emesis and gastric lavage should be instituted. Charcoal should be used because of the likelihood of enterohepatic recirculation. Oral overdose is characterized by the early onset of gastric and intestinal toxicity, similar to what can occur with "normal" dosing in sensitive individuals. Hypotension may occur from continued gastrointestinal volume losses. An initial leukocytosis may be followed several days later by profound leukopenia and pancytopenia. Disseminated intravascular coagulopathy (DIC) has been reported. Multi-organ failure with adult respiratory distress syndrome (ARDS), seizures, polyneuropathy, rhabdomyolysis, and cardiac arrhythmias including asystole may occur (19).

The use of intravenous colchicine is controversial, some authors argue that its use should be banned due to a poor risk-benefit ratio, especially since it is used to treat non-life threatening diseases. Deaths have been reported following intravenous administration, generally following miscalculation of the dose. Errors include giving too many doses, giving the drug to patients on chronic oral therapy prior to or concomitantly with the intravenous therapy, or use in the presence of significant renal or hepatic dysfunction. Dosing guidelines, based on expert opinion, include single doses not exceeding 3 mg (20). Additionally it was suggested that in the elderly and those patients with hepatic or renal dysfunction the total dose should be further reduced. Others have suggested that the drug be avoided altogether in the setting of end stage renal disease. These recommendations, although quite rational, have never been validated prospectively. It is critical to note that the premonitory gastrointestinal signs of toxicity, which accompany oral dosing, do not generally occur with the intravenous route of administration.

There have been three retrospective reviews of the use of intravenous colchicine in 261 unselected, evaluable hospitalized patients. One was published (3), and two were presented at national meetings (21,22). Despite the facts that many patients had factors denoting an increased risk for adverse effects and higher than suggested doses were frequently given, there were no serious adverse effects. In one series, 7% of 71 patients developed leukopenia with white blood cell counts less than 3500 cells/mm^3 (21). But in a second study (22), none of 90 patients experienced decreased white blood cell count to this degree. In up to 79% of patients, the symptoms of gout resolved to the point that no additional therapy was given. Therefore, intravenous colchicine is effective and was, in at least these three retrospective studies, a reasonably tolerated therapy. In hospitalized (particularly perioperative) patients, there may still be occasional situations where this route of administration would be useful. These could include when oral therapy is not feasible and contraindications exist for the use of a nonsteroidal anti-inflammatory agent or systemic or intra-articular corticosteroid. Nonetheless, significant care should be given in choosing an intravenous dose, remembering that bioavailability of the oral versus intravenous dose is approximately 50%, that previously administered colchicine therapy may persist intracellularly, and that toxicity may develop without warning signs. Finally, if colchicine is given intravenously, it should be appropriately diluted in normal saline and administered through a secure intravenous access. Colchicine is extremely caustic if infiltrated into soft tissue. Extravasation results in severe tissue necrosis.

Thirteen patients with familial Mediterranean fever refractory to oral colchicine were administered 1 mg of colchicine intravenously weekly for 12 weeks in addition to their daily oral colchicine dose of 2 to 3 mg each day in an open label study (23). No significant adverse effects were observed, and the investigators believed that efficacy was enhanced. Whether these individuals who were unresponsive to oral colchicine had poor gastrointestinal absorption of the drug is not clear. This sample population is too small to generalize any safety conclusions for this therapeutic approach, and dosing in this manner cannot be endorsed.

DRUG INTERACTIONS

Colchicine affects the intestinal absorption of many drugs and compounds via direct mucosal toxicity. Colchicine can cause or exacerbate lactose intolerance. Likely of greater significance is its potential effect on levels of drugs that are metabolized by Cytochrome P450 isoform CYP3A4. A partial list is presented in Table 1. Despite a myriad of potential drug interactions, reports of serious toxicity are relatively infrequent. This may be due to under-recognition of these drug-drug effects.

Table 1 Selected Drugs that Interfere with CYP3A4-Mediated Colchicine Metabolism

Corticosteroids	Ketoconazole
Cyclosporine	Nifedipine
Dapsone	Quinidine
Diltiazem	Statins (not fluvastatin)
Erythromycin	Terfenadine
Estrogen	Verapamil

Other drug interactions may involve the P-glycoprotein multiple resistance efflux transporter. This membrane transporter actively pumps colchicine (and some other drugs) out of cells. Cyclosporine and most statins are actively transported by this protein, and can interfere with the cellular efflux and hepatic biliary excretion of colchicine (18,24). Therefore, full dose colchicine should be used with great caution in organ-transplant patients who are taking cyclosporine. This interaction is also of concern for the many patients with gout who are prescribed statins (25) because of the high prevalence of hyperlipidemia, atherosclerotic cardiovascular disease, and the metabolic syndrome in this population.

MECHANISM OF ACTION

Colchicine binds to intracellular tubulin and inhibits microtubule polymerization and is a potent antimitotic agent. In high concentrations, colchicine intercalates into cell membranes and may nonspecifically perturb cell functions. These anti-proliferative and membrane effects may account for some toxic and in vitro effects of the drug, but are not likely responsible for its anti-inflammatory activity that renders it useful in the treatment of crystal-induced arthritis.

A critical issue in understanding the mechanism of action of colchicine is the specificity of its anti-inflammatory effect. If this agent truly has an effect limited to crystal-induced inflammation, familial Mediterranean fever, and a few other disorders, then this suggests that its primary mechanism does not target a ubiquitously necessary pathway of inflammation such as cell motility. That is unless in other inflammatory conditions there are redundant pathways which bypass or overwhelm the colchicine block. Small studies have assessed the efficacy of colchicine in conditions such as rheumatoid arthritis, psoriatic arthritis, psoriasis, sarcoid arthritis, Behçet's syndrome, and cutaneous lupus. Although definitive results have not been attained, the clinical impression is that colchicine is not particularly effective in these disorders. Efficacy in treating chronic pericarditis and small vessel cutaneous vasculitis has been reported.

In vitro, colchicine exhibits pleiotropic cellular effects which are dependent upon concentration, time of cell exposure to the drug, and the specific assay utilized. Effects on chemotaxis may differ in micropore and agarose gel migration assays. Degranulation effects can be demonstrated using relatively high concentrations of the drug. Modulation of some receptor-mediated biochemical pathways can be affected by blocking microtubule assembly and disassembly. However, certain of these effects can be readily demonstrated only by employing high colchicine concentrations.

Results of several in vivo studies suggest that colchicine does not directly affect cell influx into an inflammatory site, but instead blunts an amplification phase of cytokine generation. Specific cytokines may play variably significant roles in different disorders at different times in the course of the inflammatory response; this may account for the apparent clinical specificity of the drug.

In a model of experimental arthritis in rabbits, colchicine, in nonleukopenia-inducing doses, suppressed the inflammatory response (neutrophil influx) to the intra-articular injection of urate crystals, but did not blunt the response to intra-articular injection of a neutrophil-derived chemotactic factor or other chemotactic factors, including zymosan-activated plasma and formylated peptides (26). Using the abraded skin assay in humans for measurement of in vivo cell migration, it was demonstrated that patients with familial Mediterranean fever who had been treated with colchicine had a normal initial cellular influx, but a delayed late response (27). These results are consistent with a suppressive effect of colchicine on cellular release of cytokines and/or other mediators including leukotriene B4. It has also been suggested from several studies that colchicine has a relatively specific ability to block cellular activation by urate and some other crystals, while leaving untouched or even augmenting activation by other stimuli (28). Colchicine has also been demonstrated to alter the expression of membrane-associated proteins including adhesion molecules on inflammatory and endothelial cells (29).

INDICATIONS

It is generally accepted that colchicine is efficacious for the treatment of acute gouty arthritis, and for prophylaxis against recurrent attacks. There are also reports that it may be similarly effective in treating and preventing calcium pyrophosphate crystal-associated arthritis (30). Anecdotal experience suggests efficacy in treating calcific periarthritis and the inflammatory phase of calcinosis associated with myositis and scleroderma. There are a number of observational studies suggesting efficacy in reducing the frequency of attacks in patients with recurrent pericarditis (31). It may also be useful in the treatment of methotrexate-associated rheumatoid nodulosis (32). Colchicine has also been employed to treat autoimmune thrombocytopenia, Behçet's syndrome, palmar pustulosis, psoriatic arthritis, aphthous stomatitis, and leukocytoclastic vasculitis with variable results (33).

CONTRAINDICATIONS

Because colchicine is not a life saving therapy, a conservative approach should be utilized in assessing its risk benefit ratio prior to initiating therapy. Mixed and somewhat controversial recommendations exist regarding the absolute and relative contraindications for its administration. Patients with biliary obstruction or severe hepatic dysfunction should probably not be treated with colchicine. Although renal insufficiency and end-stage renal disease are relative contraindications to chronic colchicine use, the alternatives for prophylactic and acute gout therapy are often extremely limited in patients with these conditions. Thus, in such circumstances, efforts to prevent attacks with very low dose colchicine combined with urate-lowering therapy and careful monitoring for toxicity may at times be a reasonable option.

There are no evidence-based data to support specific chronic dosing guidelines, and it is best to err on the side of conservative dosing (20). Patients with hepatic disease, renal insufficiency, or taking medications that interfere with the metabolism of colchicine (Table 1) or its transport by P glycoprotein should be monitored by taking a careful history regarding symptoms of toxicity and periodic laboratory testing.

The use of colchicine should be avoided during pregnancy, and probably during times where conception is being attempted. Although there are few data to use for guidance, prudence dictates limiting the use of the drug in the setting of leukopenia, bone marrow disease, concurrently with other drugs likely to induce leukopenia, or by the intravenous route.

REFERENCES

1. Ahern MJ, Reid C, Gordon TP, et al. Does colchicine work? The results of the first controlled study in acute gout. Aust NZ J Med 1987; 17:301–304.
2. Paulus HE, Schlosstein LH, Godfrey FG, et al. Colchicine therapy of intercritical gout. A placebo-controlled study of probenecid treated patients. Arthritis Rheum 1974; 17:609–614.
3. Maldonado MA, Salzman A, Varga J. Intravenous colchicine use in crystal-induced arthropathies: a retrospective analysis of hospitalized patients. Clin Exp Rheumatol 1997; 15:487–492.
4. Wallace SL, Omokoku B, Ertel NH. Colchicine plasma levels: implications as to pharmacology and mechanisms of action. Am J Med 1970; 48:443–448.
5. Chappey O, Niel E, Wautier JL, et al. Colchicine disposition in human leukocytes after single and multiple oral administration. Clin Pharmacol Ther 1993; 54:360–367.
6. Ben-Chetrit E, Levy M. Does the lack of the P-glycoprotein efflux pump in neutrophils explain the efficacy of colchicine in familial mediterranean fever and other inflammatory diseases? Med Hypoth 1998; 51:377–380.
7. Rochdi M, Sabouraud A, Girre C, et al. Pharmacokinetics and absolute bioavailability of colchicine after IV and oral administration in healthy human volunteers and elderly subjects. Eur J Clin Pharmacol 1994; 46:351–354.
8. Ferron GM, Rochdi M, Jusko WJ, Scherrmann JM. Oral absorption characteristics and pharmacokinetics of colchicine in healthy volunteers after single and multiple doses. J Clin Pharmacol 1996; 36:874–883.

9. Thomas G, Girre C, Scherrmann JM, et al. Zero-order absorption and linear disposition of oral colchicine in healthy volunteers. Eur J Clin Pharmacol 1989; 37:79–84.
10. Tateishi T, Soucek P, Coraco Y, et al. Colchicine biotransformation by human liver microsomes. Biochem Pharmacol 1997; 53:111–116.
11. Caraco Y, Putterman C, Rahamimov R, Ben-Chetrit E. Acute colchicine intoxication-possible role of erythromycin administration. J Rheumatol 1992; 19:494–496.
12. Boger RH. Drug interactions of the statins and consequences for drug selection. Int J Clin Pharmacol Ther 2001; 39:369–382.
13. Guillonneau M, Aigrain EJ, Galliot M, et al. Colchicine is excreted at high concentrations in human breast milk. Eur J Ob Gyn Reprod Biol 1995; 61:177–178.
14. Kuncl RW, Duncan G, Watson D, et al. Colchicine myopathy and neuropathy. N Engl J Med 1987; 316:1562–1568.
15. Pirzada NA, Medell M, Ali, II. Colchicine induced neuromyopathy in a patient with normal renal function. J Clin Rheumatol 2001; 7:374–376.
16. Debie K, Conraads V, Vrints C. Colchicine-induced rhabdomyolysis in a patient with chronic heart failure. Acta Cardiol 2003; 58:561–562.
17. Tanios MA, El Gamal H, Epstein SK, Hassoun PM. Severe respiratory muscle weakness related to long-term colchicine therapy. Respir Care 2004; 49:189–191.
18. Simkin P, Gardner GC. Colchicine use in cyclosporine treated transplant recipients: how little is too much? J Rheumatol 2000; 27:1334–1337.
19. Murray SS, Kramlinger KG, McMichan, Mohr DN. Acute toxicity after excessive ingestion of colchicine. Mayo Clin Proc 1983; 58:528–532.
20. Wallace SL, Singer JZ. Review: Systemic toxicity associated with the intravenous administration of colchicine—guidelines for use. J Rheumatol 1988; 15:495–499.
21. Blanco A, Hutchinson G. Safety of intravenous colchicine: Patterns of use and complication rate in a hospitalized cohort. Arthritis Rheum 2004; 50:S339.
22. Khurana PS, Mandell BF. The safety and efficacy of intravenous colchicine: a retrospective review of 90 patients. Presented at Society of General Internal Medicine Annual Meeting, San Diego, CA. 1999.
23. Lidar M, Kedem R, Langevitz P, et al. Intravenous colchicine for treatment of patients with familial mediterranean fever unresponsive to oral colchicine. J Rheumatol 2003; 30:2620–2623.
24. Speeg KV, Maldonado AL, Liaci J, Muirhead D. Effect of cyclosporine on colchicine secretion by a liver canalicular transporter studied in vivo. Hepatology 1991; 14:899–903.
25. Wallace CS, Mueller BA. Lovastatin-induced rhabdomyolysis in the absence of concomitant drugs. Ann Pharmacother 1992; 26:190–192.
26. Spilberg I, Mandell B, Mehta J, et al. Mechanism of action of colchicine in acute urate crystal-induced arthritis. J Clin Invest 1979; 64:775–780.
27. Dinarello CA, Chusid MJ, Fauci AS, et al. Effect of prophylactic colchicine therapy on leukocyte function in patients with familial mediterranean fever. Arthritis Rheum 1976; 19:618–622.
28. Roberge CJ, Gaudry M, Gilbert C, et al. Paradoxical effects of colchicine on the activation of human neutrophils by chemotactic factors and inflammatory microcrystals. J Leuk Biol 1996; 59:864–871.

29. Cronstein BN, Molad Y, Reibman J, et al. Colchicine alters the quantitative and qualitative display of selectins on endothelial cells and neutrophils. J Clin Invest 1995; 95:994–1002.
30. Spilberg I, McLain D, Simchowitz L, Berney S. Colchicine and pseudogout. Arthritis Rheum 1980; 23:1062–1103.
31. Imazio M, Bobbio M, Cecchi E, et al. Colchicine as first-choice therapy for recurrent pericarditis: results of the CORE trial. Arch Int Med 2005; 165:1987–1991.
32. Abraham Z, Rozenbaum M, Rosner I. Colchicine therapy for low-dose-methotrexate-induced accelerated nodulosis in a rheumatoid arthritis patient. J Dermatol 1999; 26:691–694.
33. Sullivan TP, King LE, Boyd AS. Colchicine in dermatology. J Am Acad Dermatol 1998; 39:993–999.

21

The Use of Nonsteroidal Anti-inflammatory Drugs for the Treatment of Gouty Arthritis

Bruce N. Cronstein

Divisions of Clinical Pharmacology and Rheumatology, Department of Medicine, NYU School of Medicine, New York, New York, U.S.A.

INTRODUCTION

Gout and gouty arthritis are among the most common of rheumatic disorders. The medical community is fortunate to have a variety of medical approaches available to treat acute gouty arthritis and acute arthritis induced by other crystals. Although corticosteroids, colchicine, opiates, and other analgesics and anti-inflammatory drugs are effective therapies for acute crystal-induced arthritis, non-aspirin, nonsteroidal anti-inflammatory drugs (NSAIDs) remain the most commonly used agents for the therapy of gout and pseudogout. As a class, NSAIDs have been in widespread clinical use for many years; their mechanism of action is well understood, and their limitations and toxicities are widely known and appreciated by both primary care and specialist physicians. Both patients and physicians feel comfortable with the use of NSAIDs for the treatment of acute gouty arthritis as these drugs are used in the treatment of so many other rheumatic and non-rheumatic conditions. Indeed, textbooks of medicine and rheumatology suggest using NSAIDs as first-line therapy for most patients with acute gouty arthritis and reserve high-dose oral and intravenous colchicine, oral and intra-articular corticosteroids, and injections of ACTH for patients who are not likely to tolerate or respond to NSAIDs (1–4). This chapter reviews the pharmacologic basis for the anti-inflammatory effects of NSAIDs on acute pain and inflammation and the evidence supporting their use in the treatment of acute gouty arthritis.

MECHANISMS OF ACTION

Salicylates derived from plants have been used to treat various ailments for nearly 3000 years. Aspirin, a more tolerable semisynthetic salicylate, was developed in the late 19th century for the treatment of pain, fever, and inflammation. The mechanism by which aspirin suppressed these symptoms was not understood until 1971 when Vane first proposed the hypothesis that aspirin inhibits inflammation by diminishing prostaglandin synthesis (5). Subsequent experiments further established this hypothesis and laid the basis for the development of a new class of anti-inflammatory drugs, NSAIDs.

Prostaglandins are derived from the phospholipase A2-mediated hydrolysis of membrane phospholipids to arachidonic acid (Fig. 1), which is subsequently metabolized to prostaglandin H_2 (PGH_2) by the action of a family of isoenzymes collectively known as cyclooxygenases (COX, PGH synthases). PGH_2 is further metabolized in a tissue-specific fashion to active agents with unique and critical

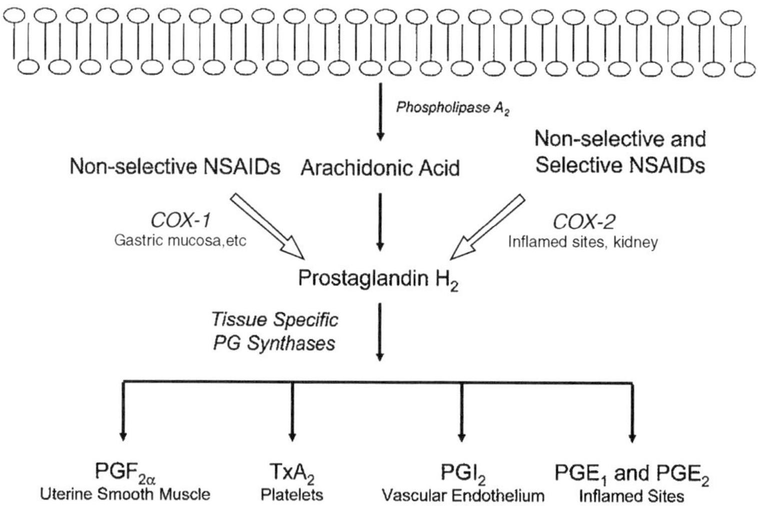

Figure 1 Production of prostaglandins from membrane phospholipids. Shown are the pathways for prostaglandin production. Although the production of substrates required for synthesis of prostanoids is common in all cells, the specific end products produced by a given cell type depend upon the terminal enzymes present in a particular cell. COX-1 and COX-2 differ with respect to the cells in which they are expressed and the stimuli for their production. Enzymes are denominated in italics; substrates and products are in plain type.

physiologic properties. Thus, platelets produce thromboxane A_2, a prostaglandin that is critical for platelet aggregation following ADP-stimulation. Vascular endothelium secretes prostacyclin (PGI_2), a potent inhibitor of platelet aggregation and stimulus for vasodilation. Inflammatory cells produce prostaglandins of the E series (PGE_1 and PGE_2) which are critical regulators of numerous processes involved in inflammation (vasodilation, edema, stimulation of leukocyte accumulation and functions, promotion of pain). Prostaglandins of the F series are potent stimuli for smooth muscle contraction (i.e., uterine contraction during labor).

Appropriate triggering, such as occurs at inflamed or injured sites, leads to rapid and sustained production of prostaglandins, providing a rapid amplification step for increasing inflammation. In response to infection, such amplification of the inflammatory response is appropriate. However, at sites of pathologic inflammation, amplification steps, such as that mediated by prostaglandins, provide a target for anti-inflammatory drug action. Thus, inhibition of prostaglandin production is a useful target for drugs capable of inhibiting acute inflammation and its symptoms, most notably pain, swelling, and erythema.

As with many physiologic actions, inhibition of prostaglandin production at inflamed sites is not without cost. Prostaglandins, as noted above, are produced in most tissues and subserve a myriad of physiologic functions. Inhibition of prostaglandin synthesis by pharmacologic agents thus has the potential to inhibit the production of prostaglandins required for critical physiologic processes. The best documented toxic effects of NSAIDs, gastric ulceration and salt and water retention, clearly result from diminished production of prostaglandins involved in maintaining a protective barrier for the mucosa of the stomach or those involved in regulation of nephron function. Inhibition of platelet function by aspirin and other NSAIDs is useful for the prevention of atherosclerosis and thrombosis but may present a therapeutic dilemma when treating patients who have developed acute gouty arthritis postoperatively.

By the early 1990s it became clear that in some tissues cyclooxygenase activity was inducible during inflammation and that the production of prostaglandins under inflammatory conditions seemed to differ from constitutive prostaglandin production (6). These observations rapidly led to the demonstration that there are at least two different cyclooxygenase isoforms termed COX-1 and COX-2, the latter of which of which is induced at inflamed sites (6). COX-2 rapidly became a target for new anti-inflammatory drugs with the hope that selective inhibition of this enzyme could selectively inhibit inflammatory prostaglandin production without interfering with production of prostaglandins required for maintenance of homeostasis in the stomach, kidney, or platelets. Although selective COX-2 inhibitors are associated with less GI toxicity, the salt and water retention associated with inhibition of prostaglandin synthesis in the kidneys remains a significant clinical problem for patients taking these drugs.

USE OF NSAIDs IN THE TREATMENT OF ACUTE GOUTY ARTHRITIS

The goal of therapy in acute gouty arthritis is to rapidly and safely control pain and inflammation in the affected joint. Interestingly, none of the NSAIDs used in the treatment of acute gouty arthritis have undergone a randomized, placebo-controlled trial in the therapy of acute gouty arthritis. Indeed, it is unlikely that any drugs will ever undergo this sort of evaluation for treating crystal-induced arthritis because the benefits of NSAIDs in treating acute gouty arthritis, like the benefits of penicillin in the treatment of pneumococcal pneumonia, are so clear that it is morally unacceptable to subject patients to treatment with placebo. Nonetheless, the natural history of untreated gouty arthritis has been documented in the modern era and it is clear that resolution of an attack of acute gouty arthritis within seven days is unlikely and little improvement is noted in the affected joints in many patients over this period of time (7). Thus, a historical comparison to the course of acute gouty arthritis in untreated patients can be used in evaluating the effectiveness of all of the drugs discussed below. New drugs are, in fact, usually tested against older medications in the therapy of acute crystal-induced arthritis. Interestingly, none of the newer drugs in this category appear to be any more efficacious in treating acute gout than any of the older drugs, although some of them are much better tolerated than others.

Probably any NSAID, with the exception of salicylates, may be used in the treatment of acute gouty arthritis, and evidence supporting this has been published for most of these drugs. Although the first members of this class of drugs, aspirin and other salicylates are not used in the therapy of acute gouty arthritis because of their paradoxical effects on renal uric acid excretion (diminished excretion at low doses and enhanced excretion at high doses and serum concentrations). Indomethacin, a non-selective NSAID, was reported to be useful in the treatment of acute gouty arthritis nearly 40 years ago even before its mechanism of action had been elucidated (8). Many other non-selective NSAIDs have been used successfully in the treatment of acute gouty arthritis, including: diclofenac, meloxicam, ketorolac, etodolac, ketoprofen, ibuprofen, flurbiprofen, meclofenemate, sulindac, piroxicam, and naproxen (9–20). All of these drugs were tested alone or in comparison to indomethacin or phenylbutazone. There seems to be little difference in the reported efficacy, with most patients reporting substantial improvement within 24 hours of initiating therapy and most having complete resolution of the acute gouty arthritis within a week.

Although unacceptable side effects were not a major issue for any of the drugs studied in the published trials, non-selective NSAIDs commonly cause gastrointestinal distress and ulceration and salt and water retention. The risk of side effects for this class of drugs increases with age, and many elderly patients cannot tolerate NSAIDs because of gastrointestinal side effects. In addition, exacerbation of other medical conditions (i.e., congestive heart failure or chronic renal insufficiency) may result from the high doses of NSAIDs used to treat acute gouty arthritis. The elderly are often taking other medications to treat concomitant medical conditions, and therefore care must be exercised to avoid drug ınteractions with medications that patients may already be taking. In addition to these common mechanism-related toxicities, each NSAID has its own spectrum of unique side effects, enumeration of which is beyond the scope of this review.

Many patients do not tolerate high doses of non-selective NSAIDs because of the gastrointestinal distress, ulceration, and bleeding. Selective inhibitors of COX-2 may be better tolerated by patients who suffer unacceptable gastrointestinal distress when taking NSAIDs, and recent studies indicate that selective COX-2 inhibitors (rofecoxib and etoricoxib) are also safe and effective therapy for acute gouty arthritis (20–23). However, salt and water retention is not an uncommon problem in patients taking rofecoxib. Etoricoxib may share this property. Thus, care must be exercised in use of these drugs in patients with comorbid conditions that may be exacerbated by salt and water retention.

In general, both the older non-selective NSAIDs and the more recently developed selective COX-2 inhibitors are safe and effective for the treatment of acute gouty arthritis. Although the cost of COX-2 selective agents is significantly greater than the cost of the older non-selective agents, their use may be justified in those patients who are unable to tolerate the non-selective agents due to gastrointestinal toxicity. NSAIDs and selective COX-2 inhibitors remain the starting point for therapy for most patients with acute gouty arthritis. For patients who are unable to tolerate these agents for any reason, other therapeutic options include high-dose oral or intravenous colchicine, oral and intra-articular corticosteroids, and injections of ACTH.

REFERENCES

1. Reginato AJ. Gout and other crystal arthropathises. In: Kasper DL, Braunwald E, Fauce AS et al., eds. Harrison's Textbook of Medicine. 16th ed. New York: McGraw-Hill, 2005:2046–2047.
2. Wortmann RL, Kelley WN. Gout and hyperuricemia. In: Harris ED, Jr., Budd RC, Firestein GS et al., eds. Kelley's Textbook of Rheumatology. 7th ed. Philadelphia: Elsevier Saunders, 2005:1405–1429.
3. Hahn PC, Edwards NL. Management of hyperuricemia. In: Koopman WJ, Moreland LW, eds. Arthritis and Alied Dconditions. 15th ed. Philadelphia: Lippincott, Williams & Wilkins, 2005:2341–2356.
4. Emerson BT. The management of gout. In: Hochberg MC, Silman AJ, Smolen JS et al. eds. Rheumatology. 3rd ed. Edinburgh: Mosby, 2003:1929–1936.
5. Vane JR. Inhibition of prostaglandin synthesis as a mechanism of action for aspirin-like drugs. Nature 1971; 231:232–235.
6. Needleman P, Isakson PC. The discovery and function of COX-2. J Rheumatol 1977; 24:6–8.

7. Bellamy N, Downie WW, Buchanan WW. Observations on spontaneous improvement in patients with podagra: implications for therapeutic trials of non-steroidal anti-inflammatory drugs. Br J Clin Pharmacol 1987; 24:33–36.
8. Emmerson BT. Regimen of indomethacin therapy in acute gouty arthritis. BMJ 1967; 2:272–274.
9. Willkens RF, Case JB, Huix FJ. The treatment of acute gout with naproxen. J Clin Pharmacol 1975; 15:363–366.
10. Sturge RA, Scott JT, Hamilton EB, et al. Multi-centre trial of naproxen and phenylbutazone in acute gout. Adv Exp Med Biol 1977; 76B:290–296.
11. Schweitz MC, Nashel DJ, Alepa FP. Ibuprofen in the treatment of acute gouty arthritis. JAMA 1978; 239:34–35.
12. Weiner GI, White SR, Weitzner RI, Rubinstein HM. Double-blind study of fenoprofen versus phenylbutazone in acute gouty arthritis. Arthritis Rheum 1979; 22:425–426.
13. Tweddell ED, Willcocks WA. An evaluation of piroxicam, a new non-steroidal anti-inflammatory agent. A multicentre trial. S Afr Med J 1981; 59:915–916.
14. Karachalios GN, Donas G. Sulindac in the treatment of acute gout arthritis. Int J Tissue React 1982; 4:297–299.
15. Eberl R, Dunky A. Meclofenamate sodium in the treatment of acute gout. Results of a double-blind study. Arzneimittelforschung 1983; 33:641–643.
16. Butler RC, Goddard DH, Higgens CS, et al. Double-blind trial of flurbiprofen and phenylbutazone in acute gouty arthritis. Br J Clin Pharmacol 1985; 20:511–513.
17. Altman RD, Honig S, Levin JM, Lightfoot RW. Ketoprofen versus indomethacin in patients with acute gouty arthritis: a multicenter, double blind comparative study. J Rheumatol 1988; 15:1422–1426.
18. Maccagno A, Di Giorgio E, Romanowicz A. Effectiveness of etodolac ('Lodine') compared with naproxen in patients with acute gout. Curr Med Res Opin 1991; 12:423–429.
19. Shrestha M, Morgan DL, Moreden JM, et al. Randomized double-blind comparison of the analgesic efficacy of intramuscular ketorolac and oral indomethacin in the treatment of acute gouty arthritis. Ann Emerg Med 1995; 26:682–686.
20. Cheng T, Lai HM, Chiu CK, Chem YC. A single-blind, randomized, controlled trial to assess the efficacy and tolerability of rofecoxib, diclofenac sodium, and meloxicam in patients with acute gouty arthritis. Clin Ther 2004; 26:399–406.
21. Rubin BR, Burton R, Navarra S, et al. Efficacy and safety profile of treatment with etoricoxib 120 mg once daily compared with indomethacin 50 mg three times daily in acute gout: a randomized controlled trial. Arthritis Rheum 2004; 50:598–606.
22. Schumacher HR, Jr., Boice JA, Daikh DI, et al. Randomised double blind trial of etoricoxib and indomethacin in treatment of acute gouty arthritis. BMJ 2002; 324:1488–1492.

22

Corticosteroids in the Treatment of Crystal-Induced Arthropathies

R. Swamy Venuturupalli and Michael H. Weisman
Division of Rheumatology, Department of Medicine, Cedars Sinai Medical Center and David Geffen School of Medicine at UCLA, Los Angeles, California, U.S.A.

INTRODUCTION

Therapeutic use of corticosteroids is an important but controversial issue in rheumatology. In 1949, Hench and others, who subsequently shared the Nobel Prize for their pioneering work, demonstrated the dramatic effects of cortisone for treating rheumatoid arthritis. Subsequent recognition of the side effects that may develop from long-term use of supraphysiologic doses dampened enthusiasm for its use. As late as the 1990s, corticosteroids were not universally recommended for the treatment of crystal-induced arthritis because of fears of side effects and concerns about rebound attacks of arthritis after the agents were discontinued. Although controversies about the use of corticosteroids continue to this date, these agents remain very effective treatments for many patients with serious rheumatic diseases. In gout and the crystal-induced arthritides, corticosteroids are potent and extremely useful therapeutic agents, and, in certain circumstances, are the agents of choice.

CORTICOSTEROID STRUCTURE

Corticosteroids are 21 carbon steroid molecules, with hydrocortisone the major endogenous biologically active glucocorticoid. Synthetic corticosteroids that

Table 1 Comparative Approximate Potencies, Duration of Action, and Equivalent Doses of Glucocorticoids

Drug	Duration of action	Glucocorticoid potency	Mineralocorticoid potency	Equivalent dose (mg)
Short acting				
Cortisol (hydrocortisone)	8–12 hour	1	1	20
Cortisone	8–12 hour	0.8	0.8	25
Intermediate acting				
Prednisone	12–36 hour	4	0.8	5
Prednisolone	12–36 hour	4	0.8	5
Methylprednisolone	12–36 hour	5	0.5	4
Long acting				
Dexamethasone	36–72 hour	25–30	0	0.7

Source: From Ref. 1.

have an 11-ketone group, such as cortisone and prednisone, are biologically inactive until reduced in the liver to their 11-hydroxyl derivatives, hydrocortisone and methylprednisone, respectively. Because these medications require bioactivation, they can only be used systemically. For local effects, biologically active glucocorticoids such as methylprednisolone or triamcinolone are used (1). Manipulation of the chemical structure has yielded preparations with useful differences in potency, mineralocorticoid activity, and pharmacokinetic profiles (Table 1).

CORTICOSTEROID PHYSIOLOGY

Corticosteroid hormones are essential for normal development and maintenance of homeostasis during both basal and stress states and are important components of the hypothalamic-pituitary-adrenal axis. The production of cortisol by the adrenal cortex is regulated by adrenocorticotropic hormone (ACTH or corticotropin) secreted by the anterior pituitary gland. ACTH release, in turn, is regulated by a hypothalamic product corticotropin-releasing hormone. Under basal conditions, the body produces 10 to 20 mg of cortisol daily, with secretion following a diurnal pattern, except under conditions of stress. With severe stress, as much as 200 mg of cortisone can be secreted in 24 hours. Inflammatory cytokines, such as TNF-α and IL-6, secreted in inflammatory states cause increased steroid release, which in turn exerts negative feedback on the cytokine levels. Intriguingly, defects in the interaction between peripheral inflammatory pathways and the hypothalamic-pituitary-adrenal axis have been postulated to contribute to the development of many rheumatic diseases (2).

MECHANISM OF ACTION OF CORTICOSTEROIDS

The pathways through which corticosteroid treatment leads to anti-inflammatory effects in disease are complex and involve multiple steps. These include expression of the corticosteroid receptor (GR) by its gene, GR activation by steroid hormone, and regulation of anti-inflammatory and pro-inflammatory gene transcription (Fig. 1). Corticosteroid receptors are present in virtually all cells and mediate the anti-inflammatory and metabolic actions of corticosteroids. They are members of a supergene family that includes receptors for other steroid hormones such as estrogen and vitamin D (3). The corticosteroid receptor is associated with two molecules of heat shock protein. After corticosteroid has bound to the receptor (GR), the ligand-receptor complex dissociates from the heat shock protein, allowing the coticosteroid-receptor to migrate to the nucleus where it causes expression of corticosteroid responsive

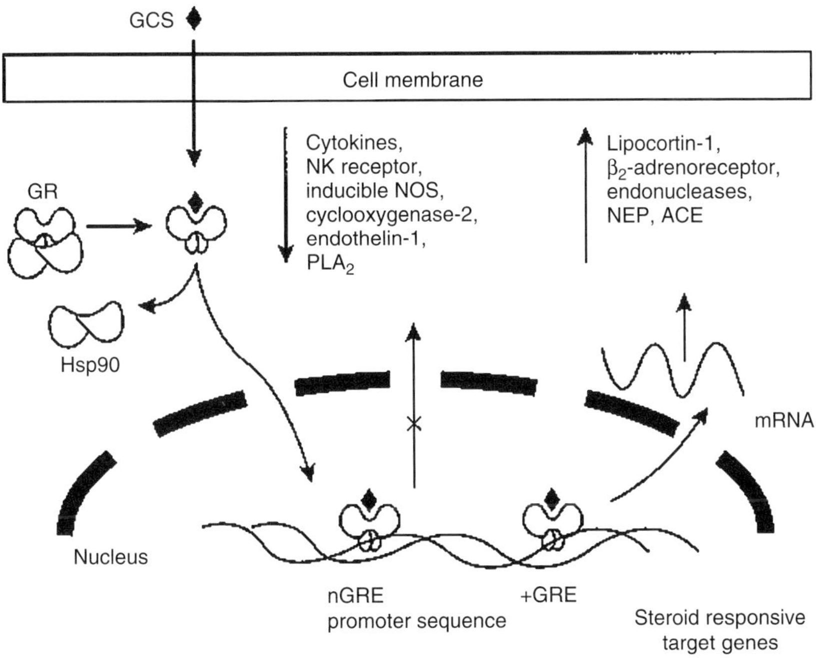

Figure 1 Corticosteroid effects on gene transcription. Corticosteroids (GCS) bind to cytosolic corticosteroid receptors (GR), which are associated with two molecules of heat shock protein 90 (Hsp90). The GCS-GR complex translocates to the nucleus and binds to glucocorticoid response elements (GRE and nGRE) in the promoter sequence of target genes, resulting in increased (GRE) or decreased (nGRE) transcription. *Source*: Adapted from Ref. 1.

genes. These effects on gene expression are complex and involve recruitment of a large number of coactivator or repressor proteins into an extensive transcriptional complex that remodels chromatin and influences transcription in both a gene-specific and cell type-specific manner. A more detailed account of these steps is beyond the scope of this chapter and is reviewed elsewhere (4).

Some of the regulatory actions of corticosteroids include competitive inactivation of c-fos:c-jun complexes and induction of the inhibitory factor I-κB which decreases NF-κB activity. NF-κB and c-fos:c-jun complexes are important transcriptional activating factors that have prominent roles in driving the cellular production of most proinflammatory cytokines and other mediators (5). Corticosteroids also enhance the production of cyclic adenosine monophosphate and destabilize several classes of mRNAs.

Glucocorticoid receptors have alpha and beta forms. The alpha form mediates the classic anti-inflammatory effects of corticosteroids whereas the beta form inhibits corticosteroid action and competes with the alpha form. The ratio of the alpha form to beta form is hypothesized to modulate the cellular effects of steroids and is one potential mechanism for corticosteroid resistance (3,6). Corticosteroid resistance can occur at a number of points in the cascade of events necessary for these agents to exert their effects.

It is postulated that corticosteroid action at the cellular level involves suppression of inflammatory and immune cascades at multiple levels (3). These include neutrophil and monocyte migration into the inflammatory site, antigen processing and presentation to lymphocytes, and cellular activation and differentiation. Corticosteroids are especially active against T lymphocytes, NK cells, and immature B cells, but have little effect on mature B cells. These agents also suppress the production of proinflammatory cytokines such as TNF-α and IL-1 and related mediators such as γ-interferon, prostaglandin E2, and leukotrienes (7).

ADVERSE EFFECTS

Adverse effects of the use of systemic corticosteroids result primarily from exposure to high doses over an extended period of time. In crystal-induced arthritis, corticosteroids are used in the management of the acute inflammatory flare, typically for short periods of time. Consequently, long-term steroid side effects are rarely seen. Side effects from intra-articular steroid injection are discussed below. Adrenal suppression from a single dose of intramuscular triamcinolone acetonide has been described but is quite rare (8). Increased blood glucose levels (especially in diabetic patients), hypokalemia, fluid overload, and facial flushing following systemic steroids are well known and can occur even with short term use (9). A detailed discussion of adverse reactions from long-term use of corticosteroids is provided elsewhere (1,3).

CORTICOSTEROIDS IN THE TREATMENT OF GOUT

Intra-articular Corticosteroids

Intra-articular corticosteroids have been used to treat gout since 1951 (10). Initially, hydrocortisone acetate was used, but now longer-acting compounds such as betamethasone phosphate and acetate, methylprednisolone acetate, triamcinolone, and triamcinolone hexacetonide are widely used for the treatment of all forms of acute crystal-induced arthritis.

The molecular mechanism of intra-articular corticosteroid action is not entirely clear, but several theories have been proposed. Transient decreases in synovial fluid complement, total leukocyte counts, polymorphonuclear leukocytes, and acid phosphatase levels have been reported following intra-articular corticosteroids. Although it has been postulated that intra-articular steroids diminish synovial vascular permeability, this has not been consistently demonstrated in studies. The possibility that corticosteroids increase the release of lubricating synovial surfactant has been suggested (11).

Intra-articular steroids are not free of side effects. Charcot-like arthropathy resulting from corticosteroid injections was first described in the late 1950s. However, the concept of corticosteroid arthropathy is based largely on subprimate animal studies and anecdotal case reports. Studies of primate models have shown no long-term adverse effect on cartilage, and intra-articular corticosteroids appear to have no net effect on bone resorption and only a transient effect on bone formation. Other rare but potential complications include iatrogenic infection, tendon rupture, tissue atrophy, fat necrosis and calcification, nerve damage, post-injection flare, uterine bleeding, pancreatitis, erythema, warmth, diaphoresis of face and torso, and posterior subcapsular cataracts (11). More serious complications such as osteonecrosis have also been reported in the literature. Highly insoluble microcrystalline preparations decrease the duration of an acute attack. However, a crystal-induced synovitis or soft tissue atrophy may occur if the preparation is not injected into a joint space. Hence, highly insoluble preparations, such as triamcinolone hexacetonide, are not recommended for use in small joints of the hands or feet unless one is confident the injection will be into the joint space.

Despite the hundreds of thousands of intra-articular corticosteroid injections that have been performed in the last half-century, there is a dearth of high quality clinical studies demonstrating their efficacy. A Medline literature search did not recover any quality published trials on the effects of intra-articular steroids in gout or other crystal-induced arthropathies. Thus, the basis for the use of intra-articular steroids in these diseases remains empiric and anecdotal. Regardless, it is believed that the aspiration of the inflammatory fluid alone can provide some relief from an acute attack of crystal-induced arthritis, but an intra-articular corticosteroid injection can provide greater and more sustained relief and is usually followed by resolution of synovitis (8).

The effectiveness of different intra-articular steroid preparations have been assessed in a rat subcutaneous air pouch model of inflammation produced by monosodium urate crystals (10). Betamethasone, which has a soluble steroid component, had a rapid but mild anti-inflammatory effect. In contrast, both prednisolone tebutate and triamcinolone hexacetonide dramatically suppressed inflammation. However, these agents also caused atrophy and necrosis of the membrane, yielding a very thin membrane with almost no vessels. More alarmingly, increased monosodium urate aggregates and tophus-like structures were seen on the synovial surface after using corticosteroid injections.

Thus, while intra-articular corticosteroids remain one of the easiest and putatively safest means to provide relief from crystal-induced joint inflammation, questions remain concerning their mechanisms of action, the optimal preparation to use, and long-term effects on the joints. Short duration conditions such as bursitis may be treated adequately with betamethasone preparations, but this specific preparation may not be optimal in more chronic synovitis (10). Although the Charcot-like arthropathy mentioned above has not been substantiated by prospective experience, the finding of membrane necrosis, atrophy, and tophus formation observed in the rat pouch model merit further study.

Systemic Corticosteroid Therapy

Although intra-articular steroids are recommended for treating acute mono-articular gout, systemic corticosteroids have not been uniformly endorsed for use in this setting. Among concerns cited are variability of response, the occurrence of rebound attacks upon corticosteroid withdrawal, and the potential for adrenal suppression (12).

Several published studies lend support for the use of systemic corticosteroids as a viable option when first line agents cannot be used or are ineffective. Although lower doses of corticosteroids (equivalent to 10 mg of prednisone) may be safe and effective in treating acute gout (13), these doses may be not be sufficient in all patients. The prevalence of gout attacks in patients being treated with cyclosporine despite their being on an average of 7.5 to 15 mg of prednisone daily suggests that a larger dosage is required (14). Therefore, doses of steroids equivalent to 20 or 30 mg of oral prednisone are generally recommended for acute gout attacks. This has been supported by multiple reviews and authors (8,15).

A prospective evaluation of the use of oral corticosteroids for the treatment of acute gout involving 13 patients treated with 20 to 50 mg of oral prednisone (or intravenous prednisolone when more than one joint was involved) given in a single daily dose on a tapering schedule resulted in complete resolution of signs and symptoms within 7 to 10 days (8). The study, however, was neither blinded nor controlled.

In a randomized, unblinded comparison trial, intramuscular triamcinolone acetonide (60 mg) was compared with indomethacin (50 mg three times a day) in 27 patients with acute gout enrolled within 5 days of onset of symptoms (12). Resolution of all symptoms occurred at an average of 7 days for the triamcinolone group and an average of 8 days in the indomethacin group. No side effects or episodes of rebound gout attacks were reported with steroid therapy.

In another prospective but non-controlled study, 14 patients with pseudogout diagnosed by crystal identification were given 60 mg of intramuscular triamcinolone and examined for improvement over a 30-day period (12). Most patients had a complete resolution of their symptoms by day 4, and all patients had complete resolution with a greater than 50% improvement in physician and patient global assessments by day 30. Six of the patients needed an additional corticosteroid injection on day 2. No rebound attacks or medication toxicity was reported. In another trial, intramuscular triamcinolone was found to be more effective than intravenous ACTH for acute gout in a controlled comparison of the two drugs (16).

Based on evidence in the literature, then, systemic corticosteroid agents employed in moderately high doses appear effective in the treatment of acute gout and pseudogout. Systemic corticosteroids are therefore indicated in patients with polyarticular arthritis, renal insufficiency, congestive heart failure, peptic ulcer disease, and multiple medical co-morbidities or when NSAIDs or colchicine are either contra-indicated, ineffective, or not tolerated.

ACTH

The use of ACTH in acute gouty arthritis was described in two separate publications in 1950 (17,18). Additional studies have confirmed its efficacy. A retrospective chart review of 38 patients with crystal-induced arthritis, including five patients with pseudogout, revealed positive outcomes. Indications for ACTH use included history of congestive heart failure, chronic renal insufficiency (creatinine >1.7 mg/dL), upper or lower gastrointestinal bleeding, and unresponsiveness to NSAIDs or colchicine. Most patients were treated initially with 40 units intravenously every 8 hours, with doses tapered according to the clinical response. All of the patients with pseudogout had a complete resolution of their symptoms, and 97% of patients with gout responded. Symptom resolution began within one day of treatment, and the mean time to complete remission was 5.5 days. The average duration of treatment with ACTH in this trial increased with the number of joints involved. There was an 11% relapse rate as ACTH doses were tapered, even though concomitant colchicine was used. Adverse effects included hypokalemia (11%), worsening of glycemic control in diabetic patients (11%), and mild fluid overload (11%) (9). The facts that this was a retrospective chart review and that colchicine was used while tapering ACTH may have influenced the results.

In a single-blind prospective evaluation, 29 patients aged 42 to 81 years with acute gouty arthritis with a median of two joints involved were randomly assigned to a single dose of 40 units of intramuscular ACTH without colchicine, or oral indomethacin 50 mg three times a day (tapered over two weeks) with concomitant colchicine 0.6 mg a day (19). Mean time to relief was shorter for the

ACTH group (8 hours vs. 48 hours), as was the time to complete resolution of symptoms (3 days vs. 7 days). Over six months of follow-up, only two patients in the ACTH group and three in the indomethacin group had a relapse in symptoms. No adverse effects were noted in the ACTH group. In the indomethacin group, three patients (21%) developed dyspepsia requiring treatment, two patients (14%) had an increase in blood pressure, and one individual (7%) had changed mentation. Thus, compared with indometahacin, a single dose parenteral ACTH was more effective, was associatied with fewer side effects, and demonstrated a higher benefit to toxicity ratio.

In another investigation, 76 patients with acute gouty arthritis with the diagnosis confirmed by crystal identification in synovial fluid were evaluated in an unblinded trial (20). Thirty-six patients were randomly assigned to receive ACTH, 40 units as a single intramuscular injection, and 40 patients received oral indomethacin, 50 mg four times daily with food until pain subsided. Subsequent attacks were treated with the assigned study medication. The mean time to pain relief was 3 hours in the ACTH group and 24 hours in the indomethacin group. In follow-up, 5.6% of the ACTH-treated patients and 7.5% of the indomethacin-treated patients experienced recurrent attacks. No adverse events were noted in the ACTH group, but 14 patients did not complete the study for reasons unrelated to therapy. In the indomethacin group, 22 patients reported abdominal discomfort, 15 reported headaches, and 12 reported difficulty with mentation.

Finally, 31 patients with acute gout of less than five days duration were randomly assigned to receive either a single dose of intramuscular ACTH (n = 14) or intramuscular triamcinolone acetonide (n = 16) (16). The study was not blinded, and patients were followed at regular intervals for 30 days. Nine patients in the ACTH group required a second injection, and three needed a third. Two individuals did not respond to ACTH and were given triamcinolone, which completely resolved their symptoms. In contrast, five patients in the triamcinolone group required reinjection and only one required a third injection. Thus in this study, triamcinolone was more effective than ACTH, perhaps because of the shorter half life of intramuscular ACTH (24–48 hours) versus depot triamcinolone, which is gradually released into the circulation for 14 to 21 days.

It appears that ACTH may have a direct effect on the immune system, independent of its ability to stimulate secretion of adrenal steroids. ACTH-binding sites are present on the membrane surfaces of peripheral blood mononuclear leukocytes (21). This receptor is functional and may serve as a component in a regulatory circuit between the immune and the neuroendocrine systems. The effects of ACTH in gout are probably mostly independent of its effect on the adrenal cortex and are mediated by the melanocortin 3 receptor that is present in peripheral immune cells (22).

Therefore, intramuscular ACTH may be an appropriate and effective therapy for acute gout and pseudogout, particularly in patients in whom therapy with NSAIDs or colchicine is ineffective, not tolerated, or potentially harmful.

Use of ACTH is limited by its short half-life, by reports of rebound attacks of crystal arthritis, and difficulty in obtaining this drug in the United States (8).

REFERENCES

1. Stein CM, Pincus T. Glucocorticoids. In: Harris E, Budd Rr, Ruddy S, Sledge CB, eds. Kelly's Textbook of Rheumatology. Philadelphia: W.B. Saunders Company, 2001:823–840.
2. Chrousos GP. The hypothalamic-pituitary-adrenal axis and immune-mediated inflammation. N Engl J Med 1995; 332:1351–1362.
3. Wilder R. Corticosteroids. In: Klippel JF, Stone JH, Weyland CM, eds. Primer on the Rheumatic Diseases. Atlanta, GA: Arthritis Foundation, 2001:593–598.
4. Leung D, Bloom J. Update on glucocorticoid action and resistance. J Allergy Clin Immunol 2003; 111:3–22.
5. Scheinman RI, Cogswell PC, Lofquist AK, et al. Role of transcriptional activation of I kappa B alpha in mediation of immunosuppression by glucocorticoids. Science 1995; 270:283–286.
6. Bamberger CM, Bamberger A, de Castro M, et al. Glucocorticoid receptor beta, a potential endogenous inhibitor of glucocorticoid action in humans. J Clin Invest 1995; 95:2435–2441.
7. Wilder R. Corticosteroids. In: Klippel JF, Wortmann RL, Weyand C, eds. Primer on the Rheumatic Diseases. Atlanta, GA: Arthritis Foundation, 1997:427–431.
8. Groff GD, Franck WA, Raddatz DA. Systemic steroid therapy for acute gout: a clinical trial and review of the literature. Semin Arthritis Rheum 1990; 19:329–336.
9. Ritter J, Kerr LD, Valeriano-Marcet J, et al. ACTH revisited: effective treatment for acute crystal induced synovitis in patients with multiple medical problems. J Rheumatol 1994; 21:696–699.
10. Rull M, Clayburne G, Sieck M, et al. Intra-articular corticosteroid preparations: different characteristics and their effect during inflammation induced by monosodium urate crystals in the rat subcutaneous air pouch. Rheumatology 2003; 42:1093–1100.
11. Owen D. Aspiraton and injection of joints and soft tissues. In: Harris E, Budd R, Ruddy S, Sledge CB, eds. Kelly's Textbook of Rheumatology. Philadelphia: W.B. Saunders Company, 2001:583–603.
12. Alloway JA, Moriarty MJ, Hoogland YT, Nashel DJ. Comparison of triamcinolone acetonide with indomethacin in the treatment of acute gouty arthritis. J Rheumatol 1993; 20:111–113.
13. Silveira L, Vargas A, Medina M. Use of low dose prednisone in the treatment of acute gouty attack. Arthritis Rheum 2003; 48:S535.
14. Clive DM. Renal transplant-associated hyperuricemia and gour. J Am Soc Nephrol 2000; 11:974–979.
15. Hench PS. The reversibility of certain rheumatic and nonrheumatic conditions by the use of cortisone or of the pituitary adrenocotropic hormone. Ann Intern Med 1952; 36:1–38.
16. Siegel LB, Alloway JA, Nashel DJ. Comparison of adrenocorticotropic hormone and triamcinolone acetonide in the treatment of acute gouty arthritis. J Rheumatol 1994; 21:1325–1327.

17. Wolfson WQ, Hunt HD, Cohn C, et al. ACTH and colchicine in the clinical treatment of acute gouty arthritis; physiological considerations and review of therapeutic results in 51 attacks. J Mich State Med Soc 1950; 49:1058–1064.
18. Gutman A, Yu T-F. Effects of ACTH in gout. Am J Med 1950; 9:24–26.
19. Mikdashi J, Hochberg M, Moy E, et al. Single-dose parenteral ACTH in the treatment of acute gouty arthritis: a high benefit to toxicity ratio. Arthritis Rheum 1994; 37:428.
20. Axelrod D, Preston S. Comparison of parenteral adrenocorticotropic hormone with oral indomethacin in the treatment of acute gout. Arthritis Rheum 1988; 31:803–805.
21. Smith E, Brosnan P, Meyer WJ, et al. An ACTH receptor on human mononuclear leukocytes. Relation to adrenal ACTH-receptor activity. N Engl J Med 1987; 317:1266–1269.
22. Getting SJ, Christian HC, Flower RJ, et al. Activation of melanocortin type 3 receptor as a molecular mechanism for adrenocorticotropic hormone efficacy in gouty arthritis. Arthritis Rheum 2002; 46:2765–2775.

23

Uricosuric Therapy

Fernando Perez-Ruiz and Iñaki Hernando
Rheumatology Section, Hospital de Cruces, Baracaldo, Vizcaya, Spain
Ana M. Herrero-Beites
Rehabilitation Division, Hospital de Gorliz, Vizcaya, Spain

INTRODUCTION

Among the classes of drugs and biological agents employed to reduce serum urate levels, uricosuric drugs are those that share the property of increasing renal uric acid excretion (1). In this chapter, we review drugs prescribed specifically for their uricosuric properties, including sulfinpyrazone, probenecid, and benzbromarone, as well as those used as adjuvants in treating hyperuricemia, such as losartan and fenofibrate. Specific attention is given to the practical issues regarding uricosuric agents: who should take them and how they should be prescribed.

HISTORICAL BACKGROUND

Although salicylates, which show a paradoxical effect on the renal handling of uric acid (decreasing renal clearance of uric acid at low analgesic or anti-aggregating doses but displaying uricosuric properties at high doses) (2,3), have the potential for use in treating hyperuricemia, high doses unfortunately have a low benefit to risk ratio and are not practical for this purpose. Consequently uricosuric drugs were the first urate-lowering drugs to be used in clinical practice (4).

Half a century ago, probenecid and sulfinpyrazone became available for clinical use (1,5). This was an incredible advance, because for the first time, all signs and symptoms of gout could be eliminated. Unfortunately the effectiveness of these drugs was blunted in subjects with moderate renal functional impairment (6). In contrast, the newest uricosuric agent, benzbromarone, which is a very potent drug with pharmacokinetic and pharmacodynamic properties substantially different from those of probenecid and sulfinpyrazone, is effective even in the presence of moderate renal insufficiency (7–10). Benzbromarone has been widely used in Europe and Japan. Since the advent of allopurinol over forty years ago, uricosuric drugs have been relegated to a secondary role in the therapy of hyperuricemia and gout (11).

Recently, losartan, an angiotensin II receptor antagonist, and fenofibrate, a lipid-lowering drug, have been shown to have mild uricosuric properties (12,13). These agents may prove useful as adjuvants for urate-lowering therapy.

TARGETS FOR THE EFFECTS OF URICOSURIC DRUGS

Nearly four decades ago, it was recognized that most agents possessing authentic uricosuric properties, such as probenecid, sulfinpyrazone, or salicylates, were organic acids (1). On this basis, it was proposed that these drugs were all secreted by the same organic acid system of renal tubular transport in common with uric acid and that the likely mechanism explaining their uricosuric action was inhibition of tubular reabsorption of uric acid.

In recent years, some of the members of the organic anion transport (OAT) family have been identified and studied at the molecular level (14,15). Mutations in URAT1, a highly specific uric acid and organic anion transporter, have been identified in patients with renal hypouricemia, a condition resulting from impaired tubular reabsorption of urate (16). In these patients, the effect of potent uricosuric drugs is blunted. Also, uric acid reabsorption by URAT1 is suppressed by most of the currently available uricosuric drugs, and conversely enhanced by furosemide (14).

Newly identified molecules involved in the tubular transport of the urate anion could be the targets for the development of uricosuric drugs in the future (17).

PHARMACOKINETICS AND CLINICAL USE

Probenecid

Probenecid was developed as a drug to inhibit renal clearance of penicillin but was noted to lower serum urate levels through an increase of urinary uric acid excretion (18). Although sparingly soluble in water, probenecid is well absorbed from the gastrointestinal tract. The drug appears in plasma within one hour after oral ingestion, and peak plasma levels are achieved in approximately four hours. Probenecid is about 90% bound to proteins, showing a dose-dependant half-life of 6–12 hours (1). Biotransformation of probenecid occurs mainly through glucuronide conjugation and oxidation with the main derivative being probenecid acyl monoglucuronide. Hydroxylated and carboxylated derivatives are also produced. All of the derivatives are excreted by renal clearance. Probenecid use at doses greater than 2 g a day increases in the renal excretion of uric acid by amounts that do not usually exceed 50% of baseline (1).

Probenecid is orally administered in a twice daily schedule, but it may have to be given three times a day to be most effective. Dosing often begins with 250 mg twice a day and increased step-wise fashion. A dose of 250 mg twice a day will bring the serum urate below 7.0 mg/dL in approximately 10% of patients. A total dose of 1 g a day will bring half the patients to target urate levels, 1.5 to 2 g are required for 25%, and 2.5 to 3.0 g a day are necessary for the remaining 15% (19,20).

The uricosuric effect of probenecid is reduced in patients showing moderate to severe reduction of the glomerular filtration rate. Therefore, its use is not recommended in such individuals (6,21). Although salicylates may interfere with the uricosuric effects of probenecid, low dose aspirin used for vascular prophylaxis does not (22).

Side effects are not frequent, but cutaneous eruptions and gastrointestinal intolerance do occur. Side effects cause up to 20% of patients to discontinue probenecid use (1).

Sulfinpyrazone

Sulfinpyrazone is a derivative of phenylbutazone that has a more potent uricosuric effect, but no analgesic or anti-inflammatory properties. Sulfinpyrazone is approximately five times more potent than probenecid on a weight basis. It is rapidly absorbed after oral administration, reaching peak levels after one hour. More than 95% of the drug is bound to proteins, and it has a short half-life of 1 to 3 hours. One-third of the drug ingested is excreted unaltered in urine (1,23,24).

Dosage is started at 100 mg a day in orally divided doses in a twice daily schedule. Doses may be increased if necessary up to 400 mg/day. At a daily dose of 400 mg/day, sulfinpyrazone induces a uricosuric response comparable to that of 1.5 to 2.0 g of probenecid (1). Like probenecid, sulfinpyrazone is less efficacious in patients with renal insufficiency, although an additive effect is observed in this setting when both drugs are simultaneously administered (1). Sulfinpyrazone has been used in combination with allopurinol (25).

Adverse events are not common with sulfinpyrazone. Like probenecid, skin reactions and gastrointestinal intolerance are the most frequently observed side effects. Because of its anti-aggregating effect on platelets, sulfinpyrazone is a less suitable drug for patients also receiving anti-coagulation therapy.

Benzbromarone

Benzbromarone is a benzofuran derivative with a very potent uricosuric effect. Its plasma concentration peak is reached at 2 to 4 hours after administration. Bioavailability after non-micronized oral administration is approximately 50% (26). Benzbromarone is excreted primarily through the bile after undergoing dehalogenation in the liver to bromobenzarone and benzarone. A longer half-life than those of other uricosuric agents permits once-a-day oral administration.

Dosing may start at 50 mg a day, increasing to 100 mg, and up to 200 mg per 24 hours. The uricosuric properties of benzbromarone are maintained in patients with moderate to severe renal insufficiency. Accordingly, this drug is effective even in patients with glomerular filtration rates of 20 mL/min and despite diuretic or cyclosporine therapy (9,10).

Unfortunately, there are few studies comparing the efficacy of uricosuric drugs or of uricosuric drugs with other xanthine oxidase inhibitors. Benzbromarone was, however, found to superior to allopurinol in a randomized, open-label study of patients with renal insufficiency, in a large cohort of renal transplant patients, and in non-randomized studies (9,10,27–29).

The combination of allopurinol plus benzbromarone may be useful in gout patients with serum urate levels not sufficiently reduced with single-drug therapy (29). This approach may be especially useful in patients with severe tophaceous gout, in whom rapid mobilization of body urate deposits may be desirable. It is important to recall that uricosuric drugs enhance renal oxypurinol clearance (30), so that higher than usual doses of allopurinol may be required if concomitant uricosuric therapy is prescribed (29).

Gastrointestinal intolerance is the most common limiting adverse effect of benzbromarone. Although the pharmacokinetic profile of benzbromarone at doses up to 100 mg a day is not substantially altered in patients with mild liver function impairment, severe hepatic toxicity, although infrequently reported, has been considered a limitation to the use of benzbromarone (31).

Adjuvant Uricosuric Agents

Other drugs with uricosuric properties may be of interest in clinical practice. The usefulness of fenofibrate, in daily doses over 200 mg/day, either in single therapy or in combination with allopurinol in patients, has been recently highlighted (13,32,33). This approach may be of interest especially in patients with coexisting hyperlipidemia, especially those whose serum urate levels exceed those likely to reduce the body serum urate pool despite taking allopurinol.

Losartan exerts a mild uricosuric effect that may be clinically useful in gout patients with hypertension (33,34). This drug may be especially useful in the presence of on-going thiazide therapy or if hyperuricemia persists after thiazide withdrawal.

CANDIDATES FOR URICOSURIC THERAPY

Uricosuric therapy can be very effective (Table 1). The optimal candidate for uricosuric therapy is the gout patient with no history of renal stones (1,6,21) and inefficient renal handling of uric acid (9,10,35). Recommendation for therapy with probenecid or sulfinpyrazone will generally be limited in those subjects with moderate renal functional impairment (creatinine clearance <50 mL/min). Therapy with benzbromarone is limited by availability of the agent (benzbromarone is not available in the United States, Canada, and a number of other countries).

Overproduction of urate is not, per se, a formal contraindication for uricosuric therapy. Indeed, until allopurinol became available, all gouty patients were treated with uricosuric drugs. If a uricosuric drug is prescribed in this setting, special care should be taken in order to avoid renal uricosuric-induced nephrolithiasis.

Table 1 A Practical Approach to Therapy with Uricosuric Drugs in 10 Items

1) Be sure that there is a real indication for prescribing urate-lowering therapy.
2) Select patients showing inefficient renal excretion of uric acid (underexcretion). Patients with tophi may be eligible for uricosuric therapy.
3) Patients with overproduction or previous lithiasis, but no other choice for urate-lowering therapy, may be treated with uricosuric drugs, but serial monitoring of spot urine and blood samples should be emphasized in order to avoid lithiasis.
4) Patients with unsatisfactory reduction of uric acid levels while on allopurinol may benefit from combination with uricosuric agents.
5) Moderate renal functional impairment may interfere with the efficacy of probenecid and sulfinpyrazone therapy. Benzbromarone shows efficacy in patients with moderate renal functional impairment (creatinine clearance >20 mL/min). Patients with hyperlipidemia may benefit from single or combined therapy with fenofibrate.
6) Renal function should be estimated in any patient with gout, either with 24-hour urine sample clearances or by the Cockroft-Gault equation.
7) Start with small doses. Adjust dosage up to that necessary to achieve serum urate under 6 mg/dL or to maximal doses of the uricosuric agent.
8) Follow-up monitoring can be accomplished using spot blood and urine samples. Along with serum urate and creatinine, urine sediment, and the concentration of uric acid and creatinine should be evaluated at each control visit. Renal response to uricosurics may be evaluated by estimating the increase of the excretion of uric acid (Table 2).
9) Monitor undissociated urinary uric acid (Fig. 1). Increase fluid intake or prescribe urine alkalinizing agent, if necessary.
10) If high levels of undissociated urinary uric acid persist, consider withdrawing uricosuric therapy.

Identifying Inefficient Handling (Underexcretion) of Uric Acid

Inefficient renal handling of uric acid (also termed renal underexcretion) results from an impairment to adapt renal excretion to a given filtered load of uric acid (36). This altered capacity to excrete the filtered load of urate may be primary or secondary to renal functional impairment or drugs. Drugs most likely to alter uric acid excretion include, most commonly, diuretics, as well as cyclosporin-A, tacrolimus, pyrazinamide, ethambutol, didanosine, and ritonavir.

Table 2 lists several methods currently used to identify patients with inefficient renal excretion of uric acid (41). These include the 24-hour urinary uric acid excretion (11); the clearance of uric acid (6); uric acid to creatinine ratio in urine samples; Simkin's Index (SI)—uric acid excretion per glomerular filtration volume (42); and fractional excretion of uric acid. The first two require a 24-hour urine collection, whereas the three latter may be calculated using spot, midmorning urine samples. Several studies have addressed the issue of the optimal method to identify and quantitate renal uric acid underexcretion. Consensus has not been achieved to date, largely because the results of applying different methods to measure the same function have differed widely (43–45).

Most of the methods described in Table 2 are useful in clinical research, especially the clearance of uric acid (39). Some are, however, impractical for use by clinicians in practice. The most practical approach may be calculating SI (41). If the SI is less than 0.6 mg/dL, then the patient may be classified as a uric acid underexcretor. In contrast, if the SI is greater than 0.6 mg/dL, the patient would have normal renal handling of urate and indicate overproduction, unless there is a reduction in glomerular filtration rate. In patients with impaired renal function, the Pcr/Ucr quotient rises and the patient may show a SI greater than 0.6 mg/dL, leading to a false positive result and misclassification as a uric acid over-producer (37,40). This situation arises in some patients who, despite normal serum creatinine levels (under about 1.5 mg/dL), may have a reduction in the glomerular filtration rate. In such instances, one must resort to methods using 24-hour urine collections (11) or estimating the clearance of creatinine with the Cockroft-Gault equation (37).

The primary reason to classify a patient with gout as an underexcretor or an overproducer is more for the identification of patients with inefficient excretion than those with overproduction. By doing so, one identifies patients who may ideally benefit from uricosuric therapy and decrease the risk of renal stones.

Identifying Risk of Nephrolithiasis

During uricosuric therapy, the risk of developing renal stones may increase due to the enhancement of uric acid excretion (1). Uric acid stones are more frequent in gouty patients than in non-gouty patients (46). In addition, patients who excrete large quantities of uric acid in the urine are at risk for calcium oxalate stones (47). These points might lead us to conclude that uric acid overproduction and accompanying hyperuricosuria would be the cause for the increased prevalence

Table 2 Most Commonly Used Methods to Classify Gouty Patients According to Renal Handling of Uric Acid, and Also to Monitor the Efficacy of Uricosuric Drugs

	Urine samples	Calculation/limit	Usefulness and limitations	References
24-hr urinary uric acid (24h-Uur)	24-hr	Uvol*Uur (mg/24 h) 880 mg/1.73m2	Absolute measure Good correlation with uric acid clearance False underexcretion in patients with near normal serum urate levels 24-hr urine collections	(37,38)
Clearance of uric acid (Cur)	24-hr	Uvol*Uur/Sur/14.4 (mL/min) 6 mL/min/1.73m2	More physiological that 24-hr Uur, measures capacity of renal uric acid handling Allows classifying patients despite allopurinol therapy (even with normal serum uric acid levels) 24-hr urine collections	(6,37,39,40)
Simkin's Index (SI)	Spot	Uur*Scr/Ucr (mg/dL GF) 0.6 mg/dL GF	Easy to apply in clinical practice False overproduction in patients with decreased glomerular filtration rate	(37,38,40)
Fractional excretion	Spot	Uur*Scr/Ucr/Sur 7%	Clearance of creatinine should be calculated (or estimated with the Cockroft-Gault equation) in such cases	

Abbreviations: Uvol, urinary volume (dL/24 h); Uur, urinary uric acid (mg/dL); Sur, serum uric acid (mg/dL); Scr, serum creatinine (mg/dL); Ucr, urinary creatinine (mg/dL); GF, glomerular filtration.

of renal stones in gout patients. In fact, urinary uric acid excretion is low in patients with pure uric acid stones, and much lower than in patients with calcium oxalate stones (47). In addition, the urinary pH is lower in gouty uric acid stone formers than in patients with calcium oxalate stones. So, both urinary uric acid concentration and urine acidity are involved in the pathogenesis of uric acid urolithiasis (48).

Urine pH is an important and perhaps the most important factor in uric acid crystal precipitation in urine (49). The solubility of uric acid in urine, in turn, depends on the concentration of the highly insoluble undissociated form of uric acid. At pH 5.5, 50% of the uric acid in urine is in the form of undissociated uric acid (50). Supersaturation of urine with uric acid at this pH requires a total uric acid concentration of only 20 mg/dL. In contrast, at pH 6.5, supersaturation of urine with uric acid occurs at a total uric acid concentration of almost 120 mg/dL (50). That is, saturation of urine with uric acid varies nearly six-fold over a range of 1 pH unit. This fact underscores the risk for crystallization in gouty individuals, many of whom have an apparently inherent deficit leading to excretion of an acid urine. In any case, supersaturation does not necessarily lead to crystallization, and, even in the case of crystal formation, crystalluria is not a decisive step for stone formation. Indeed, crystalluria is much more prevalent than stone formation (51).

The presence of tophi has not been reported in the literature to be associated with a higher risk of renal stones during uricosuric therapy. Dissolution of the solid pool of urate is a slow process. Patients with tophi have a higher total body pool of urate. Accordingly, they show a trend to maintain that higher urinary uric acid output induced by uricosuric therapy longer than patients without tophi. In patients without visible tophi, a reduction of the uricosuric effect, but not the effect of lowering serum urate levels, is observed not long after initiating uricosurics (1).

Therefore, the availability to provide the requisite long-term monitoring of uric acid excretion and pH may be the only limiting factor for prescribing uricosuric therapy in patients with tophaceous gout.

Patients taking uricosuric therapy whose urinary pH is in the lower range would appear to be at the highest risk for developing renal stones, if high urinary uric acid concentration is observed during follow-up.

The practical issue is, what is the point at which supersaturation is likely to induce lithiasis? To address that fact in clinical practice, the monitoring of undissociated urinary uric acid is likely to be important. The nomogram shown in Figure 1 allows estimation of the concentration of undissociated urinary uric acid in a fasting, first morning urine. In fact, the same urine sample can be used to monitor the course and safety of uricosuric therapy by measuring the increase in fractional excretion of uric acid (requires a blood sample a swell) and examining the urine for uric acid crystalluria and microscopic blood (52,53).

The estimated concentration of undissociated uric acid in urine was the only independent predictive factor of lithiasis in over 200 gouty patients treated with benzbromarone who were not treated with urine alkalinization. The rate of lithiasis, either calcium or uric acid stones, was less than one to 100 patient-years of therapy in patients with undissociated urinary uric acid concentrations less than 20 mg/dL. In contrast, the rate of lithiasis was eight to 100 patient-years in patients with undissociated urinary uric acid greater than 20 mg/dL. When indicated, reduction in the concentration of undissociated uric acid can be accomplished with either urine alkalinization or increased fluid intake or both.

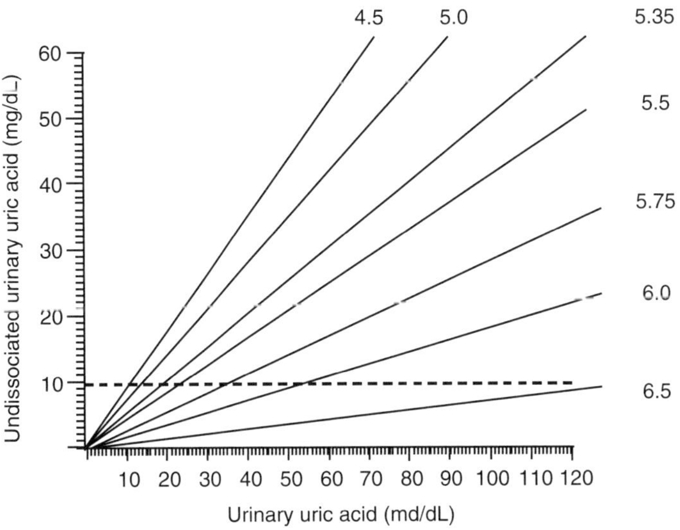

Figure 1 Nomogram used to estimate the concentration of undissociated uric acid (*y axis*) depending on (total) urinary uric acid concentration (*x axis*) and urinary pH. The physicochemical—not necessarily clinical—limit for saturation of uric acid is shown with dotted line.

Benzbromarone has also been used to treat a series of patients with previous lithiasis who had suffered severe side effects during allopurinol therapy. High fluid intake and alkali were prescribed along with close monitoring of serial urine samples and renal ultrasonography. Patients on this protocol were maintained on uricosuric therapy without side effects (Perez-Ruiz, unpublished data).

REFERENCES

1. Gutman AB. Uricosuric drugs with special reference to probenecid and sulfinpyrazone. Adv Pharmacol 1966; 4:91–142.
2. Yü TF, Gutman AB. Paradoxical retention of uric acid by uricosuric drugs in low dosage. Proc Soc Exp Biol Med 1955; 90:542–547.
3. Caspi D, Lubart E, Graff E, et al. The effect of mini-dose aspirin on renal function and uric acid handling in elderly patients. Arthritis Rheum 2000; 43:103–108.
4. Cohen H. Gout. In: Copeman WSC, ed. Textbook of the Rheumatic Diseases. 1st ed. Edinburgh: E&S Livingstone, 1948:249–305.
5. Yü TF. Milestones in the treatment of gout. Am J Med 1974; 56:676–685.
6. Emmerson BT. The management of gout. N Engl J Med 1996; 334:445–451.
7. Sinclair DS, Fox IH. The pharmacology of hypouricemic effect of benzbromarone. J Rheumatol 1975; 2:437–445.

8. Yü TF. Pharmacokinetic and clinical studies of a new uricosuric drug—benzbromarone. J Rheumatol 1976;305–312.
9. Perez-Ruiz F, Gomez-Ullate P, Amenabar JJ, et al. Long-term efficacy of hyperuricaemia treatment in renal transplant patients. Nephrol Dial Transplant 2003; 18:1–4.
10. Perez-Ruiz F, Calabozo M, Fernandez-Lopez MJ, et al. Treatment of chronic gout in patients with renal function impairment. An open, randomized, actively controlled study. J Clin Rheumatol 1999; 5:49–55.
11. Wortmann RL. Gout and hyperuricemia. Curr Opin Rheumatol 2002; 14:281–286.
12. Minghelli G, Seydoux C, Goy JJ, Burnier M. Uricosuric effect of the angiotensin II receptor antagonist losartan in heart transplant recipients. Transplant Proc 1998; 66:268–271.
13. Feher MD, Hepburn AL, Hogarth MB, et al. Fenofibrate enhances urate reduction in men treated for hyperuricemia and gout. Rheumatology 2003; 42:321–325.
14. Enomoto A, Kimura H, Chairoungdua A, et al. Molecular identification of a renal urate anion exchanger that regulates blood urate levels. Nature 2002; 417:447–452.
15. Kojima R, Sekine T, Kawachi M, et al. Immunolocalization of multi specific organic anion transporters, OAT1, OAT2, and OAT3, in rat kidney. J Am Soc Nephrol 2002; 13:848–857.
16. Ichida K, Kosoyamada M, Hisatome I, et al. Clinical and molecular analysis of patients with renal hypouricemia in Japan—influence fura T1 gene on urinary urate excretion. J Am Soc Nephrol 2004; 15:164–173.
17. Bieber JD, Terkeltaub RA. Gout. On the brink of novel therapeutic options for an ancient disease. N Engl J Med 2004; 350:2400–2414.
18. Bishop C, Rand R, Talbott JR. Effect of Benemid (p-[di-n-propylsufamyl]-benzoic acid) on uric acid metabolism in one normal and one gouty subject. J Clin Invest 1951; 30:889–895.
19. Gutman AB. Medical management of gout. Postgrad Med 1972; 51:61–66.
20. Gutman AB, YU TF. Protracted uricosuric therapy in tophaceous gout. Lancet 1957; 2:1258–1260.
21. Terkeltaub RA. Gout. N Engl J Med 2003; 13:240–244.
22. Harris M, Bryant LR, Danaher P, Alloway J. Effect follow dose daily aspirin on serum urate levels and urinary excretion in patients receiving probenecid for gouty arthritis. J Rheumatol 2000; 27:1873–1876.
23. Lecaillon JB, Souppart C, Schller JP, et al. Sulfinpyrazone kinetics after intravenous and oral administration. Clin Pharmacol Ther 1979; 26:611–617.
24. Dieterle W, Faigle JW, Mory H, et al. Biotransformation and pharmacokinetics of sulfinpyrazone (Anturan) in man. Eur J Clin Pharmacol 1975; 9:135–145.
25. Goldfarb E, Smyth CJ. Effects of allopurinol, a xanthine oxidase inhibitor, and sulfinpyrazone, upon the urinary and serum urate levels in eight patients with tophaceous gout. Arthritis Rheum 1966; 9:414–423.
26. Heel RC, Brogden RN, Speight TM, Avery OS. Benzbromarone: a review of its pharmacological properties and therapeutic use in gout and hyperuricemia. Drugs 1977; 14:349–366.
27. Schepers GW. Benzbromarone therapy; comparison with allopurinol and probenecid. J Int Med Res 1981; 9:511–515.

28. Perez-Ruiz F, Alonso-Ruiz A, Calabozo M, et al. The efficacy of allopurinol and benzbromarone for the control of hyperuricemia. A pathogenic approach to the therapy of chronic primary gout. Ann Rheum Dis 1998; 57:545–549.
29. Perez-Ruiz F, Calabozo M, Ruibal A, et al. Influence of urate-lowering therapy on the velocity of reduction of tophi in chronic gout. Arthritis Rheum 2002; 47:356–360.
30. Yamamoto T, Moriwaki Y, Takahashi S, et al. Effects of sulfinpyrazone, probenecid, and benzbromarone on renal excretion of oxypurinol. Ann Rheum Dis 1991; 50:631–633.
31. Walter-Sack I, de Vries JX, von Bubnoff A, et al. Biotransformation and uric acid lowering effect of benzbromarone in patients with liver cirrhosis—evidence for active benzbromarone metabolites. Eur J Med Res 1995; 1:16–20.
32. Hepburn AL, Kaye SA, Feher MD. Long-term remission from gout associated with fenofibrate therapy. Clin Rheumatol 2003; 22:73–76.
33. Takahashi S, Moriwaki Y, Yamamoto T, et al. Effects of combination treatment using anti-hyperuricaemic agents with fenofibrate and/or losartan on uric acid metabolism. Ann Rheum Dis 2003; 62:572–575.
34. Ohnishi K, Kohno M, Yukiiri K, et al. Influence of the angiotensin II receptor antagonist losartan on diuretic-induced metabolic effects in elderly hypertensive patients: comparison with a calcium channel blocker. Int J Clin Pharmacol Ther 2001; 39:417–422.
35. Simkin PA. The treatment of hyperuricemia: allopurinol and beyond. J Clin Rheumatol 1999; 5:45–46.
36. Simkin PA. New standards for uric acid excretion and evidence for an inducible transporter. Arthritis Rheum 2003; 49:735–736.
37. Perez-Ruiz F, Nolla JM. Usefulness of Simkin's Index and the Cockroft-Gault equation to classify patients with gout using spot blood and urine samples. Arthritis Rheum 2003; 48:S533.
38. Perez-Ruiz F, Calabozo M, Herrero-Beites AM, et al. Influence of serum uric acid levels and glomerular filtration on the tests used to classify patients with gout. Arthritis Rheuma 2001; 44:S129.
39. Perez-Ruiz F, Calabozo M, Garcia-Erauskin G, et al. Renal underexcretion of uric acid is present in patients with apparent high urinary uric acid output. Arthritis Rheum 2002; 47:610–613.
40. Perez Ruiz F, Calabozo Raluy M, Herrero Beites A, et al. Analysis of the methods for classifying gout according to renal excretion of uric acid (abstract in English). Rev Esp Reumatol 1998; 25:335–339.
41. Simkin PA. When, why, and how should we quantify the excretion rate of urinary uric acid? J Rheumatol 2001; 28:1207–1210.
42. Simkin PA, Hoover PL, Paxon CS, Wilson WF. Uric acid excretion: quantitative assessment from spot, midmorning serum and urine samples. Ann Intern Med 1979; 91:44–47.
43. Wortman RL, Fox IH. Limited value of uric acid to creatinine ratios in estimating uric acid excretion. Ann Intern Med 1980; 93:822–825.
44. Moriwaki Y, Yamamoto T, Takahashi S, et al. Spot urine uric acid to creatinine ratio used in the estimation of uric acid excretion in primary gout. J Rheumatol 2001; 28:1207–1210.

45. Yamamoto T, Moriwaki Y, Takahashi S, et al. A simple method of selecting gout patients for treatment with uricosuric agents, using spot urine and blood samples. J Rheumatol 2002; 29:1937–1941.
46. Krame HM, Curham GC. The association between gout and nephrolithiasis: the National Health and Nutrition Examination survey III, 1988-1994. Am J Kidney Dis 2002; 40:37–42.
47. Pak CYC, Poindexter JR, Peterson RD, et al. Biochemical distinction between hyperuricosuric calcium urolithiasis and gouty diathesis. Urology 2002; 60:789–794.
48. Yü TF, Gutman AB. Uric acid nephrolithiasis in gout. Predisposing factors. Ann Intern Med 1966; 67:1133–1148.
49. Asplin JR. Uric acid stones. Semin Nephrol 1996; 16:412–424.
50. Moe OW, Abate N, Khashayar S. Pathophysiology of uric acid nephrolithiasis. Endocrinol Metab Clin N Am 2002; 31:895–914.
51. Kok DJ. Clinical implications of physicochemistry of stone formation. Endocrinol Metab Clin N Am 2002; 31:855–867.
52. Perez-Ruiz F, Calabozo M, Herrero-Beites AM, et al. Usefulness of spot, first-morning urine samples during therapy with uricosuric drugs (abstract in English). Rev Esp Reumatol 2001; 28:57–61.
53. Perez-Ruiz F, Nolla JM. Nephrolithiasis during uricosuric therapy: usefulness of monitoring undissociated urinary uric acid. Arthritis Rheum 2004; 50:S341–S342.

24

Xanthine Oxidase Inhibitors

Adel G. Fam

Sunnybrook and Women's College Health Sciences Centre, University of Toronto, Toronto, Ontario, Canada

INTRODUCTION

Xanthine oxidase catalyzes the final reactions in the purine catabolic cascade in humans that result in the production of urate. The development of allopurinol, a potent inhibitor of xanthine oxidase activity, provided an effective treatment for many patients with gout. Additional xanthine oxidase inhibitors have subsequently been developed. The purpose of this chapter is to review the pharmacology of these agents and to discuss strategies and alternative therapies for patients who are unable to tolerate allopurinol.

XANTHINE OXIDASE

Xanthine oxidase is a complex iron-sulfur molybdenum flavoprotein enzyme that oxidizes a wide variety of purines and pyrimidines, including the conversion of hypoxanthine to xanthine, and of xanthine to urate (Fig. 1) (1–4). Urate synthesis is largely a hepatic process. Xanthine oxidase is present in high activity in hepatic sinusoidal lining cells and small intestinal mucosa. Lesser activities are found in capillary endothelium, mammary gland epithelium, skeletal muscle, heart, and kidney. No xanthine oxidase activity is present in leukocytes, erythrocytes, or cultured fibroblasts.

Xanthine oxidase exists in dehydrogenase- and oxidase-forms (1,3–5). The dehydrogenase-form is readily converted to the oxidase-form by oxidation of

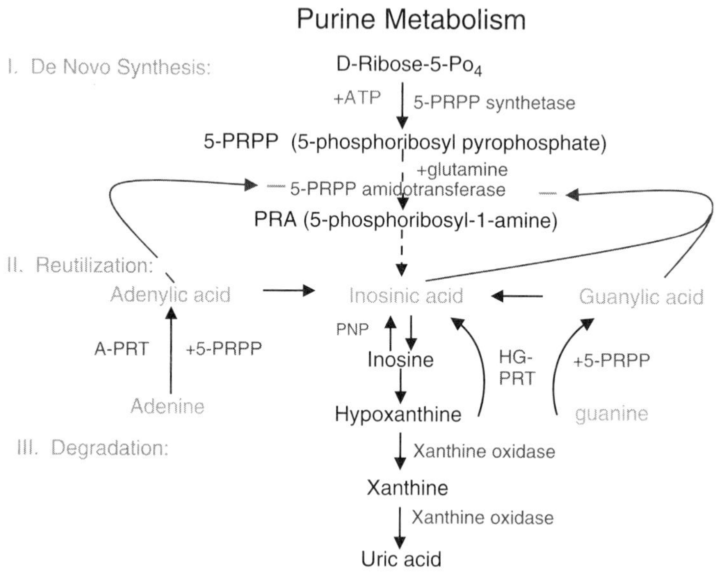

Figure 1 Purine metabolism. *Abbreviations*: ATP, adenosine triphosphate; 5-PRPP, 5-phosphoribosyl pyrophosphate; APRT, adenine phosphoribosyl transferase; HPRT, hypoxanthine guanine phosphoribosyl transferase; PNP, purine nucleoside phosphorylase.

sulfhydryl groups in the protein resulting in loss of the NAD-binding site. The oxidase-form of xanthine oxidase mediates the conversion of hypoxanthine to xanthine and xanthine to urate. In the process, superoxide anion and H_2O_2 are generated, with further conversion of H_2O_2 to free hydroxyl radicals.

XANTHINE OXIDASE INHIBITORS

Xanthine oxidase inhibitors, the most effective and widely prescribed urate-lowering drugs, can be divided into two groups: purine analogues and non-purine compounds (Table 1). The former include allopurinol and oxipurinol which are analogues of hypoxanthine and xanthine, respectively (1,3,5,6). Allopurinol inhibits the oxidized form of xanthine oxidase, whereas oxipurinol inhibits the reduced or dehydrogenase-form of xanthine oxidase (5–7). These drugs compete with both hypoxanthine and xanthine at the molybdenum-pterin active site of the enzyme protein (6–8). Both allopurinol and oxipurinol are considered "non-selective" for xanthine oxidase as they inhibit other enzymes involved in purine and pyrimidine metabolism.

Non-purine inhibitors include two newer agents; febuxostat and Y-700. Febuxostat is a 2-arythiozole derivative. It is a selective inhibitor of xanthine oxidase with no significant effects on other purine or pyrimidine enzymes (5,9–11).

Table 1 Urate-Lowering Agents

Inhibitors of uric acid synthesis (xanthine oxidase inhibitors)
Purine analogues
Allopurinol[a]
Oxipurinol[b]
Non-analogue xanthine oxidase inhibitors
Febuxostat[b]
Y-700
Uricosuric agents
Probenecid[a]
Sulfinpyrazone[a]
Benzbromarone[b]
Losartan
Fenofibrate
Ascorbic acid
Uricolytic agents (uricases)
Recombinant uricases:
A. flavus uricase (rasburicase)[c]
C. utilis uricase (uricase-PEG 20)[b]
Porcine PEG-uricase (puricase)[b]

[a]Proven drug.
[b]Limited clinical experience, not commercially available in the United States or Canada.
[c]Adjunct prophylaxis and treatment of malignancy-associated hyperuricemia and tumor lysis syndrome.

Febuxostat inhibits both the oxidized and reduced forms of xanthine oxidase by binding with high avidity to a channel on the dimeric protein leading to the molybedenum-pterine active site of the enzyme, hence blocking substrate (hypoxanthine and xanthine) access and binding (5). This high affinity binding results in a more potent and prolonged urate-lowering effect. Y-700, 1-(3-cyano-4-neopentyloxyphenyl) pyrazole-4-carboxylic acid, is a novel, non-purine, xanthine oxidase inhibitor which causes dose-dependent, long-lasting urate-lowering, and is currently under clinical evaluation for the treatment of gout (12,13).

Allopurinol

Historical Aspects

Recognition that hereditary xanthinuria, a rare disorder resulting from deficiency of xanthine oxidase, was associated with marked hypouricemia drew attention to the importance of xanthine oxidase in urate production. Allopurinol [4-hydroxypyrazolo (3,4-d) pyrimidine, or 4-HPP], a structural analogue of hypoxanthine, was initially developed by Hitchings and Elion in 1956 as an adjuvant agent to enhance the therapeutic effectiveness of 6-mercaptopurine in the treatment of leukemia (1). Xanthine oxidase inhibition by allopurinol retards oxidation of 6-mercaptopurine to the inactive metabolite,

6-thiouric acid, and thereby potentiates anti-tumor and immunosuppressive effects of the drug as well as its toxicity. In the course of development, it was noted that allopurinol consistently lowered serum urate and urinary uric concentrations, and in 1963, allopurinol was introduced for the treatment of hyperuricemia and gout (1).

Mechanism of Action

Allopurinol is both a substrate and a potent inhibitor of xanthine oxidase activity. About 70% of allopurinol is metabolized to oxipurinol [4,6-dihydroxypyrazolo (3, 4-d) pyrimidine, alloxanthine or 4,6-DHPP], which is also a potent xanthine oxidase inhibitor (1,3,7,8). Allopurinol is cleared mainly by glomerular filtration. Oxipurinol is reabsorbed in the renal tubules in a fashion similar to the reabsorption of uric acid (1,14). With normal renal function, the half-life of allopurinol is one to four hours whereas that of oxipurinol is 14 to 26 hours. Therefore, the urate-lowering effect of allopurinol is largely due to its conversion to oxipurinol and the longer half-life of this active metabolite (1). Thus, allopurinol need not be given in divided doses, and can be administered as a single daily dose (15).

Allopurinol and oxipurinol interfere with the conversion of hypoxanthine to xanthine and of xanthine to urate (Fig. 2 and 3), resulting in reductions of serum urate and urinary uric acid concentrations. These reductions are accompanied by increases in serum and urinary xanthine and, to a lesser extent, hypoxanthine concentrations. The solubilities of hypoxanthine, xanthine, and urate are independent. Renal clearances of hypoxanthine and xanthine exceed that of urate. Xanthine is about as soluble as urate and that of hypoxanthine is greater. Thus, despite the presence of increased amounts of hypoxanthine and xanthine in the urine in patients receiving allopurinol, xanthine stone formation is rare. On a molar basis, however, the increases in urinary hypoxanthine and xanthine in allopurinol-treated subjects are not equivalent to the reduction in urinary uric acid (1,16). This paradox results from salvage of hypoxanthine and conversion into IMP in a phosphoribosylpyrophosphate (PRPP)-requiring reaction catalyzed by hypoxanthine guanine phosphoribosyltransferase (HPRT) (1,8,16). Either generation of purine nucleotide inhibitors of purine synthesis de novo or depletion of the purine synthesis accelerator PRPP (or both) results in inhibition of rates of purine synthesis, reflected in a decrease in the overall urinary excretion of hypoxanthine plus xanthine plus uric acid in the urine of allopurinol-treated individuals.

Both allopurinol and oxipurinol are considered "non-selective" xanthine oxidase inhibitors, since these agents inhibit other purine and pyrimidine pathway enzymes, such as purine nucleoside phosphorylase and orotidylate decarboxylase [orotidine-5'- monophosphate decarboxylase (OMPDC)] (1,8,16–20). Allopurinol administration also results in inhibition of de novo pyrimidine nucleotide synthesis (1,8,17). Oxipurinol ribonucleotides inhibit orotidylate decarboxylase,

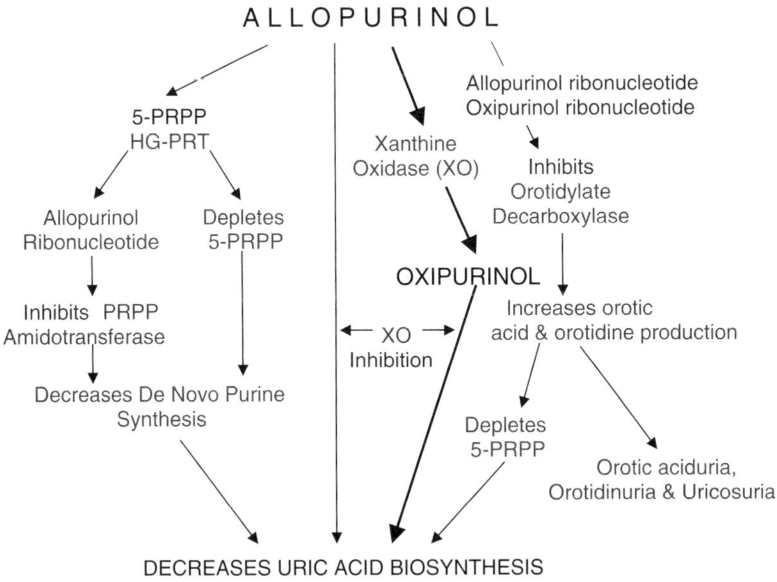

Figure 2 Mechanism of action of allopurinol. *Abbreviations*: 5-PRPP, 5-phosphoribosyl pyrophosphate; HGPRT, hypoxanthine guanine phosphoribosyl transferase.

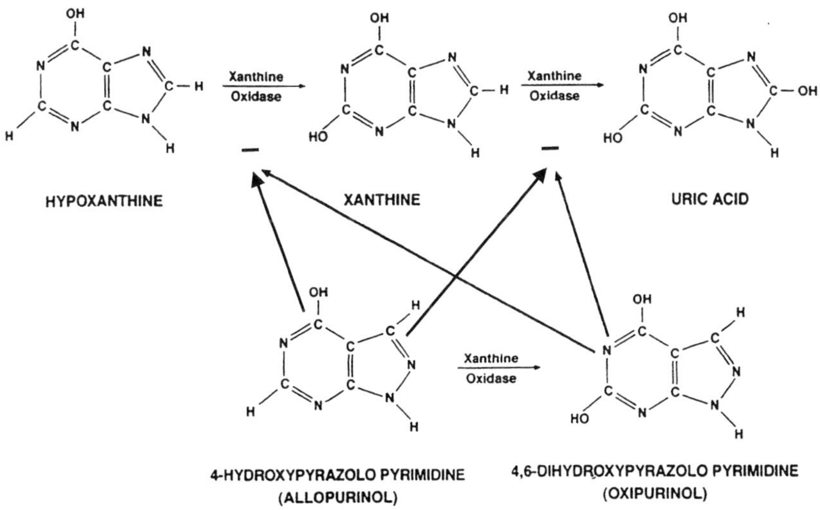

Figure 3 Structure of hypoxanthine, xanthine, uric acid, allopurinol, and oxipurinol.

the enzyme catalyzing conversion of orotidylic acid to uridylic acid, resulting in excesses of urinary orotic acid and orotidine.

Pharmacokinetics

Allopurinol is rapidly absorbed from the gastrointestinal tract, with a peak plasma level within 30 to 60 minutes. Its half-life ranges between 30 minutes to 4 hours. Most of the drug is rapidly oxidized to its principal metabolite; oxipurinol, which is also a potent xanthine oxidase inhibitor (21). Oxipurinol has a prolonged half-life of 14 to 28 hours. Both allopurinol and oxipurinol show no binding to plasma proteins, are freely distributed in the extracellular fluid, and are readily dialyzable. In dialysis patients with gout, the dose of allopurinol is, therefore, administered after dialysis. Oxipurinol is poorly absorbed from the gastrointestinal tract and has a relatively poor solubility, limiting its therapeutic usefulness in the treatment of gout (1,8,16,22). Renal insufficiency reduces and uricosuric drugs increase oxipurinol excretion (1,14).

The major route of allopurinol metabolism (60% to 70%) is oxidation to oxipurinol (1,8,17,19,22). Alternatively, about 20% of ingested allopurinol is excreted in feces, and a smaller proportion is converted by HPRT to allopurinol ribonucleotide 5'-monophosphate. The latter can be dephosphorylated to allopurinol ribonucleoside, which can also be formed directly from allopurinol by means of the purine nucleoside phosphorylase reaction.

Drug Interactions

Azathioprine and 6-mercaptopurine are inactivated by xanthine oxidase, and inhibition of this enzyme by allopurinol increases the toxicity of these drugs (1,23–25). For this reason, close monitoring of white blood cell counts and reduction of the dose of azathioprine or 6-MP by at least 50% are recommended in patients already receiving allopurinol (25). There is increased bone marrow suppression in patients concomitantly taking cyclophosphamide, cyclosporine, or vidarabine, although the mechanism is not entirely clear (26). Concurrent administration of ampicillin or amoxicillin in patients taking allopurinol is associated with a threefold increase in the incidence of skin rash (23,24). Allopurinol reduces the activity of hepatic microsomal drug-metabolizing enzymes, and can thereby potentiate the actions of warfarin, theophylline, phenytoin, and other drugs.

Indications and Therapeutic Effects

Allopurinol has been the mainstay for the treatment of hyperuricemia and gout for the last 40 years (Table 2) (1,21,22,27,28). Allopurinol is administered orally in a single daily dose of 100 to 800 mg with the most often prescribed dose being 300 mg daily. Serum urate reduction is noted within 24 to 48 hours of starting treatment. The maximum effect of a particular dose is seen within 3 to 21 days. Gouty attacks often cease within 3 to 6 months of continuous maintenance of subsaturation levels of urate in the serum (less than 6.0 mg/dL), but complete

Table 2 Indications for Allopurinol

Gout
Both "underexcretor" and "overproducer" gout patients with greater than two attacks/year
Chronic tophaceous gouty arthritis (clinical and "silent" tophi by X-rays, MRI, CT, or ultrasound)
Uric acid overproduction: primary gout (<10%), ↓ HPRT, ↑ PRPP synthetase, ↓ glucose-6-phosphatase; glycogen storage diseases III, V, VII; and ↓ fructose-1-PO_4 aldolase
Contraindication, intolerance, or failure of uricosuric drugs in urate overproducers; persons with prior uric acid nephrolithiasis or renal insufficiency aspirin greater than 325 mg/day
Non-gout
Adjunct to cytolytic therapy for hematologic malignancies
Uric acid and oxalate nephrolithiasis
Other
Cardiomyopathy, congestive heart failure
Leishmaniasis, trypanosomiasis
Allopurinol mouthwash and "iceballs" for cancer chemotherapy-induced stomatitis

Abbreviations: CT, computed tomography; HPRT, hypoxanthine guanine phosphoribosyl transferase; MRI, magnetic resonance imaging; PRPP, phosphoribosyl pyrophosphate.

resolution of gout flares and reductions in tophus size may take 6 to 24 months in individuals with higher total body urate pools. Discontinuation of allopurinol is followed by a rapid rise of serum urate to pre-treatment levels (within 2 to 3 days), although recurrence of acute gouty attacks may not occur for long periods (29).

Because oxipurinol is excreted principally by the kidney, its half-life is prolonged in patients with renal insufficiency. The increased incidence of adverse effects of allopurinol in patients with renal impairment is hypothesized to result from the prolonged oxipurinol half-life. Because of the way it is metabolized and cleared, lower doses of allopurinol are usually effective in controlling serum urate levels in patients with chronic renal insufficiency (Table 3). Patients who do not

Table 3 Guidelines for Allopurinol Dose According to Renal Function

Creatinine clearance: mL/min	Maintenance dose of allopurinol
>100 mL/min	300 mg/day
80 mL/min	250 mg/day
60 mL/min	200 mg/day
40 mL/min	150 mg/day
20 mL/min	100 mg/day
<10 mL/min	50–100 mg q 2–3 days

adequately lower serum urate levels while receiving creatinine clearance-adjusted reduced doses of allopurinol may require cautious titration to higher doses of allopurinol (30).

Long-term control of hyperuricemia with a concomitant reduction in total body urate is necessary to prevent recurrent gouty attacks, chronic tophaceous gout, urate nephropathy, and uric acid nephrolithiasis. For the agent to be effective, the dosage must be titrated to reach and maintain the target level of less than 5.0 or 6.0 mg/dL (21,22,27,28,31). Failure to sufficiently reduce serum urate to the target level will result in persistence of joint tophi and intraarticular urate crystals with cumulative joint damage (32–37).

Criteria for allopurinol use are listed in Table 2. Once initiated, allopurinol therapy is continued indefinitely. Studies have demonstrated that intermittent administration of allopurinol is less effective in controlling gout symptoms than continuous therapy (38). Failure of allopurinol to reverse the gouty process is usually the result of poor patient compliance or lack of titration to the necessary dosage (39).

Adverse Reactions

Adverse events occur in about 5% to 20% of patients who take allopurinol (21–24,27,28). These consist mainly of precipitation of gouty attacks in about 20% to 30% of subjects, and a minor pruritic maculopapular rash in 2% to 3.5% (Fig. 4). The latter reaction is sometimes associated with fever, leukocytosis, eosinophilia, and swelling of the face or tongue.

Allopurinol hypersensitivity syndrome is a rare, life-threatening reaction that occurs in about 0.4% of patients receiving allopurinol (40–42). The average time of onset of allopurinol hypersensitivity syndrome after starting allopurinol is

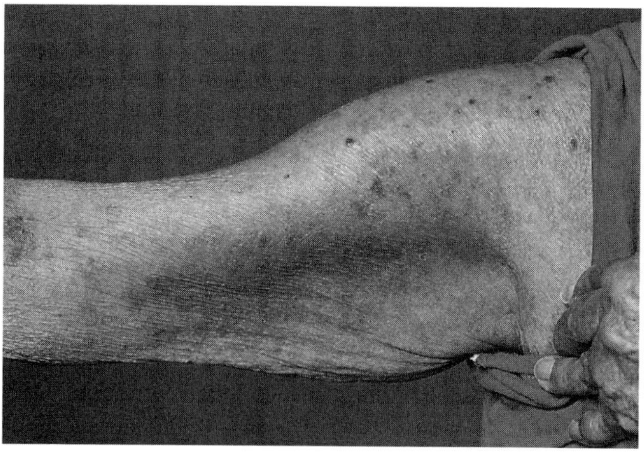

Figure 4 Allopurinol-induced maculopapular eruption.

Table 4 Criteria for the Diagnosis of Allopurinol Hypersensitivity Syndrome

A clear temporal sequence following administration of allopurinol
Lack of exposure to another drug that may cause similar symptoms
A clinical presentation meeting two major or one major + one minor criteria
Major criteria
Rash: TEN, SJS, ED
Acute hepatic necrosis
Acute interstitial nephritis + renal failure
Minor criteria
Fever
Eosinophilia
Leukocytosis
Death, often from sepsis, in about 25%

Abbreviations: TEN, toxic epidermal necrolysis; SJS, Stevens-Johnson syndrome; ED, exfoliative dermatitis.

3.5 weeks (range 2 days to 8 weeks). The syndrome is characterized by fever, severe dermatitis (toxic epidermal necrolysis, Stevens-Johnson syndrome, or exfoliative dermatitis), acute hepatitis, and acute interstitial nephritis with renal insufficiency, eosinophilia, and leukocytosis (Table 4). Mortality in allopurinol hypersensitivity syndrome is about 26% to 30%, largely the result of severe renal failure, hepatic necrosis, sepsis, gastrointestinal bleeding, or skin exfoliation.

Elevated plasma concentrations of oxipurinol, such as may develop in patients with renal insufficiency and in whom the dose of allopurinol has not been reduced appropriately, appear to correlate with the development of allopurinol hypersensitivity syndrome (20,40–46). The mechanism underlying allopurinol hypersensitivity syndrome is unknown, but an immune-mediated hypersensitivity reaction to high serum levels of oxipurinol (due to renal failure, hydrochlorothiazide coadministration, or old age) has been suggested (40–43). A CD 4+T cell-mediated immune hypersensitivity reaction to oxipurinol rather than allopurinol has been postulated (40–43). Reactivation of human herpes virus-6, as a costimulatory signal, has also been implicated (47,48). An in vitro allopurinol-induced release of interferon-gamma (IFN-γ) from patient's peripheral blood T lymphocytes may be a useful test in the diagnosis of Stevens-Johnson syndrome and other drug hypersensitivity reactions (49). Skin patch testing with either allopurinol or oxipurinol is less specific and has yielded conflicting results (43). Current treatment of allopurinol hypersensitivity syndrome consists of early recognition, withdrawal of allopurinol, and appropriate supportive therapy (40–42). The use of corticosteroids is controversial. Intravenously corticosteroids (40 to 200 mg prednisolone/day or pulse methylprednisolone 500 to 1000 mg daily for 3 days) have been tried, but proof of efficacy is lacking (42).

Other, less common side-effects of allopurinol include gastrointestinal disturbance (nausea, vomiting, abdominal pain, and diarrhea), centrilobular hepatic necrosis, granulomatous hepatitis, neurologic symptoms (somnolence, vertigo, ataxia, depression, neuritis), and resorption of intraosseous digital tophi resulting in structural instability with "telescoping" of the digits (22–24). Myelotoxicity (leukopenia, thrombocytopenia and/or aplastic anemia) is very rare, but may occur more commonly in patients with hepatic or renal impairment and in those receiving concomitant azathioprine, 6-mercaptopurine, or cyclophosphamide (23,24). Xanthine crystalluria or calculus, due to increased urinary xanthine excretion, is very rare and more likely to occur in patients with significant urate overproduction due to a purine enzyme defect, or cytolytic chemotherapy for lymphoma, lymphosarcoma, or leukemia.

Measurement of plasma concentrations of oxipurinol has been used to monitor allopurinol therapy, particularly in patients with gout and chronic renal failure. A plasma oxipurinol level between 30 to 100 μmol/L at 6 to 9 hours after allopurinol dosing is considered within the optimal therapeutic range (50,51). However, among patients with gout, there is no consistent correlation between plasma oxipurinol levels, effectiveness of allopurinol doses, and serum urate concentrations. The latter is determined by body urate stores, diet, and concomitant drugs as well as by allopurinol dose (46,52). Plasma oxipurinol levels, by comparison, are more dependent on allopurinol dose and renal function (41,50–52). Thus, serum urate levels may remain elevated in patients with plasma oxipurinol levels greater than 100 μmol/L. Currently, the major role of measuring plasma oxipurinol levels is to identify non-compliant patients or compliant individuals with a low plasma oxipurinol levels in whom the allopurinol dose may be increased (46).

Measurements of plasma concentrations of oxipurinol and xanthine may also be useful in patients with gout who are still hyperuricemic despite seemingly adequate allopurinol therapy (50). Oxipurinol concentrations in the therapeutic range (30 to 100 μmol/L) and plasma xanthine concentrations of 6 to 9 μmol/L indicate effective xanthine oxidase inhibition. In that setting, further increases in allopurinol doses are less likely to control the hyperuricemia and may lead to toxic reactions (50). Under these circumstances, additional or alternate therapies, such as a uricosuric drug, strict dietary control, and restriction of alcoholic beverages, should be considered.

True refractoriness to allopurinol is rare (Table 5). A minority of patients, particularly those with renal impairment and large tophaceous deposits, may continue to experience gouty flares associated with persistent hyperuricemia (53–56). Refractoriness is most commonly due to a lack of patient compliance, a failure of physician-patient communication, or prescription of allopurinol dose too low to reduce and maintain serum urate levels to 4 to 6 mg/dL (53). Continued high alcohol intake is associated with suboptimal response to allopurinol, because ethanol contributes to hyperuricemia and its use may lead to poor compliance (54). Renal insufficiency with impaired ability to eliminate urate despite sufficient xanthine oxidase inhibition is an important cause of refractoriness to allopurinol (55). Poor gastrointestinal absorption can on rare

Table 5 Refractoriness to Allopurinol

Sub-therapeutic plasma oxipurinol level: <30–100 μmol/L
Poor compliance
Insufficient allopurinol dose
Continued high alcohol intake
? Reduced gastrointestinal absorption
Therapeutic or above-therapeutic plasma oxipurinol level: >30–100 μmol/L
Renal insufficiency

occasions lead to subtherapeutic plasma oxipurinol levels and insufficient xanthine oxidase inhibition (56).

Management of the Allopurinol-Intolerant Patient

Therapeutic options for the management of hyperuricemia in these patients are listed in Table 6. Nonpharmacologic measures that lower serum urate levels should be maximized. These include diet, alcohol abstinence, and attention to other medications the patient may be taking (reviewed in Chapter 19) (37,35,57–59). For patients with coexistent hypertension, the mild uricosuric effect of losartan, unique among angiotensin II converting enzyme receptor antagonists, may be exploited (35,60). For those with concomitant hyperlipidemia, fenofibrate, a lipid-lowering fibric acid derivative and a modest uricosuric, may be prescribed (35,60). Obviously it is worth trying to see if a uricosuric agent will be effective (35,61,62). Newer agents such as a xanthine oxidase inhibitor that is not a purine analogue or recombinant uricase could be effective (63,64). However, recombinant uricases have not been evaluated in allopurinol-allergic patients (31).

Cautious administration of oxypurinol (100 to 600 mg per day) has been tried. However, this agent is available only for compassionate use from the manufacturer, and a significant percentage of patients who are unable to tolerate allopurinol are also sensitive to oxipurinol (35).

Table 6 Therapeutic Options in the Management of Hyperuricemia in Allopurinol Allergic Patients

Uricosuric drugs
Normal renal function: probenecid, sulfinpyrazone
Mild to moderate renal insufficiency: benzbromarone (if available)
Oxipurinol
Allopurinol desensitization
Recombinant A. flavus uricase (rasburicase) for prevention and treatment of tumor lysis syndrome
Newer agents
Febuxostat
Uricase-PEG 20

Table 7 Indications for Allopurinol Desensitization in Patients with Allopurinol-Induced Pruritic Maculopapular Eruptions

Patients with gout and renal impairment rendering uricosuric drugs ineffective
Patients with gout, underexcretion hyperuricemia, and allergy or intolerance to both probenecid and sulfinpyrazone
Patients with gout and overproducer/overexcretor hyperuricemia and those with uric acid nephrolithiasis in whom uricosuric use can increase the risk of renal stones
Transplant patients with renal insufficiency and severe debilitating gout
Prevention of malignancy-associated hyperuricemia and tumor lysis syndrome due to cytolytic therapy for hematologic malignancies; the resulting massive uricosuria precludes the use of uricosuric drugs

Therefore, allopurinol desensitization provides an important option for the allopurinol-intolerant individual in whom the above measures are not effective.

Desensitization to allopurinol has been successful by using a method of slow oral administration as well as with intravenous protocols (43,65–70). A retrospective study of slow oral administration of allopurinol to 32 intolerant patients revealed this method to be effective for most (43). Thirty of the 32 patients had gout. Of those, 26 had concomitant renal insufficiency, three were intolerant to uricosuric drugs, and one had nephrolithiasis and hyperuricosuria, contraindicating uricosuric therapy (Table 7). Using a suspension of allopurinol, unit doses containing 10 μg, 25u μg, 50 μg, 100 μg, 200 μg, 500 μg, 1 mg, 5 mg, 10 mg, and 25 mg are prepared. Fifty milligrams (one-half of a 100 mg tablet) and 100 mg (a whole tablet) are then used. The standard desensitization protocol consisted of an initial dose of 50 μg allopurinol daily, followed by slow, dose increment increases every three days (Table 8). A modified desensitization

Table 8 Standard Allopurinol Desensitization Protocol

Daily dose	Preparation[a]	Days (approx.)
50 μg	0.25-ml suspension (1 mg/5 mL)	1–3
100 μg	0.5-ml suspension (1 mg/5 mL)	4–6
200 μg	1-ml suspension (1 mg/5 mL)	7–9
500 μg	2.5-ml suspension (1 mg/5 mL)	10–12
1 mg	5-ml suspension (1 mg/5 mL)	13–15
5 mg	2.5-ml suspension (10 mg/5 mL)	16–18
10 mg	5-ml suspension (10 mg/5 mL)	19–21
25 mg	12.5-ml suspension (10 mg/5 mL)	22–24
50 mg	One-half a 100-mg tablet	25–27
100 mg	One 100-mg tablet	28+

[a]Two concentrations of allopurinol suspension are used: 1 mg/5 mL (200 μg/mL) and 10 mg/5 mL (2 mg/mL) depending on the dose required.

protocol with initial allopurinol daily doses of 10 µg and 25 µg, and a dose increase every 5 to 10 days or longer, is recommended for high-risk patients (Table 9).

Overall, desensitization was successful in 78% of patients, enabling patients to tolerate long-term allopurinol therapy (up to 92 months), with reduction or cessation of gouty attacks in 92% and partial or complete resolution of tophi in 89% of patients (43).

Other investigators reported similar results, including rapid intravenous desensitization in 2 subjects (66,67), successful re-desensitization to allopurinol after initial failure in another patient (68), desensitization of two siblings with allopurinol-induced rash (69), and desensitization to allopurinol-induced fixed drug eruptions (70). In addition, success has been reported using accelerated oral desensitization in another subject (65).

Before initiating therapy, it is important to discuss with each patient the details of allopurinol desensitization protocol, and its long-term benefits and potential risks. The procedure can be carried out in the outpatient clinic under close monitoring, because transient pruritic rashes and sensitivity to the drug may recur both during (in about one-third) and after desensitization (in approximately one-fourth of patients). Most of these cutaneous reactions can be managed by temporary withdrawal of allopurinol until the rash subsides, followed by cautious reintroduction of the drug at half the previously tolerated dose, and a slower rate of incremental dose change. Medication compliance is essential because it is unclear whether the loss of sensitivity in these individuals is temporary or permanent. The desensitization procedure can occasionally result in life-threatening reactions (68,71). To minimize such a risk, timely recognition of any sign of intolerance (pruritus, cutaneous erythema, fever, or oral ulcers) and prompt withdrawal of allopurinol are crucial. Given the potential morbidity and mortality of allopurinol hypersensitivity syndrome, re-exposure to the drug through desensitization is not recommended in those with a history of toxic epidermal necrolysis, Stevens-Johnson syndrome, or other catastrophic reactions. Finally, a slower incremental dosing regimen increases the likelihood of successful desensitization, and is recommended for high-risk patients (Table 9).

Table 9 Modified Allopurinol Desensitization Protocol

Lower initial doses: 10 µg and 25 µg
Slower rate of dose escalation: every 5–10 days or longer
Indications: high-risk patients
Frail elderly patients with comorbid medical conditions
Widespread, confluent allopurinol eruption, particularly when associated with facial/tongue swelling, stomatitis, fever, or eosinophilia
Recurrent rashes during desensitization
Interruption of therapy after successful desensitization to allopurinol

Oxipurinol

Oxipurinol, the active metabolite of allopurinol, is also a xanthine oxidase inhibitor. Gastrointestinal absorption of oxipurinol is inferior to that of allopurinol, and the drug is not commercially available in the United States or Canada, except direct from the manufacturer. Doses ranging from 100 to 600 mg a day have been proposed for those sensitive to allopurinol (57–74). However, owing to their structural similarities, allergic reactions similar to those of allopurinol have been observed in about 40% of patients treated with oxipurinol (Fig. 3) (73,74). Although the gastrointestinal absorption of rapid-release oxipurinol sodium (384 mg/day equivalent to allopurinol 300 mg/day) is superior to that of standard oxipurinol (75), its usefulness in allopurinol-allergic patients with gout has not been evaluated.

Febuxostat

Febuxostat, 2-(3-cyano-4-isobutoxyphenyl)-4-methyl-5-thiazolecarboxylic acid, also known as TEI-6720 or TMX-67, is a new potent xanthine oxidase/dehydrogenase inhibitor (5,9–11). In contrast to allopurinol and oxypurinol, febuxostat has no significant effects on the activities of other purine or pyrimidine enzymes and, therefore, has been termed a selective xanthine oxidase inhibitor (76). As would be predicted, febuxostat treatment results in dose-related reduction of both serum urate and urinary uric acid with concomitant increases in serum and urinary xanthine and hypoxanthine. To date, there are no reports of urinary xanthine crystals or calculi among a small number of patients treated with febuxostat for up to 3 years.

Metabolism

Febuxostat is rapidly absorbed in the gastrointestinal tract, and is extensively metabolized in the liver by both glucuronidation, and to a lesser extent, oxidation (77). Oxidation metabolites, including 67M-1, 67M-2, 67M-3, and 67M-4, are also active as xanthine oxidase inhibitors. Excretion is both biliary and renal. Mild-to-moderate hepatic disease and renal impairment (creatinine clearance greater than 20 mL/min) do not seem to alter the urate-lowering effects of febuxostat.

Therapeutic Uses

Febuxostat is a promising new drug for the treatment of hyperuricemia and gout. It is administered in a single daily dose and the onset of action is within 1 to 2 days, with a peak effect in about one week. The efficacy and safety of febuxostat in the treatment of hyperuricemia and gout have been demonstrated in a number of clinical studies (11,78–80). In a phase II dose-response clinical trial that was randomized, double-blind, and placebo-controlled, participants received febuxostat in single daily doses of 40 mg, 80 mg, and 120 mg or placebo for 28 days. At day 28, none of the patients taking placebo had a serum urate less than 6.0 mg/dL, whereas that target was reached in 56% of those taking 40 mg, 76% of those taking 80 mg, and 94% of those taking 120 mg of febuxostat. Adverse events were mild and similar in the placebo and febuxostat groups (79).

A phase III trial involving 760 patients with gout and serum urate levels greater than 8.0 mg/dL compared the effects of febuxostat (80 mg or 120 mg) to those of allopurinol (300 mg) once daily for 52 weeks (80). The primary endpoint of this trial was the proportion of subjects with all three of the last three monthly serum urate levels being below 6.0 mg/dL. The targeted end point of a serum urate less that 6.0 mg/dL was achieved in 53% of those on febuxostat 80 mg, 62% on febuxostat 120 mg, and 21% on allopurinol 300 mg ($p<0.001$ for each febuxostat group vs. allopurinol). Treatment-related adverse events were similar across the groups.

Febuxostat appears to be an effective agent for patients who are either intolerant or refractory to allopurinol. Because of differences in chemical structures, it is unlikely that patients who are hypersensitive to allopurinol would have similar reactions with febuxostat. This has been true for a small number of patients who had discontinued allopurinol because of adverse reactions and were enrolled in clinical trials of febuxostat (5). In addition, febuxostat may be

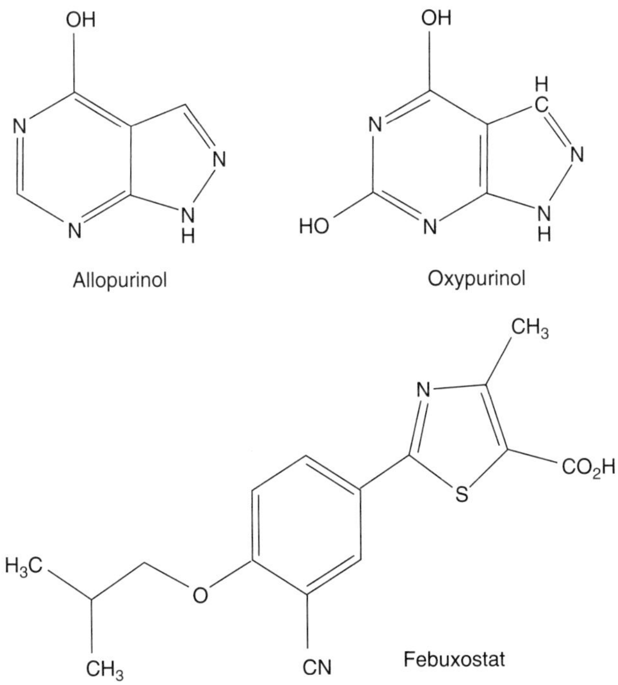

Figure 5 Structure of allopurinol, oxipurinol, and febuxostat.

especially useful in patients with mild to moderate renal failure, because dose adjustment is not required for those with a creatine clearance above 20 mL/min.

Adverse Events

Febuxostat use has generally been associated with only mild and self-limiting side effects (9–11,79,80). These include gout flares, headache, backache, arthralgia, nasopharyngitis, respiratory infections, nausea, vomiting, diarrhea, rash, and elevation of liver function tests. Other rare adverse events occurring in febuxostat-treated subjects have included: Guillain-Barré syndrome, suicidal tendency, exacerbation of heart failure, coronary artery disease, chronic obstructive lung disease, and cerebrovascular events.

No significant drug interactions have been reported with febuxostat. However, the caution employed when allopurinol is used concomitantly with azathioprine or 6-mercaptopurine should be observed (Fig. 5).

REFERENCES

1. Rundles RW. The development of allopurinol. Arch Intern Med 1985; 145:1492–1503.
2. Enroth C, Eger BT, Okamoto K, et al. Crystal structures of bovine milk xanthine dehydrogenase and xanthine oxidase: structure-based mechanism of conversion. Proc Natl Acad Sci 2000; 97:10723–10728.
3. Wortmann RL, Kelley WN. Gout and hyperuricemia. In: Ruddy S, Harris ED, Jr., Sledge CB, eds. Kelley's Textbook of Rheumatology. 6th ed. Philadelphia: W.B. Saunders Co, 2001:1339–1377.
4. Jarasch E-D, Grund C, Bruder G, et al. Localization of xanthine oxidase in mammary gland epithelium and capillary endothelium. Cell 1981; 25:67–82.
5. Okamoto K, Eger BT, Teshino T, et al. An extremely potent inhibitor of xanthine oxidoreductase. Crystal structure of the enzyme-inhibitor complex and mechanism of inhibition. J Biol Chem 2003; 278:1848–1855.
6. Cappola TP, Kass DA, Nelson GS, et al. Allopurinol improves myocardial efficiency in patients with idiopathic dilated cardiomyopathy. Circulation 2001; 104:2407–2411.
7. Massey V, Komai H, Palmer G, Elion GB. On the mechanism of inactivation of xanthine oxidase by allopurinol and other pyrazolo [3,4-d] pyrimidines. J Biol Chem 1970; 245:2837–2844.
8. Elion GB. Drugs in the treatment of hyperuricemia. Adv Nephrol 1974; 3:51–57.
9. Komoriya K, Osada Y, Hasegawa M, et al. Hypouricemic effect of allopurinol and the novel xanthine oxidase inhibitor TEI-6720 in chimpanzees. Eur J Pharmacol 1993; 250:455–460.
10. Yamamoto T, Moriwaki Y, Fujimura Y, et al. Effect of TEI-6720, a xanthine oxidase inhibitor, on the nucleoside transport in the lung cancer cell line A549. Pharmacology 2000; 60:34–40.
11. Schumacher HR, Jr., Wortmann RL, Eastace D, et al. Phase II, dose-response, safety and efficacy clinical trial of new oral xanthine oxidase inhibitor TMX-67(febuxostat) in subjects with gout. Arthritis Rheum 2002; 47:S142.

12. Osajima T, Kamezawa M, Fukunari A, et al. Pharmacokinetics and pharmacodynamics of Y-700, a potent and non-renal excretion type of xanthine oxidase inhibitor, in healthy male volunteers. Arthritis Rheum 2003; 48:S530.
13. Noma S, Verlio M, Iwane J, et al. Safety, tolerability, pharmacokinetics, and lowering uric acid effect of repeated daily dosing with Y-700, a novel xanthine oxidase inhibitor, in healthy male volunteers. Arthritis Rheum 2003; 48:S530.
14. Elion GB, Yu T-F, Gutman AB, Hitchings GH. Renal clearance of Oxipurinol, the chief metabolite of allopurinol. Am J Med 1968; 45:69–77.
15. Rodnan GP, Robin JA, Tolchin SF, Elion GB. Allopurinol and gouty hyperuricemia: efficacy of a single daily dose. JAMA 1975; 231:1143–1147.
16. Chalmers RA, Kromer H, Scott JT, Watts RWE. A comparative study of the xanthine oxidase inhibitors allopurinol and oxipurinol in man. Clin Sci 1968; 35:353–362.
17. Beardmore TD, Kelley WN. Mechanism of allopurinol-mediated inhibition of pyrimidine biosynthesis. J Lab Clin Med 1971; 78:696–700.
18. Nishida Y, Kamatani N, Tanimoto K, Akaoke I. Inhibition of purine nucleoside phosphorylase activity and of T-cell function with allopurinol-riboside. Agents Actions 1979; 9:549–552.
19. Nelson DJ, Elion GB. Metabolic studies of high doses of allopurinol in humans. Adv Exp Med Biol 1984; 165:167–170.
20. Horiuchi H, Ota M, Nishimura S-I, et al. Allopurinol induces renal toxicity by impairing pyrimidine metabolism in mice. Life Sci 2000; 66:2051–2070.
21. Fam AG. Strategies and controversies in the treatment of gout and hyperuricemia. Ballieres Clin Rheumatol 1990; 42:177–192.
22. Khawaja AT, Diamond HS. Hypouricemic drugs. In: Smyth CJ, Holers VM, eds. Gout, hyperuricemia, and other crystal-associated arthropathies. New York: Marcel Dekker, 1999:219–240.
23. Frisch JM, Lovatt GE, Sproit ARM, Turmer P. The adverse reaction profile of allopurinol. In: Frontiers of Int Med. Basel: Karger, 1974:412–419.
24. McInnes GT, Lawson DH, Jick H. Acute adverse reactions attributed to allopurinol in hospitalized patients. Ann Rheum Dis 1981; 40:245–249.
25. Cummins D, Sekar M, Halil O, Bannar N. Myelosuppression associated with azathioprine-allopurinol interaction after heart and lung transplantation. Transplantation 1996; 61:1661–1662.
26. Boston Collaborative Drug Surveillance Program. Allopurinol and cytotoxic drugs. Interaction in relation to bone marrow depression. JAMA 1974; 227:1036–1040.
27. Emmerson BT. The management of gout. N Engl J Med 1996; 334:445–451.
28. Terkeltaub RA. Gout. N Engl J Med 2004; 349:647–655.
29. Leishout-Zuidema MFV, Breedveld FC. Withdrawal of long-term antihyperuricemic therapy in tophaceous gout. J Rheumatol 1993; 20:1383–1385.
30. Vasquez-Mellado J, Morales EM, Pacheco-Tena C, Burgos-Vargas R. Relation between adverse events associated with allopurinol and renal function in patients with gout. Ann Rheum Dis 2001; 60:981–983.
31. Mikuls TR, MacLean CH, Olivieri J, et al. Quality of care indicators for gout management. Arthritis Rheum 2004; 50:937–943.
32. McCarthy GM, Barthelemy CR, Veum JA, Wortmann RL. Influence of antihyperuricemic therapy on the clinical and radiographic progression of gout. Arthritis Rheum 1991; 34:1489–1494.

33. Yamanaka H, Togashi R, Hokada M, et al. Optimal range of serum urate concentrations to minimize risk of gouty attacks during anti-hyperuricemic treatment. Adv Exp Med Biol 1998; 431:13–18.
34. Li-Yu J, Clayburne G, Sieck M, et al. Treatment of chronic gout. Can we determine when urate stores are depleted enough to prevent attacks of gout? J Rheumatol 2001; 288:577–580.
35. Fam AG. Alternate urate-lowering drugs and the management of hyperuricemia in allopurinol-intolerant patients. Int J Adv Rheumatol 2003;122–130.
36. Shoji A, Yamanaka H, Kamatani N. A retrospective study of the relationship between serum urate level and recurrent attacks of gouty arthritis: evidence for reduction of recurrent gouty arthritis with antihyperuricemic therapy. Arthritis Care Res 2004; 51:321–325.
37. Beutler AM, Rull M, Schlesinger N, et al. Treatment of allopurinol decreases the number of acute gout attacks despite persistently elevated serum uric acid levels. Clin Exp Rheumatol 2001; 19:595.
38. Bull PW, Scott JT. Intermittent control of hyperuricemia in the treatment of gout. J Rheumatol 1989; 16:1246–1248.
39. Riedel AA, Nelson M, Joseph-Ridge N, et al. Compliance with allopurinol therapy among managed care enrollees with gout: a retrospective analysis of administrative claims. J Rheumatol 2004; 31:1575–1581.
40. Hande KR, Noone RM, Stone WJ. Severe allopurinol toxicity. Description and guidelines for prevention in patients with renal insufficiency. Am J Med 1984; 76:47–56.
41. Singer JZ, Wallace SL. The allopurinol hypersensitivity syndrome. Unnecessary morbidity and mortality. Arthritis Rheum 1986; 29:82–87.
42. Arellano F, Sacristan JA. Allopurinol hypersensitivity syndrome: a review. Ann Pharmacother 1993; 27:337–343.
43. Fam AG, Dunne SM, Iazetta J, Paton TW. Efficacy and safety of desensitization to allopurinol following cutaneous reactions. Arthritis Rheum 2001; 44:231–238.
44. Bellamy N, Gilbert JR, Brooks PM, et al. A survey of current prescribing practices of anti-inflammatory and urate lowering drugs in gouty arthritis in the Province of Ontario. J Rheumatol 1988; 15:1841–1847.
45. Zell SC, Carmichael JM. Evaluation of allopurinol use in patients with gout. Am J Hosp Pharm 1989; 46:1813–1816.
46. Stamp L, Sharples K, Gow P, Raill B. The optimal use of allopurinol: an audit of allopurinol use in South Auckland. Aust NZ J Med 2000; 30:567–572.
47. Naisbitt DJ, Pirmohamed M, Park BK. Immunopharmacology of hypersensitivity reactions to drugs. Curr Allergy Asthma Rep 2003; 3:22–29.
48. Masaki T, Fukunaga A, Tohyama M, et al. Human herpes virus 6 encephalitis in allopurinol-induced hypersensitivity syndrome. Acta Derm Venereol 2003; 83:128–131.
49. Halevy S, Cohen AD, Livni E. The diagnostic role of the in-vitro drug-induced interferon-γ release test. Int J Dermatol 1999; 38:835–840.
50. Emmerson BT, Gordon RB, Cross M, Thomson DB. Plasma oxipurinol concentrations during allopurinol therapy. Br J Rheumatol 1987; 26:445–449.
51. Day RO, Miners JO, Birkett DJ, et al. Allopurinol dosage selection: relationships between dose and plasma oxipurinol and urate concentrations and urinary urate excretion. Br J Clin Pharmac 1988; 26:423–428.

52. Peterson GM, Boyle RR, Francis HW, et al. Dosage prescribing and plasma oxipurinol levels in patients receiving allopurinol therapy. Eur J Clin Pharmacol 1990; 39:419–421.
53. Pal B, Foxall M, Dysart T, et al. How is gout managed in primary care? A review of current practice and proposed guidelines. Clin Rheumatol 2000; 19:21–25.
54. Ralston SH, Capell HA, Sturrock RD. Alcohol and response to treatment of gout. BMJ 1988; 296:1641–1642.
55. Migita K, Sakai M, Aratake K, et al. Effects of hemodialysis on advanced bony tophi in a tophaceous gout patient with chronic renal failure. Clin Exp Rheumatol 2001; 19:358–359.
56. Fam AG. Managing problem gout. Ann Acad Med Singapore 1998; 27:93–99.
57. Dincer HE, Dincer AP, Levinson DJ. Asymptomatic hyperuricemia: to treat or not to treat. Cleve Clin J Med 2002; 69:594–608.
58. Dessein PH, Shipton EA, Stanwix AE, et al. Beneficial effects of weight loss associated with moderate calorie/carbohydrate restriction, and increased proportional intake of protein and unsaturated fat on serum urate and lipoprotein levels in gout: A pilot study. Ann Rheum Dis 2000; 59:539–543.
59. Fam AG. Gout, diet and the insulin resistance syndrome. J Rheumatol 2002; 29:1350–1355.
60. Bardin T. Fenofibrate and losartan. Ann Rheum Dis 2003; 62:497–498.
61. Zurcher RM, Bock HA, Thiel G. Excellent uricosuric efficacy of benzbromarone in cyclosporine-A-treated renal transplant patients: a prospective study. Nephrol Dial Transplant 1994; 9:548–551.
62. Perez-Ruiz F, Gomez-Ullate P, Amenbar JJ, et al. Long-term efficacy of hyperuricemia treatment in renal transplant patients. Nephrol Dial Transplant 2003; 18:603–606.
63. Goldman SC, Holcenberg JS, Finkelstein JZ, et al. A randomized comparison between rasburicase and allopurinol in children with lymphoma or leukemia at high risk for tumor lysis. Blood 2001; 97:2998–3003.
64. Becker MA, Schumacher R, Wortmann R, et al. Febuxostat, a novel non-purine selective inhibitor of xanthine oxidase, therapy in allopurinol intolerant patients. Arthritis Rheum 2004; 50:S336.
65. Nitti F, Fumagalli M, Incorvaia C. Rush desensitization to allopurinol. Allergy 2003; 58:690.
66. Walz-LeBlanc BAE, Reynolds WJ, MacFadden DK. Allopurinol sensitivity in a patient with chronic tophaceous gout: success of intravenous desensitization after failure of oral desensitization. Arthritis Rheum 1991; 34:1329–1331.
67. Schumacher MJ, Copeland TG. Intravenous desensitization to allopurinol in a heart transplant patient with gout. Ann Allergy Asthma Immunol 2004; 92:374–376.
68. Tanna SB, Barnes JF, Seth SK. Desensitization to allopurinol in a patient with previous failed desensitization. Ann Pharmacother 1999; 33:1180–1183.
69. Melson RD. Familial hypersensitivity to allopurinol with subsequent desensitization. Rheumatology 1999; 38:1301.
70. Kelso JM, Keating RM. Successful desensitization for treatment of a fixed drug eruption to allopurinol. J Allergy Clin Immuno 1996; 97:1171–1172.
71. Unsworth J, Black DR, D'Assis Fonseca AE, Beswick DI. Desensitization to allopurinol: a cautionary tale. Ann Rheum Dis 1987; 46:646.

72. Lockard O, Jr., Harmon C, Nolph K, Irvin W. Allergic reaction to allopurinol with cross- reactivity to oxipurinol. Ann Intern Med 1976; 85:333–335.
73. Earll JM, Saavedra M. Oxypurinol therapy in allopurinol allergic patients. Am Fam Phys 1983; 28:147–148.
74. O'Duffy JD. Oxipurinol therapy in allopurinol-sensitive patients. Arthritis Rheum 1993; 36:S159.
75. Walter-Sack I, de Vries JX, Ernst B, et al. Uric acid lowering effect of oxipurinol sodium in hyperuricemia patients—therapeutic equivalence to allopurinol. J Rheumatol 1996; 23:498–501.
76. Zhao L, Takano Y, Horiuchi H. Effect of febuxostat, a novel non-purine, selective inhibitor of xanthine oxidase (NP-SIXO), on enzymes in purine and pyrimidine metabolism pathway. Arthritis Rheum 2003; 49:S531.
77. Febuxostat Investigator Brochure, TAP Pharmaceutical Products Inc., Lake Forest, IL 2003: 176 pages.
78. Kamatani N, Fujimori S, Hada T, et al. Febuxostat, a novel non-purine selective inhibitor of xanthine oxidase, in an allopurinol-controlled phase III clinical trial in Japanese subjects with gout or hyperuricemia. Arthritis Rheum 2004; 50:S336.
79. Becker MA, Schumacher HR, Wortmann RL, et al. Febuxostat, a novel nonpurine selective inhibition of xanthine oxidase A twenty-eight day, multicenter, phase II, randomized, double-blind, placebo-controlled, dose-response clinical trial examining safety and efficacy in patients with gout. Arthritis Rheum 2005; 52:916–923.
80. Becker MA, Schumacher HR, Wortmann RL, et al. Febuxostat versus allopurinol in patients with hyperuricemia and gout. N Engl J Med 2005; 353:2450–2461.

25

Urate Oxidase (Uricase)

Michael S. Hershfield
Division of Rheumatology and Immunology, Departments of Medicine and Biochemistry, Duke University School of Medicine, Durham, North Carolina, U.S.A.

John S. Sundy
Division of Rheumatology and Immunology, Department of Medicine, Duke University School of Medicine, Durham, North Carolina, U.S.A.

INTRODUCTION

Most mammals dispose of uric acid via the urate oxidase (uricase) catalyzed reaction:

$$\text{Uric acid} + O_2 + H_2O \rightarrow \text{allantoin} + CO_2 + H_2O_2$$

This conversion is advantageous since allantoin is much more soluble and more efficiently excreted than urate. However, humans and some closely related primates lack uricase (1,2) owing to uricase gene mutations acquired during their evolution (3–5). Because of this deficiency, urate levels in extracellular fluids are relatively high in humans. In some individuals these levels may exceed solubility (values greater than 6.8 mg/dL at pH 7.4 and 37°C), posing a risk for gout, nephropathy, and nephrolithiasis caused by urate crystals or precipitated uric acid. Uricase was first isolated almost a century ago (6). About 50 years ago improved methods for protein purification led to early clinical investigation of parenteral uricase as a potential means to control hyperuricemia and prevent acute uric acid nephropathy (7,8).

The efficacy and widespread use of allopurinol after its introduction in 1964 dampened interest within the pharmaceutical industry for testing novel agents for controlling hyperuricemia, and may also have diminished awareness among physicians of a subset of gout sufferers for whom such agents might be needed. Recently, however, there has been a growing appreciation of the lack of adequate therapy for patients with chronic, tophaceous gout and who are allergic or refractory to allopurinol. This chapter reviews the experience with parenteral uricase for treating malignancy-associated hyperuricemia and summarizes the current status of polyethylene glycol (PEG) modified uricase as a potential therapy for refractory gout.

MICROBIAL URICASES

Purified Aspergillus Flavus Uricase

During the 1960s, clinical studies were initiated in France with urate oxidase isolated from an industrialized strain of the fungus *Aspergillus flavus* (8–13). Through the 1990s an estimated one kilogram of this material (Uricozyme, Sanofi Winthrop) was produced yearly and used to treat 15,000 patients, mainly in France and Italy (14). The primary use was for short term control of hyperuricemia to prevent or treat tumor lysis-associated acute uric acid nephropathy in patients with hematologic malignancies. In this setting Uricozyme was usually infused daily for up to 12 days, and was shown to be more effective than allopurinol (15). Thus, in 30 children with acute leukemia treated with intravenous uricase, mean serum urate fell to levels below 3 mg/dL within 24 hours, and to less than 2 mg/dL for the remainder of the 4 to 5 day treatment period. In 30 patients treated with allopurinol (15 mg/kg/day orally), mean serum urate remained at levels greater than 4 mg/dL over the same period. More recent studies in the United States have confirmed the efficacy of Uricozyme in children with leukemia (16).

Uricozyme was generally well tolerated. However, about 5% of patients experienced hypersensitivity reactions, including bronchospasm, urticaria, and more rarely angioedema. These reactions often occurred within 20 minutes of the first infusion and were attributed in part to impurities in the non-recombinant enzyme preparation (17). Methemoglobinemia and hemolytic anemia, due apparently to the H_2O_2 derived from uricolysis, have occurred in patients with glucose-6-phosphate (G6PD) dehydrogenase deficiency, which is considered a contraindication to treatment with uricase.

Recombinant Aspergillus Flavus Uricase

In the 1990s the gene for A. flavus uricase was cloned and the three dimensional crystal structure of the expressed recombinant enzyme was determined (14,18). The homotetrameric (subunit MW $\sim$34,000) enzyme had an unusual "porin-like" structure and contained no metal or prosthetic groups (14,19). Clinical trials with recombinant A.flavus uricase produced in a strain of Saccharomyces cerevisiae (rasburicase, Sanofi Synthelabo) have been conducted in the United States and Europe in patients with hematologic malignancies (16,17,20–26). The half-life of rasburicase after intravenous administration was 18 hours, and the volume of distribution suggested confinement to the vascular space. Clearance of rasburicase was independent of renal or hepatic function. The rate of urate degradation was dose-dependent. In children and adults with lymphoma or leukemia, intravenous rasburicase (0.15 or 0.2 mg/kg daily for 5 to 7 days) was far more rapid in onset and produced greater and more sustained lowering of serum urate than did oral allopurinol (27,28). In a retrospective analysis of multiple studies in patients with advanced B cell malignancies, 20% of 230 allopurinol-treated patients developed acute renal failure, compared with only 3% of 219 rasburicase-treated patients (17).

According to the product labeling information, antibodies to rasburicase were detected by ELISA in 61% of 28 healthy volunteers in a Phase I trial within 6 weeks of a single infusion, or after 5 daily infusions (20). Most of these antibodies were neutralizing. Despite this finding, there have been few side effects associated with clinical use of rasburicase. About 5% of children with leukemia and lymphoma developed antibodies to rasburicase and about 1% had hypersensitivity reactions. A single adult patient with non-Hodgkin's lymphoma developed acute neurotoxicity thought to be related in some unknown way to rasburicase (26). Rasburicase was approved for clinical use in the United States in 2002 for lowering plasma urate levels in pediatric cancer patients undergoing cytolytic therapy. According to the package insert, the safety and efficacy of rasburicase was established for a single 5-day course of daily infusions begun just prior to chemotherapy.

URICASES AND GOUT

Purified Microbial Uricases

During the period when Uricozyme was in use, some experience was gained with daily, alternate day, or less frequent intravenous infusions or intramuscular injections. Drug was administered for up to several months in patients with tophaceous gout and chronic renal failure and in some gout patients who were receiving azathioprine therapy following organ transplantation (7,8,13,29). In some cases, Uricozyme interrupted acute gout attacks and decreased the volume of tophi. Gout flares were precipitated in other patients, and prophylaxis with colchicine was recommended.

Several drawbacks prevented wider acceptance of fungal uricase for treating gout. A sustained hypouricemic effect required frequent (i.e., daily) dosing, and efficacy diminished quickly in some patients, who developed anti-uricase antibodies (7,8,30–32). Though uncommon, serious allergic reactions, including anaphylaxis, were also encountered (33). The recombinant fungal enzyme rasburicase is also immunogenic, and as noted, has only been approved for short term use in patients with malignancies who are at risk of developing uric acid nephropathy. However, weekly infusions of rasburicase have been used to treat a single patient with allopurinol-resistant tophaceous gout (34).

The Development of Polyethylene Glycol–Modified Uricase

Covalent attachment of PEG to proteins can prevent proteolysis and block cellular uptake, resulting in a prolonged circulating life and reduced immunogenicity (35,36). The first clinical product of this technology was the Orphan Drug, PEGylated adenosine deaminase (PEG-ADA; Adagen, manufactured by Enzon Pharmaceuticals, Inc.), which was approved in 1990 for treating children with severe combined immunodeficiency due to adenosine deaminase deficiency (37). Enzymatic control of hyperuricemia was also among the first applications envisioned for protein PEGylation (38). Shortly after initiating the clinical trial of PEG-ADA, permission was obtained for a compassionate trial of a PEGylated bacterial uricase, prepared by the same manufacturer, for a markedly hyperuricemic patient with relapsed lymphoma who had developed uric acid nephropathy and was allergic to allopurinol. Intramuscular injections of this material controlled his hyperuricemia, allowing him to receive additional chemotherapy (39).

After these results were reported in 1988, many physicians requested PEG-uricase to treat allopurinol-hypersensitive patients with severe gout or those whose disease was refractory to allopurinol and uricosuric agents. The growing experience with chronic PEG-ADA therapy for ADA deficiency indicated the potential value of PEG-uricase for treating severe gout. Thus, when industry plans to produce a microbial PEGylated uricase were abandoned in 1993, one of the authors (MSH) obtained an NIH Small Business Technology Transfer (STTR) grant to develop PEG-uricase as an "orphan drug" for treating patients with refractory gout, for whom available therapy was contraindicated or had been ineffective. The use of a recombinant mammalian rather than a microbial enzyme was proposed, in part, because of the closer similarity of the amino acid sequence deduced from the vestigial human uricase gene to the sequences of functional pig and baboon uricases.

In initial studies, recombinant porcine uricase proved to be more active than the baboon enzyme. A cDNA encoding a protein greater than 98% identical to porcine uricase, but with an extra lysine residue found in baboon uricase, was constructed. Earlier studies showed that introducing novel lysines, which are potential sites for PEG attachment, could enhance the ability of PEGylation to reduce the immunogenicity of foreign protein (40). After expression in Escherichia coli and purification, the resulting mammalian uricase had activity comparable to that of Uricozyme. Optimal conditions for PEGylating this enzyme were then developed by Mountain View Pharmaceuticals, Inc., which had become the small business component of the STTR grant when it was renewed in 1996. PEGylation did not substantially reduce its activity or stability, and it enhanced its solubility compared with that of unmodified mammalian uricases (41).

Using the resulting PEG-uricase, a proof-of-principle study was conducted in uricase knockout mice, which are highly susceptible to fatal uric acid nephropathy (42,43). Weekly intraperitoneal PEG-uricase normalized plasma urate and urinary uric acid levels in these mice prevented the development of uric acid nephropathy, and did not elicit anti-uricase antibodies (43). Savient Pharmaceuticals, Inc., (formerly BioTechnology General Corp.) licensed this PEG-uricase in 1998 and is developing it for human clinical trials. In December 2001 the FDA Office of Orphan Product Development awarded Orphan Drug Designation to this "mammalian" PEG-uricase for treatment of patients with refractory gout.

A PEG-uricase, prepared with a yeast recombinant enzyme, has been described and its potential use in treating gout has been speculated upon (44). However, this latter material was not studied in uricase deficient animals, and it has Orphan Drug Designation for treatment of hyperuricemia associated with malignancies, but not for gout. The status of clinical testing is unclear.

Clinical Studies of Mammalian PEG-Uricase

Two open-label, single injection, dose escalation Phase I clinical trials of PEG-uricase, sponsored by Savient Pharmaceuticals, were conducted at Duke University Medical Center in 2002 and 2003. Subjects in these trials had symptomatic gout, defined as at least one flare in the previous 6 months, chronic arthropathy due to gout, or tophi, and had a serum urate greater than 7 mg/dL. Exclusion criteria included renal failure requiring dialysis, the use of immunosuppressive agents other than prednisone at ≤ 10 mg per day to control attacks of arthritis, a deficiency of G6PD dehydrogenase, or co-morbidities that might complicate evaluation of safety. In both trials, allopurinol and uricosuric drugs were withheld 1–2 weeks before and for 21 days after the administration of PEG-uricase. Dosing was by subcutaneous injection in the first trial, and by intravenous infusion in the second trial. The pharmacokinetic behavior of PEG-uricase was assessed by measuring urate oxidase activity in plasma. Efficacy was assessed by the magnitude of decrease in plasma urate concentration and in the ratio of uric acid to creatinine (UA/Cr) in urine. Antibodies to PEG-uricase and to PEG were detected by ELISA.

Subcutaneous PEG-Uricase

The first Phase I trial involved 13 subjects with refractory gout (11 had tophi) and a mean plasma urate concentration of 11.2 mg/dL (45). Four subjects each received single injections of 4, 8, or 12 mg of PEG-uricase, and 1 subject received 24 mg. Within 7 days of dosing, mean plasma urate fell by almost 8 mg/dL, and normalized in 11/13 subjects at a mean of 2.8 mg/dL. Absorption of PEG-uricase was slow and variable. In 8 subjects, the enzyme circulated in plasma for 21 days after injection, maintaining pUAc at ≤6 mg/dL. In 5 subjects clearance was more rapid and the effect on plasma urate was shorter. This was associated with the appearance of IgM and IgG antibodies that, unexpectedly, reacted with PEG rather than with the uricase protein. Subcutaneously injected PEG-uricase caused transient local pain in some subjects, and 3 subjects had allergic skin reactions associated with antibody development. The only other significant adverse reactions were gout flares in 6 subjects (45).

Intravenous PEG-Uricase

Twenty four subjects were treated, consisting of 6 cohorts of 4 subjects each who received single intravenous infusions of 0.5 mg, 1 mg, 2 mg, 4 mg, 8 mg, or 12 mg of PEG-uricase. The chief findings were as follows:

1. Following intravenous infusion the circulating half life (T1/2) of PEG-uricase ranged from about 6 to almost 14 days, averaging about 10 days (i.e., much longer than the 18 hour half life observed with unmodified Aspergillus flavus uricase). There was proportionality between the dose infused and plasma uricase activity, both the Cmax and AUC.
2. The decline in plasma urate levels was proportional to the dose of PEG-uricase. The mean baseline plasma urate for all 24 subjects was approximately 11 mg/dL and was similar for all 6 dose cohorts. At all but the lowest dose, mean urate level fell to less than 5 mg/dL (nadir). The mean plasma urate level fell to less than 2 mg/dL within 24 hours for subjects in the 3 highest dose cohorts (4, 8, and 12 mg). The average plasma urate levels calculated over the entire 3-week post-infusion period was less than 6 mg/dL for each of these 3 dose groups. The decline in the UAc/Cr ratio in urine correlated with that for plasma urate levels.
3. Single intravenous infusions of PEG-uricase were well tolerated, and there were no serious adverse events. All other adverse events were considered to be mild to moderate. Fourteen subjects experienced gout flares during the 3-week period following intravenous infusion of PEG-uricase.
4. Nine of the 24 subjects developed antibody to PEG-uricase, but this did not appear to be associated with adverse events.

Based on the results summarized, Phase II clinical trials are being performed with IV PEG-uricase. An open-label, multi-center Phase II trial has been carried out, in which about 40 subjects with gout received doses of 4 or 8 mg every two weeks, or 8 or 12 mg every four weeks, over a 12-week period. In addition, an Orphan Product Development grant to conduct a separate Phase II open label multidose trial at Duke University Medical Center has been awarded. In this trial, subjects with refractory gout will receive 5 infusions of 8 mg of PEG-uricase over 12 weeks. This trial is expected to involve some subjects who have developed refractory gout following organ transplants, as well as some with gout due to rare inherited diseases, including glucose-6-phosphatase deficiency and familial juvenile hyperuricemic nephropathy.

The ability to maintain a plasma urate level below 6 mg/dL will be evaluated in both of these trials, as well as the immunologic response to PEG-uricase. It will be important to determine whether, with repeated administration, immunogenicity will limit utility, or whether tolerance might develop, as has been observed in some animal studies of PEGylated proteins (46,47).

CONCLUSION

Uricolytic therapy may have a distinct advantage over xanthine oxidase inhibitors in clinical situations where a rapid lowering of plasma urate levels is essential, or where the accumulated burden of uric acid is very great. Recombinant A. flavus uricase (rasburicase) has been shown to be significantly more effective than allopurinol, and to be well tolerated, as an agent for preventing uric acid nephropathy in the setting of malignant disease. The more prolonged action of PEG-uricase might be an additional advantage for this indication, since it would require fewer infusions, but its primary utility may be in patients with tophaceous gout who have failed to benefit adequately from other forms of treatment.

REFERENCES

1. Keilin J. The biologic significance of uric acid and guanine excretion. Biol Rev Camb Philos Soc 1959; 34:265–296.
2. Christen P, Peacock WC, Christen AE, Wacker WEC. Urate oxidase in primate phylogenesis. Eur J Biochem 1970; 12:3–5.
3. Wu X, Lee CC, Muzny DM, Caskey CT. Urate oxidase: primary structure and evolutionary implications. Proc Natl Acad Sci USA 1989; 86:9412–9416.
4. Wu X, Muzny DM, Lee CC, Caskey CT. Two independent mutational events in the loss of urate oxidase. J Mol Evol 1992; 34:78–84.
5. Oda M, Satta Y, Takenaka O, Takahata N. Loss of urate oxidase activity in hominoids and its evolutionary implications. Mol Biol Evol 2002; 19:640–653.
6. Battelli F, Stern L. Untersuchung uber die urikase in den tiergeweben. Biochemische Zeitung 1909; 19:219–253.
7. London M, Hudson PM. Uricolytic activity of purified uricase in two human beings. Science 1957; 125:937–938.
8. Brogard JM, Stahl A, Stahl J. Enzymatic uricolysis and its use in therapy. In: Kelley WN, Weiner IM, eds. Uric Acid. New York: Springer-Verlag, 1978:515–524.
9. Kissel P, Lamarche M, Royer R. Modification of uricemia and the excretion of uric acid nitrogen by an enzyme of fungal origin. Nature 1968; 217:72–74.
10. Kissel P, Schmitt J, Streiff F, et al. L'urate oxydase: son intérêt dans la prévention des hyperuricemies therapeutiques en hematologie. Ann Med Nancy 1972; 11:519–535.

11. Zittoun R, Dauchy F, Teillaud C, et al. Le traitement des hyperuricemies en hematologie par l'urate-oxydase et l'allopurinol. Ann Med Interne 1976; 127:479–482.
12. Brogard JM, Coumaros D, Frankhauser J. Enzymatic uricolysis: a study of the effect of a fungal urate-oxydase. Eur J Clin Biol Res 1972; 17:890–895.
13. Potaux L, Aparicio M, Maurel C, et al. Uricolytic therapy. Value of urate oxidase in the treatment of hyperuricemias. Nouv Presse Med 1975; 4:1109–1112.
14. Colloc'h N, El Haji M, Bachet B, et al. Crystal structure of the protein drug urate oxidase-inhibitor complex at 2.05 Å resolution. Nat Struct Biol 1997; 4:947–952.
15. Masera G, Jankovic M, Zurlo MG, et al. Urate-oxidase prophylaxis of uric acid-induced renal damage in childhood leukemia. J Pediatr 1982; 100:152–155.
16. Pui C-H, Relling MV, Lascombes F, et al. Urate oxidase in prevention and treatment of hyperuricemia associated with lymphoid malignancies. Leukemia 1997; 11:1813–1816.
17. Navolanic PM, Pui CH, Larson RA, et al. Elitek-rasburicase: an effective means to prevent and treat hyperuricemia associated with tumor lysis syndrome, a meeting report, Dallas, Texas, January 2002. Leukemia 2003; 17:499–514.
18. Legoux R, Delpech B, Dumont X, et al. Cloning and expression in Escherichia coli of the gene encoding aspergillus flavus urate oxidase. J Biol Chem 1992; 267:8565–8570.
19. Retailleau P, Colloc'h N, Vivares D, et al. Complexed and ligand-free high-resolution structures of urate oxidase (Uox) from Aspergillus flavus: a reassignment of the active-site binding mode. Acta Crystallogr D Biol Crystallogr 2004; 60:453–462.
20. Mahmoud H, Leverger G, Patte C, et al. Advances in the management of malignancy-associated hyperuricaemia. Br J Cancer 1998; 77:18–20.
21. Leach M, Parsons RM, Reilly JT, Winfield DA. Efficacy of urate oxidase (uricozyme) in tumour lysis induced urate nephropathy. Clin Lab Haematol 1998; 20:169–172.
22. Ribeiro RC, Pui CH. Recombinant urate oxidase for prevention of hyperuricemia and tumor lysis syndrome in lymphoid malignancies. Clin Lymphoma 2003; 3:225–232.
23. Pui CH. Rasburicase: a potent uricolytic agent. Expert Opin Pharmacother 2002; 3:433–442.
24. Pui CH, Mahmoud HH, Wiley JM, et al. Recombinant urate oxidase for the prophylaxis or treatment of hyperuricemia in patients with leukemia or lymphoma. J Clin Oncol 2001; 19:697–704.
25. Pui CH. Urate oxidase in the prophylaxis or treatment of hyperuricemia: the United States experience. Semin Hematol 2001; 38:13–21.
26. Pitini V, Bramanti P, Arrigo C, et al. Acute neurotoxicity as a serious adverse event related to rasburicase in a non-Hodgkin's lymphoma patient. Ann Oncol 2004; 15:1446.
27. Goldman SC, Holcenberg JS, Finklestein JZ, et al. A randomized comparison between rasburicase and allopurinol in children with lymphoma or leukemia at high risk for tumor lysis. Blood 2001; 97:2998–3003.

28. Coiffier B, Mounier N, Bologna S, et al. Efficacy and safety of rasburicase (recombinant urate oxidase) for the prevention and treatment of hyperuricemia during induction chemotherapy of aggressive non-Hodgkin's lymphoma: results of the GRAAL1 (Groupe d'Etude des Lymphomes de l'Adulte Trial on Rasburicase Activity in Adult Lymphoma) study. J Clin Oncol 2003; 21:4402–4406.
29. Rozenberg S, Koeger AC, Bourgeois P. Urate-oxidase for gouty arthritis in cardiac transplant. J Rheumatol 1993; 20:2171.
30. Escudier B, Leclercq B, Tandonnet F, Nitenberg G. Hyperuricemia resistant to urate oxidase. Efficacy of high doses. Presse Med 1984; 13:1340.
31. Mourad G, Cristol JP, Chong G, et al. Role of precipitating anti-urate oxidase antibodies in urate oxidase-resistant hyperuricemia. Presse Med 1984; 13:2585.
32. Sibony G, North ML, Bergerat JP, et al. Hyperuricemia resistant to urate oxidase. Role of anti-serum urate oxidase precipitating antibodies. Presse Med 1984; 13:443.
33. Montagnac R, Schillinger F. Anaphylactic complication tied to intravenous injection of urate oxidase in a dialysis patient. Nephrologie 1990; 11:259.
34. Moolenburgh JD, Reinders MK, Jansen TL. Rasburicase treatment in severe tophaceous gout: a novel therapeutic option. Clin Rheumatol 2005; 1–4.
35. Abuchowski A, McCoy JR, Palczuk NC, et al. Effect of attachment of polyethylene glycol on immunogenicity and circulating life of bovine liver catalase. J Biol Chem 1977; 252:3582–3586.
36. Abuchowski A, van Es T, Palczuk NC, Davis FF. Alteration of immunological properties of bovine serum albumin by covalent attachment of polyethylene glycol. J Biol Chem 1977; 252:3578–3581.
37. Hershfield MS, Buckley RH, Greenberg ML, et al. Treatment of adenosine deaminase deficiency with polyethylene glycol-modified adenosine deaminase. N Engl J Med 1987; 316:589–596.
38. Davis S, Park YK, Abuchowski A, Davis FF. Hypouricaemic effect of polyethylene glycol modified urate oxidase. Lancet 1981; 2:281–283.
39. Chua CC, Greenberg ML, Viau AT, et al. Use of polyethylene glycol-modified uricase (PEG-uricase) to treat hyperuricemia in a patient with non-Hodgkin lymphoma. Ann Int Med 1988; 109:114–117.
40. Hershfield MS, Chaffee S, Koro-Johnson L, et al. Use of site-directed mutagenesis to enhance the epitope shielding effect of covalent modification of proteins with polyethylene glycol. Proc Natl Acad Sci USA 1991; 88:7185–7189.
41. Conley TG, Priest DG. Purification of uricase from mammalian tissue. Prep Biochem 1979; 9:197–203.
42. Wu X, Wakamiya M, Vaishnav S, et al. Hyperuricemia and urate nephropathy in urate oxidase-deficient mice. Proc Natl Acad Sci USA 1994; 91:742–746.
43. Kelly SJ, Delnomdedieu M, Oliverio MI, et al. Diabetes insipidus in uricase deficient mice: a model for evaluating therapy with poly (ethylene glycol)-uricase. J Am Soc Nephrol 2001; 12:1001–1009.
44. Bomalaski JS, Holtsberg FW, Ensor CM, Clark MA. Uricase formulated with polyethylene glycol (uricase-PEG 20): biochemical rationale and preclinical studies. J Rheumatol 2002; 29:1942–1949.

45. Ganson NJ, Kelly SJ, Scarlett E, Sundy JS, Hershfield MS. Control of hyperuricemia in subjects with refractory gout, and induction of antibody against poly(ethylene glycol) (PEG), in a phase I trial of subcutaneous PEGylated urate oxidase. Arthritis Res Ther 2005; 8:R12.
46. Wilkinson I, Jackson CJ, Lang GM, et al. Tolerance induction in mice by conjugates of monoclonal immunoglobulins and monomethoxypolyethylene glycol. Transfer of tolerance by T cells and by T cell extracts. J Immunol 1987; 139:326–331.
47. Sehon AH. Suppressor T cells induced in vivo by tolerogenic conjugates of a given antigen and monomethoxypolyethylene glycol downregulate antibody formation also to a second antigen, if the latter is presented as a covalent adduct with the former. Adv Exp Med Biol 1991; 303:199–206.

26

Therapeutic Strategies for Calcium-Containing Crystal Arthropathies

Herman S. Cheung
Department of Biomedical Engineering, University of Miami and Miami VA Medical Center, Miami, Florida, U.S.A.

INTRODUCTION

The deposition of basic calcium phosphate (BCP) and calcium pyrophosphate dihydrate (CPPD) crystals in articular tissues is probably an under-recognized event. Clinical observations indicate that exaggerated and uniquely distributed cartilage degeneration is associated with these deposits. Measurements of putative markers of cartilage breakdown suggest that these crystals magnify the degenerative processes that occur in osteoarthritis. Recent studies suggest that there are three potential mechanisms by which crystals can cause degeneration. The first two involve the induction of mitogenesis in synovial fibroblasts and the secretion of matrix metalloproteinases by cells that phagocytose these crystals. The third potential mechanism involves changes in joint biomechanics. Articular calcification may lead to altered loading of the joint causing injury to the cartilage matrix, which fails under normal loading, and chondrocytes respond by elaborating matrix metalloproteinases and developing inappropriate repaired responses (1,2). Therefore, the general therapeutic strategy should include formulation of compounds that block the formation of new crystals by inhibition of nucleation, formation, and growth of the primary crystals and can also target crystal-stimulated intracellular responses. Unfortunately, more definitive investigations of therapeutic agents are impeded by the lack of a suitable animal model for studying non-inflammatory aspects of crystal deposition, and the slow pace of degeneration (3,4).

CURRENT STATUS

Our present understanding of the mechanisms of pathological calcification is limited. Therefore, no reliable method exists to prevent calcium crystals deposition (5). If crystals promote chondrolysis, then removal of crystals from the joint would be therapeutic. This can be accomplished in gout where a systemic accumulation of urate can be targeted and eliminated with urate-lowering therapy. Unfortunately, no systemic defect has been specifically recognized underlying most cases of calcium-containing crystal deposits.

Once crystals form, they may be solubilized by enzymatic or chemical methods. For example, magnesium promotes dissolution of CPPD and BCP crystals. Oral magnesium has been reported to lessen symptoms in CPPD crystal deposition disease, although no proof of decreased deposits was identified (6). In one remarkable case, small Mg supplements and low doses of oral colchicine markedly improved shoulder effusions in a patient who had synovial fluid BCP and CPPD crystals (7). Lavage of the joint or repeated aspiration, as during treatment with hyaluronan, may promote crystal dissolution. Such removal may account for the observation that knees containing CPPD crystals responded better to treatment with hyaluronan than did osteoarthritic knees without these crystals (8). Alkaline phosphatase has significant pyrophosphatase activity at physiologic pH. It dissolved CPPD crystals in vitro and would be expected to do such if it were inducible in vivo (9,10). Of course, treatments directed at dissolving crystals bear the risk of provoking acute arthritis if they result in partial dissolution and shedding of crystals from the capsule or cartilage into the synovial fluid. Accordingly, it was not surprising that acute attacks of pseudogout occurred following magnesium and $^{+}$ EDTA lavage of knee joints containing CPPD crystals (11).

β-interferon was examined as a possible modulator of the biologic effects of BCP crystals. Simultaneous addition of β-interferon with either BCP crystals or platelet-derived growth factor (PDGF) in vitro resulted in delayed c-myc message accumulation and entry into S phase (12). Since β-interferon delayed, but did not inhibit, BCP-induced cellular events, no further work was done on β-interferon.

A chondroprotective effect of prostaglandins (PG) with regards to calcium-containing crystal arthropathies has been suggested. The effect of PGE_1 and its analog, misoprostol, on BCP crystal-induced mitogenesis and collagenase induction in human fibroblasts has been investigated (13). A dose-dependent inhibition of BCP crystal-induced mitogenesis and collagenase mRNA accumulation was demonstrated. Subsequent studies confirmed that PGE_1 inhibits crystal-induced mitogenesis and collagenase induction through a cyclicAMP transduction pathway (14). In this context, non-steroidal drugs, such as indomethacin, by blocking PGE_2 synthesis, may minimize inflammation. However, a matrix protective effect for PG has also been proposed. Obliteration of that matrix protective effect, however, might worsen the outcome from long-term nonsteroidal agent treatment.

Because bisphosphonates are known to be strong inhibitors of biomineralization, the effect of bisphosphonates on crystal-induced mitogenesis and matrix metalloproteinase synthesis was examined. The three bisphosphonates were dichloromethylene diphosphonate (Cl_2MDP), aminopropylidene, and the tetra-ethyl ester of Cl_2MDP. Cl_2MDP and aminopropylidene have an anti-resorptive effect on bone with little anti-mineralizing effect, and they bind strongly to hydroxyapatite, inhibiting crystal growth and dissolution. The tetra-ethyl ester of Cl_2MDP was used as a control because the substitution of the acid groups blocks the binding of the compound to hydroxyapatite. Like Cl_2MDP and aminopropylidene, this compound still exhibits anti-inflammatory activity, suggesting that anti-inflammatory effect of these bisphosphonates is not dependent on the binding of the compounds to hydroxyapatitie.

Using concentrations ranging from 10^{-4} to 10^{-8}, none of the three bisphosphonates blocked BCP crystal-induced collagenase and stromelysin synthesis. At concentration of 10^{-4} M, both Cl_2MDP and aminopropylidene had a slight inhibitory effect (less than 20%) on crystal-induced mitogenesis. Since intracellular crystal dissolution is one of the requirements for crystal-induced mitogenesis, the anti-resorptive properties of the two diphosphonates may account for this effect (15).

PHOSPHOCITRATE: A POTENTIAL THERAPEUTIC AGENT

Phosphocitrate ($C_6H_9O_{10}P$) is a naturally occurring compound, which has been identified in mammalian mitochondria (16). Phosphocitrate may protect mitochondria from mineral formation expected as a result of the high intra-mitochondrial concentrations of phosphate, calcium, and inorganic pyrophosphate (PPi), and it may prevent mineral interaction with the vulnerable mitochondrial membranes. Phosphocitrate is a potent in vitro inhibitor of hydroxyapatite crystal formation (16). Phosphocitrate also prevents soft tissue calcification in vivo and does not produce any significant toxic side effect in rats or mice when given in doses up to 150 μmol/kg/day (17,18). More recently, a new chemical formulation of phosphocitrate, a mixed salt of calcium and sodium of phosphocitrate $[CaNa(PC)_2(H_20)]_n$ (CaPC), has been synthesized (19). Like its precursor sodium phosphocitrate, calcium phosphocitrate is a potent and specific inhibitor of the biological effects of the calcium-containing crystals. However, in comparison, the anti-mineralization property of this new formulation is at least ten-fold more potent.

PHOSPHOCITRATE INHIBITS THE BIOLOGIC EFFECTS OF CRYSTALS

Phosphocitrate is the only agent recognized to date that specifically interferes with many biological effects of calcium-containing crystals (5,15,20). In vitro, crystal-induced proto-oncogenes (c-fos, c-jun, and c-myc), matrix metalloproteinase synthesis and mitogenesis, and P44/42 MAPK activation are inhibited by phosphocitrate, although it has no effect on similar processes when they are induced by growth factors or serum (21–25). Additionally, phosphocitrate blocks both CPPD and BCP crystal formation in matrix vesicles and intact cartilage in an in vitro model of chondrocalcinosis (26), nitric oxide-induced calcification of cartilage and cartilage-derived apoptotic bodies (27), and crystal-induced cyclo-oxygenase (28) and endocytotic activities (29). In addition to blocking the deleterious biologic effects of crystals, phosphocitrae also prevents further crystal formation in vitro (15).

IN VIVO THERAPEUTIC EFFECTS OF PHOSPHOCITRATE ON IN VIVO MODELS

The murine progressive ankylosis model of abnormal calcification is a manifestation of an autosomal recessive mutation. This mutation produces an inflammatory joint disorder associated with intra-articular BCP crystal deposition and culminates in fusion of the joints. Phosphocitrate inhibits disease progression in this model if it is given before evidence of disease is established (30).

The Hartley strain guinea pigs develop an arthropathy that histologically mimics human osteoarthritis (31–33). The arthritis typically begins in the knee joints at 3 months of age, and reaches an advance stage by 12 months. Significant ossification of medial menisci appears to correlate with the disease and age. Bone remodeling and cartilage degeneration is evident in the medial compartment as well (1,2). Preliminary data showed that phosphocitrate treatment caused the resorption of calcification in the meniscus and arrested the progress of the osteoartrhritis (1).

In summary, phosphocitrate is the only compound tested so far that blocks crystal-induced mitogenesis and matrix metalloproteinase synthesis, events that initiate the deleterious biologic effects. It also prevents further crystal formation both in vitro and in the articular tissue (15,22,26). On the basis of these findings, phosphocitrate is a potential therapeutic agent for calcium-containing crystal deposition diseases.

USE OF MOLECULAR MODELING TO DESIGN THE NEXT GENERATION OF THERAPEUTIC AGENTS

Molecular modeling together with scanning electron microscopy of crystals grown in the presence of inhibitors can be used to elucidate the stereospecificity of known inhibitors and to design more efficient inhibitors. Scanning electron microscopy provides information on crystal morphology changes induced by interactions with adsorbate molecules. Expression of specific faces of the crystals indicates possible interactions between the inhibitor and the atomic pattern of those particular crystal surfaces. Such interactions are often based upon the stereospecificity of inhibitor-surface recognition. Morphology of the crystal can be changed by selective adsorption of inhibitors on specific crystal faces leading to slower growth in the direction perpendicular to these planes and frequently to the cessation of crystal growth. Molecular modeling can provide valuable insight into energetic and spatial feasibility of inhibitor-crystal surface interactions, and in the development of potent stereospecific compounds to control, and if possible, to eliminate the crystallization and aggregation of undesirable crystalline phase.

Application of this computer-modeling technology to study the crystal-phosphocitrate interaction and crystal-membrane interaction led to the discovery that the [011] face of CPPD crystals binds to phosphocitrate and to the plasma membrane (34–36). The binding of the [010] CPPD crystal surface to phosphocitrate is associated with retardation and cessation of crystal growth (34). Binding to plasma membranes results in crystal-induced membranolysis (36). This finding suggests the potential strategy that may be used to design the next generation of therapeutic agents for calcium crystal arthropathy.

In designing the next generation of crystal inhibitors, it is important to understand that each crystallite (e.g., BCP or CPPD) has its own unique structure in terms of stereochemistry and ionic properties. The crystallite is formed by multiple reproduction of the rigid unit structure as specified by the relevant incorporated ions linked by contributing bonds. Therefore, a compound expressing strong inhibitory activity toward one crystallite may not necessarily display the same potency toward another. It is, therefore, essential to understand how a compound is interacting with a crystal in order to design the ultimate drug to benefit the disease (Fig. 1).

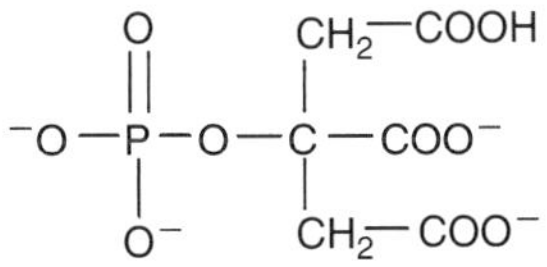

phosphocitrate

Figure 1 At physiological pH, phosphocitrate has four negative charges.

REFERENCES

1. Cheung HS, Sallis JD, Demadis KD, Wierzicki A. Phosphocitrate blocks calcification-induced articular joint degeneration. Arthritis & Rheum. In Press.

2. Kapadia RD, Badger AM, Levin JM, et al. Meniscal ossification in spontaneous OA in guinea pig. OA & Cartilage 2000; 8:374–377.
3. Cheung HS. Calcium crystal effects on the cells of the joint: implications for pathogenesis of the disease. Curr Opin Biol 2000; 12:223–227.
4. Ryan LM, Cheung HS. Role of crystals in osteoarthritis. In: Brandt KD, ed. Rheumatic Disease of America. Philadelphia: W.B. Saunders Co., 1999:257–267.
5. Sallis JD, Cheung HS. Inhibitors of articular calcium crystals. Curr Opin Biol 2003; 15:321–325.
6. Doherty M, Dieppe PA. Double blind, placebo controlled trial of magnesium carbonate in chronic pyrophosphate arthropathy. Ann Rheum Dis 1983; 42:106–107.
7. Patel KJ, Weidensaul D, Palma C, Ryan LM, Walker SE. Milwaukee shoulder with massive bilateral cysts: Effective therapy for hydrops of the shoulder. J Rheumatol 1997; 24:2479–2483.
8. de Medicis R, Lussier A. Osteoarthritis: influence of CPPD crystals on the clinical response to hylan. OA & Cartilage 1997; 5:146.
9. Shinozaki T, Pritzker KPH. Polyamines enhance calcium pyrophosphate dihydrate dissolution. J Rheumatol 1995; 22:1907–1912.
10. Xu Y, Cruz TF, Pritzker KPH. Alkaline phosphate dissolves CPPD crystals. J Rheumatol 1991; 18:1606–1610.
11. Bennett RM, Lehr JRM, McCarty DJ. Crystal shedding and acute pseudogout: an hypothesis based on a therapeutic failure. Arthritis Rheum 1976; 19:93.
12. Cheung HS, Mitchell P, Pledger WJ. Induction of expressions of c-fos and c-myc proto-oncogenes by BCP crystals: effect of beta-interferon. Cancer Res 1989; 49:134–138.
13. McCarthy GM, Mitchell P, Cheung HS. Misoprostol, a PGE_1 analogue, inhibits basic calcium phosphate crystal-induced mitogenesis and collagenase accumulation in human fibroblasts. Calc Tiss Res 1993; 52:434–437.
14. McCarthy GM, Cheung HS. The role of cAMP in prostaglandin-mediated inhibition of BCP crystal-induced mitogenesis and collagenase synthesis. Biochim Biophys Acta 1994; 1226:97–104.
15. Cheung HS. Phosphocitrate as a potential therapeutic strategy for crystal deposition disease. Curr Rheumatol Rep 2001; 3:24–28.
16. Tew WP, Mahle CD, Benavides J, Howard JE, Lehninger AL. Synthesis and characterization of phosphocitric acid, a potent inhibitor of hydroxylapatite crystal growth. Biochemistry 1980; 19:1983–1988.
17. Brown MR, Sallis JD. In: Schwille PO, Smith LH, Robertson WG, Vahlensieck W, eds. Urolithiasis and Related Clinical Research. New York: Plenum Press, 1985:891–894.
18. Cheung HS. Mechanism of destructive arthropathy and its prevention with phosphocitrate. Rev Bras Rheum 1994; 34:S117–S119.
19. Demadis KD, Sallis JD, Raptis RG, Baran P. A Crystallographically characterized nine-coordinated calcium-phosphocitrate complex as calcification inhibitor in vivo. J Am Chem Soc 2001; 123:10129–10130.
20. Shankar R, Crowden S, Sallis JD. Phosphocitrate and its analogueN-sulpho-2-aino tricarballylate inhibit aortic calcification. Atherosclerosis 1985; 50:191–198.
21. Cheung HS, Sallis JD, Mitchell P, Struve JA. Inhibition of basic calcium phosphate crystal-induced mitogenesis by phosphocitrate. Biochem Biophys Res Commun 1990; 171:20–25.

22. Cheung HS, Sallis JD, Struve JA. Specific inhibition of BCP and CPPD crystal-induced collagenase and stromelysin synthesis by phosphocitrate. Biochem Biophys Acta 1996; 1315:105–111.
23. Nair D, Misra RP, Sallis JD, Cheung HS. Phosphocitrate inhibits a basic calcium phosphate and calcium pyrophosphate dihydrate crystal-induced mitogen-activated protein kinase cascade signal transduction pathway. J Biol Chem 1997; 272:18920–18925.
24. Reuben P, Brogley M, Sun Y, Cheung HS. Molecular mechanism of the induction of metalloproteinases 1 and 3 in human fibroblasts by basic calcium phosphate crystals. Role of calcium-dependent protein kinase C-α. J Biol Chem 2002; 277:15190–15198.
25. Reuben PM, Wenger L, Cruz M, Cheung HS. Induction of metalloproteinase-8 in human fibroblasts by basic calcium phosphate crystals: effect of phosphocitrate. Connective Tissue Res 2001; 42:1–12.
26. Cheung HS, Kurup IV, Sallis JD, Ryan LM. Inhibition of CPPD crystal formation in articular cartilage vesicles and cartilage by phosphocitrate. J Biol Chem 1996; 271:28082–28085.
27. Cheung HS, Ryan LM. Phosphocitrate blocks nitric oxide-induced calcification of cartilage and chondrocyte-derived apoptotic bodies. OA & Cartilage 1999; 7:409–412.
28. Morgan MP, Whelan LC, Sallis JD, McCarthy CJ, Fitzgerald DJ, McCarthy GM. Basic calcium phosphate crystal-induced prostaglandin E2 production in human fibroblasts: role of cyclooxygenase 1, cyclooxygenase 2, and interleukin-1beta. Arthritis Rheum 2004; 50:1642–1649.
29. Sun Y, Zeng XR, Wenger L, Cheung HS. Basic calcium phosphate crystals stimulate the endocytotic activities of cells—inhibition by anti-calcification agents. Biochem Biophys Res Commun 2003; 312:1059.
30. Krug HE, Mahowald ML, Halverson PB, Sallis JD, Cheung HS. Phosphocitrate prevents disease progression in murine progressive ankylosis. Arthritis Rheum 1993; 36:1603–1611.
31. Bendele AM, Hulman JF. Spontaneous cartilage degeneration in guinea pigs. Arthritis Rheum 1988; 31:561–565.
32. Bendele AM, White SL, Hulman JF. Osteoarthritis in guinea pigs: histopathologic and scanning electron microscopic features. Lab Animal Sci 1989; 39:115–121.
33. Watson PJ, Hall LD, Malcolm A, Tyler JA. Degenerative joint disease in the guinea pig: use of MRI to monitor progression of bone pathology. Arthritis Rheum 1996; 36:1327–1337.
34. Wierzbicki A, Cheung HS. Molecular modeling of inhibition of crystals of CPPD by phosphocitrate. J Molecular Struct THEOCHEM 1998; 454:287–291.
35. Wierzbicki A, Cheung HS. Molecular modeling of inhibition of hydroxyapatite crystal by phosphocitrate. J Molecular Struct (Theochem) 2000; 529:73–82.
36. Wierzbicki A, Dalal P, Madura JD, Cheung HS. Molecular dynamics simulation of crystal induced membranolysis. J Phys Chem B 2003; 107:12346–12351.

Index